W9-BLM-079

EXCITATION-CONTRACTION COUPLING AND
CARDIAC CONTRACTILE FORCE

Excitation-Contraction Coupling and Cardiac Contractile Force

Second Edition

by

DONALD M. BERS

Professor and Chair Department of Physiology,
Loyola University Chicago,
Maywood, IL, U.S.A.

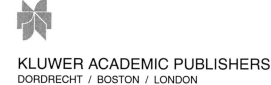

KLUWER ACADEMIC PUBLISHERS
DORDRECHT / BOSTON / LONDON

A C.I.P. Catalogue record for this book is available from the Library of Congress.

ISBN 0-7923-7157-7

Published by Kluwer Academic Publishers,
P.O. Box 17, 3300 AA Dordrecht, The Netherlands.

Sold and distributed in North, Central and South America
by Kluwer Academic Publishers,
101 Philip Drive, Norwell, MA 02061, U.S.A.

In all other countries, sold and distributed
by Kluwer Academic Publishers,
P.O. Box 322, 3300 AH Dordrecht, The Netherlands.

Printed on acid-free paper

Printed in the Netherlands.

PREFACE TO FIRST EDITION

The main aim of this monograph is to provide an overview of calcium regulation in cardiac muscle cells, particularly with respect to excitation-contraction coupling and the control of cardiac contractile force. It is my hope that this book will be useful to students of the cardiovascular system and muscle at all different levels and in different disciplines (such as physiology, biochemistry, pharmacology and pathophysiology). I also hope that it will find use for those studying developmental, comparative and disease processes as well as more integrative phenomenon. I kept several goals in mind in writing this monograph. First, it should be easily readable. Second, I chose to include numerous illustrations and tables to help integrate results from numerous investigators in practical formats and also present key figures from important papers. Thus, this monograph may serve as a resource of information for people working in the areas described herein. Third, the presentation is a very personal one, and I have necessarily drawn extensively on my personal experience in this field over the past 15 years. This, I think, helps maintain a certain continuity of thought from chapter to chapter. Fourth, I have made serious attempts to make each chapter "up to date", despite the breadth of topics covered. I have also tried to be equitable in choosing references while not intending to be comprehensive or exhaustive. Neither of these aims can be perfectly matched, and I apologize to the many investigators whose papers I have not cited, but should have.

While I thank all of my colleagues who make this a stimulating area in which to work, I would especially like to thank those who contributed by helpful discussions, providing original figures, sending preprints of manuscripts, and by commenting on drafts of individual chapters. These individuals include: S. Baudet, B.P. Bean, J.R. Berlin, J.H.B. Bridge, A. Fabiato, S. Fleischer, J.S. Frank, C. Franzini-Armstrong, M.M. Hosey, L.V. Hryshko, N. Ikemoto, L.R. Jones, W.J. Lederer, D.H. MacLennan, G. Meissner, M. Morad, K.D. Philipson, J.D. Potter, E. Ríos, R.J. Solaro, J.R. Sommer, J.G. Tidball, J. McD. Tormey, W.G. Wier, A. Williams, D.T. Yue.

I also thank my many research collaborators over the years who have joined me in making some contributions to this field, including: G.A. Langer, K.D. Philipson, D. Ellis, A. Peskoff, J.L. Sutko, C.O. Malécot, K.T. MacLeod, J.H.B. Bridge, J.G. Tidball, M.J. Shattock, S.M. Harrison, P. Hess, K.W. Spitzer, L.V. Hryshko, W.J. Lederer, J.R. Berlin.

Finally, a very special thanks are due to my wife, Kathryn E. Bers, whose combination of patience and assistance have made this book possible.

PREFACE TO THE SECOND EDITION

I have been delighted that so many people have found the 1st edition of this book to be valuable. That has encouraged me to prepare a completely revised and entirely updated 2nd edition. I have tried to maintain the flavor of the first edition, including some historical points and classic observations, while integrating a large amount of new information into this frame-work. The main aim is the same (to provide an overview of Ca regulation in cardiac muscle cells, particularly with respect to excitation-contraction coupling and contraction). I have still kept my initial four goals from the first edition in mind (readability, useful tables & illustrations, up to date references and personal perspective). I have made every effort to integrate the wealth of new data from various disciplines and perspectives from the past ten years with other work in a seamless manner. I have added a tremendous amount of new material, but have really tried to stay well focused, and limit the inevitable expansion of the volume. Nevertheless, this edition is longer, but I hope to the true benefit of the reader. The new edition is organized in the same overall sequence, but I have inserted one major new chapter on the action potential and ion channels in the heart (Chapter 4, between Ca sources and sinks and Ca channels). I have also included more discussion of heart failure and other pathophysiological issues. These aspects, I felt, were lacking in the first edition and they make the book more complete. There are 178 figures, 27 tables and 2509 references in this edition. The number of references sounds like a lot, but it was actually a challenge to keep it from getting longer. It is a tough trade-off in trying to be equitable in choosing key references while not being exhaustive. I apologize again to the many investigators whose excellent papers I have not cited, but well could have.

I hope that those people who embraced the first edition will appreciate the new edition and the extensive rewriting. I hope this second edition will also be of value to new students of the cardiovascular system at all levels, from medical/graduate students through the senior investigators in the related fields which are discussed.

I want to thank all of my colleagues who continue to make this a stimulating field in which to work. This is clearly a case where my own vision of how the heart works is built on the shoulders and minds of a series of great scientists over the years. To those, too many to be named, I thank you. I would especially like to thank those who contributed by helpful discussions, providing original figures or data, sending preprints of manuscripts, by commenting on drafts of individual chapters and collaborating with me to make some primary contributions in this arena. These individuals are listed alphabetically on the next page.

I want to give very special thanks to a few coworkers who have helped me very directly in preparing the final camera-ready manuscript. Ken Ginsburg, Tom Shannon and Lars Maier patiently read and proofread every chapter and were constant companions. Teresa Carrillo, Lars Maier and Klaus Schlotthauer did most of the painstaking work of preparing the extensive reference list and checking it. Chris Weber prepared the very useful Index and Betty Weiss helped in scanning some images from which I developed some of the figures. Finally, a very special thanks is due to my wife, Kathryn E. Bers, whose tremendous patience, understanding and encouragement have made this book possible.

ACKNOWLEDGEMENTS

These are the people who have really helped me learn about how the heart works. Thank you.

Julio Altamirano
Mike Artman
José Bassani
Rosana Bassani
Stephane Baudet
Bruce Bean
Josh Berlin
Lothar Blatter
Rolf Brandes
John Bridge
Joan Brown
Mark Cannell
Peace Cheng
Simon Chu
Lea Delbridge
Jaime DeSantiago
Sanda Despa
David Eisner
David Ellis
Alex Fabiato
Mike Fill
Sid Fleischer
Joy Frank
Clara Franzini-Armstrong
Ken Ginsburg
Ana Gómez
Peter Haddock
Simon Harrison
Gerd Hasenfuss
Marlene Hosey
Leif Hove-Madsen
Steve Houser

Larry Hryshko
Noriaki Ikemoto
Larry Jones
Hideki Katoh
Arnie Katz
Litsa Kranias
Glenn Langer
Jon Lederer
Li Li
Yanxia Li
Steve Lipsius
David MacLennan
Ken MacLeod
Claire Malécot
Lars Maier
Andy Marks
Abdul Matlib
Alicia Mattiazzi
Eileen McCall
Gerhard Meissner
Rafael Mejia-Alvarez
Ruben Mestril
Greg Mignery
Martin Morad
Rick Moss
Mark Nelson
Jeanne Nerbonne
Clive Orchard
Ed Perez-Reyes
Art Peskoff
Ken Philipson
Valentino Piacentino

Burkert Pieske
Steve Pogwizd
Jim Potter
Pepe Puglisi
Ming Qi
John Reeves
Eduardo Ríos
Allen Samarel
Mike Sanguinetti
Hirosi Satoh
Martin Schneider
Tom Shannon
Mike Shattock
Klaus Schlotthauer
Karin Sipido
John Solaro
Jo Sommer
Ken Spitzer
John Sutko
Jim Tidball
Andy Trafford
Dave Warshaw
Chris Weber
Gil Wier
Alan Williams
Ping Xiao
Weilong Yuan
David Yue
Zhuan Zhou
Mark Ziolo

Finally, I thank the American Heart Association and National Institutes of Health, without whose financial support this would not have been possible.

INTRODUCTION TO THE FIRST EDITION

How is the heartbeat generated? What controls the strength of contraction of heart muscle? What are the links between cardiac structure and function? How does our understanding of movement in skeletal and smooth muscle and in non-muscle cells influence our thinking about the development of force in heart muscle? Are there important species differences in how contraction is regulated in the heart? While these important questions have been asked many times, exciting results in many areas of mammalian biology have set the stage for this refreshing new book on *Excitation-Contraction Coupling and Cardiac Contractile Force*. This informative and quantitative book always remains readable. Don Bers explains how contraction arises in heart and how it is controlled. Furthermore, he presents insightful and stimulating discussions of apparently disparate results that will inform and delight both students and "experts". In many ways, Don paints a modern "portrait" of how the heart works and in this picture he shows a close-up of the structural, chemical and physiological links between excitation and contraction.

The recent molecular investigations of excitation-contraction coupling in skeletal and heart muscle have brought together cell physiologists, molecular biologists and physicians in numerous research projects that form the background for this book. These new investigations have led to the explosion of information that would challenge the individual who only seeks to read the primary sources. Don simplifies our task by bringing much of this material together in a single coherent presentation. Exciting questions abound and this book introduces and/or lays the foundation for many of them. Some are stated explicitly by Don while others depend on Don's presentation and the reader's background. For example, the five questions below are among the ones that jump out at me. (1) In heart and skeletal muscle cells, the sarcolemma (SL) has been reported to have many more dihydropyridine receptors than functional calcium channels. Is this apparent excess real or an artifact? If it is real, what does this excess mean? (2) Another question also centers on the dihydropyridine receptor (DHP-R) which is the L-type calcium channel in heart and skeletal muscle. Recent cDNA sequence information along with investigations of structure and function using DHP-R chimeras from heart and skeletal muscle have suggested that a specific cytoplasmic domain or loop of the DHP-R can confer important properties on this receptor/channel. With the skeletal muscle loop in place, E-C coupling in skeletal muscle is "normal" (SL voltage-sensor-dependent calcium release) but when the cardiac loop is in place, the E-C coupling resembles that normally seen in heart (calcium-induced calcium-release). This raises the question of how this particular cytoplasmic loop normally interacts with the SR calcium release channel (i.e. ryanodine receptor) in skeletal muscle. In heart muscle the question is whether there is any interaction at all between the cytoplasmic loop of the DHP-R and the SR calcium release channel. Furthermore, I must wonder if this interaction (if any exists) changes during calcium overload or during maneuvers that change the inotropic state of the heart muscle cell. (3) While calcium-induced calcium release (CICR) appears to be the dominant factor in explaining the link between excitation and contraction in heart muscle, a question lurks just below the surface. How is CICR modulated? What is the relationship between Ca influx and Ca release from the SR? It would appear that all elements of CICR can be modified by intracellular calcium, drugs and neurohormones -- including calcium channels, Na-Ca exchangers, Ca-ATPases, and calcium release channels. Furthermore the release process also seems subject to modulation by intra-SR calcium and may also involve calsequestrin. (4) Do the T-tubular membrane and the non-invaginated SL membrane participate in a similar manner in E-C coupling? Do they have similar densities of DHP-Rs? Do they possess the same CICR elements? (5) How can one make use of our knowledge of E-C coupling and Cellular Ca regulation to develop improved inotropic agents? Many questions are raised by the book, and each reader will undoubtedly focus on different ones. Although Don does not answer or directly address all of our questions, he provides an improved vantage point for us to view the issues important to each of us and to the field in general.

In his portrait of E-C coupling in heart, Don Bers presents many new findings commingled with "established" truth and paints a new picture of how contraction arises and is controlled in the heart. The picture is sharper and contains many new details. He assembles important measurements in new and useful tables, presents figures from recent and more classical publications and shows new figures to supplement his presentation. While integrating new observations with traditional "facts", Don is able to retain both the excitement of discovery and the inevitable controversy arising when important questions cannot be fully answered. This book, written by an active research scientist, therefore provides a critical state-of-the-art report on how the heart works as an electrically and chemically regulated contractile machine.

W.J. Lederer

Baltimore, Maryland

January 1991

INTRODUCTION TO THE SECOND EDITION

Since *Excitation-Contraction Coupling and Cardiac Contractile Force* was published 10 years ago, it has become a classic. The impact of the first edition was great. It was probably greatest on those of us who work in the field because it has become an invaluable tool for us in our work. Furthermore, it has become an important component in our teaching and research programs. The lofty "classic" status of the first edition is well deserved but that presents a daunting challenge for a second edition. It is difficult for a new version of any book to equal that kind of high achievement. The book had become so valuable to those of us working in heart muscle, that we had it at hand during the writing of papers and grants and during teaching. Students, postdoctoral fellows and visitors to our labs have come to expect to have copies as departing gifts. Thus, when the word spread that the second edition was due soon, it was greeted with excitement and trepidation. How can one best a classic? Would the new version be as useful as the first edition? Would it be as comprehensive? How would current controversies be addressed? Would it be as improved as were the updates of classic works by Bernard Katz (*Nerve, Muscle and Synapse*) or Bertil Hille (*Ionic Channels of Excitable Membranes*)?

The second edition of *Excitation-Contraction Coupling and Cardiac Contractile Force* is stunning. It retains the zest and compact form of the first edition, contains the wealth of information and analysis that has become the Bers' hallmark and it is well written. It is easy and delightful to read. While the work does draw heavily from Don Bers' own work, it is appropriately and modestly done. The data from all sources that is presented in the book is well chosen and new material is tightly integrated with the old. The book presents important evolving topics, classic material and issues that are now hotly debated. All of this is done in a scholarly and evenhanded manner. The book does its best at integrating information from multiple sources and providing thoughtful commentary and discussion. It is hard to pick a favorite chapter because the weaker ones were significantly improved and all were made current. The ten chapters cover the field of EC coupling and cardiac contractility with the eye of the classicist but the viewpoint of a modern biologist. I cannot help wondering if it should be called "Functional Genomics and Proteomics of Heart Muscle" since novel molecular findings are so well integrated with cellular and tissue function.

There is a theme that has been developing over the last 10 years that is of particular interest to me and nicely treated by the second edition: local, subcellular, signaling. Virtually every presentation in the second edition invokes, to some extent, "local control" as an element important to the overall signaling. Such discussions include those on Ca^{2+} sparks, mitochondrial signaling, extracellular matrix, channel gating and modulation, transporter function, ryanodine receptor organization and signaling, behavior of the sarcoplasmic reticulum, inotropic mechanisms, and many, many others.

On behalf of the many readers, contributors and colleagues of Donald M. Bers, I must end with a note of appreciation and thanks. The revised version of *Excitation-Contraction Coupling and Cardiac Contractile Force* is a magnificent work and will nicely replace our well-worn copies.

W. J. Lederer
Baltimore, Maryland
March, 2001

TABLE OF CONTENTS

TABLE OF TABLES

D.M. Bers.
Excitation-Contraction Coupling and Cardiac Contractile Force.
2nd Ed., Kluwer Academic Publishers, Dordrecht, 2001

1

CHAPTER 1

MAJOR CELLULAR STRUCTURES INVOLVED IN EXCITATION-CONTRACTION COUPLING

Numerous cellular structures are involved with the process of excitation-contraction coupling (E-C coupling) in cardiac muscle cells. This chapter serves to introduce some of these components from an ultrastructural perspective, and key functional components will be discussed in greater detail in subsequent chapters. Figures 1 and 2 are schematic drawings of the structure of amphibian skeletal muscle (Fig 1) and mammalian ventricular muscle (Fig 2) from a classic ultrastructural study by Fawcett & McNutt (1969; also based on the work of Peachey, 1965).

Despite important differences between skeletal and cardiac muscle which will be discussed below, the *general* scheme of E-C coupling is similar. Electrical excitation of the surface membrane leads to an action potential which propagates as a wave of depolarization along the surface and along the transverse tubules (T-tubules). The depolarization of the T-tubule (or sarcolemma) overlying the terminal cisternae (or subsarcolemmal cisternae) of the sarcoplasmic reticulum (SR) induces the release of Ca from the SR. The details of how this sarcolemmal depolarization is able to induce SR Ca release will be the subject of much ensuing discussion. The Ca released from the SR then binds to the Ca-binding subunit of the thin filament protein troponin which serves to activate contraction. Cellular Ca movement is also complicated (especially in heart muscle) by the presence of Ca channels and transport systems in the sarcolemmal membrane which may transport substantial quantities of Ca and may play an important role in mediating or modulating Ca release from the SR.

There is a recurring theme that skeletal muscle contraction depends almost exclusively on Ca released from the SR with quantitatively insignificant Ca entry across the sarcolemma during a normal twitch. Cardiac muscle contraction, on the other hand, depends on both Ca entry across the sarcolemma and Ca release from the SR (and the relative importance may vary, e.g. Bers, 1985, 1991; see Chapter 9). While these conclusions are based mainly on physiological experiments to be discussed later, it is notable that ultrastructural differences (Figs 1 and 2) are consistent with this conclusion. That is, skeletal muscle has an extensive and well organized SR network with large capacious terminal cisternae abutting the narrow T- tubules. In contrast, cardiac muscle typically has a more sparse and less rigidly organized SR system with smaller saccular enlargements at the cell surface and at junctions. with the much larger diameter T-tubules (200 nm in heart *vs.* 30-40 nm in skeletal muscle). In addition, cardiac myocytes are typically < 20 μm thick, whereas the diameter of skeletal muscle fibers can be many times larger (up to 200 μm). The smaller diameter of heart cells makes diffusion from the extracellular space (and T-tubule matrix) to the myocyte interior more plausible with respect to diffusional limitations than would be the case for skeletal muscle. The larger volume:surface ratio in cardiac

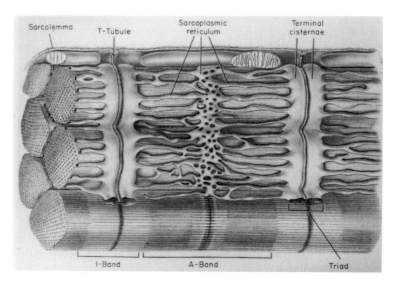

Figure 1.   Schematic diagram of T-tubules and SR associated with several myofibrils in frog skeletal muscle. Each myofibril is surrounded by the meshwork of SR. The SR is greatly enlarged at the terminal cisternae where it comes into close contact from both sides with the relatively narrow T-tubule forming the *triad* at the Z-line.   In mammalian skeletal muscle, T-tubules and triads are normally at the A-I band junction. (From Fawcett & McNutt, 1969, by copyright permission of the Rockefeller University Press).

muscle T-tubules also means that a given ion flux across this membrane will produce smaller depletions and accumulations of ions in the T-tubules. Thus, the structure of the cardiac myocyte is consistent with a quantitatively more important role of transsarcolemmal Ca fluxes.

SARCOLEMMA AND TRANSVERSE TUBULES

The surface sarcolemma is physically continuous with the membrane of the T-tubule and as such the two combine to form the permeability barrier between the inside of the cell and the extracellular medium. Thus, from this functional perspective it is suitable to refer to the complex simply as "the sarcolemma". As a point of semantic distinction it seems reasonable to use the terms "surface sarcolemma" or "external sarcolemma" if one means to exclude the T-tubule when referring to sarcolemma. Another semantic point is that the T-tubules are not strictly transverse, but have many longitudinal and oblique components (Sommer & Waugh, 1976; Soeller & Cannell, 1999), such that the term sarcolemmal tubule network would also be apt.

The ultrastructural organization of the cardiac sarcolemma is important for several reasons. First, it is the site at which Ca enters (and leaves) the cell, so the localization of the relevant transport systems is of functional importance. This is particularly the case because there is differential distribution of ion channels, pumps and other membrane specializations. For example, Almers & Stirling (1984) point out that the densities of Na channels (Jaimovitch *et al.*, 1976), delayed rectifier K channels (Kirsch *et al.*, 1977) and Na/K-ATPase pump sites (Venosa & Horowicz, 1981) are considerably lower in skeletal muscle T-tubules than on the surface sarcolemma, while the density of Ca channels is >4 times higher in T-tubules (Almers. *et al.*, 1981). Indeed, vesicles isolated from skeletal muscle T-tubules have very high densities of

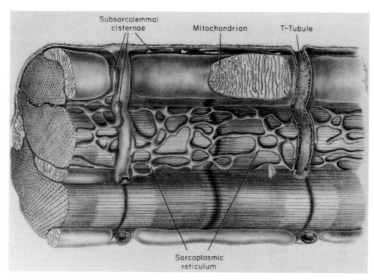

Figure 2. Schematic diagram of T-tubules, SR and myofilaments in mammalian cardiac muscle. Compared to skeletal muscle, cardiac T-tubules are much larger in diameter and the SR is more sparse, but includes junctional couplings with the external sarcolemma as well as the T-tubules. Mitochondria are plentiful and myofibrils are also more irregular in heart. (From Fawcett & McNutt, 1969, with permission from Rockefeller University Press).

dihydropyridine receptors (DHPRs), which are Ca channels. Jorgensen *et al.* (1989) immuno-localized skeletal muscle DHPRs in clusters, primarily in T-tubules. Brandt (1985) separated SR-associated sarcolemmal vesicles from rabbit heart (a presumed T-tubular fraction). This fraction had a high density of DHPRs (*vs.* muscarinic receptors), when compared to the non-SR associated sarcolemmal fraction (i.e. presumed to be surface sarcolemma). Wibo *et al.* (1991) also showed that DHPRs were 3 times more concentrated in a rat T-tubule *vs.* a surface sarcolemmal fraction. Kawai *et al.* (1999) found that sealing off of rat ventricular T-tubules reduced membrane capacitance by 26% (consistent with the 21-33% of sarcolemma being T-tubular; Table 1) and that 75% of Ca channels were in T-tubules. This implies that Ca channel density is ~9 times higher in T-tubule *vs.* external sarcolemma. Doyle *et al.*, (1986) found lower density of DHPRs (*vs.* saxitoxin receptors) in putative T-tubular fractions than in surface sarcolemma fractions from sheep or bovine hearts. Immunofluorescence studies by Carl *et al.* (1995) indicated that in rabbit ventricle DHPRs co-localize with both ryanodine receptors and triadin at dyads in T-tubules. In rabbit atrium and ventricle surface DHPRs were discretely localized over junctional SR containing ryanodine receptors (see also pg 15). This is also the case in chicken heart v here all dyads are superficial (Sun *et al.*, 1995). Thus E-C coupling sites where the SR comes into close contact with the sarcolemma are 1) almost exclusively in T-tubules in skeletal muscle (Spray *et al.*, 1974), 3) mostly in T-tubules in mammalian ventricle or 2) primarily at the surface sarcolemma in mammalian atrium and avian heart.

Table 1 lists some quantitative ultrastructural data of surface areas of sarcolemma and SR components in several cardiac and skeletal muscle preparations. Peachey (1965) reported that in frog skeletal muscle the T-tubular area is ~7 times the area of the external sarcolemma. In mammalian skeletal muscle T-tubular area is somewhat less dominant, but still relatively large.

D.M. Bers Cardiac E-C Coupling

Table 1
Cellular Elements: Surface Area/Cell Volume ($\mu m^2/\mu m^3$)

	Sarcolemma					SR		
	External SL	TT	% of SL in TT	Junct Ext SL	Junct TT	Junct SR	Free SR	Tot SR
Finch V [a]	0.56	0	0	-	-	0.18	0.57	0.75
Mouse V [a]	0.28	0.22	44%	-	-	0.20	0.64	0.84
Mouse V [b]	0.324	0.34	51%	-	-	0.22	0.65	0.84
Mouse V [c]		0.55						1.85
Mouse A [c]		0.26						2.69
Mouse LA [b]	0.65	0.10	13%	-	-	0.09	1.48	1.57
Mouse RA [b]	0.62	0.08	11%	-	-	0.06	1.63	1.69
GP A [d]	-	0.014	-	-	-	0.08[†]	2.21	2.29
GP V [d]	-	0.42	-	-	-	0.13[†]	1.83	1.96
Rat V [e]	0.27	0.07	21%	0.038	-	0.16	1.3	1.46
Rat V [f]	0.31	0.15	33%	0.023	0.069	0.19	1.0	1.19
Rabbit V [f]	0.33	0.23	41%	0.010	0.042	-	-	-

	External SL	TT	% of SL in TT	Junct Ext SL	Junct TT	Junct SL Tot	% of SL as dyad Ext SL	TT
Rabbit V [g]	0.35	0.25	42%	0.016	0.051	0.068	4.6%	21%
Rat V [g]	0.31	0.15	33%	0.023	0.069	0.093	7.7%	48%
Mouse V [g]	0.31	0.17	37%	0.020	0.070	0.090	6.5%	40%
Rat V [h]	0.24	0.44	64%					

	External SL	TT	% of SL in TT	Junct Ext SL	Junct TT	Junct SR	Free SR	Tot SR
Frog V [i]	1.19	0	0	-	-	0.014	0.26	0.27
Frog A [i]	1.32	0	0	-	-	0.018	0.44	0.46
Lizard V [i]	1.14	0	0	-	-	0.045	0.46	0.50
Lizard A [i]	1.25	0	0	-	-	0.056	0.89	0.94
Frog Sartorius [j]	0.04	0.28	88%	-	-	1.4	4	5.4
Frog Sartorius [k]	0.064	0.22	77%	-	-	0.54	1.5	2.0
GP soleus [l]	0.116	0.064	36%	-	-	0.24	0.73	0.97
GP white vastus [m]	0.097	0.146	60%	-	-	0.41	0.91	1.32
GP red vastus [m]	0.097	0.148	60%	-	-	0.33	0.65	0.98
Sheep Purkinje [n]	0.037	0.423*	92%*	-	-	-	-	-
Dog Purkinje [o]	0.096	0.041*	30%*	-	-	-	-	-

[a] Bossen et al., 1978; Sommer & Johnson, 1979
[b] Bossen et al., 1981
[c] Forbes & Sperelakis, 1995
[d] Forbes & Van Niel, 1988
[e] Page et al., 1971, [f] Page, 1978
[g] Page & Surdyk-Droske, 1979; Soeller & Cannell, 1999
[i] Bossen & Sommer, 1984
[j] Peachey, 1965
[k] Mobley & Eisenberg, 1975
[l] Eisenberg et al., 1974
[m] Eisenberg & Kuda, 1975, 1976
[n] Mobley & Page, 1972
[o] Eisenberg & Cohen, 1983

Ventricle (V), Atrium (A), Guinea Pig (GP), External sarcolemma (Ext SL), T-tubule (TT), Junctional (Junct), Total (Tot). Mammalian skeletal muscle can be classified into slow (soleus), fast/glycolytic (white vastus) and fast/oxidative/glycolytic (red vastus). *Intercellular clefts or folds for Purkinje fibers, which lack TT. [†] Excluding corbular SR. In some cases right (R) and left (L) heart data were averaged.

There also seems to be a difference between fast (vastus) and slow (soleus) muscle which may have a functional correlate (Eisenberg, 1983). In mammalian ventricle about 30-50% of the sarcolemmal area is in the T-tubules and in mammalian atrium this fraction is < 15%. This may be an upper limit since anecdotal reports often claim to see no T-tubules in mammalian atrium, and Tidball *et al.* (1991) reported ~20 times less T-tubular area in rabbit atrium *vs.* ventricle (and also greater cell to cell variability in atrium). Bird, amphibian and reptilian hearts lack T-tubules entirely. The ratio of external sarcolemma/cell volume is also inversely related to the cell diameter (i.e. 2/radius if one assumes a cylindrical shape). The cell diameters in frog and lizard hearts and mammalian atria are smaller than those of mammalian ventricular muscle. For these smaller cells (with high surface to volume ratio), T-tubules are less important for inward spread of activation (or Ca diffusion) than in mammalian ventricle or the even larger diameter cells in skeletal muscle. Cardiac Purkinje fibers are cells which are specialized for electrical conduction, and the large cross-sectional area decreases the longitudinal internal resistivity and hence increases the rate of propagation of electrical impulses.

Soeller & Cannell (1999) used 2-photon fluorescence microscopy in intact rat ventricular myocytes and found T-tubules to occupy 3.6% of the cell volume and a surface area of 0.44 $\mu m^2/\mu m^3$, *vs.* 0.24 $\mu m^2/\mu m^3$ for the external sarcolemma (i.e. 64% of sarcolemma in T-tubules). They also found that 60% of the T-tubular area is within 0.55 μm of the Z-line and includes many non-transverse elements, leading them to suggest that T-tubules be renamed the sarcolemmal Z-rete. Perhaps the term sarcolemmal tubule network is simpler and still de-emphasizes the transverse component, but today T-tubule remains the standard term.

The complexity of the T-tubule network also means that when one changes extracellular solutions around a myocyte there is a delay between bulk concentration changes and diffusion in and out of the T-tubules (Blatter & Niggli, 1998). Shepherd & McDonnough (1998) measured the functional time dependence of rapidly changing $[Na]_o$ or $[Ca]_o$ on Na or Ca current (I_{Na} or I_{Ca}) in guinea-pig myocytes. In atrial myocytes (which lack T-tubules) I_{Na} and I_{Ca} changed with a single fast time constant (τ) of 20-30 msec (i.e. >90% complete in 85 ms, reflecting bulk solution flow). For ventricular myocytes, 36% of the I_{Ca} and I_{Na} also changed rapidly (reflecting surface SL channels), but 64% changed more slowly ($\tau \sim 200$ msec) indicating that ~64% of functioning Na and Ca channels are in T-tubules (in agreement with data discussed on pg 3). If these channels are concentrated in T-tubules, this value ought to be higher than the percent of sarcolemmal area in T-tubules (21-51% in Table 1), but Soeller & Cannell (1999) remarkably got the same number (64%). This T-tubule diffusional problem also requires >500 msec for an abrupt change in surface $[Ca]_o$ or $[Na]_o$ to be fully transmitted to the T-tubules.

The surface:volume ratios in Table 1 are also valuable (see Chapter 3) in quantitative evaluations of trans-sarcolemmal ion fluxes (e.g. Ca current) in terms of how they alter cellular ion concentrations. Indeed, Satoh *et al.* (1996) measured cell volume and membrane capacitance simultaneously in myocytes from several cardiac preparations and determined surface to volume ratios (in pF/pL). These results in Table 2 are particularly useful for translating electrophysio-logical measurements of ion flux (in pA/pF or pmol/pF) to fluxes per unit cell volume (μM).

A major structural specialization of the sarcolemma is coupling with the SR (e.g. triads and dyads). Figure 1 suggests that in skeletal muscle, most of the T-tubular membrane is

Table 2

Electrophysiological Surface: Volume measures

	Rabbit	Rat		Ferret
		3 mo.	6 mo.	
V_{Cell} (pL)	30.4	30.9	36.8	30.9
C_M (pF)	138	207	324	162
Length (μm)	143	124	140	138
Width (μm)	32	34	33	31
Depth (μm)	12	13	14	14
% V_{cell} Mitochondrial[†]	71	68	68	68
Surface:Volume Ratios				
C_M/V_{Cell} (pF/ pL cell)	4.58	6.76	8.88	5.39
C_M/V_{Cyt} (pF/ pL cytosol)	6.44	9.94	13.0	7.96
$μm^2/μm^3$ (as in Table 1)	0.46	0.68	0.89	0.54

Data from Satoh *et al.* (1996) and [†] Barth *et al.* (1992). Note that surface:volume ratio in units of pF/pL are 10 times larger than in $μm^2/μm^3$. Thus, using 1 $μF/cm^2$, 4.58 pF/pL would translate to 0.46 $μm^2/μm^3$ in Table 1.

involved in junctional, triadic complexes with the SR (Peachey, 1965). The triad refers to the coupling of two SR terminal cisternae to either side of a T-tubule. In cardiac muscle these junctions are more apparent as dyads and can occur either at the surface sarcolemma or with T-tubular membrane. In mammalian ventricular muscle Page & Surdyk-Droske (1979) found that 4-8% of the external sarcolemma is involved in junctional complexes whereas 20-50% of the T-tubular membrane is so involved. They also reported that rabbit ventricle had a smaller sarcolemmal fraction involved in SR junctions (4.6% of surface and 20.6% of T-tubule) compared to rat or mouse ventricle (6.5-7.7% of surface and 40-48% of T-tubule). This structural observation correlates with physiological data, indicating that ventricular contraction in rat is more SR Ca-dependent than in rabbit, which is more SR Ca-dependent than frog (where junctional couplings are sparse and mainly sub-sarcolemma; Fabiato & Fabiato, 1978; Bers *et al.*, 1981; Fabiato, 1982; Bers 1985 and see Chapter 9). That is, twitches in frog and to a lesser degree rabbit (but not rat) can be supported largely by Ca entry from the extracellular space.

The sarcolemma also exhibits caveolae, which are flask-shaped invaginations (50-80 nm in diameter) and contribute significantly (~10%) to the surface area of both surface and T-tubular sarcolemma (Levin & Page, 1980; Anderson, 1993). Caveolae are probably neither pinocytotic nor reservoirs of membrane for recruitment during physical stress (Sommer & Johnson, 1979; Langer *et al.*, 1982, Forbes & Sperelakis, 1995). They do seem to be the preferential location of the scaffolding protein caveolin-3 and signaling molecules such as nitric oxide synthase and protein kinase C (Song *et al.*, 1996; Feron *et al.*, 1996; Rybin *et al.*, 1999).

The other major specialization of the sarcolemma is the region where cells are closely apposed end to end, known as the intercalated disk. The ends of cardiac muscle cells generally interdigitate (as in Fig 3) and the classic work of Sjöstrand *et al.* (1958) described three differentiations in this region known as 1) the nexus or gap junction, 2) fascia adherens or intermediate junction and 3) macula adherens or desmosome. The fascia and macula adherens appear to be of central importance in the mechanical connection of one cell to the next and the macula adherens is sometimes likened to a spot-weld between cells. Intermediate and actin

Table 3

Cellular Elements: As % of Cell Volume

	MF	Mito	Nucleus	TT	Junct SR	Free SR	SR tot	SR:TT
Finch V [a]	57.3	34	-	0	0.21	0.62	0.83	-
Mouse V [a]	54.3	37.5	-	0.8	0.22	0.65	0.87	0.75
Mouse V [b]	54.3	37.5	-	0.95	0.22	0.65	0.87	0.92
Mouse L.A [b]	53.0	20.3	-	0.25	0.10	1.62	1.73	6.92
Mouse R.A [b]	52.6	19.8	-	0.20	0.06	1.69	1.76	8.80
Mouse V [c]	43.3	37.0	1.32	3.19			6.9	2.16
Mouse A [c]	44.6	25.7	2.1	1.52			12.3	8.09
Guinea Pig A [d]	43.2	17.9	3.8	0.08	0.46[†]	9.47	9.93	124
Guinea Pig V [d]	45.2	25.3	2.8	2.62	0.56[†]	7.37	7.93	3.03
Guinea Pig A [e]	41.4	14	4	-	0.5	1.7	2.2	-
Guinea Pig V [f]	50	25	-	~2	-	-	-	-
Rat V [g]	48.1	34	-	1.2	0.3	3.2	3.5	2.9
Rat V [h]	46.7	36	2	-	0.3	3.2	3.5	-
Frog V [i]	46.1	13.8	-	0	0.03	0.35	0.38	-
Frog A [i]	42.4	12.0	-	0	0.03	0.53	0.56	-
Lizard V [i]	50.1	25.8	-	0	0.09	0.6	0.69	-
Lizard A [i]	41.1	18.7	-	0	0.11	1.12	1.22	-
Frog V [j]	-	-	-	0	0.2	0.3	0.5	-
Frog Sartorius [k]	82.6	1.6	-	0.32	4.1	5	9.1	28.4
Guinea Pig								
Soleus [l]	86.7	4.9	0.9	0.14	0.9	2.2	3.1	22.1
White Vastus [m]	82.0	1.9	0.15	0.27	1.6	3.0	4.6	17.0
Red Vastus [n]	80.3	8.2	0.9	0.28	1.2	2.0	3.3	11.8
Sheep Purkinje [o]	23.4	10.3	1	0.23*	-	-	-	-

[a] Bossen *et al.*, 1978	[h] Page, 1978
Sommer & Johnson, 1979	[i] Bossen & Sommer, 1984
[b] Bossen *et al.*, 1981	[j] Page & Niedergerke, 1972
[c] Forbes &Sperelakis, 1995	[k] Mobley & Eisenberg, 1975
[d] Forbes & Van Niel, 1988	[l] Eisenberg *et al.*, 1974
[e] Frank *et al.*, 1975	[m] Eisenberg & Kuda, 1975
[f] Eisenberg, 1983	[n] Eisenberg & Kuda, 1976
[g] Page *et al.*, 1971	[o] Mobley & Page, 1972

Myofilaments (MF), Mitochondria (Mito), Nucleus (Nuc), Ventricle (V), Atrium (A), T-tubule (TT), Junctional (Junct). Mammalian skeletal muscle can be classified into slow (soleus), fast/glycolytic (white vastus) and fast/oxidative/glycolytic (red vastus). *Intercellular clefts or folds for Purkinje fibers. [†]Excluding corbular SR. The SR volumes estimated by Forbes & Van Niel were acknowledged to be artifactually high due to a contrast effect. In some cases right (R) and left (L) heart data were averaged.

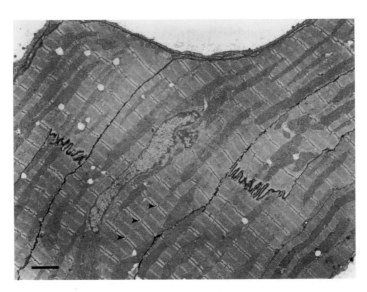

Figure 3. Finch cardiac muscle stained with colloidal lanthanum hydroxide as extracellular marker. Note the interdigitation of cell ends and the lack of T-tubules. Arrowheads indicate structures identified at higher magnification as extended junctional SR. Bar = 2 µm. (From Sommer & Waugh, 1976, with permission).

filaments also insert at the intercalated disk (Price & Sanger, 1983), emphasizing the mechanical function of this cytoskeletal structure (see pg 17-18).

Gap junctions are predominantly on parts of the intercalated disk parallel to the long axis of the cell (edges of interdigitations, Spray & Burt, 1990; Severs, 1990, 1997). Page & Shibata (1981) estimated that gap junctions make up only 0.7-1% of the total sarcolemmal area in rat and rabbit ventricle (~3% in dog Purkinje Strand, Eisenberg & Cohen, 1983). Chen *et al.*, (1989), however, suggested that these values in rat ventricle may underestimate the gap junctional area by 3-4 fold (based on comparison of classical cross sections *vs. en face* sections of the transverse cell borders). These gap junctions serve as the low resistance electrical pathways that allow the heart to function as an electrical syncytium. Revel & Karnovsky (1967) first demonstrated that the membranes of the two cells did not fuse, but were separated by a narrow 2 nm gap at the nexus and also observed hexagonal arrays, now known to be the functional units. A general working model of the gap junction has evolved (e.g. Unwin & Zampighi, 1980; Makowski *et al.*, 1977) in which one hexameric unit with a central pore (or connexon) from each cell meet within the gap and form a pore which allows direct connection between the cytoplasms of the two cells. The molecular weight of the "connexin" monomers which make up the connexon differ in liver (mw ~28,000, Henderson *et al.*, 1979; Hertzberg & Gilula, 1979) lens (mw = 26,000, Goode-nough, 1979) and cardiac cells (mw = 43,000, known as connexin-43, Kensler & Goodenough, 1980; Manjunath *et al.*, 1982; Beyer *et al.*, 1987). The cardiac protein appears to have an extra polypeptide on the cytoplasmic side which may contribute to functional differences in channel properties (Manjunath & Page, 1985). Each connexin molecule has 4 transmembrane spanning regions, an intracellular loop and a carboxy tail. Six connexins come together to form a connexon with a central pore whose conductance can be regulated. While connexin-43 is the dominant ventricular (and vascular smooth muscle) isoform, connexin-40 is abundant in the A-V node, bundle branches, Purkinje fibers and some atrial cells. Connexin-45 is also expressed in heart at much lower levels and connexin-37 and 40 are expressed in the vascular endothelium (Beyer *et al.*, 1989; Gourdie *et al.*, 1993; Kanter *et al.*, 1993; Severs, 1997; Spray, 1998). The diameter of the pore has been estimated to be 1.6-2.0 nm by the cell-to-cell diffusion of fluorescent tracers (Flagg-Newton *et al.*, 1979). Notably, this allows ions such as Ca and K to pass, as well as small signaling molecules like cyclic AMP and inositol phosphates. The single channel conductance of connexin-43 (60 pS) is lower than that of connexin-40 (150-200 pS).

Cardiac gap junction permeability is decreased by high [Ca]$_i$ (DeMello, 1975; Weingart, 1977) and intracellular acidification (Reber & Weingart, 1982). This has the functional advantage of uncoupling metabolically compromised cells. While the interaction of these effects is complex and synergistic (Burt, 1987), Spray *et al.*, (1982) concluded that the pH sensitivity exceeds the Ca sensitivity. This may protect healthy cells from neighboring cells which have either pathologically high [Ca]$_i$ or low pH$_i$ (or depolarization). The down-side may be that diverting the normal electrical conduction pathway can also be pro-arrhythmic (see pg 99-100).

So far, sarcolemma has been used in reference to the phospholipid/cholesterol bilayer with the integral proteins (e.g. ion channels and pumps) which are floating in it. The sarcolemma as such has clear regional specialization (e.g. dyads & gap junctions), where the bilayer surfaces are in close contact with special structures and where special proteins are located. The outer surface of muscle sarcolemma is also invested with a layer abundant in acidic mucopoly-saccharides (Bennett, 1963). Frank *et al.* (1977) divided this glycocalyx (or "sweet husk") functionally into a surface coat (a less dense 20 nm layer adjacent to the sarcolemma) and an external lamina (a more dense outer 30 nm layer at the interstitial interface). This glycocalyx is rich in sialic acid residues, which may account for fixed negative charges in this region and explain the observation that pretreatment with neuraminidase decreases the labeling of the glycocalyx with cationic electron-dense markers (lanthanum, ruthenium red and colloidal iron, Frank *et al.*, 1977). Langer *et al.* (1976) found that such neuraminidase treatment greatly increased cellular Ca exchange and suggested that sialic acid in the surface coat may importantly regulate sarcolemmal Ca permeability. Exposure of cells to Ca-free solution causes the external lamina to lift away from the surface coat (Fig 4, Frank *et al.*, 1977). They attributed this to break-down of sugar-Ca-sugar bridges and suggested that this might be involved in damage associated with readmission of Ca (i.e. the Ca paradox described by Zimmerman & Hülsmann, 1966; see also Frank *et al.*, 1982; Chapman & Tunstall, 1987; Bhojani & Chapman, 1990).

This separation of external lamina in Ca-free solution creates surface blebs which span from T-tubule to T-tubule, such that the external lamina remains anchored by its extension into the T-system. This also points to the fact that these surface layers remain associated with the sarcolemma within T-tubules in cardiac muscle. This contrasts with skeletal muscle where the glycocalyx does not appear to extend into the narrower T-tubules (Fawcett & McNutt, 1969).

EXTRACELLULAR SPACE

Knowledge of the contents of the extracellular space is important for understanding their possible direct participation in cardiac function (above), but also for correcting measurements made in intact preparations in terms of intracellular *vs.* extracellular concentrations. Frank & Langer (1974) characterized the extracellular space in arterially perfused rabbit intraventricular

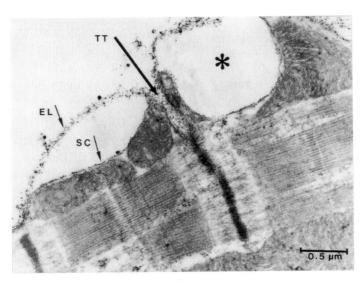

Figure 4. Rabbit ventricular muscle stained with colloidal iron. The muscle had been perfused in Ca-free solution for 20 min. Note the separation of the external lamina (EL) from the surface coat (SC) forming a bleb (*). The EL is anchored where it penetrates into the T-tubule (TT). (From Frank *et al.*, 1977, by permission of the American Heart Association, Inc.).

septum and also measured extracellular space volume by both morphological and chemical means. They found that 59% of the extracellular space is vascular, 23% ground substance (resembling the glycocalyx material described above), 7% connective tissue cells, 6% empty space and 4% collagen. They also demonstrated that 36% of the cell circumference at its widest point is within 200 nm of a capillary. This close proximity to capillaries is illustrated in Fig 5 and emphasizes the fact that in vascularly perfused ventricular muscle, the myocyte has rapid access to the vascular contents (rather than requiring a strictly series model for diffusion through a large intervening interstitial compartment).

Frank & Langer (1974) estimated tissue extracellular space morphometrically (27.6% including T-tubules) and chemically (35.7% using ^{14}C-sucrose and 36.2% using ^{35}S-sulfate). Lee & Fozzard (1975) reported a similar value (32.9%) for the ^{35}S-sulfate space in superfused rabbit papillary muscle. Bridge *et al.* (1982) measured a similar value for the extracellular space in rabbit heart *in vivo* using ^{14}C-sucrose (0.303 ml/g) and CoEDTA (0.294 ml/g), but found much larger values in the isolated aqueous perfused intraventricular septum (0.51 ml/g for CoEDTA and 0.46 ml/g for ^{14}C-sucrose). While most extracellular space values for mammalian ventricle are in the 25-35% range, the higher value reported by Bridge *et al.* (1982) for the intraventricular septum may reflect tissue edema due to the low oncotic pressure of the aqueous vascular perfusion. Thus, the extracellular space volumes used to correct tissue contents to intracellular or extracellular contents should be measured under the same experimental conditions.

SARCOPLASMIC RETICULUM

The SR is an entirely intracellular, membrane bounded compartment which is not continuous with the sarcolemma. The main function of this organelle in muscle appears to be sequestration and release of Ca to the myoplasm. The volume of SR varies among cell types

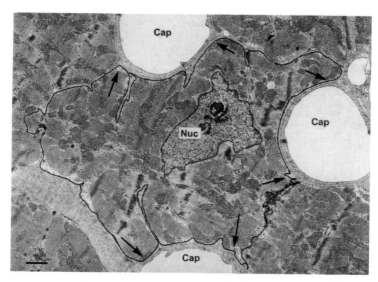

Figure 5. Rabbit interventricular septal cell in transverse section. Note that ~36% of the cell surface is within 200 nm of a capillary (cap), as indicated by the borders between arrowheads. Bar = 1 μm. (From Frank & Langer, 1974, by copyright permission of the Rockefeller University Press).

(e.g. Table 3) being most abundant in skeletal muscle, less abundant in mammalian heart and least abundant in frog ventricle. This may reflect functional differences in the relative importance of SR Ca in the activation of contraction (See Chapter 9). The SR in skeletal muscle is very highly organized. This allowed Winegrad (1965) to perform his classical auto-radiographic study in which he directly confirmed the terminal cisternae as the site of Ca release from the SR. This was a very important conclusion because it indicated anatomical segregation of transport functions within the SR. Except for the junctions between the SR and sarcolemma, the SR membrane appears fairly homogeneous and contains mainly the SR Ca-ATPase pump protein (Stewart & MacLennan, 1974; Katz *et al.*, 1986) which is manifest as intramembrane particles ~8 nm in diameter and 3000-5000/μm^2 of SR membrane (Franzini-Armstrong, 1975). These particles are also observed in isolated SR vesicles and the density may be slightly lower in cardiac *vs.* skeletal muscle SR vesicles (Baskin & Deamer, 1969). Even the major part of the terminal cisternae appear to have Ca-pump protein. Thus, the vast majority of the surface of the SR is likely to function primarily to remove Ca from the cytoplasm. The relative area of the SR surface involved in couplings with the sarcolemma also varies substantially from one muscle type to another (see Junct SR in Table 1). Again, skeletal muscle has the greatest relative area of junctional SR, with mammalian heart less, and frog heart the least.

The junctions of SR with sarcolemma (surface or T-tubule, see Fig 2) are highly specialized and feature bridging structures or spanning proteins which have been called "feet" by Franzini-Armstrong (1970, see Fig 6), and also pillars, spanning proteins, bridges and junctional feet. Similar structures are seen in cardiac muscle at the junction of SR with either surface or T-tubular sarcolemma (see Fig 7). Caldwell & Caswell (1982) showed biochemical evidence for a high molecular weight protein which could be the junctional feet (see Chapter 7).

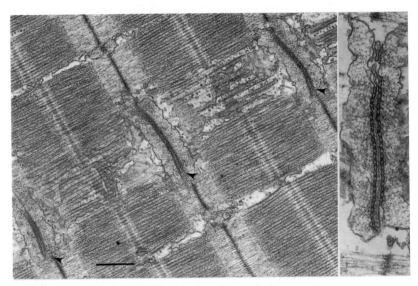

Figure 6. Tangential view of 3 triads from frog sartorius (arrowheads) showing periodic junctional "feet" at the site where the SR and T-tubule come into close contact. Bar = 0.5 μm; inset is at 2.2× higher magnification. (From Franzini-Armstrong, 1970, by copyright permission of the Rockefeller University Press).

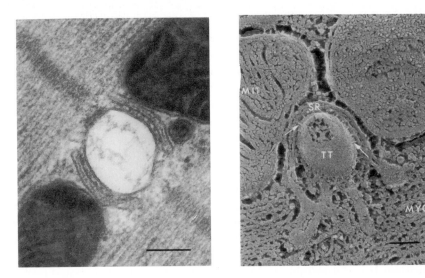

Figure 7. Rat papillary muscle in a thin section electron micrograph (left) and freeze-etched electron microscopy after ultra-rapid freezing without fixation (right). Junctional "feet" between the SR and T-tubule (TT) can be seen to periodically span the gap. Bar=0.2 μm. (From Frank, 1990 with permission).

Based on their distinctive morphology and high affinity for the neutral plant alkaloid, ryanodine, feet were purified and identified as the SR Ca-release channel in skeletal (Inui *et al.*, 1987a; Lai *et al.*, 1987) and cardiac muscle (Lai *et al.*, 1988a; Inui *et al.*, 1987b). This ryanodine receptor protein is so large (560 kDa for the monomer; Takeshima *et al.*, 1989), that the

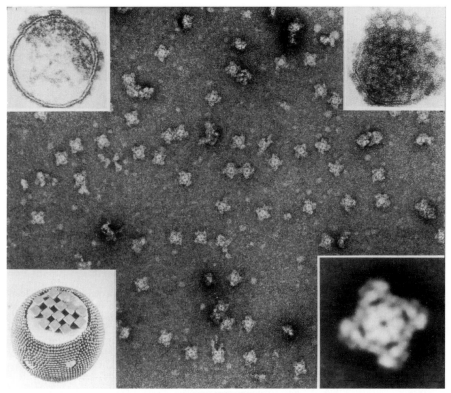

Figure 8. Morphology of the foot protein/ ryanodine receptor/ Ca release channel of skeletal SR. Center) Electron micrograph of negatively stained receptors showing the 4-fold symmetry, square shape (~27 nm/ side) and computer average of 240 images (bottom right). The foot protein extends ~12 nm from the SR surface of SR vesicles originating from terminal cisternae (top left) and the same square array can be seen in tangential sections of these vesicles (top right, see also Fig 99). A model of the terminal cisternal membrane (bottom left) shows a junctional face membrane with feet, and the remainder of the SR surface covered largely by the Ca-pump protein. (From Fleischer & Inui, 1989, with permission).

functional tetramer can be seen at the electron microscopic level (Fig 8; Saito *et al.*, 1988; Wagenknecht *et al.*, 1989, 1994, 1995; Seresheva *et al.*, 1995, 1999; Samsó *et al.*, 1999). This channel will be discussed in detail in Chapter 7 (see pg 189).

In addition Block *et al.* (1988) demonstrated that these feet are organized in a distinct pattern on the SR underneath the T-tubular membrane in skeletal muscle and are matched by an organized array of particles in the T-tubule membrane which are likely to be the sarcolemmal Ca channel protein (or DHPR, see Fig 9). This arrangement is consistent with a stoichiometry of 1 ryanodine receptor tetramer (RyR) to 2 DHPR as measured in skeletal muscle, whereas in mammalian ventricle the RyR:DHPR ratio is 4-10, depending on species (Bers & Stiffel, 1993; Wibo *et al.*, 1991, see Table 25, pg 287). That constrains the organization of the junctional coupling as indicated in Fig 10 (and observed experimentally by Franzini-Armstrong & Protasi, 1997). Since the ryanodine receptors are clustered at these junctions, it may be important to consider how many tetramers (or feet) there are in a typical array. Franzini-Armstrong *et al.* (1999) estimated that these domains (referred to as couplons) in skeletal muscle contain from 17 feet (in guinea-pig slow soleus) to 38 feet (in fast rat extensor digitorum longus). In dog and

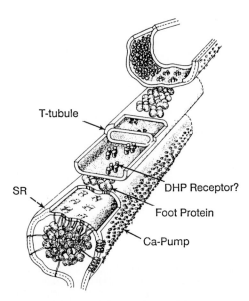

T-tubule

SR

DHP Receptor?

Foot Protein

Ca-Pump

Figure 9. Three-dimensional reconstruction of the relative positions of key proteins at the skeletal muscle triad. The SR is filled with calsequestrin and the non-junctional surface is covered with the Ca-pump protein. The RyR feet are organized in two parallel rows and protrude from the SR. A similar array of proteins (dihydropyridine receptor) exists in the T-tubular membrane, but the axis of fourfold symmetry is rotated and they lie only over alternating foot structures (see also Fig 109). Based on toadfish swim-bladder muscle (from Block *et al.*, 1988, by copyright permission of the Rockefeller University Press).

mouse ventricle the couplon size was 90-128 feet for internal dyads, and 61-150 for surface couplings (rat ventricle T-tubule couplons averaged 267 feet). Given the packing array, 100 ryanodine receptors would occupy a 60-100 nm diameter circle. So a typical cardiac couplon may have about 100 RyR and 10-25 DHPR. They also measured the minimum transverse distance between couplons (300-400 nm along mouse and rat T-tubules). The implications of this arrangement for E-C coupling will be considered more specifically in Chapter 8. The SR also contains calsequestrin, a low affinity, high capacity Ca binding protein (Ostwald & MacLennan, 1974) which is especially concentrated in the terminal cisternae (Meissner, 1975). Calsequestrin is crucial to the Ca buffering capacity of the SR (Chapter 7, pg 172).

Sommer and colleagues have also described what seems to be junctional SR (including feet), which does not come into contact with any sarcolemma component. One specialized region (extended junctional SR) is prominent in the interior of avian cardiac myocytes which lack T-tubules (Jewett *et al.*, 1971; Sommer & Johnson, 1979). This extended junctional SR occurs along the Z-disk in bird ventricle where T-tubule/SR junctions would be prominent in mammalian ventricle (see Table 1 and Fig 3). Corbular SR (Dolber & Sommer, 1984) is a basket-like form of extended junctional SR. It exhibits the morphology of junctional SR, but it is not in the vicinity of the sarcolemma, and is normally connected to the free or network SR only at one point. Corbular SR has been described in mammalian ventricle (Dolber & Sommer, 1984), but is particularly apparent in atrium, Purkinje fibers (Sommer & Johnson, 1968; 1979) and chicken cardiac muscle (Jewett & Leonard, 1973; Jorgenson & Campbell, 1984). Jorgensen *et al.* (1985, 1993 & personal communication) found that up to 30-40 % of the calsequestrin and ryanodine receptors in rat and dog ventricular myocytes are in this sort of non-junctional SR. These "uncoupled" SR components with morphology like true junctional SR provide a functional

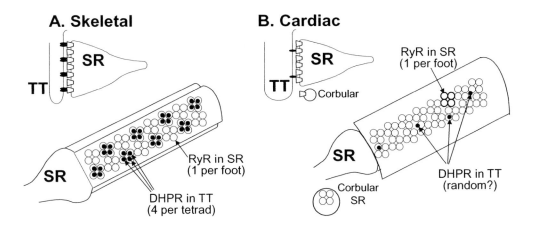

Figure 10. Diagram comparing the organizational differences between skeletal and cardiac T-tubule junctions. The upper diagrams are side views of the junction (trapezoids are ryanodine receptors, RyR and filled ovals dihydropyridine receptors, DHPR). Lower panels are views from inside the T-tubule at the junction. Note that DHPRs are sparse and less aligned in heart (modified from Bers & Stiffel, 1993).

challenge to models of E-C coupling. That is, what is the function of these SR components? Do they participate in Ca release during the activation of a normal contraction? Is the mechanism of release distinct from that of true junctional SR?

Scriven *et al.* (2000) examined the colocalization of several key proteins with respect to E-C coupling (Table 4). While all of the DHPRs were near RyRs, some RyRs were not near DHPRs (e.g. possibly in corbular SR). Notably, neither Na channels nor Na/Ca exchanger were colocalized near RyRs, nor each other. Thus, both Na channels and Na/Ca exchange appear to be excluded from the cardiac SR-sarcolemmal junctions. This may limit the role that these transporters have in E-C coupling (see pg 205, 232-237).

Table 4
Co-localization of some key Proteins in Rat Ventricular Myocytes*

| | | Co-Localization (%) ||
A (FITC Label)	B (Texas Red)	A with B	B with A
DHPR	RyR	56.7 ± 5.1	36.7 ± 4.8
Calsequestrin	RyR	61.6 ± 7.2	55.8 ±.6.2
NaCaX	RyR	5.8 ± 1.9	7.7 ± 2.3
Na Channel	RyR.	2.9 ± 0.9	3.1 ± 1.2
NaCaX	Na Channel	3.5 ± 1.5	3.6 ± 2.1
RyR	RyR	64.7 ± 5.8	61.2 ± 5.7

*Ca channel is L-type Ca channel, NaCaX is Na/Ca exchange, RyR is ryanodine receptor. Data are from Scriven *et al.* (2000) with one antibody labeled with FITC (fluorescein isothiocyanate) and the other with Texas Red. Note that maximal colocalization (last line) is ~65%.

MITOCHONDRIA

About 35% of the volume of mammalian and avian ventricular muscle cells is occupied by mitochondria (see Fig 2, Table 2 & 3 and Barth *et al.*, 1992). The mitochondria are the site of oxidative phosphorylation and the tricarboxylic acid cycle and the large mitochondrial content in mammalian ventricle bespeaks the high demands on this organelle for energy supplied by aerobic metabolism. The mitochondrial fraction of cell volume is lower in mammalian atrial muscle and Purkinje fibers as well as amphibian and reptilian hearts and skeletal muscle (Table 3). Indeed, there is substantial variation in mitochondrial volume among different types of skeletal muscles that reflects differences in the oxidative capacity of those muscle types. The surface area of the folded inner mitochondrial membrane in rat left ventricle has been estimated to be 20 $\mu m^2/\mu m^3$ of cell volume (Page, 1978). This membrane is the site of control of metabolite and ion transport (e.g. Ca and protons). The surface area is more than 10 times larger than that of the combined sarcolemmal and SR membranes, so a modest Ca transport by mitochondria could have a large impact on overall cellular Ca regulation (see Chapter 3, pg 56-62).

Cardiac mitochondria are usually cylindrical, but can flatten because of the tight packing in cells. The cristae in cardiac mitochondria are more tightly packed than those in hepatocytes, perhaps reflecting the continuous intensive energy demands of the myocardium (Sommer & Johnson, 1979). A layer of mitochondria is often found just under the plasma membrane and also between adjacent myofibrils. As mitochondria are squeezed in everywhere in cardiac cells, it is not realistic to assign a specific functional role to the cellular mitochondrial distribution.

MYOFILAMENTS

The myofilaments occupy 45-60% of the cell volume in mammalian ventricle (Table 3, Fig 2). This fraction is larger in skeletal muscle and smaller in atria and cells specialized for electrical conduction (Purkinje fibers). Myofilaments are composed of the thick (or myosin) and thin (or actin) filaments as well as associated contractile and cytoskeletal components. Myofilament bundles or fibrils are less defined in cardiac *vs.* skeletal muscle due to branching.

The myofilaments are the contractile machinery of the cell and indeed they represent the end effector responsible for transducing chemical energy into mechanical energy and work. The sarcomere is the fundamental contractile unit in striated muscle and is bounded by the Z-line (Fig 11). The thin actin filaments (~10 nm thick) extend ~1 μm from the Z-line toward the center of each sarcomere (for more detailed structure and function of the thin and thick filaments with

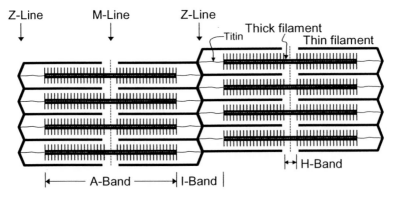

Figure 11. The organization of the sarcomere. The thin filaments meet at the Z-lines and the center of the thick filaments is known as the M-line. The I-band (or isotropic band) is the area where there are only thin filaments and the A-band (or anisotropic band) is the length of the thick filaments. The region of the thick filament where there is no overlap with thin filaments is known as the H-band (or H-zone).

respect to contraction see Chapter 2). Tropomodulin is localized at the tip of the thin filament and may be involved in regulating the length of the filament (Sussman *et al.*, 1994; Gregorio *et al.*, 1995a,b). At the Z-line α-actinin is also a crucial structural element. Connections from the Z-line to the sarcolemma include actin filaments (F-actin), α-actinin, the 7-10 nm thick intermediate filament protein desmin (Lazarides, 1980, 1982; Eriksson & Thornell, 1979) and ankyrin. Ankyrin has also been found to associate with the sarcolemma and certain membrane transporters, such as the Na/Ca exchanger (Li *et al.*, 1993).

The thick myosin filaments are ~1.6 μm long (~15 nm thick). Myosin heads protrude from the long axis every 14.3 nm, with the protrusion angle rotating 120° at each point, such that in one plane (as Fig 11) the heads seem to be spaced 43 nm apart. These myosin heads create the crossbridges that interact with actin to generate contraction. Myosin binding protein C (sometimes called C-protein) appears to wrap around the thick filament and may be important in stabilizing and modulating the thick filament (Offer, 1972; Freiburg & Gautel, 1996). C-protein appears as 10 nm bands (near the crossbridge extension away from the filament axis) every 43 nm, within two 200 nm zones on either side of the M-line separated by a 400 nm bare zone. Thick filaments are interconnected transversely at the M-line by M-protein and myomesin (Obermann *et al.*, 1995). Titin is an extremely long (3,000 kDa) structural protein that runs from the M-line, through the thick filament and all the way to the Z-line (Gautel & Goulding, 1996). Titin may be important in creating a scaffold for myosin deposition on the thick filament (Trinick, 1994), and stabilizing it structurally in association with C-protein (Freiburg & Gautel, 1996). Titin is also extremely important in determining the passive stiffness of the heart (Brady, 1991). Regulation of myofilament force will be discussed in Chapter 2.

CONNECTIONS TO THE EXTRACELLULAR MATRIX

The myofilaments develop and bear the active force within the cardiac myocyte. However, unlike skeletal muscle, cardiac myofilaments are not continuous in series from one cell to another, but must transmit force across cell-to-cell junctions. In addition, the complex mechanical stresses on cardiac myocytes require strong mechanical links between the intracellular myofilaments and cytoskeleton and the extracellular matrix. The Z-lines appear to be the anchor points where intermediate filaments of the cytoskeleton connect actin filaments to the sarcolemma (Price & Sanger, 1983; Price, 1991). The points of attachment across the sarcolemma occur at the intercalated disks (at fascia adherens and desmosomes discussed above) and also on lateral surfaces aligned with Z-lines at costamere-like focal adhesions.

Figure 12 illustrates two of the major structural complexes involved in transsarcolemmal mechanical connection to the extracellular matrix, integrins (left) and dystrophin complexes (right). The right integrin complex emphasizes important proteins involved in the mechanical connection at Z-lines (actin, α-actinin, vinculin, talin, paxillin, tensin, α- and β-integrins, laminin and collagen, Bloch, 1996; Schlaepfer *et al.*, 1999). It is increasingly clear that these complexes are also extremely important in the transduction of physical stretch of the myocardium to intracellular signaling cascades (see pg 312-316). The left integrin complex emphasizes some of the key signaling proteins so far implicated (including focal adhesion kinase or FAK, the small GTP-binding protein Ras, and the protein kinase C δ isoform with its anchoring protein RACK-1). The right side of Fig 12 shows the dystrophin complex (Campbell, 1995) which links actin to

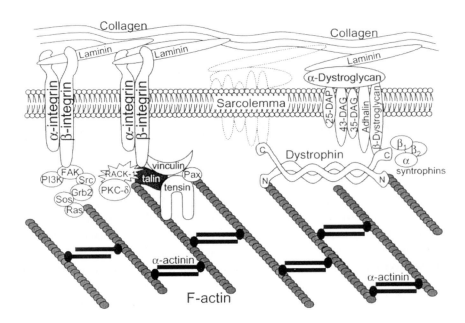

Figure 12. Schematic diagram indicating connections between the actin cytoskeleton and the extracellular matrix via integrins (left) and the dystrophin complex (right). The two integrin complexes are drawn to separately focus on the mechanically important proteins (right complex) and signaling proteins (left complex), although the proteins and functions coexist there. The integrin side was adapted from an original kindly supplied by A.M. Samarel and the dystrophin complex is based on Campbell (1995).

a complex of transmembrane proteins which link up to laminin and collagen in the extracellular matrix. The N-terminal of the large dystrophin molecule (400 kDa) binds to actin and a cysteine-rich region near the C-terminal of dystrophin links it via β-dystroglycan to the cluster of transmembrane proteins. This cluster is composed of several dystrophin-associated proteins (DAP) and glycoproteins (DAGs, & adhalin). On the outer sarcolemmal surface α-dystroglycan binds to laminin in a Ca-dependent manner (Ervasti & Campbell, 1993).

OTHER CELLULAR CONSTITUENTS

Cardiac myocytes are typically mononucleate (although some are binucleate) and contain Golgi apparatus, lysosomes, lipofuscin granules and peroxisomes (Sommer & Johnson, 1979). Lipid droplets and β-glycogen granules are also present and are more abundant than in skeletal muscle. Cardiac myocytes also have a well developed cytoskeleton, only briefly discussed above, including microtubules and microfilaments. Microtubules have also been implicated in altering cardiac mechanical properties in hypertrophy (Zile *et al.*, 1999; Tagawa *et al.*, 1998).

D.M. Bers.
Excitation-Contraction Coupling and Cardiac Contractile Force.
2nd Ed., Kluwer Academic Publishers, Dordrecht, 2001

CHAPTER 2

MYOFILAMENTS:
THE END EFFECTOR OF E-C COUPLING

When cytoplasmic [Ca] rises, the myofilaments are activated in a [Ca]-dependent manner, thereby transducing the chemical signal and chemical energy (ATP) into mechanical force or shortening. Under physiological conditions, skeletal muscle contractile force can be varied by summation of contractions, tetanus and recruitment of additional fibers. Cardiac muscle, on the other hand, functions as a syncytium such that each cell contracts at every beat. The heart must also relax between contractions. Thus, there is neither the practical possibility of recruitment of additional cells, nor summation, nor tetanization to alter the force of contraction to meet altered demands. Therefore, in cardiac muscle, the force of contraction is varied in large part by changes in the peak $[Ca]_i$ reached during systole (as well as sarcomere length).

For this reason I place considerable emphasis on the factors influencing the $[Ca]_i$ in subsequent chapters, often with implicit assumptions about the consequent effects on myofilament activation. However, since contraction is the physiological function of cardiac muscle, the fundamental characteristics of the contractile proteins and how they sense [Ca] under physiologically relevant conditions is important to consider.

MYOFILAMENT PROTEINS

Each thick filament is composed of ~300 myosin molecules, but also contains other proteins, such as titin and C-protein. Each myosin heavy chain (MW ~450,000) has a long (~130 nm) α-helical tail and a globular head (Fig 13A). The tails of the myosin heavy chain form the main axis of the thick filament. The heads form the crossbridges to actin on the thin filaments, contain the site of ATP hydrolysis, and have two light chains associated with each head. The myosin molecule is hexameric, composed of two heavy chains with their tails coiled around each other and two myosin light chains per heavy chain. Based on susceptibility to specific proteases, the myosin heavy chain has been broken down into light meromyosin (2/3 of the 150 nm tail) and heavy meromyosin (HMM). HMM is further divided into subfragment 2 (S2, the residual 50 nm tail) and subfragment 1 (S1, 20 nm of neck and long globular head). The central region of the thick filament, around the M-line (Fig 11) is devoid of crossbridges, reflecting the tail-to-tail abutment of myosin molecules there. The two myosin light chains (MLC1 and MLC2) bind to each myosin heavy chain at the base of the S1 domain or in the neck region (Fig 13A). MLC1 is also referred to as the alkali or essential light chain (ELC). MLC2 is also called the phosphorylatable or regulatory light chain (RLC). Both light chains confer physical stabilization of the thick filament (along with C-protein and titin). However, the regulatory light chain (MLC2) may also alter function in response to Ca binding or phosphorylation (see pg 34-35).

Table 5

Cardiac Contractile Proteins

	Molecular Weight[†]
Myosin Heavy Chain	223,000
Myosin Light Chain 1 (essential)	21,000
Myosin Light Chain 2 (regulatory)	19,000
Actin	41,700
α-Tropomyosin	67,000
Troponin T	38,000
Troponin I	23,500
Troponin C	18,400

[†] from Swynghedauw (1986) and Moss & Buck (2001) for mammalian ventricular muscle.

The proteins of the thin filament and their interactions (Fig 13B) have been reviewed in detail (Zot and Potter, 1987; Solaro & Rarick, 1998; Solaro, 2000). The backbone of the thin filament is composed of two chains of the globular protein G-actin, which form a helical double-stranded F-actin polymer (Fig 14). Tropomyosin (Tm) is a long flexible protein which lies in the groove between the actin strands and spans about 7 actin monomers (Fig 14). Tropomyosin is also double-stranded and mostly α-helical (coiled coil) and the two strands may be connected by a disulfide bridge. The carboxy end also overlaps the amino end of the next tropomyosin by 5-10 amino acids, contributing to thin filament functional cooperativity that spans beyond a single 7-actin span of one tropomyosin (Lehrer et al., 1997). At every seventh actin there is a troponin complex attached to tropomyosin. The troponin complex is made up of three subunits: troponin T (TnT, or the tropomyosin binding subunit), troponin C (TnC, or the Ca binding subunit), and troponin I (TnI, or the inhibitory subunit, which also binds to actin). The sites of interaction of thin filament proteins are shown in Fig 13B, while the arrangement of these subunits in the thin filament is indicated in Fig 14. TnT has a globular carboxy region and an elongated shape that lies along Tm over about 3 actin monomers (Ohtsuki, 1979; Flicker et al., 1982). This arrangement may allow TnT to better control the position of tropomyosin. TnI (near its amino terminal) interacts specifically with the carboxy ends of both TnT and TnC (Figs 13 & 14). The strong binding of the amino end of TnI to TnC depends on Ca or Mg binding to sites on the carboxy end of TnC (physiologically almost always fully occupied; see pg 21 & 46). In the resting state (low [Ca]$_i$) the carboxy end of TnI also binds specifically to actin, and this prevents the myosin head from interacting with actin. When Ca binds to the amino end of TnC, at the lower affinity physiological regulatory site, this part of TnC binds to the carboxy end of TnI causing TnI dissociation from actin. This change in TnC-TnI interaction is sensed by TnT and causes movement of tropomyosin to allow myosin to interact with actin (see Fig 14-16).

Skeletal TnC has been extensively characterized and contains 4 Ca-binding sites, two Ca-specific sites ($K_{d(Ca)}$ = 200 nM in the troponin complex) and two sites at which Ca and Mg bind competitively and with high affinity, known as Ca-Mg sites ($K_{d(Ca)}$ = 2 nM; $K_{d(Mg)}$ = 25 μM in the troponin complex). It is notable that the affinities of these sites on TnC are different when the intact system is partly or wholly disassembled (e.g. in isolated TnC the Ca-specific site has

A. Myosin

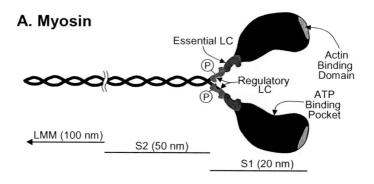

B. Thin Filament Regulatory Proteins

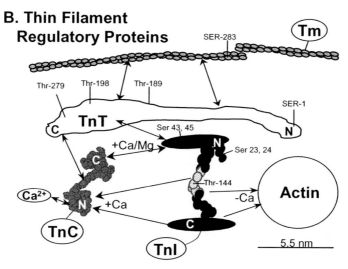

Figure 13.   Myofilament proteins. **A.** The myosin molecule is ~170 nm in overall length with two globular heads (S1) and tails (including light meromyosin LMM + S2) which exist as a coiled coil. The two light chains (LC) are indicated on the neck (Based on Warshaw, 1996). **B.** The thin filament regulatory proteins interact extensively with one another (arrows); some of the interactions are Ca-dependent. Several phosphorylation sites are indicated (Ser, Thr). (Based on a figure generously supplied by R.J. Solaro).

~10 times lower affinity for Ca than the whole troponin complex; see Table 6). The Ca-specific sites are the sites which are responsible for the regulation of contraction (Zot and Potter, 1987).

Cardiac TnC differs significantly from skeletal TnC in that the cardiac isoform has only one Ca-specific binding site at the amino end, but almost the same two Ca-Mg sites on the carboxy end. With the affinities in Table 6, resting $[Ca]_i = 100$ nM and $[Mg]_i = 1$ mM, the cardiac Ca-Mg sites would be ~97% saturated (90% with Ca and 7% with Mg). Thus, these sites would always be nearly saturated and this is probably important in the structural stability of the TnC-TnI complex (above). The Ca-specific site has a K_d ~500 nM and thus would be expected to respond to $[Ca]_i$ changes which occur physiologically (see below). Pan and Solaro (1987) measured Ca binding in detergent treated canine ventricle which was otherwise intact. They found a slightly lower affinity for the Ca-specific site of TnC during rigor compared to the

Table 6

Ca and Mg Binding Affinities of Skeletal and Cardiac Troponin

	Ca Specific Sites		Ca-Mg Sites		
	number of sites	K_{Ca} (M^{-1})	number of sites	K_{Ca} (M^{-1})	K_{Mg} (M^{-1})
Skeletal TnC	2	3.2×10^5	2	2.1×10^7	4×10^3
Skeletal TnC · TnI	2	3.5×10^6	2	2.2×10^8	4×10^4
Skeletal Tn	2	4.9×10^6	2	5.3×10^8	4×10^4
Cardiac TnC	1	2.5×10^5	2	1.4×10^7	7×10^2
Cardiac TnC · TnI	1	1.0×10^6	2	3.2×10^8	3×10^3
Cardiac Tn (reconstituted)	1	2.5×10^6	2	3.7×10^8	3×10^3
Cardiac Tn (native)	1	1.7×10^6	2	4.2×10^8	---

Values are from Holroyde *et al.* (1980) and Potter & Johnson (1982).

isolated TnC complex in Table 6 (1.2×10^6 M^{-1}) and the affinity was further reduced ~3-4 fold by adding ATP to dissociate the rigor complexes.

TnC can also bind other di- and trivalent cations (Fuchs, 1974). Kerrick *et al.* (1980) demonstrated that cardiac myofilaments could be activated similarly by Ca or Sr, but that skeletal muscle is much less sensitive to activation by Sr than Ca. Skeletal muscle can have a higher Ca-sensitivity than cardiac muscle, partly due to lower pH sensitivity (see Fig 21D & pg 32).

Cardiac muscle also exhibits different contractile protein isoforms (e.g. troponins, myosin and myosin light chains) than fast skeletal muscle and the expression of various cardiac isoforms is modulated *in vivo* (Swynghedauw, 1986; Morkin, 1987). For example, there are two main isoforms of the cardiac myosin heavy chain (α, β), sometimes referred to as fast (α) and slow (β) based on the myosin ATPase rate or muscle fiber shortening rate. Three different dimers can form ($\alpha\alpha$, or V_1, $\alpha\beta$ or V_2 and $\beta\beta$ or V_3). There are species differences (e.g. rat ventricle is mostly V_1 while rabbit and human ventricle are mostly V_3), adaptational differences (rat ventricle shifts from α to β during hypertrophy) and thyroid hormone induces a switch from β- to α-myosin heavy chain production. There are also 4-5 isoforms of TnT in rabbit and human ventricle (Anderson *et al.*, 1988, 1991, 1995) which confer different Ca sensitivities to the myofilaments. These change developmentally and also with hypertrophy or heart failure.

MECHANISM BY WHICH Ca ACTIVATES CONTRACTION

It is well established that the rise in cytoplasmic [Ca] is the event which activates the myofilaments and a fairly clear picture (though not complete) of the molecular basis for this regulation has developed, including mapping of peptide regions involved with changes in subunit interactions (Zot and Potter, 1987; Solaro & Rarick, 1998). Figures 14 (side view) and 15 (end-on view) illustrate our current understanding of some of these interactions. At rest when [Ca]$_i$ is low, the Ca-specific sites of TnC are unoccupied. In this condition the interaction between TnI (carboxy-middle) and TnC (amino) is weak and this region of TnI interacts more strongly with actin. This favors the configuration where the troponin-tropomyosin complex is shifted peripherally and more out of the axial groove of the actin filament. This position sterically

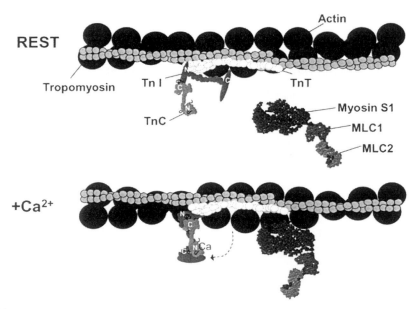

REST

Actin

Tropomyosin   Tn I   TnT

TnC

Myosin S1
MLC1
MLC2

+Ca²⁺

Ca

Figure 14. Side view of Ca-dependent regulation of acto-myosin interaction in cardiac muscle (based on diagram supplied by R.J. Solaro and see also Rayment *et al.*, 1993a,b). At rest the C-terminal domain of TnI is bound to actin, thereby anchoring the TnT-tropomyosin (Tm) complex and preventing the myosin head (S1) from binding to actin. When Ca binds to the amino terminal of TnC, this region binds strongly to the carboxy terminal of TnI, which comes off actin, allowing the TnT-Tm complex to roll deeper into the actin groove and exposing the sites on actin along the chain which interact with the myosin S1 head.

hinders the binding of the myosin S1 head to actin. When $[Ca]_i$ rises, Ca binds to the Ca-specific site of TnC. This strengthens the specific interaction of TnC with TnI and effectively destabilizes the interaction of TnI with actin. This favors the more axial location of the troponin-tropomyosin complex, and removes the steric hindrance to myosin interaction with actin, consequently allowing force production and/or shortening. The tight interaction between TnT and tropomyosin is probably important in the transmission of this conformational change along the thin filament to the actin monomers which do not have associated TnI subunits.

The movement of tropomyosin deeper into the actin groove was first suggested by x-ray diffraction studies (Haselgrove, 1973; Huxley, 1973) and the structural and biochemical results generally support this steric hindrance model of myofilament regulation. However, Chalovich *et al.* (1981) suggested that the regulatory proteins might directly block the acto-myosin ATPase reaction in the absence of Ca, without preventing interaction between myosin heads and actin. Thus, there may be weak binding interactions between actin and myosin that can still occur in the sterically blocked (rest state), but for these to become strong or force-bearing and cycle through the ATPase reaction, the interaction domains must become unblocked. Moreover, there is evidence to suggest that when the myosin S1 head binds to actin it pushes the tropomyosin deeper into the actin groove than when Ca binding to TnC switches the filament into the open state (Lorenz *et al.*, 1995). This is depicted in Fig 15A as 2 prospective Tm positions.

Figures 14 & 16 illustrate how a series of 7 actin molecules can be cooperatively activated by one troponin complex. The head to tail overlap of tropomyosin molecules in series in cardiac muscle may also allow this cooperativity to spread to neighboring tropomyosin-actin

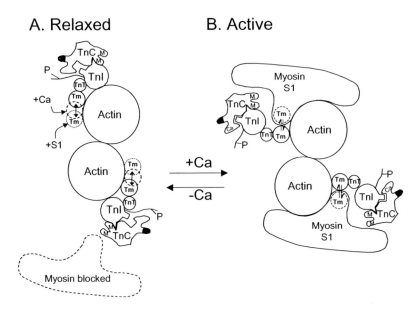

Figure 15. End-on view of Ca-dependent regulation of acto-myosin interaction in cardiac muscle (based on diagram by Warber & Potter, 1986). In the absence of Ca (**A**), TnI binds to actin thereby preventing myosin from interacting with actin. This also draws Tm out of the groove between actins, thereby extending the myosin blocking effect to adjacent actin monomers (which lack TnI). In the presence of Ca (**B**), TnI binds more firmly to TnC and not to actin. In this case Tm is also not drawn out of the groove and the interaction of myosin and actin can occur. The two dashed positions of Tm in A illustrate that Ca-dependent shifts cause partial movement into the groove, but when myosin S1 binds Tm shifts further.

units (Lehrer *et al.*,1997; Solaro, 2001). The binding of myosin heads to actin can also contribute to this sort of long-range cooperativity along the thin filament (Fig 16). This is, in part, a direct steric effect, but binding of myosin S1 heads also increases the affinity of Ca binding to TnC (Pan & Solaro, 1987; Fuchs, 1995). This would also contribute to cooperative activation. In this manner the thin and thick filaments can be viewed as more dynamically involved in their own state of activation, rather than as simply responding passively to the ambient [Ca].

ACTO-MYOSIN ATPase

In the presence of sufficient Ca, myosin can interact with actin, which greatly increases the ability of myosin ATPase to hydrolyze ATP and also allows transformation of chemical energy stored in ATP to mechanical energy and work. A physical model for this transduction known as the sliding filament theory, came from x-ray diffraction studies (Huxley, 1969) and mechanical perturbation studies (Huxley and Simmons, 1971) and is illustrated schematically in Fig 17. At rest the myosin heads (or crossbridges) extend from the thick filament perpendicular to the filament axis. Upon activation the crossbridge can interact with the thin filament and produce either force generation or relative filament movement by a rotation of the myosin head (perhaps due to a series of stable states). Isometric force would be analogous to storing the potential energy of this myosin head rotation temporarily in an elastic component of the myosin

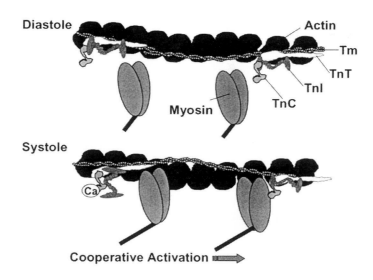

Figure 16. Cooperative spread of activation along the thin filament stimulated by myosin S1 binding to actin. When Ca binding to the left TnC complex allows myosin binding, this pushes tropomyosin further from the blocking position along the actin filament. This increases the probability of additional downstream myosin binding (right) and also increases Ca affinity at neighboring TnC molecules. (modified form of figure generously supplied by R.J. Solaro).

molecule (Fig 17C). Alternatively, the rotational movement can produce relative motion of the thick and thin filaments (i.e. shortening) if the muscle force exceeds the load (Fig 17D). The amount of force developed by a single crossbridge is 0.5-1 pN and the physical movement or filament translation from a single crossbridge cycle is 5-10 nm or 0.25-0.5% of sarcomere or muscle length (Cooke, 1997; Molloy *et al.*, 1995; Tyska *et al.*, 1999). Furthermore, Tyska *et al.* (1999) showed that both myosin heads are required to generate maximal force and displacement and nearly double both values (to 1.4 pN and 10 nm). The details of how the two heads work synergistically are not yet clear.

The chemical steps involved in the crossbridge cycle have also been extensively characterized and correlated with such physico-mechanical schemes (e.g. Goldman, 1987; Brenner, 1987). The general chemical scheme is illustrated in Fig 18. At rest myosin (M) is mostly complexed with ATP (M•ATP) or in the rapidly equilibrated M•ADP•P$_i$ where ATP is technically hydrolyzed, but the energy has not been used. As [Ca]$_i$ rises M•ADP•P$_i$ can interact with actin and phosphate is rapidly released. The acto-myosin passes through at least two energetic states where ADP remains bound (A•M•ADP* and A•M•ADP) and these transitions may encompass the so-called "power stroke" or myosin head rotation. The affinity of myosin for actin increases along this series of steps and is strongest after ADP dissociates (i.e. A•M). However, at normal [ATP]$_i$, A•M binds ATP rapidly and this induces dissociation of actin and M•ATP. The cycle can then continue until [Ca]$_i$ declines, thereby stopping myofilament interaction (in the M•ADP•P$_i$ state) or until ATP is depleted. When ATP is depleted the cycle stops in the A•M state (known as rigor) and crossbridges are firmly attached, creating the

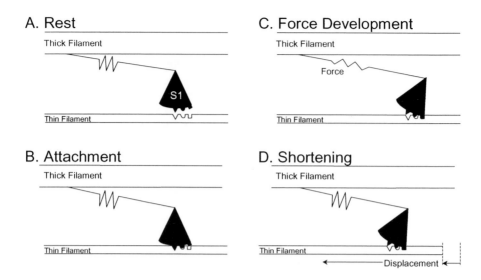

Figure 17. A mechanical model of active crossbridges based on the original diagram by Huxley and Simmons (1971). **A.** a detached crossbridge (e.g. M•ATP in Fig 18). **B.** an attached crossbridge prior to developing force (e.g. A•M•ADP•P$_i$ in Fig 18). **C.** an attached crossbridge developing force stored in the elastic component (e.g. A•M•ADP* in Fig 18). **D.** a crossbridge rotated and translated so the filaments slide relative to one another (e.g. A•M•ADP or A•M in Fig 18).

stiffness associated with rigor mortis). There may also be a small component of crossbridge cycling that occurs in the absence of elevated [Ca]$_i$ (Fabiato and Fabiato, 1975b; Goldman *et al.*, 1984; Reuben *et al.*, 1971; see also pg 32).

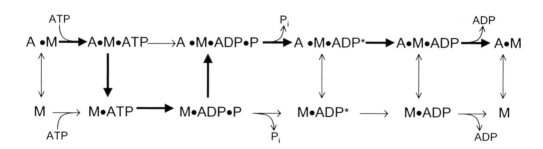

Figure 18. A chemical model of the steps in the crossbridge cycle (or acto-myosin ATPase) based on Goldman & Brenner (1987). The top row shows the states in which actin (**A**) interacts with myosin (**M**). The heavy solid lines indicate the normal reaction pathway, but all the reactions can occur and are reversible. Two energetically different states of **A•M•ADP** are indicated by the inclusion of an asterisk on one.

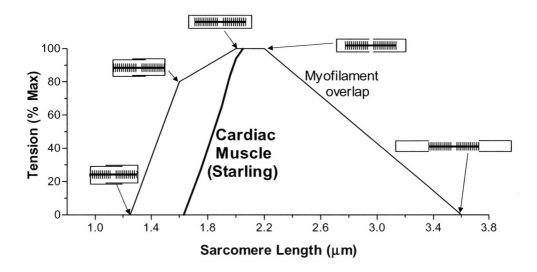

Figure 19. The length-tension relationship in frog skeletal muscle as described by Gordon *et al.* (1966) is shown along with inset diagrams. The length-tension relationship for cat cardiac muscle (Allen *et al.*, 1974) is also illustrated for the range of physiological sarcomere lengths (thick trace).

THE LENGTH-TENSION RELATIONSHIP

The relationship between sarcomere length and the maximum force which can be developed is a central issue in the above physical models of muscle contraction. The relationship was described in detail by Gordon *et al.* (1966) in frog skeletal muscle and their results are summarized in Fig 19. The fundamental assumption is that the maximal force at any sarcomere length is determined by the degree of overlap of the thick and thin filaments (i.e. how many crossbridges can cycle). Thus, as the sarcomere is stretched from its optimal overlap (2 - 2.2 μm) the force gradually declines until it is 0 at the point where there is no longer overlap (~3.6 μm). At shorter sarcomere lengths (2.0 to 1.6 μm) the thin filaments cross over and may impede effective crossbridge formation. Finally, when the thick filament collides with the Z-line (~1.65 μm) the resistance to shortening is greatly increased and externally developed force drops steeply as the thick filament is compressed.

Cardiac muscle has a strong parallel elastic component which normally prevents cardiac sarcomeres from reaching the "descending limb" of the length-tension curve (e.g. sarcomere lengths >2.3 μm). This is of course a good thing for the heart since such long sarcomere length could result in progressive decrease in contraction and failure of cardiac output. Thus the heart normally functions along the "ascending limb" of the length-tension curve, so that one would expect increased contraction with increase in sarcomere length (end diastolic volume or preload). This increase in fiber overlap is undoubtedly involved in the classic Frank-Starling law of the heart, whereby increased diastolic volume leads to increased systolic contraction. However, the length-tension relationship for cardiac muscle is considerably steeper than that for skeletal muscle at sarcomere lengths between 1.8 and 2.0 μm (Allen *et al.*, 1974; see thick curve in Fig

19). Indeed, the changes in myofilament overlap may only explain ~20% of the classic Frank-Starling effect (Moss & Buck, 2001).

Hibberd and Jewell (1982) and Kentish *et al.* (1986) demonstrated that the Ca sensitivity of the myofilaments was significantly increased at longer sarcomere lengths which would steepen the length-tension curve for a given [Ca]. Babu *et al.*, (1988) suggested that this was due to cardiac TnC, since when they reconstituted cardiac fibers with skeletal TnC they failed to see the effect. However, this finding has been challenged by more recent results from three different angles (Moss *et al.*, 1991; Fuchs & Wang, 1991; McDonald *et al.*, 1995a). Thus it cannot simply be due to cardiac *vs.* skeletal TnC. Another important factor is geometric. That is, as sarcomere length is increased the myocyte and sarcomere must become thinner to maintain constant volume. This will cause the thick and thin filaments to come closer together in the myofilament lattice, thereby enhancing the chance for crossbridges to bind to actin (see narrower interfilament gap at long sarcomere length in Fig 19 insets). Indeed, osmotic compression of the myofilament lattice can reverse the decreased Ca sensitivity and Ca binding seen at shorter sarcomere length (Hoffman & Fuchs, 1988; Wang & Fuchs, 1994, 1995; McDonald & Moss, 1995; Fuchs & Wang, 1996).

Allen & Kurihara (1982) provided evidence for this length-dependent Ca binding in intact ferret cardiac muscle where a quick release and shortening of ferret ventricular muscle was accompanied by a release of Ca from the myofilaments (measured using the Ca-sensitive photoprotein aequorin). In addition, at longer steady state sarcomere lengths, SR Ca uptake and release may be increased (Fabiato, 1980; Allen & Kurihara, 1982; Kentish & Wzosek, 1998). Thus, there are multiple protective mechanisms which increase the heart's ability to contract as it is stretched. Increased myofilament overlap, increased myofilament Ca sensitivity and increased SR Ca release may all contribute to the Frank-Starling law of the heart.

THE Ca SENSITIVITY OF THE MYOFILAMENTS

Cardiac myofilaments are activated by Ca in a graded manner, so the relationship between free [Ca] and force development is of fundamental importance. Most of the experimental results on this issue have been obtained in cardiac muscle preparations which have had their sarcolemma removed or permeabilized and are called "skinned" preparations. Since myofilaments are sensitive to submicromolar [Ca] and contaminant [Ca] is usually several micromolar, Ca chelators such as EGTA are used to buffer [Ca] in the range of interest. The solutions used for these skinned fibers usually also contain ATP, Mg and some other solutes (e.g. ATP regenerating systems, pH buffer and KCl). Computer programs (e.g. Fabiato, 1988; Bers *et al.*, 1994) are usually used to solve the multiple ion equilibria and prepare solutions of known free [Ca].

The pCa ($-\log$[Ca]) values reported for the threshold [Ca] and [Ca] at half maximal force for mammalian cardiac muscle have been reported to be 5.9-7.0 and 4.7-6.0, respectively (Solaro *et al.*, 1974; Kerrick & Donaldson, 1975; Endo & Kitazawa, 1977; Fabiato & Fabiato, 1975a; 1978; McCLellen & Winegrad, 1978; Hibberd & Jewell, 1979; Fabiato, 1981a; Miller & Smith, 1984; Harrison & Bers, 1989a). While some portion of this large variance is due to species differences and particular experimental conditions (i.e. ionic strength, temperature, pH etc.), it is also possible that it reflects inaccuracies in calculated free [Ca]. This issue has been critically

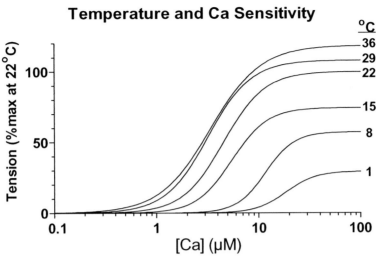

Figure 20. The influence of temperature on the Ca sensitivity of chemically "skinned" rabbit ventricular muscle (data from Harrison and Bers, 1989a have been redrawn). Both the Ca sensitivity and the maximum force are reduced at lower temperatures.

Table 7

Temperature and the Ca Sensitivity of Rabbit Ventricular Myofilaments

Temperature (°C)	pCa$_{1/2}$	Hill Coefficient	Maximum Force (%)
36	5.47 ± 0.07	1.75 ± 0.1	118.5 ± 10.0
29	5.49 ± 0.07	2.06 ± 0.1	108 ± 4.6
22	5.34 ± 0.05	2.15 ± 0.6	100
15	5.26 ± 0.09	2.49 ± 0.2	74.3 ± 6.0
8	4.93 ± 0.06	3.06 ± 0.5	57.2 ± 7.0
1	4.73 ± 0.04	2.94 ± 0.6	29.3 ± 5.4

Data (from Harrison and Bers, 1989a) were fit to a Hill equation $F=F_{max}/(1+\{K_m/[Ca]\}^n)$.

addressed (Bers, 1982; Miller & Smith, 1984; Harrison & Bers, 1989b) and the errors in [Ca] can be greater than 3-fold (i.e. 0.5 pCa units). These inaccuracies can be attributed to a) incorrect choice of (or use of) association constants, b) inappropriate modifications of the association constants for differences in ionic strength and temperature, c) small systematic errors in pH and d) overestimation of EGTA purity.

This complication makes it more difficult to compare quantitative details of Ca-sensitivity curves from one lab to another. While qualitative conclusions are probably valid, this may not always be the case. For example, based on results from 12°C and 22°C in mechanically skinned canine Purkinje cells, Fabiato (1985b) concluded that myofilament Ca sensitivity in cardiac muscle may be increased by cooling, as is the case in skeletal muscle (Stephenson &

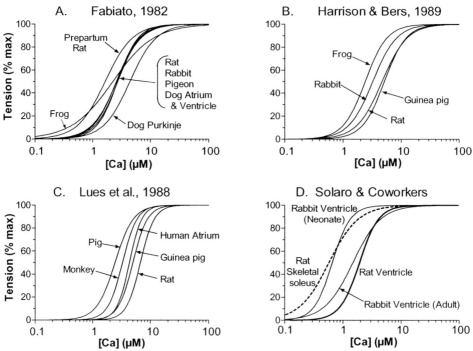

Figure 21. Myofilament Ca sensitivity in cardiac muscle preparations. Data from **A.** Fabiato (1982), **B.** Harrison & Bers (1989a), **C.** Lues *et al.* (1988) and **D.** Solaro *et al.* (1998) & Wattanapermpool *et al.* (1995a) have been redrawn (based on Hill equation fits, $100/(1+\{K_m/[Ca]\}^n)$). All data were normalized to the maximum force under the prevalent conditions and are from ventricle, unless noted. The conditions including ionic strength (Γ) are slightly different in the three panels. The major variations are (in mM):

	Temp.	pH	Γ	[EGTA]	[pH-buff]	[Mg]	[MgATP]
A.	22°C	7.1	160	10	30	3	3
B.	29°C	7.0	180	10	25	2.3	~5
C.	21°C	6.7	140	5	30	~2.5	~10
D.	23°C	7.0	160	10	60	2	~5

Williams, 1981; 1985; Godt & Lindley, 1982). However, a relatively minor adjustment of Fabiato's solution calculations, based on our studies of the influence of ionic strength and temperature on the affinity of EGTA for Ca (Harrison & Bers, 1987), greatly reduced the apparent temperature-induced shift reported by Fabiato (Harrison & Bers, 1989b). Furthermore, we found that over the temperature range 37°C to 1°C there was a progressive decrease in Ca sensitivity of the myofilaments with cooling in chemically skinned rabbit ventricular muscle (Fig 20 and Table 7, Harrison & Bers, 1989a). Similar shifts were also reported for guinea-pig, rat and frog ventricle (Harrison & Bers, 1990a). We also found that much of the difference between the influence of temperature on cardiac and skeletal muscle could be attributed to the TnC type in the muscle, based on experiments where rat ventricular TnC was extracted and replaced by either rabbit skeletal TnC or bovine cardiac TnC (Harrison & Bers, 1990b). These results indicate an interesting thermodynamic difference between cardiac and skeletal muscle regulation at the level of TnC. That is, cooling decreases the Ca sensitivity of cardiac myofilaments, but increases the sensitivity of skeletal myofilaments (largely due to the TnC type).

The foregoing indicates that minor oversights in the calculations of free [Ca] in the complex solutions used in skinned fiber studies can lead to qualitative as well as quantitative errors. It is therefore useful to obtain an independent check of the free [Ca] in the solutions used whenever possible (e.g. with a Ca-selective electrode; Bers, 1982; Bers *et al.*, 1994). With these caveats in mind some factors which alter myofilament Ca sensitivity will be discussed below.

Skinned cardiac muscle fibers also exhibit hysteresis in the force-[Ca] relationship, such that Ca sensitivity is apparently greater when [Ca] is decreasing than when [Ca] is increasing (Harrison *et al.*, 1988). This hysteresis diminishes with increasing sarcomere length and is virtually eliminated at sarcomere lengths greater than 2.2 μm. This implies that for full relaxation to occur at shorter sarcomere lengths, the $[Ca]_i$ must be lower than would be supposed from force-pCa relationships obtained in the activating direction. From a functional standpoint, this may be an important consideration, since this may limit relaxation between contractions even if $[Ca]_i$ has reached a stable diastolic level.

Figure 21 shows superimposed [Ca] *vs.* tension curves from skinned fibers from several cardiac species. The data in Fig 21A are from Fabiato (1982). Fabiato & Fabiato (1978b) reported comparative data under slightly different conditions (with 3 abscissa calibrations, illustrating the calibration problems above). In that report they found that the myofilament Ca sensitivity of human atrium and ventricle were indistinguishable from those of rat and rabbit ventricle. Figures 21B-D are from other studies. The experimental conditions in the three panels are all somewhat different. While neonatal ventricle and skeletal muscle myofilaments have somewhat higher Ca affinity, the main point is that there are only minor differences in Ca sensitivity among mammalian cardiac muscle preparations under the same conditions. The $pCa_{1/2}$ values for these skinned fiber preparations are typically between 5.2 and 5.7 (2-6 μM) with Hill coefficients 1.9-2.5 at 22-29°C, at ionic strength ~160 mM, pH~7.0 with 3-5 mM Mg ATP and 2-3 mM free Mg. These will serve as a base for the comparisons below.

FORCE-pCa RELATION IN INTACT CARDIAC MUSCLE

All of the foregoing and much of what will come below is based on experiments in muscles in which the sarcolemma has been disrupted so that the intracellular environment can be controlled. However, this has the substantial disadvantage that some cellular constituents which might affect myofilament Ca sensitivity may be lost. For example, Harrison *et al.* (1986) found that carnosine and related compounds (imidazoles), which are abundant in skeletal muscle (Crush, 1970) and may total as much as 10 mM in cardiac muscle (O'Dowd *et al.*, 1988) significantly increase cardiac myofilament Ca sensitivity. Skinning also causes osmotic swelling of the myofilament lattice in simple ionic solutions. This reduces apparent myofilament Ca sensitivity in skinned fibers (see pg 28).

Yue *et al.* (1986) estimated the steady state force-$[Ca]_i$ relationship in intact ferret ventricular muscle using aequorin to measure $[Ca]_i$ and ryanodine treatment to allow the heart muscle to be effectively tetanized. They found a mean $pCa_{1/2}$ of 6.3 and a mean Hill coefficient of 6.1. This is a remarkably steep curve and the half-maximum point is at a $[Ca]_i$ (500 nM), considerably lower than almost any skinned fiber results. The myofilament force would go from less than 5% at 300 nM $[Ca]_i$ to 95% of maximum at 800 nM $[Ca]_i$. The specific factors responsible for the disparity in Fig 22 are not entirely clear, but the intact cell myofilament Ca

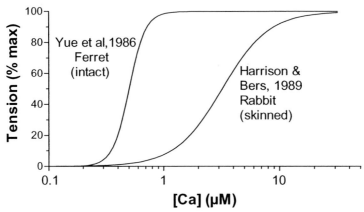

Figure 22. The myofilament Ca sensitivity in intact ferret ventricular muscle at 30°C (from Yue *et al.*, 1986) and in chemically skinned rabbit ventricular muscle at 29°C (from Harrison and Bers, 1989a). The curves are Hill curves based on the reported $pCa_{1/2}$ and n values.

sensitivity has been confirmed in subsequent studies using other Ca indicators (Gao *et al.*, 1994; Backx *et al.*, 1995). Gao *et al.* (1994) found similar myofilament Ca sensitivity before and after skinning when they used 0.5 mM free [Mg] in the skinned fiber solutions (as they measured in the intact muscle). Thus, 2 mM free [Mg], used in many skinned fiber studies, may be too high, but the difference in Fig 22 is not completely understood.

Sollott *et al.* (1996) demonstrated that even during diastole and very low [Ca]$_i$, there is appreciable acto-myosin interaction contributing to resting force. They also showed that this interaction was still Ca-dependent and correlated with very slow decline in [Ca]$_i$ (even in cells with Ca-free, EGTA containing solution). Stuyvers *et al.* (1997) also found that as diastolic [Ca]$_i$ continues to decline and sarcomere length increases, muscle stiffness increases. This may be indicative of dynamic structural changes which occur even in the apparent quiescent state.

FACTORS WHICH INFLUENCE THE FORCE-[Ca] RELATIONSHIP

A large number of factors are known to modify the relationship between [Ca] and the force generated by cardiac myofilaments and these have been most extensively studied in skinned cardiac muscle preparations (e.g. Table 8). As described above, both cooling and shorter sarcomere length decrease the Ca sensitivity and also the maximum force generated by the myofilaments (Hibberd & Jewell, 1982; Kentish *et al.*, 1986; Harrison and Bers, 1989a). Similarly, acidosis decreases both the Ca sensitivity and maximum force generated by the myo-filaments (see Fig 170; Fabiato & Fabiato, 1978a, Blanchard & Solaro, 1984). This may be particularly important during pathological conditions such as hypoxia or ischemia where intracellular pH (pH$_i$) is known to decline (Jacobus *et al.*, 1982). An interesting note is that the Ca sensitivity of myofilaments from perinatal hearts is much less affected by acidosis (Solaro *et al.*, 1986, 1988; Martin *et al.*, 1991). The results suggested that the difference in pH sensitivity was mainly due to a difference in TnI (slow skeletal TnI is expressed in the newborn heart). However, it is not due to the unique N-terminal domain in cardiac TnI (Guo *et al.*, 1994), which is crucial in modulation by phosphorylation (below). Skeletal muscle force is also less depressed by acidosis, and both skeletal TnI and TnC contribute to this effect (65 & 35% respectively, Metzger *et al.*, 1993; Ball *et al.*, 1994; Ding *et al.*, 1995).

It has been argued that the intracellular acidosis accompanying early ischemia is not sufficient to explain the mechanical dysfunction (Jacobus *et al.*, 1982; Weiss *et al.*, 1984; Allen & Orchard, 1987) especially if one only considers the effect of pH_i on the myofilaments. Ischemia also results in decreases of [creatine phosphate] and [ATP] and increases inorganic phosphate (PO_4) levels. While decreasing [ATP] (as MgATP) increases myofilament sensitivity, it also decreases the maximum force (Best *et al.*, 1977). Kentish (1986) demonstrated that the increase in PO_4 which accompanies the decline in high energy phosphates (ATP and creatine phosphate) during ischemia can dramatically decrease both Ca sensitivity and maximum force. Overall the increase in PO_4 and the decrease in pH_i in ischemia combine to produce a dramatic decrease in myofilament Ca sensitivity (with PO_4 being slightly more important). This combination plays an important role in the early decline in mechanical function (see pg 307).

Increasing the free [Mg] also decreases myofilament Ca sensitivity (Fabiato & Fabiato, 1975b; Best *et al.*, 1977). Increasing ionic strength (but not osmolality) decreases both Ca sensitivity and maximum force of the myofilaments (Kentish, 1984). Imidazoles (e.g. carnosine and *N*-acetyl histidine) which are naturally occurring in cardiac muscle cells (O'Dowd *et al.*, 1988) increase myofilament Ca sensitivity (Harrison *et al.*, 1986). These compounds are chemically related to caffeine, which is often used in the study of cardiac muscle Ca metabolism because it can deplete the SR of Ca. However, caffeine and other methylxanthines are potent myofilament Ca sensitizers (Wendt & Stephenson, 1983; Fabiato, 1981b). Interestingly, caffeine exerts its potent sensitizing effect without affecting Ca binding to the myofilaments (Powers & Solaro, 1995). This contrasts to other Ca sensitizers which exert their effect by increasing Ca affinity (e.g. pimobendan and MCI-154, Fujino *et al.*, 1988; Kitada *et al.*, 1989). Caffeine and other methylxanthines also inhibit phosphodiesterases, but the effects on the myofilaments are not mediated by cyclic AMP.

A number of inotropic agents function in part via their ability to inhibit cardiac phosphodiesterases and thereby elevate cyclic AMP (e.g. amrinone, milrinone, pimobendan and sulmazole), while some increase myofilament Ca sensitivity (Endoh, 1998, Table 8, see also pg 324-328). Ca sensitizers include levosimendan (Edes *et al.*, 1995), EMD 57033 (Solaro *et al.*, 1993; Vannier *et al.*, 1997), pimobendan (or AR-L 115-BS, Fujino *et al.*, 1988), sulmazole (or UDCG-115-BS, Solaro & Rüegg, 1982), isomazole (Lues *et al.*, 1988), BM 14.478 (Freund *et al.*, 1987), MCI-154 (Kitada *et al.*, 1987; 1989), DPI 201-106 (Scholtysik *et al.*, 1985) and perhexiline & bepridil (Silver *et al.*, 1987), but not milrinone (Fujino *et al.*, 1988). Racemic EMD-53998 has both phosphodiesterase inhibitory and Ca sensitizing actions, but these actions are selectively due to either the (−) enantiomer (EMD-57439) or (+) enantiomer (EMD-57033) respectively (see Figs 177 & 178; White *et al.*, 1993; Solaro *et al.*, 1993). Thus, myofilament effects of some of these drugs contribute to their inotropic effects.

Ray and England (1976) and Solaro *et al.* (1976) demonstrated a cyclic AMP-dependent phosphorylation of cardiac TnI in response to β-adrenergic stimulation. This phosphorylation decreases myofilament Ca sensitivity in intact ventricular muscle (Okazaki *et al.*, 1990) and in skinned fibers, a result which is mimicked by cyclic AMP (McClellan & Winegrad, 1978;

Holroyde *et al.*, 1979; Mope *et al.*, 1980; Herzig *et al.*, 1981). Phosphorylation of TnI (and the shift in Ca sensitivity) can also be reversed by cyclic GMP or cholinergic agonists (Mope *et al.*, 1980; Horowits & Winegrad, 1983). Phosphorylation of TnI at both Ser 23 & 24 appear to be essential for this effect (Zhang *et al.*, 1995a). This region is in the N-terminal extension of TnI that is not present in slow skeletal TnI. Studies with mutant cardiac TnI lacking this N-terminal extension demonstrated that this phosphorylation was both necessary and sufficient to produce the reduced myofilament Ca sensitivity seen with PKA (Guo *et al.*, 1994; Wattanapermpool *et al.*, 1995b). Transgenic mice in which cardiac TnI was quantitatively replaced with slow skeletal TnI exhibit higher myofilament Ca sensitivity, which is no longer affected by PKA phosphorylation (Fentzke *et al.*, 1999). These data provide compelling evidence that TnI phosphorylation mediates the alterations in myofilament properties induced by PKA. While PKA also phosphorylates C-protein, it is less clear wether this really alters myofilament function (Weisberg & Winegrad, 1996; Winegrad, 1999; Solaro, 2001).

For β-adrenergic stimulation to produce its well known inotropic effect, the amplitude of the intracellular Ca transient must more than compensate for the reduced myofilament Ca sensitivity (e.g. by enhancement of Ca-current and SR Ca release, see Chapters 5, 7 & 10). The decline in myofilament Ca sensitivity induced by β-adrenergic stimulation is accompanied by an increased off-rate of Ca from TnC. In principle this could contribute to the faster relaxation of contractions (or lusitropic effect) observed in the presence of β-adrenergic agonists. Studies in skinned cardiac muscle fibers using photolysis of a caged Ca chelator, diazo-2, have been equivocal, finding either enhanced (Zhang *et al.*, 1995b) or unchanged relaxation upon phosphorylation of cardiac TnI (Johns *et al.*, 1997). In intact fibers, McIvor *et al.* (1988) showed that myofilament desensitization was not necessary for faster relaxation. That is, the acceleration of relaxation could be attributed entirely to the other actions of isoproterenol (e.g. increased SR Ca uptake rate, secondary to cyclic AMP dependent phosphorylation of phospholamban, Kirchberger *et al.*, 1974; Tada *et al.*, 1974; Lindeman & Watanabe, 1985a). This could be true even though phosphorylation of TnI appears to occur at lower isoproterenol concentrations than for phospholamban (Karczewski *et al.*, 1990). Indeed, Fentzke *et al.* (1999) found that even with slow skeletal TnI (lacking the phosphorylation sites), isoproterenol greatly accelerated relaxation in myocytes. Li *et al.* (2000) also showed that in mice lacking phospholamban, PKA phosphorylation of TnI produced no change in myocyte relaxation. However, with increasing force generation in muscle (as opposed to unloaded myocyte shortening) there was a small lusitropic effect of isoproterenol in these phospholamban knockout mice. We concluded that all of the lusitropic effect on unloaded myocyte relaxation was attributable to phospholamban phosphorylation, whereas with maximal force development the TnI phosphorylation may contribute ~15% to the lusitropic effect of isoproterenol.

One of the myosin light chains (MLC2 or regulatory light chain) can also be phosphorylated by a Ca-calmodulin dependent protein kinase (Pires *et al.*, 1974). Phosphorylation of this regulatory light chain by myosin light chain kinase is crucial in the activation of smooth muscle contraction (Aksoy *et al.*, 1976; Walsh *et al.*, 1983). Yang *et al.* (1998) showed that MLC2 phosphorylation in skeletal muscle could mimic the effect of reducing filament lattice spacing (increasing the likelihood of myosin binding to actin). However, the physiological role of this phosphorylation in cardiac muscle is not clear (England, 1984; Gevers, 1984; Solaro,

Table 8

Factors which alter Cardiac Myofilament Ca Sensitivity

Factor	ref	Factor Change	Sensitivity Direction	$\Delta pCa_{1/2}$	Maximum Force Direction	$\Delta(\%)$
Temperature	a	36→ 22°C	dec	0.18	dec	16
		2→ 8°C	dec	0.20	dec	43
Sarcomere Length	b	2.0→ 2.35 μm	inc	0.21	inc	34
	c	1.75→ 2.05 μm	inc	0.25	inc	36
pH	d	7.0→ 6.6	dec	0.34	dec	10
pH	e	7.0→ 6.5	dec	0.29	dec	12
PO_4 (pH 7)	f	0→ 20 mM	dec	0.37	dec	69
MgATP (1mM Mg)	g	0.03→ 4 mM	dec	0.3	dec	31
Mg (4mM MgATP)	g	0.05→ 1 mM	dec	0.4	inc	21
Mg (3mM MgATP)	h	0.3→ 3 mM	dec	0.33-	-	
Ionic Strength (Γ)	i	0.1→ 0.2 M	dec	0.3	dec	17
TnI Phosphorylation	j	0→ ~50%	dec	0.45	-	-
Carnosine	k	0→ 15 mM	inc	0.2	inc	3
Caffeine	l	0→ 20 mM	inc	0.32	dec	6
Sulmazole (AR-L115 BS)	m	0→ 1 mM	inc	0.2	inc	7
Isomazole	n	0→ 1 mM	inc	0.1	inc	~15
Pimobendan (UDCG-115-BS)	o	0→ 50 μM	inc	~0.2	noΔ	
MCI-154	p	0→ 10 μM	inc	~0.2	noΔ	
Levosimendan	q	0→ 10 μM	inc	0.1	noΔ	
EMD 57033	r	0→ 10 μM	inc	0.3	inc	20
CGP-48506	s	0→ 10 μM	inc	0.14	inc	13
Butanedione monoxime (BDM)	t	0→ 3 mM	dec	0.15	dec	30

a) Harrison & Bers, 1989a
b) Hibberd & Jewell, 1982
c) Kentish *et al.*, 1986
d) Fabiato & Fabiato, 1978a
e) Blanchard & Solaro, 1984
f) Kentish, 1986
g) Best *et al.*,1977
h) Fabiato & Fabiato, 1975b
i) Kentish, 1984
j) Mope *et al.*, 1980

k) Harrison *et al.*, 1985
l) Wendt & Stephenson, 1983
m) Rüegg, 1986
n) Lues *et al.*, 1988
o) Fujino *et al.*, 1988
p) Kitada *et al.*, 1989
q) Edes *et al.*, 1995
r) Solaro *et al.*, 1993; Vannier *et al.*, 1997
s) Wolska *et al.*, 1996a
t) Gwathmey *et al.*, 1991

2001). Phosphorylation of this regulatory light chain by myosin light chain kinase increases the Ca sensitivity of the myofilaments in skinned pig ventricular muscle (Morano *et al.*, 1985), and increases the rate of force development (Morano *et al.*, 1995), but decreases myosin cross-bridge cycling rate (Franks *et al.*, 1984). Silver *et al.* (1986) showed a frequency dependent change in the degree of phosphorylation of myosin light chains in rabbit ventricular muscle. Thus, while phosphorylation of myosin light chains occurs and may modify acto-myosin ATPase, the details of this action and its physiological importance remain to be unequivocally established. Other myofilament sites are also targets for phosphorylation (see Fig 13B and Solaro *et al.*, 1987; Solaro, 2001 for further discussion).

FORCE VELOCITY CURVES

So far most of the discussion has focused on the development of force under isometric conditions (i.e. fixed sarcomere length) and at fixed resting force (or preload) and infinite

Force-Velocity Curve

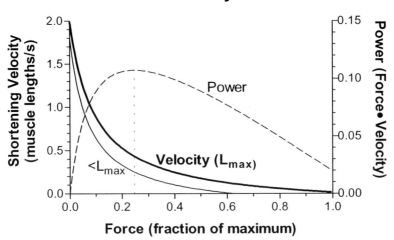

Force (fraction of maximum)

Figure 23. Force-velocity and force-power curves in cardiac muscle. The thick curve is at optimal sarcomere length for force development (L_{max}) and shortening velocity varies inversely with load (or force). At
shorter sarcomere length this curve shifts down and to the left (lower maximal force). Power (force ×
velocity) is shown for the L_{max} curve. Based on data and analysis in Moss & Buck (2001).

afterload. Indeed, ventricular filling, end diastolic pressure and volume are the preloads that set
the sarcomere length and position on the Starling curve (Fig 19) where contraction begins.
However, only the early part of ventricular contraction *in situ* is isometric (i.e. the isovolumic
phase when both the A-V valves and the aortic/pulmonic valves are closed). Once the force (or
ventricular pressure) development reaches the afterload (or aortic pressure), the aortic (or
pulmonic) valve opens and ejection begins. This is associated with shortening of individual
sarcomeres at a velocity that is related to the afterload (i.e. the force or pressure against which
the heart must perform work). Clearly physiological cardiac contraction is not isometric, nor is it
ideal to simply measure unloaded shortening (as often done with isolated cardiac myocytes).
Cardiac muscle normally shortens under a continually changing afterload (aortic pressure).

      To understand the relationship between load (or force) and velocity of shortening,
muscles have traditionally been released from a certain sarcomere length bearing different loads
and the velocity of shortening measured (Moss & Buck, 2001). According to the classic work of
Hill (1938) one expects a hyperbolic relationship of the form $(P+a)(V+b) = b(P_{max} + a)$ (where P
and V are force and velocity, P_{max} is maximal isometric P, and a and b are constants). As Figure
23 shows, this simply means that the maximum velocity (V_{max}) occurs when there is no load and
that at P_{max} the muscle cannot shorten (V =0 = isometric). This is intuitive in that the greater the
load, the slower the shortening velocity. It also means that as the muscle shortens from L_{max} and
maximal isometric force declines (Fig 19), the force-velocity relationship will fall along a lower
curve (lower solid curve in Fig 23, where P_{max} is 62% of that at L_{max}). Thus as ventricular
ejection proceeds, the velocity of ejection decreases for a given load (or pressure, or force).
Thus higher initial sarcomere length (higher preload) partly explains why the early ejection phase
is the fastest. Of course the initial ventricular ejection phase is also the time when the aortic
pressure (afterload) is minimal (which would be relatively leftward in Fig 23).

The maximum shortening velocity (V_{max}) occurs with no load and this reflects the maximum turnover rate of the myosin ATPase cycle. That is, with truly zero load, a single myosin head could (in principle) shorten the muscle at its maximal cycle rate. Moreover, the rate limiting step is thought to be ADP release, which also governs the crossbridge detachment step (Siemenkowski *et al.*, 1985) Thus, situations which alter the isoform of myosin expressed can alter V_{max} (α fast or β slow). The switch from α- to β-myosin in hypertrophic rats may be adaptive in sustaining force or pressure longer during contraction, at the expense of V_{max}. Since slower myosin splits ATP more slowly, this may also conserve energy for a given force-time integral. Figure 23 also shows that changes in sarcomere length typically produce greater changes in maximal isometric force than in V_{max}. This is because P_{max} depends on the number of crossbridges working in parallel, while V_{max} is determined mainly by the single crossbridge turnover rate. It should also be noted that even without an external load, the cardiac myocyte has internal load due both to the mass of the cell and also internal elastic elements which resist shortening (as well as lengthening). That is, even isolated myocytes spring back to a given resting length after contraction and [Ca]$_i$ decline (sarcomere length 1.85-1.95 μm; see Roos, 1997 for references and discussion). In the intact heart, where the extracellular matrix also contributes to resting sarcomere length the values tend to be a bit longer (2-2.2 μm; Roos, 1997).

Figure 23 also shows how the power output of cardiac muscle changes with afterload. Work is, of course, equal to force × distance and power (work/time) is then force × velocity. The maximal power typically occurs at 20-40% of maximal isometric force, which coincides with the typical degree of myofilament activation during a twitch (Harrison & Bers, 1990a).

A large factor in the rate of activation of the myofilaments is the rate of rise of [Ca]$_i$. However, even at a constant level of Ca activation it takes a finite time for the crossbridges to cycle and for development of force. Figure 24 shows an approach that has been used to assess this fundamental activation characteristic of the myofilaments. The muscle is initially released (by 10-20% of its initial length) such that force drops to zero. After 20-50 ms the muscle is rapidly stretched back to the initial length, instantly breaking any attached crossbridges (note the spike). The exponential rate constant of force redevelopment is indicative of the transition from weak or unbound crossbridges to the strongly bound, force generating state (k_{tr}, Brenner, 1986; Moss & Buck, 2001). Cardiac k_{tr} increases at higher steady [Ca] (Wolff *et al.*, 1995a; Palmer & Kentish, 1998; but see also Hancock *et al.*, 1996). Swartz & Moss (1992) found that this effect could be produced in skeletal muscle by either higher [Ca] or N-ethylmaleimide S1 heads (which mimic strongly bound crossbridges) and they inferred that this reflected Ca- or crossbridge-dependent cooperative activation.

Brenner & Eisenberg (1986) proposed a crossbridge model where strong crossbridge binding is regulated by the rate constant for formation (f_{app}) and dissociation (g_{app}) of the complex, such that k_{tr} depends on both f_{app} & g_{app}, but detachment depends only on g_{app}.

Palmer & Kentish (1998) showed that the rate constant of force development after flash photolysis of caged Ca and k_{tr} measured as in Fig 24 were almost identical, indicating that there is little delay due to the local rise in [Ca]$_i$, Ca binding and troponin-tropomyosin changes. Clearly it is mostly due to crossbridges going from weak (or unbound states) to strong binding states which develop force. They found that activation rate constants were much faster in rat

Quick Release and Re-stretch

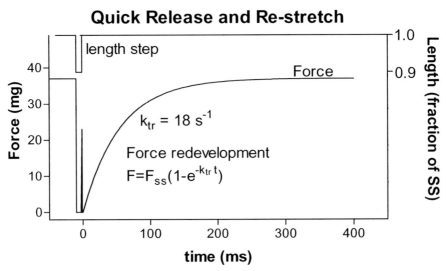

Figure 24. Redevelopment of force after release and rapid re-stretch in cardiac muscle. Force (F) drops to zero with the release and shortening. A transient spike in force occurs upon re-stretch as crossbridge attachments are stressed, then broken, allowing the re-attachment-force development to be monitored (based on data in Moss & Buck, 2000).

than guinea-pig ventricle (14 *vs.* 2.7/s). They also flash photolyzed a caged Ca-trap (NP-EGTA) to drop [Ca] extremely fast and found a similar difference in relaxation rate constants (16/s in rat *vs.* 3/s in guinea-pig), despite similar Ca-dependence for steady state force (pCa$_{1/2}$ = 5.6). These findings are consistent with the rat having 90% α-myosin (fast) and guinea-pig having 50-60% β-myosin (slow) and also emphasize that intrinsic properties of the myofilaments can contribute importantly in the kinetics of contraction and relaxation.

The control of the myofilaments by [Ca] and other factors is very complex. Furthermore, the simplifying assumption often used (e.g. in subsequent chapters) that the myofilaments respond to a given [Ca]$_i$ in a direct and simple *black box* manner is obviously incomplete. However, this implicit assumption makes it considerably easier to discuss the equally compli-cated area of [Ca]$_i$ regulation in relation to cardiac muscle function. One must retain the perspective that the relationship between [Ca]$_i$ and contraction is not fixed and it is contraction which is the physiological function of cardiac muscle cells. Indeed, even when cellular cardiac physiologists talk about contraction, we usually mean quasi-isometric contractions in papillary muscles (or muscle strips) or unloaded contractions in single isolated myocytes, rather than the more complicated *in vivo* contractions. Again, the simplifications made in the name of reductionist science should be borne in mind as we go forward.

D.M. Bers.
Excitation-Contraction Coupling and Cardiac Contractile Force.
2nd Ed., Kluwer Academic Publishers, Dordrecht, 2001

39

CHAPTER 3

SOURCES AND SINKS OF ACTIVATOR CALCIUM

GENERAL SCHEME OF Ca CYCLE IN CARDIAC MYOCYTE

Transsarcolemmal Ca influx and SR Ca release play dominant roles in the rise of $[Ca]_i$ which activates contraction in the heart. It is useful at this point to present a simple working model of cellular Ca fluxes which can serve as a background for further discussion (Fig 25).

During the cardiac action potential, Ca enters the cell via sarcolemmal Ca channels (possibly more than 1 type) and there may also be some Ca entry via Na/Ca exchange. This Ca which enters the cell can contribute directly to the activation of the myofilaments. Ca entry is also involved in the activation of SR Ca release. This is the well known Ca-induced Ca-release process described in detail in Chapter 8. Whether sarcolemmal Ca channels are, in fact, located directly over the SR Ca-release channel has not yet been proven, but enough indirect evidence (see Chapters 1, 7 & 8) consistent with this arrangement justifies inclusion in this working model. The possibility of direct electro-mechanical coupling between the sarcolemmal Ca channel protein and the SR Ca-release protein (as in skeletal muscle) is controversial and will be discussed in Chapter 8. In any event, the myofilaments are activated by the combination of Ca influx and SR Ca release. The degree of contractile activation depends on how much Ca is delivered to the myofilaments (as well as how they respond, see Chapter 2). As $[Ca]_i$ rises the regulatory TnC binding site also has to compete with other cytosolic Ca buffers.

For relaxation to occur, Ca must be removed from the cytoplasm, lowering $[Ca]_i$ such that Ca will dissociate from TnC. Four Ca transport processes may be involved in removing Ca from the cytoplasm (Bassani *et al.*, 1992). Ca can be transported: 1) into the SR by the SR Ca-ATPase pump, 2) out of the cell by the sarcolemmal Ca-ATPase pump, 3) out of the cell by the sarcolemmal Na/Ca exchange or 4) into mitochondria via the Ca uniporter. These 4 Ca transport systems are all in direct competition for cytoplasmic Ca (see below and Chapters 6 & 9).

Each of these transport systems will be discussed in considerable detail in later sections. Ca influx via Ca current and Na/Ca exchange will be discussed in Chapters 5 and 6 respectively. The SR Ca-ATPase and release channel will be the focus of Chapter 7, while Chapter 8 will focus on the details of the E-C coupling mechanism itself. Ca extrusion from the cell via Na/Ca exchange and the sarcolemmal Ca-ATPase will be discussed in Chapter 6. Mitochondrial Ca transport will be discussed below (pg 56). Discussion of how these mechanisms interact functionally will start below and recur throughout (especially in Chapters 9 & 10).

A small leak of Ca out of the SR into the cytoplasm must occur at rest. It is unimportant here whether this leak occurs via the SR Ca-release channel (Ca sparks) or not. The point is that

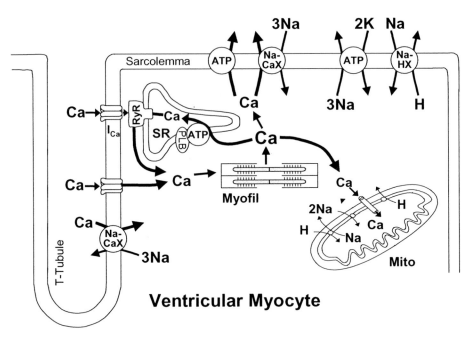

Figure 25. General scheme of Ca cycle in a cardiac ventricular myocyte. Ca can enter via Ca channels (I_{Ca}) and Na/Ca exchange (NaCaX). Ca influx controls SR Ca release by the ryanodine receptor (RyR). Ca is removed from the myofilaments (Myofil) and cytosol by the SR Ca-ATPase pump (modulated by phospholamban, PLB), sarcolemmal Ca-ATPase pump, Na/Ca exchange & mitochondrial (Mito) uniporter.

there must be some finite rate at which Ca leaks down its ~10,000-fold concentration gradient (~1 mM inside SR: ~100 nM in cytosol). This cytoplasmic Ca is then subject to the competing Ca transport systems above. If all the Ca were re-accumulated by the SR there would be no net loss of SR Ca. However, if some of that Ca leaked by the SR is extruded from the cell by Na/Ca exchange or the sarcolemmal Ca-pump, it would represent a net loss of Ca from the SR and the cell. This is the basis for the cardiac muscle phenomenon known as rest decay (Allen *et al.*, 1976; Bers, 1985), wherein most mammalian cardiac muscle preparations exhibit smaller post-rest contractions after longer rest intervals (see Chapters 6, 7 and 9). Thus, the resting muscle may not be at a true steady-state with respect to Ca fluxes for a rather long time.

A similar type of leak must exist at the sarcolemma, since the electrochemical gradient between the extracellular space and cytoplasm is even greater than between the SR and cytoplasm (due to the negative membrane potential). Again, it matters little whether this leak is via sarcolemmal Ca channels or some less specific route. This Ca influx must be balanced by Ca extrusion; otherwise such Ca entry could cause progressive gain or loss of cell (and SR) Ca. Thus, the contribution of the sarcolemma to maintaining cellular Ca content within specific limits is absolutely essential. The intracellular compartments can only buffer the changes in cell Ca driven by the sarcolemma. In addition, the intracellular cytosolic Ca buffers are in a closed system in quasi-equilibrium with free $[Ca]_i$, and consequently are of finite capacity.

This qualitative picture is useful, but it becomes apparent quickly that the actual quantities of Ca movement are extremely important. It will therefore be critical to consider Ca transport and cytosolic buffering much more quantitatively. This is the only way to address questions such as: How much Ca enters the cell via Ca current *vs.* Na/Ca exchange? How much SR Ca is released compared to Ca influx? How do the four Ca transport systems compete for Ca extrusion from the cytosol during relaxation? Thus we must consider how Ca transport is quantified and how much Ca is involved in activation of contraction.

CELLULAR VOLUME CONVENTIONS AND Ca FLUXES

A variety of different cardiac preparations and techniques have been used to measure Ca transport (with different advantages and disadvantages). This information must all be brought together in a common framework for overall quantitative consideration. We usually consider free ion concentrations in mM or μM. For the intracellular environment it makes sense then to consider $[Ca]_i$ in nM or μM and total cytosolic Ca in similar units ($\mu mol/L$ cytosol). A fundamental convention must be developed with respect to the cytosolic volume of interest.

Fabiato (1983) suggested excluding mitochondrial volume as not readily accessible. Since mitochondria occupy 30-35% of total cell volume in ventricular myocytes (see Tables 2 & 3), this constitutes a substantial decrement from total cell volume. Nuclear volume is about 2% of cell volume in rat ventricular myocytes (Table 3), but Ca probably passes through large nuclear pores such that this volume should probably not be excluded. The SR also occupies 1-3.5% of cell volume (Table 3). While the SR is clearly a separate compartment, its absolute volume is less accurately known. Partly to account for this we typically use the lower end of non-mitochondrial cell volume (65%) for cytosolic volume. The myofilament space which occupies almost 50% of the cell volume is considered to be part of the cytosol.

Ca fluxes into and out of the cytosol of ventricular myocytes have been measured in several different units, depending on the type of preparation and measurement. For example, Ca transport by SR or sarcolemmal vesicles may be reported in nmol Ca/mg SR protein, ^{45}Ca fluxes in heart tissue in $\mu mol/kg$ wet wt of whole tissue, while integrated Ca current may be reported in pCoul/pF (or fmol/pF). Table 9 shows convenient conversion factors for some of the most commonly used units and preparations. These values are not all from one species, but are generally based on values from either rabbit or rat ventricle. My choice of common units for Ca flux in Table 1 is somewhat arbitrary, but reflects the cellular focus here. Another value that comes from these calculations is the protein concentration in a ventricular myocyte (109 mg cell protein/ml cell volume) or 9.2 μl cell volume/mg protein or 5.95 μl cytosol per mg protein.

Ca BUFFERING IN THE CYTOSOL

Ca is very highly buffered in cardiac myocytes, as in all cells. Indeed, while the free [Ca] transient in cardiac myocytes may rise from 100 nM at diastole to a peak near 1 μM, it takes ~100 μM Ca added to the cytosol to produce this change (see below). Having established some convention about cytosolic volume units, we can consider the cytosolic Ca binding sites in terms of their concentrations (in $\mu mol/L$ cytosol or simply μM) and in terms of their equilibrium dissociation constants (K_d, in μM or nM).

Table 9

Ca flux (or sites): Conversion to μmol/L cytosol

Preparation	Measurement units	Multiply by this factor for units μmol/L cytosol
ventricular muscle	μmol/kg wet weight	2.43 [a]
ventricular muscle	μmol/kg dry weight	0.49 [b]
ventricular homogenate	nmol/mg homog pn	292 [c]
ventricular myocytes	nmol/mg cell pn	168 [d]
subcellular fractions (e.g. SR or SL)	nmol/mg SR pn	29.2 [e]
ventricular myocytes	fmol/pF	7046 [f]
ventricular myocytes	μmol/L cell volume	1.55 [a]

[a] using 35% of cell volume occupied by mitochondria (Table 3), 1.06 g/ml ventricular density and 33% extracellular space (Chapter 1). [1.06 kg wet wt/L vent][1 L vent/0.67 L cell][1 L cell/0.65 L non-mito volume]=2.43 kg wet wt/L cytosol, similar to 2.5 from Fabiato (1983) via a more complex calculation.

[b] similar to above, but including wet weight: dry weight = 5 (Langer et al., 1990).

[c] using [120 mg homog pn/g wet wt][2.4 kg wet wt/L cytosol] = 292 g homog pn/L cytosol.

[d] using the 1.83-fold and 1.66-fold purification of dihydropyridine and ryanodine receptors in isolated myocytes (Bers & Stiffel, 1993; Hove-Madsen & Bers, 1993a) [0.574 mg cell pn/mg vent homog pn][120 mg homog pn/g wet wt][2.43 kg wet wt/L cytosol]=168 g cell pn/L cytosol.

[e] assuming a 10-fold purification factor for SR or sarcolemma (SL). [1 mg SR pn/10 mg homog protein][120 mg homog pn/g wet wt][2.43 g wet wt/ml cytosol] = 29.2 mg SR protein/ ml cytosol]. More generically the conversion factor is 292/x, with x the purification factor for a given organelle. Mitochondrial protein is about 40 mg/g wet wt (half that reported by Scarpa and Graziotti, 1973). This limits potential purification of mitochondria to 3x (vs. 50-60x for SL or SR).

[f] using 4.58 pF/pl for rabbit ventricular myocytes (see Table 2, pg 6; Satoh et al., 1996) [4.58 pF/pl][1 l cell/0.65 l cytosol] = 7.046 pF/pl cytosol [×1000 (pl/l)(μmol/fmol)]. Satoh *et al.* (1996) found higher values for ferret (5.39 pF/pl), young rats (6.76 pF/pl) and older rats (8.88 pF/pl) and these values are slightly different than stereological measurements in Table 1 in rabbit and rat (0.6 and 0.46 $\mu m^2/\mu m^3$ respectively) which correspond to 6 and 4.6 pF/pl for 1 $\mu F/cm^2$.

Ca which enters the cytosol may bind to any of numerous Ca-binding ligands in addition to the Ca regulatory site on cardiac troponin C. Two general strategies have been used to evaluate intracellular Ca buffering: 1) calculations using the Ca binding properties of known cellular constituents based on measurements in isolated systems (Fabiato, 1983) and 2) attempts to directly measure the total Ca buffering properties in ventricular muscle or myocytes under conditions approaching those *in situ* (Pierce *et al.*, 1985; Hove-Madsen & Bers, 1993a; Berlin *et al.*, 1994; Trafford *et al.*, 1999). These approaches are described below and I will try to synthesize them into a current "best guess" composite.

The first serious effort to estimate the total Ca requirements for contractile activation was by Fabiato (1983). He collected data on known concentrations and Ca binding characteristics of the following cardiac myocyte constituents: cardiac troponin C, the SR Ca-ATPase, calmodulin, ATP, creatine phosphate and sarcolemmal sites (see curve #6 in Fig 26). This was an extremely useful first approximation and indicated that a total of ~57 μM total Ca would be required to raise free $[Ca]_i$ from 100 nM to 1 μM (or to activate 70% of maximal contraction). However, this estimated Ca buffering is likely to be low because there must be additional Ca binding sites in the cell not on Fabiato's list, and K_d values for Ca binding to

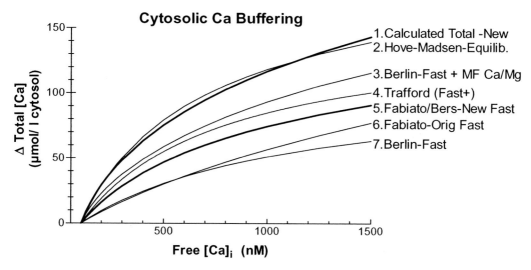

Figure 26. Ca buffering in cardiac myocytes. The data are: 1) Calculated Total using values in Table 10, 2) measured by Hove-Madsen & Bers, 1993a, 3) fast buffering measured by Berlin *et al.* (1994) plus slow myofilaments Ca/Mg binding as in Table 10, 4) from Trafford *et al.* (1999) based on integrated Ca efflux during caffeine-induced contractures, 5) Fabiato's (1983) calculations updated as described in text, 6) Fabiato's original values, 7) Fast buffering only from Berlin *et al.* (1994). The curves are all well fit by hyperbolic functions of the form: ΔCa bound $= (B_{max} /\{1+(K_m /[Ca])\})+B_{min}$, where B_{min} is the theoretical Y-intercept at $[Ca]=0$ (i.e. below diastolic $[Ca]_i$). The values below describe each curve. One can also extract total rather than ΔCa binding, by using $B_{max} -B_{min}$ as B_{max} in the classic binding hyperbola.

	1.New Calc.	2. Equilib.	3.Berlin +Ca/Mg	4. Trafford	5.Fabiato Update	6.Fabiato Orig.	7.Berlin Fast
B_{max} (μmol/L cytosol)	244	236	203	175	162	217	123
K_m(Ca) (nM)	673	498	779	590	730	2307	960
B_{min} (μmol/L cytosol)	−28	−39	−20	-25	−19	−8.8	−12

troponin C and the SR Ca-ATPase used by Fabiato (2 μM and 1 μM respectively) were probably too high (see Table 10). Curve #5 in Fig 26 is an update to the Fabiato compilation. It includes lower K_d values (0.6 μM) for both the SR Ca-ATPase and regulatory site on troponin C based on various studies (e.g. Hove-Madsen & Bers, 1993b; Mattiazzi *et al.*, 1994; Yue *et al.*, 1986; Gao *et al.*, 1994). I have also updated the sarcolemmal Ca binding to include a slightly lower total, based on more recent measurements of inner sarcolemmal sites from Post and Langer (1992; B_{max}=42 μM, K_d=13 μM) and our own data at low [Ca] (Bers *et al.*, 1986 and unpublished; B_{max}=15 μM, K_d=0.3 μM). I also refer to this calculated total estimate as fast buffering since the major contributors are expected to bind rapidly (see below concerning slow binding).

Direct Ca titration in whole ventricular homogenate (as well as particulate and soluble fractions) was first done by Pierce *et al.* (1985). This study probably overestimated intracellular Ca buffering because they include titration of sites on the external cell surface, disrupted organelle sites and additional non-myocyte sites. However, they would also include (appropriately) some intracellular sites not included by Fabiato (1983). This approach was refined by Hove-Madsen & Bers (1993a), who performed similar Ca titrations on isolated ventricular myocytes which had been permeabilized by digitonin and where the SR and mitochondrial Ca transport were blocked by thapsigargin and ruthenium red, respectively. The equilibrium binding results of Hove-Madsen & Bers (1993a; see curve #2 in Fig 26) were lower than reported by Pierce *et al.*(1985), but might still include some external sarcolemmal sites. On the other hand, this overestimate may be minor at submicromolar [Ca] because passive Ca binding to the sarcolemma is asymmetric with the Ca binding phospholipids situated almost exclusively on the inner sarcolemmal surface (Post *et al.*, 1988). As Hove-Madsen & Bers (1993a) pointed out, the SR Ca binding might also be underestimated in the presence of thapsigargin, since this agent appears to lock the SR Ca-ATPase in a Ca-free E_1 state (Kijima *et al.*, 1991; Sagara & Inesi, 1991). The results of Hove-Madsen & Bers (1993a) are curve #2 in Fig 26, and are labeled "Equilibrium" because the data were acquired on a very slow time scale which would include both rapidly and slowly equilibrating sites.

Berlin *et al.* (1994) used a single cell intracellular titration strategy to assess cytosolic Ca buffering using the fluorescent Ca indicator indo-1 and voltage clamp. We blocked Ca transport by the SR Ca-pump, Na/Ca exchange, sarcolemmal Ca-ATPase and mitochondria using thapsigargin, Na-free solutions, high [Ca]$_o$ and a mitochondrial uncoupler. Then we measured total Ca injected into the cytoplasm via I_{Ca} (using voltage clamp) and the resulting change in free [Ca]$_i$ (Fig 27A). Stepwise increases in [Ca]$_i$ accompany the I_{Ca} traces. Closer inspection of these [Ca]$_i$ steps (e.g. Fig 27B) reveals a rapid phase of [Ca]$_i$ increase followed by a slow decline. The rapid increase, which was in phase with integrated Ca influx via I_{Ca} (Fig 27B) is due to very rapid Ca buffering. Note that entry of 9 µM total Ca in Fig 27A only raises free [Ca]$_i$ by 0.1 µM, implying 90:1 Ca buffering. Focusing on this rapid phase, Berlin *et al.* (1994) used only the initial rapid Δ[Ca]$_{bound}$/Δ[Ca]$_i$ component to find a mean fast cytosolic buffering with B_{max} = 123 µM and K_d = 960 nM (curve #7 in Fig 26). These results agree well with the fast buffering in curve #6 calculated by Fabiato (1983). Trafford *et al.* (1999) used a related strategy, applying caffeine to release SR Ca and measuring the rate of total Ca removal (via Na/Ca exchange current) at the same time as recording the Δ[Ca]$_i$ (Fig 93). They found B_{max} =175 µM and K_m= 590 nM. Notably their approach would measure both fast and some slow buffering.

The slow [Ca]$_i$ decline in Fig 27B could be due to either a slower phase of Ca buffering or incomplete inhibition of Ca transport out of the cytosol. Berlin *et al.* (1994) set up and tested conditions to ensure block of such transport, so residual transport is expected to be extremely small. It is reasonable to expect slow Ca buffering by sites which are initially bound to Mg or protons. This is because bound Mg or H must first dissociate before Ca can bind. This is why EGTA is a slower Ca buffer than BAPTA (i.e. it exists mainly as H_2EGTA at neutral pH). Troponin C and myosin both have divalent cation binding sites at which Ca and Mg compete (Ca/Mg sites, see Chapter 2, Table 6; Holroyde *et al.*, 1979, 1980; Pan & Solaro, 1987). The Ca/Mg sites on troponin C and myosin are expected to bind Ca slowly because they are nearly saturated with either Ca or Mg at resting levels of [Ca]$_i$ (Robertson *et al.*, 1981 and see Table 10). Simple inclusion of these sites along with the measured fast buffering sites in the cell in Fig 27B would cause [Ca]$_i$ to fall to the level indicated by the arrow (F+S) in the figure. Inclusion of these myofilament Ca/Mg sites would also raise the overall buffering curve up as indicated by curve #5 in Fig 26 (Berlin-Fast + MF Ca/Mg). This still doesn't explain all of the equilibrium buffering measured by Hove-Madsen & Bers (1993a) or all of the apparent slow buffering in Fig 27. For example, in Fig 27A the overall increase in [Ca]$_i$ expected from the total integrated Ca

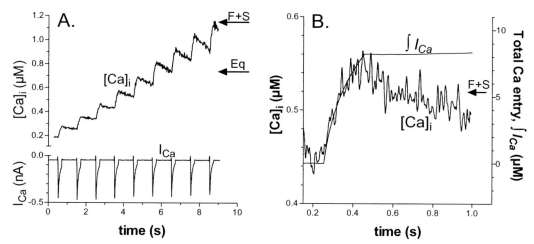

Figure 27. Fast Ca buffering titration in a voltage clamped rat ventricular myocyte. Ca transport was blocked by 10 μM thapsigargin (for SR Ca-ATPase), Na-free solutions inside and out (for Na/Ca exchange), 10 mM [Ca]ₒ (for sarcolemmal Ca-ATPase) and *1799* (for mitochondrial Ca uptake). **A.** Voltage clamp pulses (–40 to 0 mV for 200 ms) injected I_{Ca} to cause step-like increases in [Ca]ᵢ. **B.** The I_{Ca} integral from the fourth pulse in **A** ($\int I_{Ca}$) follows the kinetics of the rise in [Ca]ᵢ. F+S indicates where [Ca]ᵢ is expected to fall to based on curve #3 in Fig 26 (see text). Eq in panel **A** is the predicted final settling points for [Ca]ᵢ if curve #2 in Fig 26 (equilibrium) is used (modified from Berlin *et al.*, 1994).

influx by the end of 9 pulses would be to 1.75 μM considering only the measured fast sites (off the scale of the graph). Inclusion of the calculated myofilament Ca/Mg sites would predict a final [Ca]ᵢ of 1.15 μM, indicated by F+S in Fig 27A. Clearly free [Ca]ᵢ is falling below the F+S level, but perhaps not all the way down to the level predicted by the equilibrium buffering (Eq in Fig). There may well be additional slow Ca/Mg buffers such as Mg-sensitive Ca binding sites on the inner sarcolemmal surface (Frankis & Lindenmayer; 1984; Bers *et al.*, 1986), mitochondria or other sites that contribute to equilibrium Ca binding (Hove-Madsen & Bers, 1993a).

To better marry the empirical titration results with our knowledge about the buffering species, I have chosen the values in Table 10 (plotted as curve #1 in Fig 26). Specific values are still provisional, but this provides a practical working model for the present. Not surprisingly, the proteins which show the largest change in bound Ca between 100 nM and 1 μM are the regulatory Ca binding sites on troponin C and the SR Ca-pump (which are present at 70 and 47 μM in the cytosol). However, these sites only account for about 50% of the total overall change in bound Ca and 75% of the fast buffering. It can also be seen that even at the resting [Ca]ᵢ (100 nM) there is a substantial amount of Ca already bound (142 μM) with 83% of that at the Ca/Mg sites of troponin C. Furthermore, there are several constituents which don't make a large impact by themselves (e.g. calmodulin, ATP and sarcolemma), but collectively make a buffering contribution that is not negligible. These calculations are based on 0.5 mM [Mg]ᵢ at pH of 7-7.2 and mostly at room temperature. Obviously, changing conditions would change the buffering.

Extrapolation of data with these calculations depends on accurate knowledge of the Ca, H and Mg affinities of the various binding sites as well as what the conditions are in the cell. For example, if the Mg affinity of the Ca/Mg sites is underestimated, then the "Berlin-Fast+ Ca/Mg"

Table 10

Passive Intracellular Ca Buffering[a]

	K_d	B_{max}	Ca Bound		
			at 100 nM $[Ca]_i$	at 1 µM $[Ca]_i$	Delta
	(µM)		----- (µmol Ca/L cytosol)[b] -----		
Fast					
Troponin C	0.6	70	10	43.9	33.9
SR Ca-pump	0.6	47	6.8	29.6	22.8
Calmodulin total[c]	0.1-1	24	0.45	3.57	3.1
ATP	200	5,000	0.35	3.46	3.1
Creatine phosphate	71,073	12,000	0.02	0.17	0.2
Sarcolemma[d]	13	42	0.32	3.0	2.7
Membrane/High+[e]	0.3	15	3.7	11.5	7.8
Free $[Ca]_i$		-	0.1	1.0	0.9
Fast Total			21.7	96.2	74.5
Slow: Ca/Mg					
Troponin C: Ca[f]	0.013	140	117	137	20
Mg (Mg bound)	*1111*		*Mg 7.1*	*Mg 0.8*	
Myosin: Ca[g]	0.033	140	3	25	22
Mg (Mg bound)	*3.64*		*Mg 136*	*Mg 114*	
Slow Total			120	162.2	42
Total Ca			**142**	**259**	**117**

a these constants describe curve #1 in Fig 26. Values are mostly taken from Fabiato, 1983; Bers, 1991 and other sources noted in the text. Binding was calculated assuming [K] = 140 mM and [Mg] = 0.5 mM, where relevant (e.g. ATP, creatine phosphate, calmodulin, Ca/Mg sites).

b see Table 9 for unit conversion factors.

c calmodulin results are from four classes of binding sites which also exhibit specific affinities for H, Mg and K and these characteristics were accounted for using the constants compiled by Fabiato (1983) and Haiech *et al.* (1981).

d inner sarcolemmal binding measured by Post and Langer (1992).

e this is based on our earlier estimates of sarcolemmal Ca binding at low [Ca] with K_d ~0.3 µM. The B_{max} was reduced from our earlier estimates (Bers, 1991) because the moderate affinity sarcolemmal sites from Post and Langer (1992) are now included. This modest B_{max} value was also slightly adjusted such that calculated total buffering matched the equilibrium measurements (curve #2 in Fig 26). These sites could also include some unaccounted for high affinity sites from other sources.

f K_d values are from Pan and Solaro (1987).

g values are from Holroyde *et al.* (1979) and Robertson *et al.* (1981).

curve in Fig 26 could move up to curve #1 (Berlin *et al.*, 1994). Also, when Robertson *et al.* (1981) did detailed kinetic calculations of Ca binding to cardiac myofilaments, they assumed that diastolic $[Ca]_i$ was 10 nM and free $[Mg]_i$ was 2 mM. This led them to predict that the Ca/Mg sites on troponin C were 91% saturated with Mg with little bound Ca at rest. Based on more recent data, diastolic $[Ca]_i$ is probably between 100 and 150 nM and free $[Mg]_i$ is probably about 0.5 mM (Blatter & McGuigan, 1986; Murphy *et al.*, 1989a,b; Gao *et al.*, 1994). This means that at diastole, the troponin C Ca/Mg sites would be 84% saturated with Ca and only 5% with Mg (Table 10). Obviously the kinetics of binding will also be important to clarify further.

Table 10 reflects a Ca buffer capacity of 123 µM/pCa unit (from 0.1 to 1.1 µM $[Ca]_i$), much lower than cardiac cellular pH buffering (20-90 mM/pH unit, Ellis & Thomas, 1976;

Wallert & Fröhlich, 1989; Bountra *et al.*, 1990). This is relevant because intracellular acidosis can increase [Ca]$_i$ due to competition with Ca at intracellular binding sites (Bers & Ellis, 1982) and changes in [Ca]$_i$ can lead to intracellular acidosis (Vaughan-Jones *et al.*, 1983).

A subtle additional consideration is what constitutes accessible cytosolic volume. Our standard cytosolic volume above only excludes the cell space occupied by mitochondria (~35%). If we additionally exclude SR volume (3.5%, Table 3) and space occupied by the concentrated cytosolic protein (~10-15%), all the curves in Fig 26 would be shifted up by another 15-20%. Protein volume is based on cytosolic [protein] of 120 mg/ml cytosol and density of 1.2 g protein/ml. This would bring Curve #3 close to Curve #1 in Fig 26 and to values in Table 10. Thus, these estimates of cellular Ca buffering have caveats, but are meant as a best guess guide, subject to further clarification.

Ca REQUIREMENTS FOR ACTIVATION OF CONTRACTION

Figure 28A illustrates the impact of cooperativity (assessed by the Hill coefficient) on the [Ca] dependence of myofilament activation. As discussed in Chapter 2, measurements made in chemically skinned cardiac muscle fibers are fit with Hill coefficients (*n*) of ~2-3 (as for Ca binding) and half-maximal force at K$_m$ ~1-2 μM. Measurements of myofilament Ca sensitivity in intact ventricular muscle have given both a higher affinity (K$_m$~0.6 μM) and cooperativity (Hill coefficient = 4-6, Yue *et al.*, 1986; Backx *et al.*, 1995; Gao *et al.*, 1994). The result is a very steep force dependence on [Ca] between 300 and 800 nM (Fig 28A).

Figure 28B shows force as a function of the amount of Ca added to the cytosol from an initial free [Ca] of 150 nM using the Ca buffering from Table 10 and curve #1 in Fig 26. It can be seen that very little force is developed with the first 30 μM Ca supplied. As the amount of Ca increases the relationship is fairly steep, such that most of the force development occurs between

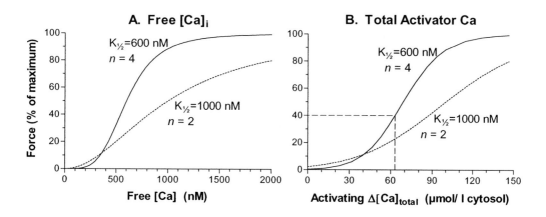

Figure 28. Total Ca requirements for myofilament activation. **A.** Myofilament Ca sensitivity over the range of relevant [Ca]$_i$, plotted as Force = F$_{max}$/(1 + (K$_m$/[Ca]$_i$)^n), where *n* is the Hill coefficient, indicative of cooperativity of both Ca binding and myofilament activation (see Chapter 2). **B.** The amount of added total cytosolic Ca required to activate contractile force (from [Ca]$_i$ =150 nM), based on Table 10.

40 and 80 µM of added Ca. The steady state twitch in mammalian ventricular muscle is typically sufficient to reach ~40% of maximal force at 25-30°C (Harrison & Bers, 1989a). This would require a free $[Ca]_i$ of ~540 nM and about 62 µM of added total Ca. To reach 600 nM $[Ca]_i$ (the K_m for force in Fig 28A) would require between 31 and 74 µM for the seven curves in Fig 26 (from diastolic $[Ca]_i$=150 nM). Thus, while some quantitative points could be known more precisely, a reasonable current estimate of the Ca which must be added to the cytosol to activate a normal ventricular twitch is ~60 µM (i.e. µmol/L cytosol).

It should also be recognized that many factors can alter cytosolic Ca buffering and Ca requirements for myofilament activation, such as pH and Mg. Under normal conditions intracellular pH is 7.1-7.2 and free $[Mg]_i$ is probably ~0.5 mM (Blatter & McGuigan, 1986; Murphy *et al.*, 1989a,b; Gao *et al.*, 1994). Both acidosis and increased $[Mg]_i$ can occur in pathophysiological situations and would be expected to reduce cytosolic Ca buffering by competition. In 10-15 min of ischemia $[Mg]_i$ can increase 3-fold as a consequence of decline in [ATP], which normally exists mostly as Mg-ATP (Murphy *et al.*, 1989b). Cytosolic Ca buffering increases developmentally (Bassani *et al.*, 1998) and there may also be temperature- and species-dependent differences, which have not been systematically addressed.

Ca DYNAMICS DURING A TWITCH

In Figures 26 and 28 I have dealt with cytosolic Ca buffering in a steady state manner, without explicit consideration of kinetic aspects. Figure 29 shows a simplified kinetic model of a myocyte Ca transient. The starting point is a generic free $[Ca]_i$ signal which starts at 100 nM, rises to a peak of 744 nM at 70 ms and falls exponentially with a time constant $\tau = 300$ ms. This $[Ca]_i$ transient is the driving function to determine Ca binding to each cytosolic ligand L in Table 11 (using the general function $d[Ca-L]/dt = k_{on}[Ca]_i [L] - k_{off}[Ca-L]$). Not all of the kinetic parameters have been directly measured, so some approximations are used. Figure 29A shows the time course of free $[Ca]_i$ as well as the change in total cytoplasmic [Ca] (ΔTotal Ca_{cyt}) after considering on- and off-rates for Ca (and Mg) binding to each cellular ligand (see Table 11). Figure 29B shows how Ca bound to different ligands varies dynamically during the Ca transient. From these figures it can be appreciated that free $[Ca]_i$ peaks earlier than total cytosolic Ca and also comes back to near initial value faster due to these intrinsic kinetics. Relatively slow buffering can also create a ratcheting up of total cytosolic Ca (e.g. see Ca/Mg sites). This would be expected to be influenced by stimulation frequency. In Figure 29 total cytosolic Ca is 6.5 µM higher at the end of 2 sec than before the pulse, with 5.3 µM of this still bound to TnC Ca/Mg sites and 1.1 µM still bound to myosin Ca/Mg sites. At the end of 10 pulses at 0.5 Hz these Ca/Mg sites gain an additional 6 µM Ca (see also Shannon *et al.*, 2000a).

Figure 29C adds a simplified consideration of Ca fluxes which may underlie the Ca transient in Fig 29A. This also serves as an introduction to the following chapters where these fluxes will be addressed more directly. Fluxes in Fig 29C were calculated as described in Table 11. Ca current (I_{Ca}) peaked at 6.8 pA/pF with rising and falling time constants of 3 and 40 ms, respectively (bringing in a total of 16 µM Ca; Yuan *et al.*, 1996). The Ca transported by the SR Ca-ATPase was calculated using a classic Michaelis-Menten relationship with a V_{max} of 210 µM/sec, a K_m of 300 nM and a Hill coefficient of 2 (Bassani *et al.*, 1994a; Balke *et al.*, 1994; see also Chapter 7). The SR Ca leak was set to counterbalance the resting SR Ca-ATPase rate (21

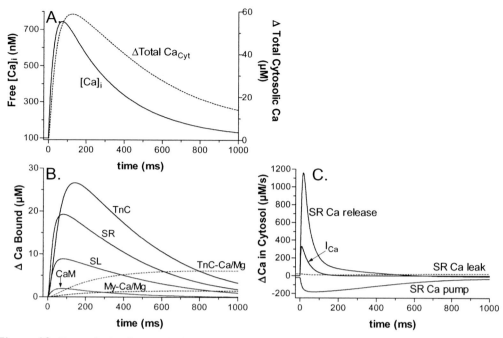

Figure 29. Dynamic Ca changes during a twitch in rabbit ventricular myocyte. **A**. Free [Ca]$_i$ and change in total cytosolic ([Ca]$_{Cyt}$). **B**. Associated changes in Ca bound to different cytosolic ligands. **C**. I$_{Ca}$, SR Ca release flux, SR Ca-pump flux and SR Ca leak. See Tables 10 & 11 and text for details.

μM/s) and was varied in direct proportion to the calculated intra-SR free [Ca] ([Ca]$_{SR}$). The initial SR Ca content was set at 100 μmol/L cytosol (Bassani & Bers, 1995) with passive intra-SR Ca buffering (B$_{max}$ = 180 μmol/L cytosol and K$_d$ = 600 μM; Shannon & Bers, 1997). The SR Ca release flux in this particular model ends up being predicted as the amount of change in total cytosolic [Ca] required for the initial free [Ca]$_i$ waveform and not accounted for by either I$_{Ca,}$ SR Ca-ATPase or SR Ca leak. Thus, the SR Ca release flux is the residual of the calculations, and is similar to other estimates (e.g. Sipido & Wier, 1991; Wier *et al.*, 1994; Shannon *et al.*, 2000b).

It is not precisely known what *normal* resting, diastolic or peak [Ca]$_i$ really is in cardiac muscle. This is largely due to questions about the *in vivo* calibration of the Ca$_i$ indicators which have been used (e.g. Ca microelectrodes, aequorin, quin2, fura-2 and indo-1, Blinks, 1986). For example, Ca microelectrodes can overestimate [Ca]$_i$ because of imperfect impalements, fura-2 and indo-1 may underestimate [Ca]$_i$ because of binding of the indicator to intracellular constituents (Konishi *et al.*, 1988, Hove-Madsen & Bers, 1992; Bassani *et al.,* 1995d; Harkins *et al.*, 1993). The situation is even more problematic when cells are loaded with the acetoxymethylester (AM) forms of these indicators (rather than direct intracellular application of the free acid form). In this case, the cellular signals are complicated by the fluorescence of incompletely de-esterified forms of the indicator (Lückhoff, 1986) and intracellular compartmentalization of the indicator (e.g. ~50 % may be trapped in the mitochondria, Spurgeon *et al.*, 1990). Bassani *et al.* (1995d) calibrated indo-1 *in situ* in ferret using null-point titrations and found that: a) the K$_d$ for Ca-indo-1 in the cell was 844 nM (*vs.* ~250 nM in aqueous solution), b) diastolic [Ca]$_i$ right after a train of beats at 0.5 Hz at 23°C was 294 nM, and c) resting [Ca]$_i$ continues to decline very slowly with rest reaching ~80 nM after 30 min. This

Table 11

Kinetic Parameters used for Figure 29[a]

	B_{max} (μM)	K_d (μM)	k_{off} (sec^{-1})	k_{on} ($\mu M^{-1}sec^{-1}$)	Reference
Troponin C	70	0.6	19.6	32.7	Robertson, Gao
Troponin C Ca/Mg	140	0.0135	0.032	2.37	Pan, Robertson
(Mg sites)		*1111*	*3.33*	*0.003*	Pan, Robertson
Myosin Ca/Mg	140	0.0333	0.46	13.8	Robertson
(Mg sites)		*3.64*	*0.057*	*0.0157*	Robertson
SR Ca-pump	47	0.6	60	100	Diffusion
Calmodulin total[b]	24	7	238	34	Haiech
Sarcolemma	42	13	1300	100	Post
Membrane/High	15	0.3	30	100	Bers

Flux Calculations

SR Ca-ATPase	$J_{SR} = (210\ \mu M/s)/(1+ \{0.3\ \mu M/[Ca]\}^2)$
Ca current	$I_{Ca} = (9\ pA/pF)\ exp(-t/40\ ms)(1-exp(-t/3\ ms))$
SR Ca leak	at t=0 set at SR Ca-ATPase rate, changes proportional to $[Ca]_{SR}$
SR Ca content	initially 100 $\mu M/L$ cytosol; $[Ca]_{SR\text{-}bound} = 180\ \mu M/(1+0.6\ mM/[Ca]_{SR})$
	SR volume taken as 3.5% of cell volume
SR Ca release	Δtotal cytosolic Ca (accounting for I_{Ca}, SR Ca-ATPase and leak)

[a] B_{max} and K_d values are generally as in Table 10. In most cases values are only available for k_{on} or k_{off} so that the other was calculated using $K_d = k_{off}/k_{on}$. If neither k_{on} or k_{off} are available, diffusion limited k_{on} (100 $\mu M^{-1}sec^{-1}$) and K_d were used. References are Robertson *et al.*, 1981; Gao et al., 1994; Pan and Solaro, 1987; Haiech *et al.*, 1981; Post and Langer, 1992; Bers *et al.*, 1986; Bers, 1991.

[b]   The 4 Ca-calmodulin binding sites were lumped as a single site. The K_d was artificially increased so that the steady state Ca-calmodulin binding was well predicted over the relevant range of $[Ca]_i$ (0.1 to 3 μM) without requiring separate kinetic calculations of H, Mg and K competition at each of the 4 sites (although these equilibrium interactions were included in Table 10 and Figs 26 and 28).

diastolic $[Ca]_i$ is probably on the upper limit of current estimates, but diastolic $[Ca]_i$ is probably in the range 80-250 nM and peak $[Ca]_i$ during a *normal* twitch probably reaches 0.5-2 μM.

       Another consideration relevant to the potential contribution of cellular sites to Ca fluxes is the rates at which they can supply Ca to and remove Ca from the cytoplasm. The peak of the Ca transient in mammalian cardiac muscle at ~30°C can be reached as early as 30 msec. Thus, the rate of total Ca rise must be able to approach 2 mmol/L cytosol/sec (60 μmol/L cytosol/30 msec). The rate of Ca removal from the cytoplasm is about 10-fold slower, i.e. ~200 μmol/L cytosol/sec (see Fig 29C). These rough estimates are given to indicate the general magnitudes that might be expected of sources and sinks of Ca underlying contraction.

SOURCES AND SINKS OF Ca

Extracellular Space: The extracellular space (ECS~30% of the tissue volume, see Chapter 1), could supply more than enough Ca (2 mmol/L ECS × 0.55 L ECS/L cytosol = 1000 μmol/L cytosol). This does not include low affinity Ca binding sites in the ECS which may at least double this value (Bers & Langer, 1979; Philipson *et al.*, 1980). Clearly, this would be more than enough Ca to activate contraction, but the critical question lies in the regulation of Ca influx. The two main routes by which Ca is known to enter the cell are by voltage-dependent Ca channels and the Na/Ca exchange system. Since there is a very large electrochemical gradient favoring Ca entry at rest (E_m $-E_{Ca}$~200 mV) any type of leak could provide an additional route of Ca entry. Ca current and Na/Ca exchange will be discussed in Chapters 5 & 6. There are also two mechanisms which contribute to Ca efflux across the sarcolemma discussed in Chapter 6: Na/Ca exchange and sarcolemmal ATP-dependent Ca-pump (or Ca-ATPase).

Inner Sarcolemmal Surface: The surface of the sarcolemmal membrane facing the cytoplasm can also bind substantial Ca; and this may be as much as 60 μmol/L cytosol (Table 10, Bers *et al.*, 1986; Mansier & Bers, 1984; Post & Langer, 1992). This is a relevant range (although 20× less than the ECS). A provocative hypothesis by Lüllman & Peters (1977, 1979) was that Ca bound to specific sites at the inner sarcolemmal surface could be released upon membrane depolarization (due to locally induced acidification and altered binding affinity). This Ca liberated upon depolarization could rebind during repolarization and relaxation. Negatively charged phospholipids (phosphatidylserine and phosphatidylinositol) which comprise 7.2% of the sarcolemmal phospholipids are exclusively on the inner sarcolemmal leaflet and would be plausible sites (Post *et al.*, 1988). Bers *et al.* (1986) measured a decrease in sarcolemmal Ca binding at 300 nM [Ca] upon membrane depolarization from –80 to 0 mV (2 nmol/mg protein, 20 μmol/L cytosol). However, the Ca binding to these sites would also increase with I_{Ca} and SR Ca release. So this depolarization-dependent decrease in bound Ca was more than offset by a rise in local [Ca] to 1-5 μM. Thus, depolarization may simply decrease the ability of these sites to buffer increases in local [Ca]$_i$. Physiological [Na]$_i$ (5-15 mM) and [Mg]$_i$ (0.5-3 mM) also decrease sarcolemmal Ca binding (Frankis & Lindenmayer, 1984; Bers *et al.*, 1986). Large rapid changes in local [Na]$_i$ subsequent to Na channel current could also displace Ca from these local sites, and may also enhance Ca entry via Na/Ca exchange (Akera *et al.*, 1976; LeBlanc & Hume, 1990), but the role of these sarcolemmal sites as a source of activating Ca is not clear.

These are provocative ideas. However, intact cell data preclude any quantitative role for these inner sarcolemmal Ca binding sites in E-C coupling. When extracellular Ca is removed very quickly (<1 sec) so that [Ca]$_i$ and stores are not altered, depolarization does not produce measurable contraction or [Ca]$_i$ rise under a wide array of conditions (Rich *et al.*, 1988; Näbauer *et al.*, 1989, see Chapter 8). Thus, in the absence of Ca influx, depolarization alone does not lead to a significant Ca release or [Ca]$_i$ rise. In conclusion, inner sarcolemmal sites are likely to serve mainly as additional intracellular Ca buffering sites.

Sarcoplasmic Reticulum: The amount of Ca held in the SR is discussed in detail in Chapter 7 (Table 21, pg 179). The bulk of values under physiological conditions are in the range of 50-250 μmol/L cytosol (e.g. Solaro & Briggs, 1974; Hunter *et al.*, 1981; Fabiato, 1983; Hove-Madsen & Bers, 1993a; Varro *et al.*, 1993; Delbridge *et al.*, 1996). Thus, there is more than enough Ca in the SR to support a single contraction. Again, the key issues are the regulation of SR Ca transport. Chapter 7 will address both the SR Ca-ATPase and the SR Ca release channel. Chapters 8 and 9 will focus on more integrated aspects of SR Ca release and Ca content.

Mitochondria: Mitochondria can accumulate massive amounts of Ca, especially when there is sufficient inorganic phosphate, which can precipitate insoluble Ca-phosphate in mitochondria, a process known as matrix loading (Lehninger *et al.*, 1967; Carafoli & Lehninger, 1971; Carafoli,

1987). Indeed, isolated mitochondria can take up 100 nmol Ca /mg mitochondrial protein (corresponding to 10,000 µmol/L cytosol, assuming 40 mg mitochondrial protein/g wet weight) and can store several times more (Carafoli, 1975). While this is a potentially enormous capacity, it appears that under conditions anticipated *in vivo*, mitochondria are likely to contain very much less (e.g. 1 nmol/mg, or 100 µmol/L cytosol, Carafoli, 1987). Thus, mitochondria are a potential source of activator Ca, but again the issue is whether the fluxes of Ca across the mitochondria on the time frame of E-C coupling make significant contributions. This issue will be dealt with in more detail in subsequent sections of this chapter.

It may be useful at this point to note that the same sites considered above as potential Ca sources are also potential Ca sinks. The important question to be addressed from here is the mechanism by which Ca is transported to and from these sources and sinks. First let us consider where Ca goes during relaxation.

Ca REMOVAL DURING RELAXATION

As mentioned earlier, four Ca transport systems can compete for cytoplasmic Ca during relaxation in cardiac muscle: 1) SR Ca-ATPase, 2) sarcolemmal Na/Ca exchange, 3) sarcolemmal Ca-ATPase and 4) mitochondrial Ca uniport system. Obviously, Ca entering the cytosol from the extracellular space or SR is mostly bound to the various Ca buffers which were discussed with respect to Figs 26-28 and Tables 10-11. Here I will consider how the four Ca transport processes described above contribute to the Ca removal which allows relaxation to proceed. In particular how do these Ca transporters compete dynamically during relaxation? Bers & Bridge (1989) addressed this first by separately blocking SR Ca reuptake or Na/Ca exchange during relaxation from rapid cooling contractures in rabbit ventricular muscle (see pg 152-155). Blocking Na/Ca exchange slowed relaxation by 30%, preventing SR Ca reuptake slowed relaxation by 70%, while inhibiting both pathways slowed relaxation by >1000%. This made it clear that the SR Ca-ATPase and to a lesser extent Na/Ca exchange could produce relaxation, but that these were the main two relevant mechanisms. This work was extended in a series of more detailed quantitative studies in isolated ventricular myocytes by Bassani *et al.* (1992, 1993a; 1994a,b, 1995a; Puglisi *et al.*, 1996) and others (see Chapter 9).

Bassani *et al.* (1992) initially evaluated this competition by using inhibition of each of the four Ca transport systems and observing the impact on the rate of $[Ca]_i$ decline and relaxation in rabbit ventricular myocytes. Figure 30 shows a summary of their results for relaxation, which were in close agreement with data from $[Ca]_i$ decline. The normal twitch relaxes with a half-time $(t_{1/2})$ of 170 ± 30 ms where all Ca removal systems are functional. Rapid and sustained application of 10 mM caffeine causes abrupt SR Ca release via ryanodine receptors, and with appropriate flow characteristics the rate of rise of $[Ca]_i$ can be comparable to that during the twitch. However, the sustained exposure to caffeine prevents net SR Ca reuptake, while the other Ca removal systems can still function. When SR reuptake was inhibited this way (or by thapsigargin, Bassani *et al.*, 1994a) relaxation was slowed by a factor of 3 $(t_{1/2} = 540 ± 70$ ms). This result makes it clear that SR Ca uptake is important in relaxation, but also that a reasonable rate of relaxation can be obtained by the other 3 systems. Then Na/Ca exchange was blocked at the same time as SR Ca reuptake, by applying 10 mM caffeine in a Na-free, Ca-free solution containing EGTA (Caff, 0Na, 0Ca). Note that this blocks Ca flux via Na/Ca exchange in both

Relaxation of Rabbit Ventricular Myocytes

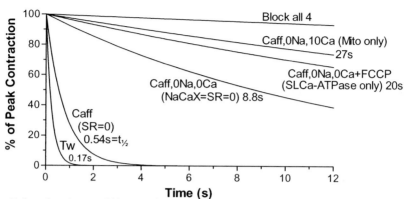

Figure 30. Relaxation in a rabbit ventricular myocyte with selective inhibition of Ca transporters. Normalized cell relaxation is shown where: 1) all Ca transporters function during a normal twitch (Tw), 2) net SR Ca uptake is prevented during a contracture induced by 10 mM caffeine (Caff), 3) SR Ca transport and Na/Ca exchange are prevented by caffeine in 0Na, 0Ca solution (Caff,0Na,0Ca), 4) only the sarcolemmal Ca-ATPase is functional (Caff,0Na,0Ca+FCCP), 5) only the mitochondrial Ca uniport is functional (Caff,0Na,10Ca) after pre-depletion of $[Na]_i$, or 6) All four Ca removal systems were blocked by combining the caffeine with 0Na, 10Ca and FCCP (after pre-depletion of $[Na]_i$). Relaxation traces are based on mean $t_{1/2}$ values (shown along traces) from Bassani *et al.* (1992).

directions. This maneuver slowed relaxation and $[Ca]_i$ decline by almost 20-fold ($t_{1/2}$ =8.8 ± 1.0 s) compared to caffeine alone. Thus Na/Ca exchange is responsible for most of the relaxation and $[Ca]_i$ decline during a caffeine-induced contracture (93%, Bassani *et al.*, 1994a).

Even when both SR Ca-uptake and Na/Ca exchange are prevented, relaxation and $[Ca]_i$ decline still proceed, albeit very slowly. This slow relaxation and $[Ca]_i$ decline, requiring tens of seconds, could be due to Ca transport by the mitochondrial Ca uniporter or the sarcolemmal Ca-ATPase. To inhibit mitochondrial Ca uptake in the intact myocyte Bassani *et al.* (1992) used application of FCCP and oligomycin (each at 1 µM) a few seconds before exposure to caffeine, 0Na, 0Ca solution. FCCP is a protonophore which dissipates the mitochondrial proton and potential gradient, thereby eliminating the driving force responsible for Ca influx into mitochondria (oligomycin was included to minimize mitochondrial ATP consumption during the brief exposure to FCCP). Inhibition of mitochondrial Ca uptake in this way slowed the mean relaxation time by about 2-fold compared to caffeine, 0Na, 0Ca (20 s *vs.* 8.8 s). Two different strategies were used to inhibit the sarcolemmal Ca-ATPase (thermodynamic and pharmacological). The thermodynamic approach used elevation of $[Ca]_o$ to 10-100 mM to impede the sarcolemmal Ca-pump by steepening the $[Ca]_i$ /$[Ca]_o$ gradient. However, to do this experiment in Na-free solution it is essential that the cells first be depleted of intracellular Na by incubation in 0Na, 0Ca. Otherwise extracellular Ca would enter in exchange for intracellular Na, greatly complicating the interpretation. As seen in Fig 30, this slowed relaxation about 3-fold with respect to caffeine, 0Na, 0Ca ($t_{1/2}$ went from 8.8 to 27 s). The second method employed carboxyeosin, a potent inhibitor of the sarcolemmal Ca-pump (Gatto & Milanick, 1993) and produced very similar results (Bassani *et al.*, 1995a). That is, carboxyeosin slowed the $t_{1/2}$ of $[Ca]_i$ decline in rabbit ventricular myocytes during caffeine, 0Na, 0Ca from 7.5 ± 0.5 s to 26.3 ± 2.1 s. When all four Ca transport systems were blocked, relaxation and $[Ca]_i$ decline were nearly

Table 12

Contributions of Different Ca Transporters to Relaxation in Rabbit Ventricular Myocytes

Transporter	Relaxation analyzed	Relaxation rate λ (s^{-1})	Percent of Ca removal Flux
SL-Ca-Pump	Caff-0Na,0Ca,FCCP	0.035	0.86%
Mito. Ca uniport	Caff-0Na,+10Ca	0.025	0.62%
Na/Ca exchange	Caff†	1.22	30.0%
SR-Ca-Pump	Twitch‡	2.79	68.5%
All 4 systems	Twitch	4.08	100.0%

SL is sarcolemmal, Mito. is mitochondrial and Caff is caffeine. Rate constants (λ) are reciprocals of time constants (ln $2/t_{1/2}$) of relaxation. †The λ value for Caff is adjusted by subtracting those for the SL Ca-ATPase + Mito (-0.06) which also function during a caffeine-induced contracture. ‡Similarly λ_{SR} is obtained by subtracting ($\lambda_{Tw} - \lambda_{NaCaX} - \lambda_{Mito} - \lambda_{SL-Ca-Pump}$). See pg 250-253 for more detailed analysis.

abolished (Bassani *et al.,* 1992, 1995a). This indicates that these are the only four Ca removal systems that need to be considered from any practical standpoint.

This series of studies allows a crude prediction of relative Ca extrusion rates in rabbit ventricular myocytes (comparing $t_{1/2}$ values). Compared to the Na/Ca exchanger, the SR Ca-ATPase was 2-3 times faster and the sarcolemmal Ca-ATPase and mitochondrial Ca transport were 37 and 50 times slower respectively (Bassani *et al.,* 1992).

Table 12 shows a more quantitative treatment of this data, considering each Ca transport system to function independently with a rate constant (λ_{SR}, λ_{NaCaX}, $\lambda_{SL-CaATP}$ & λ_{Mito}) that contributes additively to the overall relaxation rate constant (λ). This allows a breakdown of the four individual values and their percent contribution to relaxation. We find that in rabbit ventricle the relative values for SR Ca-ATPase and Na/Ca exchange are 68% and 30%, while the sarcolemmal Ca-ATPase and mitochondrial Ca uniport contribute less than 1% each. This is consistent with both prior less direct estimates above (Bers & Bridge, 1989), as well as more detailed quantitative analysis of rabbit ventricular myocyte Ca transients using integrated Ca fluxes (where 70% of the transported Ca during relaxation was via the SR Ca-ATPase and 28% via Na/Ca exchange; Bassani *et al.,* 1994a; see pg 250-253). This balance of Ca fluxes differs among species (e.g. SR Ca-ATPase contributes 92% in rat ventricle, Bassani *et al.,* 1994a; Negretti *et al.,* 1993) and in pathophysiological conditions (e.g. Na/Ca exchange contributes 50% in failing rabbit heart (Pogwizd *et al.,* 1999). This will be further addressed in Chapters 9 & 10.

Ca INFLUX *vs.* SR Ca RELEASE IN CONTRACTILE ACTIVATION

The two main sources of Ca involved in the normal activation of cardiac muscle contraction are Ca influx and SR Ca release. In the steady state the amount of Ca entry during the cardiac cycle must be the same as the amount of Ca efflux. Otherwise the cell will gain or lose Ca and not be in a steady state with respect to cellular Ca balance. The same is true for the SR. Thus the quantitative analysis of the contributions of the SR Ca-ATPase and Na/Ca exchange to relaxation should roughly reflect the fraction of activation by SR Ca release or Ca

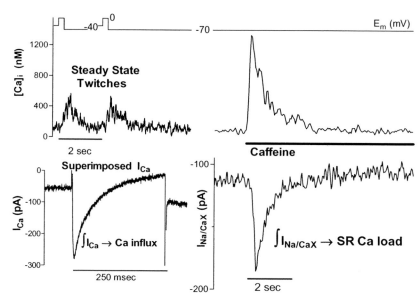

Figure 31. Ca transients, Ca influx via I_{Ca} and SR Ca content measured by integrating $I_{Na/Ca}$ in a rabbit ventricular myocyte (dialyzed with 50 µM indo-1). The last 2 steady state Ca transients and superimposed I_{Ca} traces were during voltage clamp pulses to 0 mV (left) and rapid applications of 10 mM caffeine at a holding potential –70 mV caused SR Ca release and activation of $I_{Na/Ca}$ (right). Note different scales for I_{Ca} and $I_{Na/Ca}$ (from Delbridge *et al.*, 1996, with permission).

influx respectively. Thus, based on Fig 30 we might expect Ca influx and SR Ca release to supply 25-30% and ~70% of the activating Ca respectively in rabbit ventricle.

Delbridge *et al.* (1996) assessed this electrophysiologically, by measuring Ca influx via I_{Ca}, the SR Ca content by caffeine-induced $I_{Na/Ca}$, and using the fraction of this SR Ca content released during a twitch (Bassani *et al.*, 1993b). Figure 31 shows steady state voltage clamp pulses, Ca transients and I_{Ca} (left). On the right, 10 mM caffeine is applied to release the SR Ca content and prevent net reuptake. This causes a large and rapid Ca transient and an inward current that decreases as [Ca]$_i$ declines. This inward current is Na/Ca exchange current ($I_{Na/Ca}$) because it is abolished in the absence of extracellular Na (Li substituted) and in the absence of a Ca transient (i.e. a second caffeine application did not cause a current or a [Ca]$_i$ rise; Delbridge *et al.*, 1996). Furthermore, one sustained caffeine application was sufficient to empty the SR, since a second caffeine exposure caused no further Ca release. The integral of I_{Ca} allows direct evaluation of Ca influx and the SR Ca content can be calculated from the integral of $I_{Na/Ca}$. Since Na/Ca exchange only removes 93% of the Ca during a caffeine-induced Ca transient in rabbit (Bassani *et al.*, 1994a), the SR Ca content is calculated by dividing the $I_{Na/Ca}$ integral by 0.93 (=87 µM). The other data required is the fraction of SR Ca content released during a twitch, measured to be 43% in rabbit ventricular myocytes (Bassani *et al.*, 1993b). These Ca fluxes are converted to µmol/L cytosol using appropriate surface to volume ratios (Tables 2 & 9).

We then find that during the rabbit ventricular twitch I_{Ca} brings in 9.7 µM Ca and the SR Ca release is 37 µM (0.43×87 µM). Thus 23% of the Ca comes from I_{Ca} and 77% from SR Ca release. These numbers are in rather good agreement with the data in Fig 30, Table 12 and Bassani *et al.* (1992, 1994a, 1995a), based on [Ca]$_i$ decline during relaxation. This is remarkable quantitative agreement between very different analytical methods, which have different intrinsic limitations. Again, species-, development- and condition-dependent differences in this balance of Ca fluxes will be discussed further in Chapter 9.

One may well ask whether Ca entry via Na/Ca exchange also contributes to Ca influx during the cardiac action potential. This is certainly possible, but for various reasons I think that the quantitative contribution of Ca entry via Na/Ca exchange is very small during the normal action potential (≤ 1 μmol/L cytosol) when compared to the Ca influx via I_{Ca}. This issue will be discussed in further detail in other chapters (e.g. 4, 6, 9 & 10). The amount of Ca influx via Na/Ca exchange can vary dramatically under different conditions.

In conclusion, we now have a fairly clear quantitative picture about the number of Ca ions involved in the activation of cardiac muscle contraction, including which transport pathways are involved in bringing Ca into the cytosol, what the Ca ions bind to in the cytosol (and when) and how Ca removal systems compete quantitatively during relaxation. For a typical 32 pL myocyte the amount of Ca cycling during a twitch (~60 μmol/L cytosol) corresponds to 1.25 fmol Ca/cell or 750 million Ca ions/cell. Obviously, there is continual refinement of this quantitative picture as more data become available, but we are probably much closer to reality now than 10 years ago. There are also major species differences in the balance of Ca fluxes and how these systems change during development, as well as under pharmacological and patho-physiological situations. The snapshot described in this chapter may thus serve as a reference point for much of the ensuing discussion throughout this book.

MITOCHONDRIAL Ca TRANSPORT

While the foregoing discussions indicate that mitochondrial Ca plays only a very minor quantitative role in Ca fluxes associated with E-C coupling, mitochondrial Ca fluxes may still be important with respect to mitochondrial function and energetics. Thus, mitochondrial Ca transport will be considered in more detail here, rather than in a separate chapter.

As mentioned above (pg 52), mitochondria can accumulate large amounts of Ca, but under physiological conditions the Ca content is probably on the order of 100 μmol/L cytosol. Under conditions approaching those *in vivo* Fry et al. (1984a) showed that mitochondrial Ca uptake was not appreciable in digitonin permeabilized cardiac myocytes until cytoplasmic [Ca] exceeded 1 μM (where a Ca uptake rate of 2-5 μmol/L cytosol/sec can be inferred).

Figure 32 illustrates the Ca cycle of mitochondria. Ca enters via a uniport system, down a large electrochemical gradient (about −180 mV) set up by proton extrusion linked to the passage of electrons down the cytochrome system in the respiratory chain. This Ca uniporter is blocked competitively by physiological $[Mg]_i$ (Nicholls & Ackerman, 1982), lanthanides (Mela, 1969; Reed & Bygrave, 1975), and also potently by ruthenium red (Moore, 1971) and the novel selective blocker Ru360 (Ying *et al.*, 1991; Matlib *et al.*, 1998; Zhou *et al.*, 1998). Ca entry via the uniport pathway exhibits a sigmoid dependence on [Ca] and under physiologic ionic conditions has a K_m above 30 μM Ca. Thus, at the $[Ca]_i$ associated with the cardiac cycle (0.1-1 μM) the influx rate is expected to be quite low. In particular, Crompton (1985, 1990) developed a model to describe Ca uptake by isolated mitochondria. At 0.1 and 1 μM [Ca] mitochondrial Ca uptake was 0.1 and 3.1 μmol/L cytosol/sec respectively (using 40 mg mitochondrial protein/ml

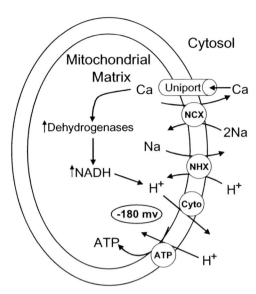

Figure 32. The Ca cycle across the inner mitochondrial membrane. Ca enters via a uniport, down an electrical gradient formed by H-pumping in the respiratory chain (Cyto). Ca is extruded by a Na/Ca antiport and Na is extruded by Na/H exchange thereby completing the cycle. Elevated cytoplasmic [Ca] can lead to elevated mitochondrial [Ca] and increased activity of mitochondrial dehydrogenases.

cell and 0.65 L cytosol/L cell). This is consistent with our data and analysis in intact myocytes at [Ca]$_i$ between 0.1 and 1 µM, where mitochondrial Ca uptake was ≤1 µmol/L cytosol/sec (Bassani *et al.*, 1994a, 1995a). The ability of mitochondria to accumulate Ca led Lehninger (1974) and Carafoli (1975) to speculate initially that it may contribute to cardiac relaxation by removing Ca from the cytoplasm, but it seems now that the quantitative contribution is almost negligible.

Ca extrusion from the mitochondria is mainly via a Na/Ca antiporter, which may be electroneutral (2:1), but might also be >2:1 (Crompton *et al.*, 1976; Crompton, 1985; Jung *et al.*, 1995). The [Na] dependence of this Na/Ca antiporter is sigmoidal with half-maximal Ca extrusion at ~5-8 mM Na, making this system quite sensitive to changes of [Na]$_i$ in the physiological range (Crompton *et al.*, 1976; Fry *et al.*, 1984b). While variations in bulk cytoplasmic [Na] during the cardiac cycle are probably insufficient to cause rapid release of mitochondrial Ca, large changes in [Na] can induce substantial mitochondrial Ca release *in vitro* (Crompton *et al.*, 1976). There is also a Na-independent extrusion of Ca from mitochondria which is less prominent in heart, but is more important in tissues where Na/Ca antiport activity is low (e.g. liver & kidney; Crompton, 1985). The inner mitochondrial membrane has an active Na/H exchange system (Mitchell & Moyle, 1967) which is the pathway for Na extrusion from the matrix and also completes the cycle. In this way the energy for Ca extrusion via Na/Ca exchange depends also on the proton movement during respiration and the consequently negative intramitochondrial potential.

Under relatively physiological conditions there is probably only a small [Ca] gradient across the inner mitochondrial membrane, with intra-mitochondrial free [Ca] ([Ca]$_M$) being slightly lower than [Ca]$_i$ (Moreno-Sanchez & Hansford, 1988; McCormack *et al.*, 1989; Miyata *et al.*, 1991; Zhou *et al.*, 1998, Fig 33). Based on the trans-mitochondrial potential (–180 mV)

$[Ca]_M$ would have to be 0.1-1 M to be at equilibrium. Ca is thus far from equilibrium and considerable energy is required to extrude Ca from mitochondria up this electrochemical gradient. While the Na electrochemical gradient may be the immediate source of energy, this gradient is created by the proton gradient. Thus the true energy source is respiration and the protonmotive force it generates. Figure 33 shows how $[Ca]_M$ responds to $[Ca]_i$ changes induced by reduction in $[Na]_o$, thereby promoting Ca entry via Na/Ca exchange, (Miyata *et al.*, 1991). As resting $[Ca]_i$ rises to 650 nM the value of $[Ca]_M$ stays below $[Ca]_i$. However, as resting $[Ca]_i$ becomes very high, mitochondrial Ca uptake appears to be activated and $[Ca]_M$ exceeds $[Ca]_i$.

There is almost no detectable fluctuation in $[Ca]_M$ during an individual twitch in ventricular myocytes (Miyata *et al.*, 1991; Griffiths *et al.*, 1997; Zhou *et al.*, 1998). Chacon *et al.* (1996) reported phasic $[Ca]_M$ transients in heart mitochondria which were kinetically identical to the cytosolic signal, but these might be due to contamination of the $[Ca]_M$ signal by $[Ca]_i$ (since the authors did not block mitochondrial Ca uptake or quench cytosolic indicator to confirm their interpretation). Gunter *et al.* (1998; Sparagna *et al.*, 1995) described a novel rapid Ca uptake mode (RaM) in isolated liver mitochondria, which produces small amplitude, but very rapid bursts of Ca uptake with Ca pulses. They found this to differ from Ca uniport flux in terms of ruthenium red, Mg and spermine sensitivity, but RaM was also different in cardiac mitochondria (Bunitas *et al.*, 1997). This could produce up to 10 µmol/L cytosol Ca flux in 1-2 sec at physiological $[Ca]_i$, but the role in cardiac myocyte Ca regulation is not yet clear.

Crompton (1985) modeled the Ca transport of isolated cardiac mitochondria to phasic changes in $[Ca]_i$ during the cardiac cycle. For a cytoplasmic [Ca] change from ~200 nM to ~2 µM and back, $[Ca]_M$ increased by only ~2% (*vs.* 1000% for the rise in $[Ca]_i$). On the other hand, both this model and cellular data show that high stimulation rate (4 Hz) or strong cellular Ca loading via the Na/Ca exchange cause a slow rise in $[Ca]_M$ over tens of seconds (Miyata *et al.*, 1991; Griffiths *et al.*, 1997; Zhou *et al.*, 1998). Zhou *et al.* (1998) demonstrated that under these conditions phasic increases of $[Ca]_M$ could be detected, but they were still slow and only observed at diastolic $[Ca]_i > 400$ nM. This is consistent with Fig 33 and the sigmoid dependence of mitochondrial Ca uptake on $[Ca]_i$ (Crompton, 1976; Fry *et al.*, 1984a,b). The 0.6% of twitch $[Ca]_i$ decline attributed to mitochondrial uptake (Table 12) would be 0.36 µmol/L cytosol, or 0.7 µmol/L mitochondria. Assuming 100:1 Ca buffering of free $[Ca]_M$, we expect mitochondrial twitch Ca transients of ~7 nM amplitude, with extremely damped kinetics compared to $[Ca]_i$.

Mitochondrial Ca transport may be more consequential for Ca transient dynamics in other cell types, such as neurons (Friel & Tsien, 1994) and adrenal chromaffin cells (Park *et al.*, 1996; Herrington *et al.*, 1996; Babcock *et al.*, 1997). These chromaffin cell studies showed that a large bolus of Ca influx via I_{Ca} produced large Ca transients which were substantially curtailed by mitochondrial Ca uptake over 10-30 sec, allowing $[Ca]_i$ to recover to low levels much more rapidly than when FCCP was present. Notably, this mitochondrial Ca uptake was only seen when $[Ca]_i$ exceeded 500 nM for a relatively long time, consistent with cardiac data above. This mitochondrial Ca in the chromaffin cell was then slowly extruded to the cytosol at a rate at which the plasma membrane Ca-ATPase and Na/Ca exchange could remove it from the cell without greatly elevating $[Ca]_i$. Using a similar analysis to Table 12, relative contributions of SR/ER: NaCaX: plasmalemmal-CaATP: mitochondrial Ca uniport were a) 68:30:1:1% in rabbit ventricle b) 0:9:16:75% in chromaffin cells (Herrington *et al.*, 1996) and c) 7% plasmalemmal extrusion

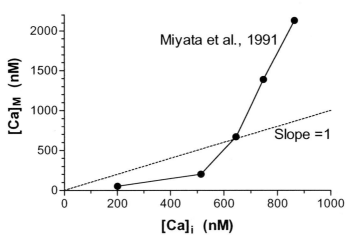

Mitochondrial [Ca] in intact cells

Figure 33. Mitochondrial free [Ca] ($[Ca]_M$) as a function of cytosolic [Ca] ($[Ca]_i$). Increases of $[Ca]_i$ in rat ventricular myocytes were induced by reducing $[Na]_o$ (i.e. via sarcolemmal Na/Ca exchange). Mean $[Ca]_i$ was measured using indo-1 (loaded as the salt form) and $[Ca]_M$ was measured using indo-1 (loaded as the AM form) with Mn quench of cytosolic indo-1. Data are redrawn from Miyata *et al.* (1991) (without error bars) and including a broken line corresponding to $[Ca]_M = [Ca]_i$ (slope = 1).

and 46% each for ER and mitochondrial Ca uptake in neurons (Friel & Tsien, 1994). The main difference in heart is probably the extremely high density and Ca transport capacity of the SR Ca-ATPase and Na/Ca exchanger. These systems cause rapid $[Ca]_i$ decline in heart which limits the opportunity for the mitochondria to contribute to $[Ca]_i$ decline. In other words, if we were to slow cardiac Na/Ca exchange and SR Ca-ATPase by 20-100-fold, the competition among the 4 Ca transporters would be more balanced. (e.g. see top traces in Fig 30).

Location is probably also important with respect to mitochondrial Ca transport. Rizzuto *et al.* (1992, 1993, 1998) showed close proximity between mitochondria and IP$_3$-sensitive Ca stores in non-cardiac cells. They also used mitochondrially-targeted recombinant Ca-sensitive photoproteins to show that mitochondria near these Ca release sites sense a much higher local [Ca] (compared to bulk $[Ca]_i$) and that $[Ca]_M$ is also higher than would be expected from bulk $[Ca]_i$. It is unclear how important this consideration is in cardiac myocytes. Parts of mito-chondria are close to junctional SR in heart. However, this is partly a consequence of these two important structures being physically excluded from the series arrangement of myofibers necessary to transmit force. Local $[Ca]_i$ near both sarcolemmal and SR Ca release channels is very high when the channels are open, and this is functionally important (see Fig 118).

Hunter & Haworth (1979) first described a large conductance pore in the inner mitochondrial membrane known as the mitochondrial permeability transition pore (MTP; see reviews by Zoratti & Szabo, 1995; Crompton, 1999). This pore allows passage of molecules up to a molecular weight of 1500 Da, is activated by high $[Ca]_M$ and is blocked by cyclosporin A. MTP is a complex of the voltage-dependent anion channel (VDAC) on the outer membrane, the ADP/ATP translocase in the inner membrane and cyclophilin D (a matrix peptidyl-prolyl *cis/trans* isomerase, which is also the receptor for cyclosporin A). The ADP/ATP translocase may serve as the actual pore in the inner mitochondrial membrane, but many details of how this complex works as the MTP are still to be worked out (Crompton, 1999). The MTP is opened by high $[Ca]_M$ (K_M ~25 µM, Al Nasser & Crompton, 1986) and oxidative stress. Openings of the MTP cause abrupt dissipation of membrane potential in individual mitochondria and these can be transient (Hüser *et al.*, 1998a). This depolarization allows Ca efflux to the cytosol, relieving the mitochondrial Ca overload. However, this is costly because other mitochondrial contents are lost, the mitochondrial F_0F_1-ATP synthase consumes ATP (rather than making it) and the large negative membrane potential must be reestablished by electron transport. Moreover, prolonged MTP opening causes further dysregulation of Ca and energetic state leading to mitochondrial run down and cell death.

Mitochondrial Ca fluxes might not be important quantitatively in E-C coupling, but the small gradual changes in mitochondrial [Ca] with heart rate changes or cellular Ca load may help to regulate mitochondrial energy production. Three key mitochondrial matrix enzymes are activated by low µM [Ca] (pyruvate dehydrogenase, α-ketoglutarate dehydrogenase and the NAD-dependent isocitrate dehydrogenase, Denton & McCormack, 1980, 1985, 1990; Hansford, 1985, 1987). Thus, increases in mitochondrial Ca via the above mechanisms could occur when cytosolic [Ca] is relatively high and the energy demands are also high (i.e. when contractile activation and Ca pumping are consuming ATP at high rates). In this way, the rise in cytoplasmic (and mitochondrial) [Ca] can increase oxidative metabolism and thereby increase ATP production to meet increased demands. A potentially interesting twist on this is that cellular Ca loading is often secondary to cellular Na loading, via sarcolemmal Na/Ca exchange (e.g. when the Na-pump is inhibited by digitalis). In this case the increase of mitochondrial Ca which *could* stimulate oxidative metabolism may be limited by the high $[Na]_i$ which would tend to minimize the gain of mitochondrial Ca. Thus, energy supply may not go up to meet demands and the cytoplasmic Ca load will be more severe. This might favor more force production, but could also elevate diastolic $[Ca]_i$ and compromise cardiac relaxation and energy balance.

Brandes & Bers (1997) demonstrated a $[Ca]_i$-dependent stimulation of mitochondrial NADH production by measuring [NADH] in intact contracting ventricular muscle (Fig 34). With a sudden increase in stimulation frequency or $[Ca]_o$ there was a transient decrease in [NADH], consistent with NADH production not keeping up with the increased ATP and NADH consumption. However, this [NADH] decline was followed by a recovery toward the initial value. This recovery was entirely dependent on increased average $[Ca]_i$. That is, a comparable increase in work by increasing sarcomere length was associated with the same initial decline, but no recovery (Fig 34C). We concluded that the increased average $[Ca]_i$ caused an increase in $[Ca]_M$ and stimulation of dehydrogenases and NADH production. Indeed, when the elevation of $[Ca]_i$ or frequency was terminated, there was an overshoot of [NADH] (again not seen when the work increase was not due to higher average $[Ca]_i$). The overshoot is probably due to slow extrusion of $[Ca]_M$ and loss of Ca-dependent dehydrogenase stimulation. The time course of this overshoot concurs with slow mitochondrial Ca efflux (20-40 sec, Bassani *et al.*, 1993a).

In an extension of the studies described in Fig 30, Bassani *et al.* (1993a) evaluated the fate of the Ca which was "forced" into mitochondria during caffeine-induced contractures with Na/Ca exchange blocked. That is, under the Caff-0Na, 0Ca condition in Fig 30 ~50% of the SR Ca load is slowly taken up by the mitochondria over 20-30 sec (with the remainder transported

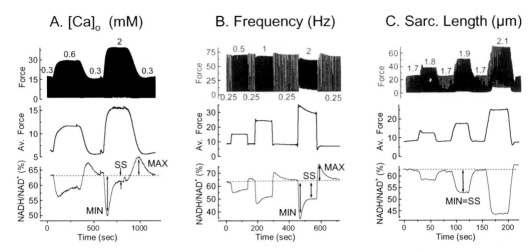

Figure 34. Mitochondrial NADH fluorescence and force measured in rat ventricular muscle. Work was increased by either elevating [Ca]$_o$ (**A**), increasing frequency (**B**) or increasing sarcomere length (**C**). Force (in mN/mm^2) was converted to time-averaged force (middle traces) as an index of work level. Increasing either [Ca]$_o$ or frequency increases average [Ca]$_i$ along with work, while increasing sarcomere length increases work without substantial change in average [Ca]$_i$. Increasing work in A & B causes NADH to decline to a minimum (MIN) then recover during sustained high work load (SS) and finally overshoot (MAX) upon return to original work level. Without [Ca]$_i$ change (C) there is no recovery and overshoot phase (from Brandes & Bers, 1997, with permission).

out by the sarcolemmal Ca-ATPase). After removal of caffeine (in sustained 0Na, 0Ca solution with EGTA) this mitochondrial Ca was transported back to the SR with a time constant of 40 sec. We concluded that this represented mainly the time constant of mitochondrial Ca efflux (with relatively rapid reuptake into the SR, because [Ca]$_i$ remained low). Furthermore, the rate of Ca redistribution from mitochondria back to SR was slowed when intracellular Na was removed (consistent with the Na-dependence of mitochondrial Ca efflux in cardiac myocytes). Thus, it seems clear that transient increases in mitochondrial Ca may accumulate gradually over a large number of beats (e.g. during cytosolic Ca transients of higher frequency or amplitude) and [Ca]$_M$ gradually dissipates over 1-3 min when the initial steady state is resumed.

It should be noted that mitochondria use the same pool of energy to phosphorylate ADP to ATP as to drive Ca uptake (i.e. the protonmotive force). Energized, isolated mitochondria have been shown to take up Ca at the expense of making ATP (Vercesi *et al.*, 1978). This would obviously be a dangerous situation *in vivo*, but it appears that at physiological [Mg]$_i$ the uniport is inhibited strongly enough that mitochondrial energy is preferentially used to make ATP (Sordahl, 1975). This may not be the case when the cell is exposed to chronically elevated [Ca]$_i$, where mitochondrial Ca uptake gets much more active.

The ability of heart mitochondria to accumulate massive amounts of Ca under pathological conditions such as ischemia (Reimer & Jennings, 1992) may serve as an important safety device for heart cells. Cellular Ca overload is a common early component of cell injury in many cell types (Shanne *et al.*, 1979) and could quickly become disastrous in heart cells since high cytosolic [Ca] would keep energy consumption by the myofilaments and Ca-ATPases high while mitochondrial Ca uptake could limit ATP synthesis. Sustained contracture due to rigor crossbridges (induced by low ATP) could also worsen the situation by vascular compression leading to decreased local blood flow. If the mitochondria can temporarily compensate for the cellular Ca load by taking up large amounts of Ca, permanent cell damage might be avoided. Unfortunately it is a double-edged sword, since Ca accumulation by the mitochondria diminishes ATP production and eventually compromises the mitochondria. Thus the survival of the cell might depend on whether the mitochondria can survive a given degree of transient Ca loading.

In conclusion, mitochondria play a minor role in Ca movements on a beat-to-beat basis. However, with slower increases in "mean" $[Ca]_i$ mitochondrial Ca transport may be important in increasing metabolism to meet metabolic demands. In more severe Ca overload, mitochondria may provide a temporary Ca store to protect the cytoplasm from very high Ca levels.

It is worth considering the energy requirements for key ion transporters in heart. Table 13 shows that the Na/K-ATPase, sarcolemmal Ca-ATPase and SR Ca-ATPase all function at a very high energetic efficiency (70-80%). The ΔG required for the generation of normal ionic concentration gradients is valuable to keep in mind, since anything that reduces ΔG_{ATP} (i.e. lower [ATP] or higher [ADP] or $[P]_i$) could also reduce the ionic gradients. The ATP required to transport 60 µM Ca into the SR, 15 µM Ca out of the cell via Na/Ca exchange (which requires 3 Na, and 1 ATP/ 3 Na via Na/K-ATPase) and 15 µM Na from I_{Na} out via Na/K-ATPase, would be 50 µmol ATP/L cytosol/beat or ~300 µL O_2/kg wet wt/beat (or 1% of the cellular [ATP]/beat). At a heart rate of 1 Hz and cardiac O_2 consumption of 100 ml O_2/kg wet wt/min Na and Ca transport would require 15-20% of the total O_2 consumption for the heart, with the myofilaments accounting for most of the rest. Thus the myocyte uses ~5-7% of its ATP for each beat.

Table 13

Energy Requirements for Cardiac Ion Transporters

Transporter	Transport & Stoichiometry	$[X]_{Low}/[X]_{Hi}$ (mM)	E_m (mV)	ΔG_X (mV)	ΔG_X (kJ/mol)	Efficiency (%)
Na/K-ATPase	3Na out + 2K in	$10Na_i/140Na_o$ $5K_o/120K_i$	−80	461	44.5	76.4
SL Ca-ATPase	1 Ca out	0.0001/ 2	−80	425	41.0	70.3
SR Ca-ATPase	2 Ca in	0.0001/ 1	0	492	47.5	81.5
F_0F_1-ATP synthase	2.5 H in[†]	pH 7.1/8.1	−180	−604	−58.3	100[†]

ΔG_X was calculated from $\Delta G_X = RTln([X]_{Low}/[X]_{Hi}) - zFE_m$. [†]it is assumed that generation of 1 ATP requires 2.5 protons to flow through the mitochondrial F_0F_1-ATP synthase, such that the energy available is $\Delta G_{ATP} = -58.3$ kJ/mol. This is defined as 100% for comparison to energy use by the ATPases. However, it may take 3 protons to generate this ΔG_{ATP} making F_0F_1-ATP synthase efficiency 83%.

This chapter has provided a general framework and some quantitative values for the processes involved in Ca regulation in cardiac myocytes. This sets the scene for more detailed discussion of these key mechanisms and their interrelationships in the subsequent chapters.

D.M. Bers.
Excitation-Contraction Coupling and Cardiac Contractile Force.
2nd Ed., Kluwer Academic Publishers, Dordrecht, 2001

CHAPTER 4

CARDIAC ACTION POTENTIAL
AND ION CHANNELS

The initiating event in cardiac E-C coupling is the action potential (AP). The AP is the membrane potential (E_m) waveform that is determined by a complex interplay of many ion channels and transporters, and the Ca transient itself. The AP is also the driving E_m waveform that influences ion channels and transporters, and results in the genesis of the Ca transient. The AP is also responsible for the propagation of excitation information from cell to cell in the heart and allows the heart to function as a syncytium (electrically and mechanically). The underlying ionic currents also contribute to initiating pacemaker activity as well as arrhythmogenic delayed- and early afterdepolarizations (DADs & EADs) and conditions for re-excitation and reentry. This chapter is only a basic overview of cardiac ion channels and the cardiac AP. A comprehensive treatment of this topic could readily fill another book of this type. For additional depth and references I recommend some excellent recent reviews by Weiss (1997), Roden & George (1997), Yellen (1998), Carmeliet (1999) and Nerbonne (2000, 2001). The main focus here will be on the ventricular myocyte AP and basic understanding of the ionic currents which contribute to its shape and modulation.

ACTION POTENTIAL & HETEROGENEITY

Figure 35 demonstrates the classical phenotypes of APs in different regions of the heart. The normal heartbeat initiates in the sino-atrial (SA) node since the cells in that region normally have the fastest intrinsic pacemaker activity. The maximum diastolic polarization in these cells is typically about –50 to –60 mV and a gradual pacemaker depolarization leads to an AP with a slow rate of rise and consequently slow rate of local propagation. As will be clear from the ensuing discussion, Na channels are almost entirely inactivated and don't participate in the rapid depolarization phase (in these cells Ca channels serve this role). In the atrio-ventricular (AV) node, the AP resembles that in the SA node. In atrial and ventricular muscle cells the resting E_m is near –80 mV and the AP has a very fast upstroke attributable to Na current, and overshoots 0 mV to reach a peak at +30-50 mV. Repolarization is much faster in atria than in ventricular myocytes and Purkinje fibers. Thus in ventricular cells there is a more prominent plateau. Moreover, the ventricular AP duration (APD) is shortest in epicardial cells, longer in endocardial cells and longest in mid-myocardial cells (reflecting in part differential ion channel expression). The longer endocardial AP also explains why T waves in the ECG are typically in the same direction as the QRS complex (repolarization vector is in opposite direction of depolarization).

The long APD in ventricular myocytes serves two functions. First, it prevents electrical re-excitation, by keeping the membrane depolarized (and thus Na and Ca channels inactivated). This inhibits aberrant conduction pathway development. Second, it allows contraction to relax

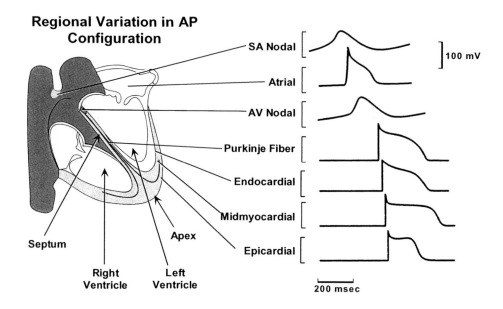

Figure 35. Regional variation in action potential configuration. The APs at right are representative of the different shapes typically observed for the cardiac regions indicated. The position along the time axis for AP upstrokes reflect the different delays from SA node firing. For example, the delay between atrial and Purkinje fiber firing reflects slow transmission through the AV node (and the P-R interval in the ECG). Atrial and ventricular myocyte AP upstrokes are responsible for the P wave and QRS complex in the ECG (Fig kindly supplied by J. Nerbonne).

before the next beat (since the APD is almost as long as the Ca transient and contraction). This also prevents tetanization of cardiac muscle, which would not be advantageous for cardiac function in the way that it is for skeletal muscle function (i.e. The heart must fill between beats).

From the SA-node the wave passes to atrial muscle (fast propagation 0.1-1 m/s) and the AV node, where conduction slows again progressively from atrial end (AN) to the central node region (N; 0.01-0.05 m/sec), before slightly speeding through the last part of the node (NH). As the wave gets through the His bundle, bundle branches and Purkinje fibers, propagation becomes very rapid (2-4 m/sec) and it remains very fast through ventricular muscle (0.3-1 m/sec). At this point I will consider the resting E_m, how ionic channels influence E_m and propagation.

RESTING E_m, NERNST POTENTIAL & PROPAGATION

The resting cardiac myocyte membrane is preferentially permeable to K (due mainly to I_{K1} channels, see below). The Na/K-ATPase generates the ionic concentration gradients for Na and K, but K-channels dictate the negative resting E_m in myocytes (and virtually all cells). How does this come about? Let's consider the simplest case of a generic cell (Fig 36) which has high $[K]_i$ and low $[K]_o$, but the membrane is impermeable with E_m initially at 0 mV. If the membrane is only permeable to K, then K will tend to flow down its concentration gradient, but as positive charge leaves the cell a membrane potential is created (inside negative). This negative E_m limits further K efflux, so an electrical driving force opposes the driving force of the chemical gradient ($[K]_i$ /$[K]_o$). So at what point are these forces equal and opposite? This is easiest to consider

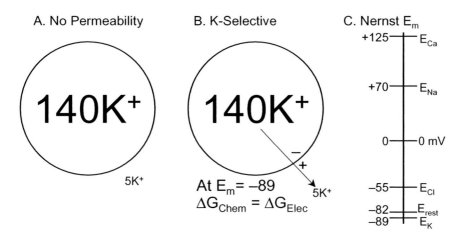

A. No Permeability   **B. K-Selective**   **C. Nernst E$_m$**

140K$^+$

5K$^+$

140K$^+$

At E$_m$= –89
ΔG_{Chem} = ΔG_{Elec}

5K$^+$

+125 —— E$_{Ca}$

+70 —— E$_{Na}$

0 —— 0 mV

–55 —— E$_{Cl}$

–82 —— E$_{rest}$
–89 —— E$_K$

Figure 36. Resting membrane potential and Nernst potentials. The Na/K ATPase generates a [K] gradient across the cell membrane even if there are no functional channels (A). The presence of only K-selective channels (B) causes an E$_m$ to develop (E$_K$) at which the K concentration gradient is exactly balanced (thermodynamically) by a negative transmembrane E$_m$ (Nernst or equilibrium potential). Nernst potentials for other ions (x) are also shown (C) according to (RT/zF) ln([x]$_o$/[x]$_i$). The Goldman-Hodgkin-Katz equation uses relative permeabilities for monovalent ions to estimate E$_m$ =(RT/F) ln{([K]$_o$+ P$_{Na}$/P$_K$ [Na]$_o$+ P$_{Cl}$/P$_K$ [Cl]$_i$) /([K]$_i$+ P$_{Na}$/P$_K$ [Na]$_i$ + P$_{Cl}$/P$_K$ [Cl]$_o$)}.

quantitatively with the free energy equation: ΔG = RT ln([K]$_o$/[K]$_i$) – zFE$_m$ where the two terms reflect the energy in the chemical and electrical gradient respectively. When these are equal and opposite ΔG =0 and E$_m$ = (RT/zF) ln([K]$_o$/[K]$_i$) or 61.5 log$_{10}$([K]$_o$/[K]$_i$), which is the Nernst or equilibrium potential for K (E$_K$). For [K]$_o$ = 5 mM and [K]$_i$ = 140 mM, E$_K$ = –89 mV. This means that at an E$_m$ of –89 mV there will be no net K flux and the system will be stable.

Obviously this is too simple for a myocyte where there are many channels and even the selectivity of K channels for K over Na is not absolutely 100%. Similar Nernst potentials can be calculated for Na, Ca and Cl and are indicated in Fig 36C (+70, +125 and –55 mV respectively). So, if the membrane becomes more permeable to a given ion, the E$_m$ will move closer to the Nernst potential for that ion (due to an increase in flux of that ion down its electrochemical gradient). Thus, the opening of only a few Na selective channels (or finite Na permeability in K or leak channels) will cause inward Na current and a more positive E$_m$ than –89 mV. The relative permeability can be used to predict the actual E$_m$ using the Goldman-Hodgkin-Katz equation or its more generalized forms (see Fig 36 legend; Hille, 1992; Campbell *et al.*, 1988). To keep it simple, the resting E$_m$ in myocytes reflects only slight permeability to Na (~100 times smaller than for K), such that resting E$_m$ is close to E$_K$ (–82 *vs.* –89 mV). In pacemaker cells, which have less resting K permeability, other conductances move diastolic E$_m$ further from E$_K$ and closer to E$_{Na}$ so that E$_m$ is considerably more positive (e.g. –50 to–60 mV).

To jump ahead a little in this simple permeability framework, when Na channels open Na ions will come in (an inward current) causing E$_m$ to move toward E$_{Na}$. The amount of current flowing can be considered using Ohm's law: I = GΔV or I$_{Na}$ =G$_{Na}$(E$_m$ – E$_{Na}$), where G$_{Na}$ is the Na conductance. Of course as E$_m$ gets closer to E$_{Na}$ the driving force for current through the Na

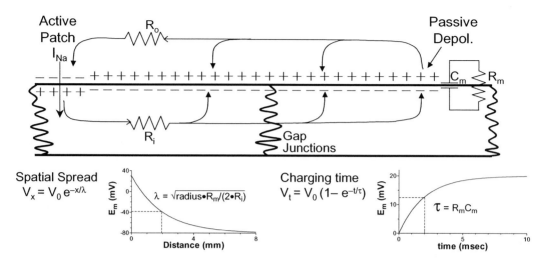

Figure 37. Propagation of depolarization in cardiac myocytes. Inward ionic current (I_{Na}) in the active patch at left causes passive spread of depolarization longitudinally through resistance (R_i and R_o) which includes gap junctions. The flow of positive charge (K ions) down the cell can charge the membrane capacitance (C_m) and leak out via R_m (K channels). The degree and rate of spatial spread are dictated by the length (or space) constant (λ) and time constant (τ) as indicated in insets. Technically λ should use $R_o + R_i$ in place of R_i, but R_o is usually small in comparison. This same cable model can be extended to the transverse and depth dimensions in the real heart, and space constants differ in different directions. Insets show expressions for passive spatial and temporal E_m spread.

channel ($E_m - E_{Na}$) declines and the driving force for K current ($E_m - E_K$) gets larger. At the point where inward I_{Na} and outward I_K are equal and opposite, net current is zero and this marks the AP peak. As Na channels turn off (G_{Na} approaches 0), outward K current repolarizes the cell back to the initial diastolic E_m.

The wave of AP depolarization proceeds via gap junctions and depolarizing current spreads from one cell to the next, bringing E_m in the latter cell beyond the threshold for an AP. Figure 37 shows how electrotonic spread of current contributes to this activation. At the left a patch of membrane where Na channels are open has a positive E_m. This results in passive spread of current through the cytoplasm and gap junctions (carried mainly by K ions), causing the downstream regions to depolarize. Current flow in the reverse direction occurs in the extracellular space (where Na and Cl carry the charge). This current charges up the membrane capacitance to depolarize the downstream membrane electrotonically, without ions passing through the membrane *per se*. This downstream membrane is thus being depolarized *passively* as opposed to *actively* (as in the case where Na channels are open and ionic current causes depolarization). This passive depolarization can bring the neighboring membrane closer to threshold to trigger an AP at that point by opening E_m-dependent Na channels (see below). This passive current spread shows no refractoriness and conducts in both directions. An AP would also propagate in both directions from an initial focal depolarization. However, if Na channels in the region to the left are refractory (due to recent inactivation) retrograde AP is prevented.

The ability of the membranes to propagate passive depolarization is extremely important in determining the rate and fidelity of the wave of excitation that spreads through the heart. If the active zone depolarizes faster and to more positive E_m, this will spread faster and farther to excite downstream regions with a faster conduction velocity. This is partly why atrial and ventricular conduction are much faster than in the SA and AV node. The cellular geometry and characteristics, especially resistance, also play a big role. As the passive current in Fig 37 proceeds down the cell and across gap junctions a limiting factor in how far it will reach is how easily it flows longitudinally *vs.* across the membrane. Thus if the membrane resistance (R_m in Ω-cm^2) is high compared to the longitudinal resistivity (R_i in Ω-cm) more current will stay intracellular and charge membrane capacitance further downstream. R_i also gets smaller with increasing cell diameter (like a larger diameter copper wire). The usual quantitative measure of how well passive current spreads along a fiber is the *space* or *length constant* λ = (radius $\times$ $R_m/(2R_i))^{1/2}$ which is on the order of 2 mm in cardiac muscle. This means that at one point in time it takes 2 mm for the impact of a local active depolarization to decay to 37% of its peak value. More generally E_m at a distance x from a point where it is V_0, is given by $V_x = V_0 e^{-x/\lambda}$. While external resistivity (R_o) should also be added to R_i in the λ equation, its value is usually small in comparison to R_i. Thus large diameter cells with many gap junctions and high R_m would have the largest space constant and be best at high propagation velocity. Indeed, these factors contribute directly to the slow propagation in AV nodal cells (small diameter) and the very high rates of propagation in Pukinje fibers which have high diameters (large radius & small R_i), no T-tubules (hence higher R_m) and many longitudinal gap junctions (lowering R_i). The membrane capacitance (C_m) is also important in determining the time constant ($\tau = R_m C_m$) for charging up the membrane to the AP threshold. The equation describing this charging at time t is $V_t = V_0(1-e^{-t/\tau})$. Thus, smaller τ values will enhance propagation velocity.

The heart is normally well tuned in terms of its propagation network, so that APs are activated in all cells in a progressive and synchronized manner. Local alterations in channel function or passive properties (R_m, R_i, λ & τ) can upset the normal activation pattern and contribute to altered conduction patterns and reentrant arrhythmias.

BASIC STRUCTURE & FUNCTION OF ION CHANNELS

The overall structure of most of the ion channels discussed here (and in Fig 38) fall into two main categories: 1) Na, Ca and many K channels and 2) inward rectifier K channels. Na and Ca channels have four homologous domains (I-IV), each of which has 6 transmembrane spans (S_1-S_6). In each domain there is also a pore (or P) loop between S_5 and S_6 which dips back into the membrane and is thought to line the actual permeation pore and be involved in channel selectivity. The pore is created by one P-loop from each domain around the center with the remaining transmembrane regions layered around this S_5-P-loop-S_6 core. The S_4 span in each domain has a highly conserved stretch where every third amino acid is positively charged. These S_4 spans are thought to move within the electric field in response to changes in E_m. That is, they function as the E_m-sensor of voltage sensitive channels (Yang *et al.*, 1996; Mannuzzo *et al.*, 1996). Most E_m-dependent K channels (and the pacemaker channel that produces I_f) have the same overall structure except that each of the four domains is a separate protein, which assembles into a tetramer that is analogous to the Na and Ca channel. Inward rectifier K channels have a related structure, but are only ~400 amino acids long with only two trans-membrane domains (M_1 and M_2) which are analogous to S_5 and S_6 above, including a pore loop between them. These channels also function as tetramers with a central pore. These inward rectifiers lack the S_4 domain of E_m-activated channels, and some are ligand-activated. The first relevant ion channel crystal structure in Fig 39A (from Doyle *et al.*, 1998) is from a bacterial K channel that is similar in structure to these inward rectifier channels. They describe the shape as an inverted teepee (more apparent in other structural views). The P loops converge to a very narrow region at the outside mouth of the pore (and notably do not span the whole membrane bilayer). This region contains the selectivity filter and can be occupied by 2 K ions in single file. This pore is so narrow that these ions must shed all of their associated water molecules to fit. After the selectivity filter there is an aqueous cavity which may serve to lower the electrostatic barrier and ensure a low resistance and high throughput of ions. The inner mouth of the pore is lined by the S_6 or M_2 domain, and where they converge at the inner end may also be the site of the activation gate (Yellen, 1998; Perozo *et al.*, 1999).

The activation gate for E_m-dependent channels has long been expected to be at the inner mouth of the channel (Armstrong, 1971, 1975; Yeh & Narahashi, 1977, Cahalan & Almers, 1979; Yellen, 1998). This is mainly because channel blockers can only enter the pore from the inside when the channel is activated. Blockers can either inhibit closure of the activation gate (foot in the door effect) or be trapped in the channel by activation gate closure (Yellen, 1998).

Permeation and Selectivity

Many ion channels are highly selective for one physiological ion and as such are called Na, Ca or K channels. This selectivity is essential for their specific physiological function. Selectivity is usually measured in a relative sense and P_{Na}/P_K for Na channels are ~50-100:1. P_K/P_{Na} varies for different K channels, but are also in a similar range (Hille, 1992). Other channels (e.g. I_f) show little discrimination among monovalent cations. Ca channels do not discriminate very well among Ca, Ba and Sr, but P_{Ca}/P_K and P_{Ca}/P_{Na} are ~1000 and 3000 (see Table 17; Hess *et al.*, 1986; Tsien *et al.*, 1987). The channels gain selectivity because of binding sites in the pore formed by the 4 P-loops coordinately binding one type of ion preferentially. For K channels a signature 'GYG' sequence in the P loop seems to be essential. For Ca channels a ring of four negatively charged amino acids (one glutamate from the P-loop of each domain) forms the Ca-selective site (see Fig 53; Kim *et al.*, 1993; Yang *et al.*, 1993). Na channels are similar to Ca channels except that the analogous positions in domains III and IV are lysine and alanine rather than glutamate. Heinemann *et al.* (1992) replaced either one or both of these amino acids in the Na channel with glutamate and the resulting channel showed a remarkable shift in selectivity toward that of a Ca channel (including block by μM Ca). Thus, the P-loops dictate the channel selectivity and probably do so by creating selective binding sites with appropriate chemical coordination. These issues will be discussed more explicitly for Ca channels in Chapter 5. Ion channels can pass ~10^6 ions/sec and one may wonder how they can attain such high throughput if ions bind with high affinity in the pore. One answer to this is that many channels have multiple binding sites, such that a second charged ion entering the region can help propel the first ion through the channel by electrostatic repulsion (i.e. destabilizing its binding; see Chapter 5).

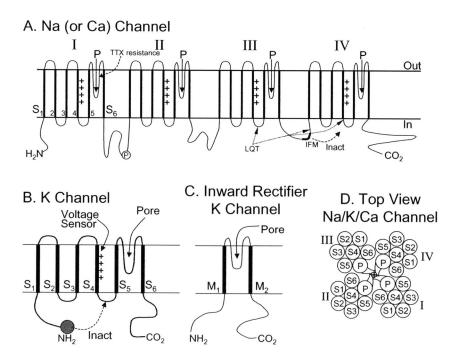

Figure 38. Overall structure of some ion channels. **A**. The Na channel has four domains (I-IV) each of which has 6 homologous repeating transmembrane regions (S_1-S_6) and a pore loop (P). Repeating positively charged gating region in S_4 is indicated by +. Other noted sites are 1) the site responsible for low cardiac TTX sensitivity (and high Cd sensitivity) compared to neuronal or skeletal muscle Na channels, 2) PKA phosphorylation site (P), 3) site implicated in inactivation gate (IFM) and 4) sites mutated in congenital long QT syndromes (LQT). The Ca channel has a similar topology (see Fig 51 Chapter 5). **B**. E_m-dependent K channels have similar overall structure, but 4 monomers (of S_1-S_6) are required to form the channel. N-type inactivation domain and receptor region are indicated. **C**. The M_1-P-M_2 region in inward rectifier K channels is analogous to just the S_5-P-S_6 region of E_m-dependent K channels. **D**. A top view of an E_m-dependent channel showing a likely organization of transmembrane regions around the pore (+ indicates K ion in the selectivity filter; based on Durell *et al.*, 1998).

CHANNEL GATING

Ion channels can be activated and inactivated by changes in E_m (e.g. depolarization or hyperpolarization), binding of ligands (e.g. acetylcholine, ATP) or mechanical deformation (e.g. cell swelling). At the single channel level, the opening and closing transitions of most channels are very abrupt ($\ll$ 1 ms), so that current through a channel changes in a square or seemingly instantaneous manner between open and closed states (see Fig 40A). At the whole cell level one measures a current which is the ensemble of all of the individual channel events and thus a smoother function. This represents the average behavior of all Na channels and reflects statistical or stochastic differences in latencies of opening, closing and reopening of individual channels. Table 14 lists many of the most important cardiac ion channels, categorized by their type of gating. At this point it is fair to say that we know the most about voltage-gated ion channels in the heart, somewhat less about ligand-gated channels and least about mechano-sensitive channels. Thus our appreciation of the different channels and their importance is still evolving. Before discussing each individual channel it is useful to consider some general aspects of channel gating, focused here on voltage-dependent channels.

E_m-dependent Activation

Most E_m-dependent channels are activated by depolarization, and this implies that there is part of the channel which moves in response to a change in E_m. The S_4 region has been a prime candidate since Noda *et al.* (1984) noted the repeating positive charge motif in the first cloned Na channel.   Depolarization would tend to move these charges outward across the membrane electrical field, and this charge movement can be measured (Fig 40A) as a non-linear component of capacitative current (Armstrong & Bezanilla, 1973). A key feature of such gating current is that the total 'on-charge' which moves upon depolarization (outward current) must be equal to the 'off-charge' moved upon repolarization (inward current). A complication in this point is that some charge can become immobilized (or inactivated) and recover on a much slower time frame, making it difficult to measure experimentally (when compared to the large phasic component as depicted in Fig 40A) . It should be noted that one usually has to block all ionic currents across the membrane, in order to reliably detect gating currents (which are charge movements confined within the membrane).   Moreover, it is particularly difficult to measure gating current attributable to a specific channel in cardiac myocytes because there are so many channels with overlapping activation ranges (see Fig 40C).

The amount of charge moved per channel can be estimated in two ways. First, one can measure the number of channels by either ligand binding experiments (e.g. ^{3}H-STX binding) or by measuring whole cell current, divided by the single channel current and open probability measured under the same conditions ($N=I_x/(i_x \times P_o)$). Then the number of charges per channel is a simple quotient. The steepness of the E_m-dependence of conductance (current activation curves) can also provide an estimate of charges moved per channel (but only the initial part or limiting slope should be used; Hille, 1992). A steeper slope implies more charges/ channel. Activation curves as in Fig 40 are normally described by a Boltzmann relation ($1/\{1+ \exp((E_{0.5} - E_m)/S)\}$) where $E_{0.5}$ is the E_m for half-maximal activation and S is a slope factor (RT/zF), which gives the slope in e-fold per S mV. Since RT/F is 25-26 mV, an S value of 4 would correspond to 6 charges moved across the membrane field. This is typical of many experimental estimates for different channels. Values as high as 12-15 charges per channel (or 2.7-fold change in current in 2 mV) have been reported for Na, Ca and K channels (Schoppa *et al.*, 1992; Hirschberg *et al.*, 1995; Noceti *et al.*, 1996). This could be due to 12 charges moving all the way through the membrane electric field or 24 charges moving halfway etc. With ≥ 4 positive charges on each S_4 region, there are >16 of these candidate charges in E_m-dependent channels. Indeed, mutations in the S_4 which neutralize or reverse charges produce reductions in charge movement consistent with this idea (Aggarwal & MacKinnon, 1996).

The physical charge movement was initially considered to be a vertical outward translation of S_4 domains in Fig 38. However, more recent data suggests that the S_4 may be tilted and also interacts with amino acids on S_2 and S_3 (Papazian *et al.*, 1995; Tiwari-Woodruff *et al.*, 1997; Durell *et al.*, 1998). The cartoon in Fig 39B shows how a modest degree of rotation of S_4 along S_2 may effectively move several positive charges from inside to outside, without dramatic vertical movement (Yang *et al.*, 1996; Yellen, 1998). It is less clear how the gating charge

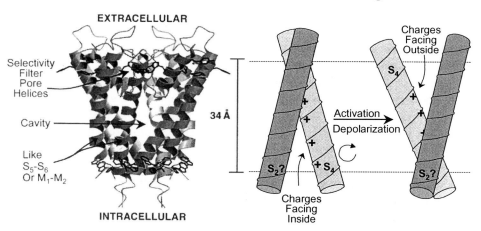

A. K Channel Structure   **B. Possible Gating Movement**

Figure 39. Channel crystal structure and possible gating movement. **A.** Structure of the bacterial Ksca channel which is analogous to inward rectifier K channels in heart (Doyle *et al.*, 1998). Four M_1-P-M_2 regions form a narrow selectivity filter, internal aqueous cavity and inner narrowing which may be the activation gate (reproduced from Doyle *et al.*, 1998, with permission). **B.** Possible mechanism of charge movement in E_m-dependent channels (note that the K channel in A does not have S_1-S_4 regions). Rather than moving vertically through the membrane field, the charged S_4 domains may rotate with respect to other helices (e.g. S_2) to effectively move the charges from inside to outside during gating charge movement (based closely on a figure by Yellen, 1998).

movement physically couples to the channel activation gate on S_6 at the inner mouth. Presumably this S_2-S_4 movement causes movement of the S_5-S_6 to allow opening of the channel.

Figure 40B shows the E_m-dependence of charge movement and current activation. It is clear that charge movement occurs at significantly more negative E_m values, and this is seen for most channels. This is consistent with the channel having one or more E_m-dependent transitions prior to the channel opening step. Indeed, most state models of channel gating suggest that the final closed to open transition is not intrinsically E_m-dependent, and all of the E_m-dependence comes from transitions between closed states leading up to the opening step. This also makes physical sense if the S_4 (& S_2) bears the intrinsic E_m-dependence and this simply increases the likelihood that the S_6 (& S_5) will flip to the open state.

Figure 40C shows the E_m-dependence of activation of several cardiac ion channels. These channels all have relatively fast activation and it can be appreciated that with depolarization one would progressively activate I_{Na}, $I_{Ca,T}$, $I_{Ca,L}$ and I_{to}. Of course the activation kinetics are not identical and the impact of individual currents also depends on the overall conductance and the driving force ($E_m - E_x$). The nature of these interactions will be discussed below.

Channel Inactivation

All E_m-dependent channels exhibit deactivation, which is simply the reverse of activation and would be in principle described by the same steady state activation curves as in Fig 40C. Many E_m-dependent channels also exhibit *inactivation*, which is a separate process from activation and this is an important semantic distinction. Inactivation of I_{Na} is illustrated in Fig 40A by the reduction in current amplitude under sustained depolarization. Inactivation rate is generally found to be E_m-dependent, getting faster with stronger depolarization. However, for Na and some other channels, inactivation is not intrinsically very E_m-dependent. The apparent E_m-dependence of inactivation derives from the strong E_m-dependence of activation and the property that the channel readily undergoes inactivation only from the activated state (Patlak, 1991). Thus these processes are linked, but the linkage can be broken. Proteolytic enzymes applied intracellularly or truncation/mutation of intracellular loops can remove inactivation (Armstrong *et al.*, 1973; Hoshi *et al.*, 1990; McDonald *et al.*, 1994; Stümer *et al.*, 1989; West *et al.*, 1992). Based on their early work Armstrong & Bezanilla (1977) proposed that inactivation was mediated by a 'ball-and-chain' mechanism (see Fig 38B). Elegant confirmation of this hypothesis comes from molecular studies with *Shaker* K channels (Hoshi *et al.*, 1990; Zagotta *et al.*, 1990) which are related to I_{to} in heart. They found that removal of the 46 N-terminal amino acids (the ball) could prevent inactivation, and that this mutant channel could still be inactivated by exogenous ball-peptide dialyzed into the cell from a patch pipette. This latter observation is also important in showing that the process of inactivation depends on activation. That is, the ball-peptide did not produce inactivation of channels until they were activated (but then it was almost normal), implying that the activation process must present a target for the inactivation ball. Isacoff *et al.* (1991) demonstrated that the ball binds to the S_4-S_5 region to block the channel. MacKinnon *et al.* (1993) also showed that the length of the chain connecting to the ball dictates the speed of inactivation (shorter chain, faster inactivation) and also that binding of one ball from one K channel subunit was sufficient to block the tetrameric K channel. The key portion of the ball (20 amino acids) has 11 hydrophobic and 4 positively charged amino acids, and both characteristics are probably functionally important. Notably, more positive charge hastens inactivation (Murell-Lagnado & Aldrich, 1993) and this may confer some E_m-dependence to inactivation or recovery therefrom.

This mode of channel inactivation is referred to as N-type inactivation. Inactivation of some components of I_{to} in heart almost surely works this way (e.g. Kv1.4). There are also several variations on this ball-and-chain scheme of inactivation. In some K channels a β channel subunit appears to provide the ball (Rettig *et al.*, 1994; Morales *et al.*, 1995) and in the Na channel it appears to be more of a hinged lid formed by the intracellular loop between domain III and IV, containing a critical 'IFM' sequence (Ile, Phe, Met; Fig 38A, West *et al.*, 1992). There is also a second general type of inactivation referred to as C-type, which again comes from work with *Shaker* K channels (Hoshi *et al.*, 1990, 1991). This type of inactivation appears to be due to a constriction in the P-loop region of the pore and is linked to activation, but is generally a much slower process than N-type inactivation, taking seconds, rather than msec (Yellen, 1998). The rapid inactivation of cardiac I_{Kr} (HERG) appears to be an unusually fast variant of C-type inactivation (Smith *et al.*, 1996). Ca channels also show Ca-dependent inactivation which will be discussed in Chapter 5 (see pg 116-119 & 122).

Once activated and inactivated, membrane repolarization is required for the channels to recovery from inactivation. The rate of recovery from inactivation also depends on how negative the E_m is (faster at more negative E_m). Figure 40B shows a Na channel availability curve (sometimes referred to as a steady state inactivation curve). This is measured by holding E_m at

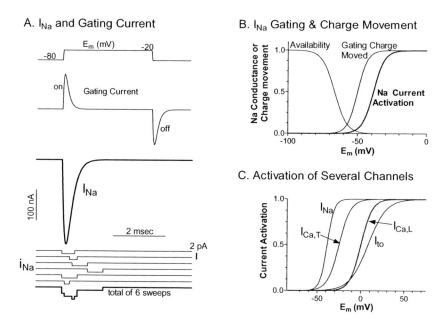

Figure 40. E_m-dependent gating of ion channels. **A**. Schematic diagram illustrating outward gating charge movement upon depolarization, activation & inactivation of whole cell I_{Na} and 6 simulated single channel sweeps (with their total, ensemble current). **B**. Steady state E_m-dependence of I_{Na} activation, gating charge movement and inactivation (or availability). **C**. E_m-dependence of current activation in several cardiac channel types.

different values to allow a state steady state condition and then depolarizing to test what fraction of channels are available for activation. As E_m becomes more positive Na channel availability decreases. Thus if diastolic E_m is more positive (e.g. due to membrane leak) fewer Na channels are available and the rate of rise of the AP and the rate of propagation will be decreased.

I_{Na} activation and inactivation (or availability) curves in Fig 40B overlap such that there is almost no availability when E_m is held at values where activation is appreciable. This ensures that activated Na channels inactivate nearly completely whenever activated by depolarization. However, at about –52 mV there is a very small window where both channel availability and activation are ~3.5%. This would produce a steady state "window current" with a conductance of about 0.1% of maximum. Given the large I_{Na} in heart cells, small shifts in the activation and inactivation properties could result in substantial sustained Na influx via window I_{Na} at relatively negative E_m. This same type of window current exists in Ca channels (especially from –25 to +5 mV for $I_{Ca,L}$) and also in K channels. For I_{Kr} where inactivation is fast compared to activation, most of the I_{Kr} during the AP is this type of window current (see Fig 41C-D).).

Na CHANNELS

The first channel cloned was the Na channel from the elctrical organ of electric eel (Noda *et al.*, 1984). The cardiac Na channel (Rogart *et al.*,1989; Gellens *et al.*, 1992) and brain and skeletal muscle channels are highly homologous. There are also β subunits associated with Na channels, but it is somewhat controversial how these alter cardiac I_{Na} (Roden & George,

1997). The cardiac Na channel is much less sensitive to block by tetrodotoxin (TTX) and more sensitive to Cd block than other Na channels. This has been attributed to a specific cysteine (373) in the P-loop of domain I in heart *vs.* Phe or Tyr in other Na channels (Backx *et al.*, 1992; Heinemann *et al.*, 1992; Satin *et al.*, 1992a). One must use >10 μM TTX to block cardiac I_{Na}, *vs.* 10-50 nM for neuronal I_{Na}. Cardiac I_{Na} can also be blocked by type 1 antiarrhythmic agents (e.g. 1A: quinidine, procainamide; 1B lidocaine, dilantin, mexiletine; 1C flecanide, encainide, propafenone, which prolong, shorten or don't change APD respectively). Some of these bind to the S_6 region of domain IV (Ragsdale *et al.*, 1994). Most of these agents also exhibit E_m- or use-dependent block, meaning that they interact more strongly with open or inactivated channels. This produces cumulative block of I_{Na} at high frequency. They thus block I_{Na} more effectively during tachycardia and in depolarized tissue, conditions which can be pro-arrhythmic.

The function of Na channels is to generate a large and very brief inward I_{Na} and cause the rapid upstroke of the AP. This is accomplished by very brief channel openings with very short latency, normally without reopenings (e.g. Fig 40A). That is, the channel inactivates quickly into an absorbing state, requiring recovery at negative E_m. However, cardiac Na channels can also exhibit some persistent late openings (Saint *et al.*, 1992; Zilberter *et al.*, 1994) and this may contribute to a background Na leak current. An ultraslow component of I_{Na} inactivation (τ =600 ms) has also been reported in heart (Maltsev *et al.*, 1998) which could contribute to EADs. Hypoxia and lysophospholipids also cause persistent Na channel openings even at very negative E_m (Undrovinas *et al.*, 1992; Jue *et al.*, 1996).

A human congenital mutation (deletion of 3 amino acids, KPQ) in the cardiac Na channel very close to the IFM region in the III-IV loop which is crucial in inactivation) results in the long QT syndrome (Fig 38A; Bennett *et al.*, 1995). This is characterized by long ventricular APD and may predispose these individuals to arrhythmias. The mutation does not greatly alter macroscopic I_{Na}, but late bursting openings are seen at the single channel level, which could cause the APD prolongation. Two other congenital long QT mutations in the Na channel gene are in the S_4-S_5 linker region in domains III and IV and produce similar I_{Na} effects (Wang *et al.*, 1995a, 1996a; Dumaine *et al.*, 1996). This site is analogous to the ball-receptor region involved in N-type inactivation in K channels, as discussed above. The peak I_{Na} is very large (>1 nA/pF) and even minor problems in inactivation can have significant electrophysiological consequences. The amount of Na which enters the cell via I_{Na} is only 15 μM or so, but this is because I_{Na} is normally so brief (Fig 45). If inactivation were only 99.5% complete, such that 0.5% of peak I_{Na} flowed for most of the APD, this would easily double the amount of Na influx. This would increase the burden on the Na/K-ATPase to extrude Na, but could also perturb Ca balance via the Na/Ca exchange.

In the absence of [Na]$_o$ some Na channels can allow TTX-sensitive Ca influx (Cole *et al.*, 1997; Aggarwal *et al.*, 1997), but the amount of Ca current is several hundred times smaller than for Na. The selectivity of cardiac Na channels for Na relative to Ca (P_{Na}/P_{Ca}) is >3000 (Nilius, 1988), such that it not clear how much Ca influx might occur under physiological conditions. Santana *et al.* (1998; Cruz *et al.*, 1999) showed evidence that isoproterenol and digitalis glycosides cause cardiac Na channels to increase their Ca permeability such that P_{Na}/P_{Ca} approaches 1. This was based on shifts in reversal potential and also on the ability of a TTX-sensitive current to activate SR Ca release. This provocative effect, which was dubbed 'slip

Table 14

Cardiac Ion Channels

Current	Candidate Gene	Acti-vation	Inacti-vation	Role in AP	Subunits?	Blockers
Voltage gated Channels						
I_{Na}	SCN5A	VVF	VF	Rapid Depol.	β	TTX,STX
$I_{Ca,L}$	α_{1C}, α_{1D}	VF	M	Depol & Plat	$\alpha_2\delta$, β	DHP, ΦAA
$I_{Ca,T}$	α_{1G}, α_{1H}	VF	F	Depol-PMK	β	Mibefradil, Ni
$I_{to,fast}$	Kv4.2, 4.3	VF	F	Early Repol	β	4-AP, 2,3-DAP
$I_{to,slow}$	Kv1.4	VF	M	Early Repol	β	4-AP, 2,3-DAP
I_{Kr}	HERG	M	VF	Plat-Repol	MirP1	Dofetilide, E-4031
I_{Ks}	KvLQT1	VS	x	Plat-Repol	MinK	Chromanol 293
I_{Kur}	Kv1.5	F	x	Plat-Repol		μM 4-AP
I_{Kp}	Kv1.5?	F	x	Plat-Repol		Ba
$I_{K,slow}$	Kv1.2	F	VS	Plat-Repol		TEA
I_{K1}	Kir2.1 (IRK1)	VF	x	Rest E_m		Ba
I_f	HCN2, HCN4	MS	x	PMK		
Ligand Gated Channels						
$I_{K(ACh)}$	Kir 3.1:3.4	ACh		$\downarrow$ PMK		
$I_{K(ATP)}$	Kir6.2	Pinacidil		$\downarrow$APD & PMK	SUR	Glibenclamide
$I_{Cl(Ca)}$	?	$[Ca]_i$		Early Repol		DIDS,niflumate
$I_{Cl(cAMP)}$	CFTR	cAMP		$\uparrow$Repol.		9-AC, DNDS
Mechanosensitive Channels						
$I_{Cl(Swell)}$	ClC-3	Swelling		$\downarrow$APD?		Gd, DIDS
$I_{NS(stretch)}$	?	Stretch		PMK?		Gd

Abbreviations: F=fast, S=slow, M=moderate, V=very and x=none. Depol=depolarization, Repol= repolarization, Plat= plateau, PMK= pacemaker, TTX = tetrodotoxin, STX= saxitoxin, DHP= dihydropyridine, ΦAA=phenylalkylamine, TEA= tetraethylammonium, 4-AP= 4-aminopyridine, 2,3-DAP = 2,3-diamino-pyridine, DIDS= 4,4′-diisothiocyanatostilbene - 2,2′-disulphonic acid, DNDS= 4,4′-dinitrostilbene-2,2′-disulphonic acid, 9-AC= 9-aminoacridine, ACh= acetylcholine. The nomenclature for E_m-dependent K channels (Kv) is based on homology to Drosophila gene families referred to as *Shaker, Shab, Shaw* and *Shal* for Kv1.x, Kv2.x, Kv3.x and Kv4.x (Jan & Jan, 1992; Pongs, 1992).

mode conductance' has been challenged (Nuss & Marbán, 1999; Balke *et al.*, 1999) and remains controversial at present.

Na channels are modulated by cAMP-dependent protein kinase (PKA) and PKC (Cukierman, 1996). The site of phosphorylation is in the loop between domain I and II and results in an increase of I_{Na} (Murphy *et al.*, 1993; Catterrall, 1995). However, phosphorylation results in a shift of activation and availability to more negative E_m, such that fewer Na channels may be available for contribution to the AP. Activation of several receptors (e.g. muscarinic, α-adrenergic, angiotensin II, and purinergic) can stimulate PKC activity and this can also modulate I_{Na}, but the net effect on I_{Na} may depend on the specific method of activation (Ono *et al.*, 1993; Cukierman, 1996).

Na channels require repolarization to recover from inactivation before another ventricular AP can occur. The same is true for Ca channels which initiate APs in pacemaker cells. Otherwise the cell is refractory to another electrical excitation. Recovery of I_{Na} requires that the membrane be repolarized to near the diastolic level for a finite period of time ($\tau \sim$ 10 ms at −100 mV, 30 ms at −80 mV or 100 ms at −72 mV) before the cell is able to fire another AP. Thus Na channels don't recover very rapidly until repolarization is nearly complete. In this way the long AP contributes to limiting the ability of the cell to respond to an early depolarization. Ca channels have the same property (but with longer recovery times, Fig 57) and are crucial in recovery from refractoriness in SA and AV node cells

Ca CHANNELS

There are two types of Ca channels in cardiac myocytes (T- and L-type). These will be the subject of much more detailed discussion in Chapter 5 and will only be discussed briefly here. $I_{Ca,L}$ is the dominant I_{Ca} and is in all myocytes. $I_{Ca,T}$ is not detectable in most ventricular myocytes, but is present to a variable extent in atrial and conduction cells (e.g. Purkinje fibers). Both $I_{Ca,L}$ and $I_{Ca,T}$ activate rapidly upon depolarization (though not as fast as I_{Na}) and both show inactivation (again, not as fast as I_{Na}). $I_{Ca,T}$ activates at more negative E_m and inactivates more rapidly than $I_{Ca,L}$ (Fig 40C). $I_{Ca,T}$ thus contributes only to the early phases of the AP. There is some evidence to suggest that $I_{Ca,T}$ can contribute to the late pacemaker depolarization seen in some cells (Hagiwara *et al.*, 1988; Zhou & Lipsius, 1994).

$I_{Ca,L}$ inactivation is slower than $I_{Ca,T}$ and is both E_m- and Ca-dependent. The intrinsic E_m-dependent inactivation is relatively slow, so that with Ca influx and SR Ca release most of the inactivation is Ca-dependent (see Chapter 5, pg 116-119). Indeed, with larger amplitude Ca transients and I_{Ca} the inactivation is greatly accelerated. This creates a negative feedback, such that when Ca entry and release are large, less total Ca entry occurs during the AP (Puglisi *et al.*, 1999). $I_{Ca,L}$ contributes inward depolarizing current to the cardiac AP. It may not contribute much to the very rapid rising AP phase in myocytes (dictated by I_{Na}), but is the key depolarizing current responsible for the slower rising AP in SA and AV node cells. $I_{Ca,L}$ is also sustained during the plateau phase of the AP and is the primary inward current at this time that must be counterbalanced by K currents. I_{Ca} is also stimulated by PKA, which increases both amplitude and inactivation rate. Many of these points will be expanded upon in Chapter 5.

K CHANNELS

K channels in cardiac myocytes are the most diverse group and they serve numerous important functions, but of course they all produce outward current at physiological E_m values and tend to drive E_m toward E_K (Fig 36C). They are structurally grouped into two classes (Fig 38B-C, Table 14). E_m-gated K channels resemble Na and Ca channels and are activated by depolarization. Some of these show inactivation and some do not (Table 14). The second group, inward rectifiers, are generally ligand-gated and have fewer transmembrane spans (Fig 38C).

K Channel Rectification

Inward rectification means that the channel conducts inward current better than outward current. Figure 41A shows that without rectification K current would be a linear function of E_m with a reversal potential at E_K. That is, the slope or conductance (g_K) would be constant. With weak inward rectification (as shown for $I_{K(ATP)}$) the outward current at $E_m > E_K$ is less than expected. For strong inward rectification (as for I_{K1}), outward current can be completely blocked at more positive E_m. This inward rectification can be largely explained by open channel block of outward current by intracellular Mg and polyamines, such as spermine and spermidine (Vandenberg, 1987; Mazzanti & DiFrancesco, 1989; Lopatin *et al.*, 1994; Fickler *et al.*, 1994). That is, when outward current is favored ($E_m > E_K$) these positively charged species are driven into the channel and prevent K from flowing out. For I_{K1} the concentrations of Mg and polyamines required for 50% block are μM and nM respectively, and normal $[Mg]_i$ and $[polyamine]_i$ are 0.1-1 mM. This accounts for the strong inward rectification in this channel. Negatively charged amino acids in the M_2 and carboxy tail appear critical for Mg and polyamine block (Yang *et al.*, 1995). After steps to more negative E_m, inward I_{K1} shows an initial peak and slow decline, which may also be due to block of inward I_{K1} mainly by extracellular Na (Biermans *et al.*, 1987).

Inward rectification of K channels in heart is functionally important, both in a permissive sense for the long plateau phase of the AP, and also in limiting cellular K loss during activity (which would have to be re-accumulated by the Na/K-ATPase). If K conductance did not decrease during the AP there would be a huge outward K current at positive E_m due to the large electrochemical driving force (consider the extrapolation of the "no rectification" line in Fig 41A to positive E_m). Thus, inward rectification allows a stable AP plateau with relatively small and balanced inward and outward currents.

Some E_m-dependent K channels exhibit outward or delayed rectification (e.g. see I_{Ks} in Fig 41A), characterized by an increasingly positive slope at more positive E_m. This increasing slope upon depolarization constitutes apparent outward rectification. However, this conductance increase is attributable to the E_m-dependent gating of the channels rather than an intrinsic permeation property. That is, the conductance increases with depolarization because more channels are open, not because individual channels really exhibit rectification. It is referred to as delayed rectification because these channels take a finite time to be activated (e.g. I_{Ks} activation is very slow). Some K channels also exhibit negative slope regions at positive potentials due to inactivation (see I_{Kr} in Fig 41C). While the term is somewhat imprecise, these E_m-dependent K channels (I_{Kr}, I_{Ks} & I_{Kur}) are referred to as outward or delayed rectifier channels.

I_{K1} Stabilizes the Resting E_m

I_{K1} is the resting or background K channel responsible for stabilizing the resting E_m near E_K. This current is thought to be carried by the Kir2.1 (IRK1, or other Kir2.x) channel protein (Kubo *et al.*, 1993). Figure 41B shows I_{K1} on an expanded scale. Conductance (g_{K1}, slope of the curve) is very high around the resting E_m and as such I_{K1} tends to bring small depolarizing or hyperpolarizing influences back to rest. As Na channels are activated to bring E_m near threshold, g_{K1} declines allowing the positive feedback associated with the upstroke of the AP to occur. Increasing $[K]_o$ (hyperkalemia) depolarizes E_m due to a change in E_K, and also increases g_{K1} (as the square root of $[K]_o$). While this moves the resting E_m closer to a threshold for triggering an AP, two factors cause hyperkalemia to actually reduce excitability. First, the increase in g_{K1} means that more inward I_{Na} would be required to overcome the I_{K1} which tends to keep E_m near E_K. Second the depolarized E_m reduces the number of Na channels available by increasing the fraction in the inactivated state (Fig 40B). This reduces the amount of I_{Na} that can be mustered to cause depolarization in the face of increased g_{K1}. Conversely, hypokalemia causes increased excitability, but the hyperpolarization is less than expected based on the change of E_K (since g_K is reduced, allowing other currents to move E_m further away from E_K).

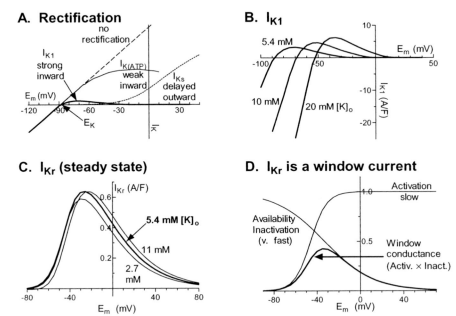

Figure 41. K channel E_m-dependence and rectification. **A.** A non-rectifying channel (dashed line) should have an ohmic conductance (constant slope I-V curve, in symmetrical solutions) reversing at E_K. Weak and strong inwardly rectifying current ($I_{K(ATP)}$ & I_{K1} respectively) show a gradual decline in slope at more positive E_m and may have a negative slope region. I_{Ks} exhibits outward rectification and is also time dependent in activation (delayed). Currents are normalized in this panel. **B.** Raising $[K]_o$ makes E_K more positive and increases conductance of I_{K1} and I_{Kr} (C). **C.** E_m-dependence of I_{Kr} at different $[K]_o$. **D.** Very rapid inactivation dictates I_{Kr} availability, so maximal conductance is proportional to the product of fractional activation and fractional inactivation.

I_{K1} density is generally very low in pacemaker cells and I_{K1} may be absent in SA node cells (Irisawa *et al.*, 1993). I_{K1} is also lower in Purkinje fibers than in ventricular myocytes (Cordeiro *et al.*, 1998). This facilitates the pacemaker induced APs in these cells. This is because there is less outward I_{K1} to be overcome by I_{Na} or I_{Ca}, to cause the regenerative AP depolarization. Indeed, these cells have much lower resting conductance (and capacitance since they lack T-tubules). Thus a small inward pacemaker current can produce a large depolarization. The low I_{K1} also explains the more positive resting E_m in these cells (further away from E_K).

I_{K1} also participates in the final stages of E_m repolarization during the AP as the E_m range is reached where channels are not blocked (see Fig 45). Based on the strong inward rectification, I_{K1} has minimal involvement during the peak and plateau phases of the AP (despite the high driving force for K efflux). This channel does not seem to be strongly modulated by PKA.

Transient Outward Current (I_{to})

Transient outward K current (sometimes called I_{to1}) as well as a Ca-activated Cl current (or I_{to2}, see below) contribute to the early repolarization phase of the AP. These K channels are E_m-dependent and exhibit rapid activation and inactivation. There appear to be two main components, one that inactivates faster than the other ($I_{to,fast}$ and $I_{to,slow}$; Nerbonne, 2000, 2001). $I_{to,fast}$ is mediated by Kv4.2 and/or Kv4.3, while $I_{to,slow}$ is attributable to Kv1.4 (Xu *et al.*, 1999a;

Bou Abboud & Nerbonne, 1999). These two currents both activate rapidly ($\tau \leq 5$ msec), but $I_{to,fast}$ inactivates with $\tau \sim 100$ msec *vs.* 200 msec for $I_{to,slow}$. Even more striking is the difference in recovery from inactivation ($\tau = 30\text{-}50$ msec for $I_{to,fast}$ *vs.* 1 sec for $I_{to,slow}$). This very slow recovery of $I_{to,slow}$ would limit its contribution to the AP, especially at higher frequencies (due to accumulating inactivation). Most mammalian myocytes exhibit $I_{to,fast}$. Guinea-pig ventricle appears to lack appreciable I_{to} of either sort, and rabbit ventricular I_{to} is more like $I_{to,slow}$ and Kv1.4 (Fedida & Giles, 1991; Wang *et al.*, 1999; Nerbonne, 2000, 2001). Slow recovery of I_{to} in rabbit limits the amount of APD shortening which occurs upon increasing frequency (due to accumulation of inactivated channels). Both $I_{to,fast}$ and $I_{to,slow}$ are blocked by mM 4-aminopyridine, but only $I_{to,fast}$ is sensitive to *Heteropodatoxins-2* and *-3* (Xu *et al.*, 1999a). PKC appears to attenuate $I_{to,fast}$ and Kv 4.2 (Apkon & Nerbonne, 1988; Nakamura *et al.*, 1997) and can also depress Kv1.4 induced currents in *Xenopus* oocytes (Murray *et al.*, 1994). CaMKII phosphorylation of Kv1.4 slows inactivation, but accelerates recovery (Roeper *et al.*, 1997).

There is also a transmural gradient of higher I_{to} amplitude with faster inactivation and recovery from inactivation in epicardial *vs.* endocardial cells in ferret and human ventricle (Näbauer *et al.*, 1996; Brahmajothi *et al.*, 1999). There is also 5-6 times more $I_{to,fast}$ in canine epicardium *vs.* endocardium (Liu *et al.*, 1993), consistent with the more rapid repolarization and shorter APD in epicardial cells (Fig 35). In mouse, there is $I_{to,slow}$ in the septum but not in the left ventricular apex (Xu *et al.*, 1999a). It is possible that in ventricular muscle which is under more mechanical stress, Kv4.2/3 (& $I_{to,fast}$) expression is lower, while Kv1.4 (& $I_{to,slow}$) is upregulated. This would be consistent with the reduction of I_{to} which is a common finding in ventricular hypertrophy and heart failure (Bénitah *et al.*, 1993; Beuckelmann *et al.*, 1993; Tomita *et al.*, 1994; Näbauer & Kääb, 1998). Lower I_{to} could also contribute to the AP prolongation typical of hypertrophy and heart failure. There is also a developmental increase in I_{to} as well as altered isoform expression. Neonatal rat ventricle shows more of an $I_{to,slow}$ phenotype which shifts to $I_{to,fast}$ in adult (Wickenden *et al.*, 1997). In rabbits as the density of I_{to} expressed increases developmentally the reverse shift occurs from $I_{to,fast}$ to $I_{to,slow}$ (Sánchez-Chapula *et al.*, 1994).

Delayed Rectifier K currents

There are at least three key delayed rectifier K channels in heart, I_{Kr}, I_{Ks} and I_{Kur} (for rapid, slow and ultra-rapid). Sanguinetti & Jurkiewicz (1990, 1991) first distinguished two different components of delayed rectifier K current in guinea-pig based on sensitivity to class III antiarrhythmic drugs. I_{Kr} is blocked by dofetilide, E-4031, almokalant and sotalol, while I_{Ks} is sensitive to clofilium, NE-10064, NE-10133, L-768,673 and HMR-1556 (Cameliet, 1993; Busch *et al.*, 1994; Lerche *et al.*, 2000; Xu *et al.*, 2001). Both currents are present in many cardiac cells types, including human ventricle with varying ratios (Beuckelmann *et al.*, 1993; Konarzewska *et al.*, 1995; Salata *et al.*, 1996). Some myocytes show only I_{Ks} (guinea-pig node, Anumonwo *et al.*, 1992), while others show only I_{Kr} (cat & rat ventricular cells, Follmer & Colatsky, 1990; Pond *et al.*, 2000). An even faster component called I_{Kur} was described in human and rat atrium (Boyle & Nerbonne, 1991; Wang *et al.*, 1993a) and a similar current (I_{Kp} for plateau) was described in ventricular myocytes (Backx & Marbán, 1993). I_{Kur} and I_{Kp} may be the same current (Nerbonne, 2000, 2001) and will be considered such here. These channels are highly selective for K, but their selectivity (P_K/P_{Na}) is not as high as for I_{K1}, and consequently the E_{rev} is slightly more positive than E_K (Carmeliet, 1999).

I_{Kr} (HERG). Sanguinetti *et al.* (1995, 1996a) and Trudeau *et al.* (1995) showed that I_{Kr} is mediated by a K channel related to the mutant *Drosophila* gene *ether-à-go-go* (eag), called human eag-related gene (or HERG). They also showed that mutations in HERG, which inhibit I_{Kr} in a dominant negative manner, are responsible for congenital long Q-T syndrome (LQT2), a reflection of increased ventricular APD. So, I_{Kr} is involved in ventricular repolarization. The ventricular AP prolongation in long Q-T syndromes can lead to the clinical ECG observation *torsades de pointes* (literally, turning of the points) and can reflect a cardiac substrate with increased arrhythmogenic potential.

I_{Kr} activates slowly, but inactivates extremely rapidly. This is unusual behavior in that inactivation is relatively divorced from, and faster than activation. It may be a consequence of a very fast variant of C-type *vs.* N-type inactivation (as mentioned above). The result is that the I-V curve for I_{Kr} in Fig 41C is bell-shaped. Here the negative slope is due to inactivation at positive E_m, which creates unavailability of channels which would otherwise be activated at those E_m (i.e. this is not true inward rectification with respect to permeation). In this sense the I_{Kr} is highly analogous to a window current (see Figs 40B & 41C-D). Once activation reaches a steady state (τ ~50 msec at $E_m = 0$ mV) I_{Kr} does not decline with time, so the time course doesn't look like classic inactivation, as in I_{Na} or I_{to}.

Single channel conductance of I_{Kr} is ~13 pS (Veldkamp *et al.*, 1993). I_{Kr} amplitude is increased by higher [K]$_o$ (like I_{K1}; as the square root of [K]$_o$, see Fig 41C). This is not expected thermodynamically, since raising [K]$_o$ would reduce the chemical driving force on K flux through the channel. It must reflect allosteric regulation by [K]$_o$. While HERG is sufficient to produce I_{Kr}, the current is modulated by MirP1 (minK related peptide 1, where minK is considered an important subunit of I_{Ks} (see below).

I_{Ks} (KvLQT1 + minK). I_{Ks} is a very slowly activating current which does not show appreciable inactivation. The gene coding I_{Ks} was identified from positional cloning studies that identified mutations in the most common congenital form of long Q-T syndrome (LQT1; Wang *et al.*, 1996b). Expression of both KvLQT1 and minK (like a β-subunit) is essential to fully recapitulate cardiac I_{Ks} (Barhanin *et al.*, 1996; Sanguinetti *et al.*, 1996b). KvLQT1 has the usual topology for E_m-dependent K channels (Fig 38B) and minK is a 130 amino acid protein with a single transmembrane domain, and was an early candidate gene by itself for I_{Ks}.

I_{Ks} activates very slowly, over several seconds under sustained depolarization (τ ~400 msec at $E_m = 0$ mV). Thus activation is never complete during an AP. I_{Ks} activation also exhibits remarkably shallow E_m-dependence (Fig 41A) with a midpoint near 0 mV and e-fold increase for 15 mV (*vs.* 2-4 mV for I_{Na}). Given the major fundamental differences between I_{Kr} and I_{Ks} it is rather surprising that the outward current carried by these channels looks similar superficially during the AP (Fig 45). This results from very slow activation of I_{Ks} and the negative slope conductance of I_{Kr} (i.e. g_{Kr} gets larger during repolarization (Fig 41D). I_{Ks} expression is two times less in canine midmyocardium than either epi- or endocardium and this may contribute to the very long APD which is characteristic of these cells (Sicouri & Antzelevitch, 1991; Liu & Antzelevitch, 1995).

I_{Ks} is strongly regulated by PKA and PKC in an E_m- and temperature-dependent manner (Walsh & Kass, 1988, 1991). β-adrenergic agonists increase I_{Ks} amplitude by 2-fold and shift activation to more negative E_m. PKC produced less increase in amplitude, but there was less shift in E_m-dependence. The PKA and PKC-mediated effects are additive, suggesting that they may be mediated by phosphorylation at different sites. In contrast to these results in guinea-pig ventricular myocytes, PKC can decrease I_{Ks} in rat and mouse myocytes, but this effect may be due to phosphorylation of a different minK which contains a serine that is not in guinea-pig minK (Varnum *et al.*, 1993). PKA-dependent phosphorylation results in increased outward I_{Ks} during the AP and contributes to the decrease in APD usually observed with sympathetic or β-adrenergic stimulation. The increase in I_{Ks} helps to offset the effect of PKA-induced increase of I_{Ca} amplitude, which would tend to increase APD. I_{Ks} is also increased by elevated $[Ca]_i$ (Toshe *et al.*, 1987) which would speed repolarization during large Ca transients.

<u>I_{Kur} (Kv1.5).</u> I_{Kur} activates more rapidly (τ=2-20 msec) than either I_{Kr} or I_{Ks}, does not inactivate and is much more sensitive to block by 4-aminopyridine (i.e. μM *vs.* mM required for I_{Kr} and I_{Ks}; Boyle & Nerbonne, 1991; Wang *et al.*, 1993b). Heterologous expression of Kv1.5 produces currents which resemble I_{Kur} and Kv1.5 message and protein is abundant in heart (see reviews by Nerbonne, 2000, 2001). This led to the suggestion that Kv1.5 underlies cardiac I_{Kur} (Fedida *et al.*, 1993; Wang *et al.*, 1993a; Barry *et al.*, 1995). Feng *et al.* (1997) and Bou Abboud & Nerbonne (1999) showed that antisense mRNA knock-down of Kv1.5 in human myocytes specifically reduced I_{Kur}, clarifying that Kv1.5 does indeed underlie I_{Kur}. Similar tests have not been reported yet to clarify whether I_{Kp} is indeed, also the product of Kv1.5. This may also be the same current some have referred to as I_{SS} (steady state) or I_{sus} (sustained). I_{Kur} may be particularly important in the early plateau phase where I_{Kr} and I_{Ks} are not yet activated (see Fig 45). Indeed, block of I_{Kur} in atrial myocytes greatly prolongs APD (Wang *et al.*, 1993b).

<u>Other Delayed Rectifiers.</u> Nerbonne (2000, 2001) discusses some additional delayed rectifier K currents, but these will only be mentioned briefly here. $I_{K,slow}$ is a rapidly activating and slowly inactivating current in mouse. It is blocked by nanomolar concentrations of α-dendrotoxin and appears to be attributable to Kv1.2 and/or Kv2.1 (Bou Abboud & Nerbonne, 1999; Xu *et al.*, 1999b,c). I_{ss} is a slowly activating current that remains at the end of 10 sec long depolarizations, and is relatively insensitive to 4-aminopyridine (Xu *et al.*, 1999a,c), but its molecular identity is not yet clear.

Other Inward Rectifier K Channels

<u>$I_{K(ACh)}$ (Kir3.1 & 3.4).</u> $I_{K(ACh)}$ is a strong inward rectifier K channel which is activated by muscarinic agonists such as acetylcholine (ACh). $I_{K(ACh)}$ is prominent in atrial myocytes and cells of the SA and AV nodes, notably the sites where vagal innervation in the heart is highest. It is also in ventricular myocytes at lower density. The parasympathetic activation of K current is centrally important in mediating the physiological mechanism of heart rate slowing. That is, the K current tends to stabilize E_m near E_K and increase the amount of inward current required to depolarize cells to the threshold of AP activation. ACh secreted from parasympathetic neurons binds to muscarinic M_2-receptors which are members of the 7-transmembrane domain G-protein coupled receptor family. This stimulates the GTPase activity of the heterotrimeric GTP binding protein G_i (with α, β & γ subunits) resulting in the dissociation of $G_{i\alpha}$-GTP from $G_{i\beta\gamma}$. While

there was initially some controversy as to whether the α or βγ subunit was responsible for activating $I_{K(ACh)}$, it is now clear that $G_{i\beta\gamma}$ is the species which binds to the carboxy terminal of the $I_{K(ACh)}$ channel protein to cause activation (Reuveny *et al.*, 1994; Inanobe *et al.*, 1995; Wickman & Clapham, 1995).

$I_{K(ACh)}$ is mediated by a heterotetrameric K channel composed of two Kir3.1 (or GIRK1) and two Kir3.4 (GIRK4 or CIR, cardiac inward rectifier) molecules (Krapivinsky *et al.*, 1995). The single channel conductance is high (~40 pS), and K selectivity is very high, as in I_{K1}. Knockout of $I_{K(ACh)}$ by targeting the Kir3.4 gene, results in a mouse with depressed resting heart rate variability and bradycardic response to vasoconstriction (Wickman *et al.*, 1998).

$I_{K(ACh)}$ can also be activated by some other agonists which couple to G-proteins, such as adenosine, ATP (purinergic P_1 & P_2), endothelin, somatostatin, calcitonin gene related peptide, and also by the generation of phosphoinositol 4,5-bisphosphate (PIP_2) via an ATP-dependent lipid kinase (Berlardinelli & Isenberg, 1983; Lewis & Clapham, 1989; Kim, 1991a,b; Matsura & Ehara, 1996; Huang *et al.*, 1998). $I_{K(ACh)}$ also demonstrates fade or desensitization, whereby sustained exposure to ACh results in a gradual decline in current. A fast phase (within 30 sec) may be due to reduced single channel open times, reflecting alteration in the G protein level (Kim, 1993a), while the slower phase over ~3 min may be due to receptor phosphorylation by a receptor kinase (Zang *et al.*, 1993; Wang & Lipsius, 1995a).

$\underline{I_{K(ATP)}}$ (Kir6.2 + SUR). A K current which is inhibited by intracellular ATP ($I_{K(ATP)}$) was first described in heart cells by Noma (1983), but it is present and functionally important in many other cell types (Ashcroft & Ashcroft, 1990). When $[ATP]_i$ falls during local ischemia these K channels become activated and can shorten the AP and also prevent excitability (Nichols *et al.*, 1991; Weiss *et al.*, 1992). This would be functionally important in conserving ATP by limiting excitation and consequent contraction in cells where ATP is low.

The [Mg-ATP] required to half maximally inhibit $I_{K(ATP)}$ in excised patches is 15-50 μM. This is much lower than the levels of $[ATP]_i$ in the normal myocyte (5-10 mM), and even in the early stages of ischemia where APD shortens and can be prevented (see pg 306). Intracellular [ADP] is also a strong modulator of $I_{K(ATP)}$ and increases of $[ADP]_i$ from normal (≤20 μM) to above 100 μM (as occurs relatively early during ischemia) can shift the apparent K_m for ATP to 100 μM. In this sense it is probably the [ADP]/[ATP] ratio which activates this channel (see pg 306-307). This makes sense teleologically, because this ratio is more directly related to the energetic state of the cell. $I_{K(ATP)}$ may also be preferentially regulated by local glycolytic enzymes which can regenerate ATP from local ADP (Weiss & Lamp, 1989).

These $I_{K(ATP)}$ channels are present at high density in cardiac myocytes and have a very high single channel conductance (~40 pS). Thus, activation of <1% of $I_{K(ATP)}$ (which can happen with little reduction in $[ATP]_i$) is sufficient to shorten APD by 50% (Nichols *et al.*, 1991; Weiss *et al.*, 1992). Mg-ATP also prevents rundown of $I_{K(ATP)}$ possibly by preventing actin depolymerization (Furukawa *et al.*, 1996) and also by stimulating PIP_2 production by a lipid kinase (Hilgemann & Ball, 1996). PIP_2 increases the [ATP] required to block $I_{K(ATP)}$. Thus, $I_{K(ATP)}$ channels are present in great functional excess with most fully inhibited, and only a small fraction must be activated to protect the cell from depletion of ATP or increase of [ADP]/[ATP]. The down side of this is that local regions of cells which are not conducting the normal AP can alter the normal conduction pathway and contribute to arrhythmogenesis. Even in cells which retain APs the APD is shorter, reducing refractory period, which can be pro-arrhythmic.

To reconstitute cardiac $I_{K(ATP)}$ requires both the sulfonylurea receptor (type 2A, SUR2A) plus the inward rectifier K channel Kir6.2 (Inagaki *et al.*, 1995, 1996; Aguilar-Bryant *et al.*, 1998). This is a heteromultimer where the inner ring and pore is made up by 4 Kir6.2 molecules and an outer ring includes 4 SUR2A molecules. SURs are members of the superfamily of ATP Binding Cassette (ABC) proteins which include the cystic fibrosis transmembrane regulator (CFTR) and multidrug resistance protein. These have 12-17 transmembrane segments and 2 characteristic nucleotide binding folds in intracellular loops. SUR2A gives the channel its characteristic sensitivity to K-channel openers (cromakalim, lemakalim, pinacidil, nicorandil & aprikalim) and blockers (glibenclamide, tolbutamide).

Work with $I_{K(ATP)}$ channel openers had suggested that $I_{K(ATP)}$ activation could be a key cardioprotective mechanism induced by brief ischemic periods (preconditioning; Yao *et al.*, 1994; Gross, 1995; Grover *et al.*, 1996). However, there is also a mitochondrial K(ATP) channel (Garlid *et al.*1996). Recent work with the selective mitochondrial $I_{K(ATP)}$ activator diazoxide and blocker 5-hydroxydecanoate has shown that the mitochondrial $I_{K(ATP)}$ is crucial in mediating cardioprotection in preconditioning, via a PKC-dependent pathway (see pg 311, Garlid *et al.*, 1997; Liu *et al.*, 1998; Sato *et al.*, 1998a; Takashi *et al.*, 1999). How opening mitochondrial $I_{K(ATP)}$ channels would be protective is not known. The loss of mitochondrial membrane potential would prevent mitochondrial Ca uptake (Holmuhamedov *et al.*, 1999). On the other hand, this would also limit ATP synthesis (see Chapter 3), so the protective mechanism remains unclear.

Na- and Fatty Acid-activated K Channels

A K channel activated by high $[Na]_i$ has been reported in cardiac muscle (Kameyama *et al.*, 1984; Luk & Carmeliet, 1990; Lawrence & Rodrigo, 1999). This channel has high K selectivity, but the K_m for activation by $[Na]_i$ is very high (66 mM). The physiological role of this current is unclear. Intracellular arachidonic acid, unsaturated fatty acids, phospholipids and stretch can also activate K-selective channels in heart (Kim & Clapham, 1989; Kim, 1993b). The specific physiological role of these currents is unclear, but they could serve the same function as $I_{K(ATP)}$ to inhibit the AP under stressful cellular conditions.

Cl CHANNELS

There are three types of Cl currents in heart which will be discussed below (see Hume *et al.*, 2000 for review): a) Ca-activated Cl current ($I_{Cl(Ca)}$), b) cAMP-activated Cl current ($I_{Cl(cAMP)}$) and c) swelling-activated Cl current ($I_{Cl(swell)}$). There is also a purinergic receptor activated Cl current (Matsura & Ehara, 1992; Levesque & Hume, 1995), but this will not be discussed further here. These Cl currents are generally blocked by disulfonic stilbenes DIDS and SITS, except for $I_{Cl(cAMP)}$ which is not sensitive to these, but can be blocked by DNDS (see Table 14). The reversal potential for Cl is positive to resting E_m in atrial and ventricular myocytes (Fig 36C) which makes the functional role of Cl channel opening less intrinsically obvious. Thus activation of Cl currents may hasten AP repolarization, but also cause diastolic depolarization.

CFTR: cAMP-Activated Cl Channel.

The PKA activated $I_{Cl(cAMP)}$ is present in ventricular myocytes, is less dense in atrial myocytes, and is not present in rabbit SA node, canine myocardium or rat ventricle (Horowitz *et al.*, 1993; Gadsby *et al.*, 1995). The current is carried by the cardiac variant of the cystic fibrosis transmembrane regulator (CFTR). CFTR has two sets of 6 transmembrane domains (not homologous to Na or K channels), separated by a large intracellular loop or regulatory domain which contains one of the two nucleotide binding domain (NBD1, with NBD2 near the intra-cellular C-terminal). Any pathway which activates PKA can cause phosphorylation in the regulatory domain and activation of CFTR. Once phosphorylated, ATP binds at NBD1 and is hydrolyzed. While ADP remains bound at NBD1 the channel is active and exhibits brief opening bursts. When a second phosphorylation occurs and ATP is bound and cleaved at NBD2, ADP bound at NBD1 is stabilized and CFTR enters an active conformation characterized by long openings (~1 sec) and brief closures (Ehara & Matsura, 1993; Gadsby *et al.*, 1995). Dephos-phorylation of CFTR or ADP dissociation from the NBDs causes channel deactivation.

$I_{Cl(cAMP)}$ does not show appreciable E_m-dependent gating and the current shows no rectification in symmetrical Cl solutions. However, since intracellular [Cl] is much lower than $[Cl]_o$ there is slight apparent outward rectification under physiological conditions. The selectivity sequence for $I_{Cl(cAMP)}$ is $NO_3 > Br \geq Cl \geq I$ (Overholt *et al.*, 1993). When $I_{Cl(cAMP)}$ is activated it constitutes a static increase in Cl conductance at the whole cell level. One consequence is that the outward $I_{Cl(cAMP)}$ during most of the AP will speed repolarization and thus tend to shorten APD. This, along with PKA activation of I_{Ks} may offset the enhanced inward I_{Ca} and contribute to the shorter APD seen with β-adrenergic agonists and sympathetic stimulation. Diastolic $I_{Cl(cAMP)}$ would tend to depolarize E_m somewhat toward E_{Cl} (about –55 mV). This effect may be minor in ventricular myocytes where I_{K1} is relatively large, but could be larger in cells with lower I_{K1} (such as pacemaker cells). However, pacemaker cells may have relatively little $I_{Cl(cAMP)}$ and since diastolic E_m in these cells is already close to E_{Cl}, the impact may be small.

Ca-Activated Cl Current $I_{Cl(Ca)}$: a Transient Outward Current.

The Ca_i-dependent component of transient outward current which used to be referred to as I_{to2} is now clearly attributable to $I_{Cl(Ca)}$, (Zygmunt & Gibbons, 1991,1992; Zygmunt, 1994; Sipido *et al.*, 1993; Kawano *et al.*, 1995). This channel does not appear to have intrinsic E_m-dependence or rectification, but is activated by the rise in $[Ca]_i$ during E-C coupling. $I_{Cl(Ca)}$ has been most extensively characterized in rabbit, ferret and dog myocytes, but is probably present in many cardiac myocytes. Current density is higher in atrium. A high temperature-dependence was indicated by the results of Puglisi *et al.* (1999) who saw almost no detectable $I_{Cl(Ca)}$ in rabbit ventricular myocytes at 25°C, despite prominent $I_{Cl(Ca)}$ at 35°C. The kinetics of $I_{Cl(Ca)}$ are much faster than the global cellular Ca transient, as is true for $I_{Na/Ca}$ and Ca-dependent inactivation of $I_{Ca,L}$ (Trafford *et al.*, 1998; Puglisi *et al.*, 1999). This is undoubtedly due to the much higher and faster local Ca transient in the submembrane space (or junctional gap) due to both Ca influx and SR Ca release, when compared to global $[Ca]_i$ sensed by Ca indicators. In this way, Ca-dependent currents ($I_{Cl(Ca)}$, $I_{Na/Ca}$ and $I_{Ca,L}$) can serve as a valuable indicators of local $[Ca]_i$. This also emphasizes that the local, rather than global $[Ca]_i$, is important in regulating these currents. These 3 Ca-dependent currents can also have substantial impact on the AP. It is not clear how much of the rapid early repolarization is due to $I_{Cl(Ca)}$ *vs.* I_{to}, but it is probably a significant fraction (N.B. $I_{Cl(Ca)}$ is not included in the Fig 45 model). At diastolic E_m (below E_{Cl}) spontaneous SR Ca release can activate inward $I_{Cl(Ca)}$, contributing to DADs (Zygmunt *et al.*, 1998).

Collier *et al.* (1996) reported that the single channel $I_{Cl(Ca)}$ is small (~1 pS) and that the apparent K_m for $[Ca]_i$ activation was 150 µM. This is relevant to the discussion above, because a slow rise in global $[Ca]_i$ to 1 µM would not activate appreciable $I_{Cl(Ca)}$, whereas submembrane $[Ca]_i$ may reach 50 µM briefly at the peak of SR Ca release (Chapter 7) and this would activate considerable $I_{Cl(Ca)}$ with the short timecourse observed. $I_{Cl(Ca)}$ can be blocked by mM DIDS, 50 µM niflumate and glibenclamide (K_m =65 µM; Yamazaki & Hume, 1997).

Swelling-Activated Cl Current

$I_{Cl(swell)}$ was first reported in dog atrium and ventricle (Tseng, 1992; Sorota, 1992) and seems to be more prominent in atrium than ventricle (Sorota, 1999). The likely candidate protein for $I_{Cl(swell)}$ is ClC-3 (Duan *et al.*, 1997a). ClC-3 is a member of a larger Cl channel family, and these channels have 10-12 transmembrane spans, function as dimers and may have double barreled pores (Jentsch *et al.*, 1999). The current is activated slowly in response to an increase in cell size (usually evoked by hypoosmotic superfusate or inflation via patch pipette). Activation can be prevented by 50 µM genestein, implicating a tyrosine kinase in the transduction pathway (Sorota, 1995), and the extent of activation can be modulated by PKA and PKC (Sorota, 1999). $I_{Cl(swell)}$ is outwardly rectifying, even in symmetrical Cl solutions and has a large unitary conductance, 49 pS (Vandenberg *et al.*, 1994; Duan *et al.*, 1997b). It can be blocked by 1 mM DIDS, 100 µM niflumate or 20 µM tamoxifen, but there are no selective inhibitors. $I_{Cl(swell)}$ can be substantial (>50 pA) and contribute to depolarization of resting E_m and shortening of APD (Vandenberg *et al.*, 1997). Clemo *et al.* (1999) found persistently activated $I_{Cl(swell)}$ in dogs with congestive heart failure and suggested that this contributes to electrophysiological dysfunction.

STRETCH-ACTIVATED CHANNELS

In addition to the $I_{Cl(swell)}$ channels described above, there are stretch-activated channels (SACs) in the heart, some of which are blocked by Gd, as reviewed by Hu & Sachs (1997). They point out that mechanical stretch *per se* is different than cell swelling in response to osmotic or hydrostatic pressure. If one wants to measure electrophysiological impact of the kind of mechanical stretch which occurs in the heart this places challenging constraints on experimental design. In rat atrial cells Kim & Fu (1993) reported a swelling-induced nonselective cation current. Hu & Sachs (1996) found that swelling chick ventricular myocytes induced $I_{Cl(swell)}$, while mechanical strain activated a nonselective cation current. Clemo & Baumgarten (1997) demonstrated a swelling-activated cationic current in rabbit ventricular myocytes. This current was relatively non-selective (P_K/P_{Na} =5.9), carried mainly inward Na flux at resting E_m and was blocked by Gd (K_m = 0.5 µM). Block of this current limited cell swelling in response to hypotonic stress, suggesting that this channel along with $I_{Cl(swell)}$ plays a role in volume regulation and can cause diastolic depolarization. Stretch or swelling can also stimulate a K-selective channel (Kim, 1992), $I_{K(ATP)}$ (Van Wagoner, 1993), increase I_{Ca} (Matsuda *et al.*, 1996), and inhibit $I_{K(ACh)}$ (Ji *et al.*, 1998). The integrated electrophysiological role of these SACs is not known, but nonselective cationic currents could contribute to arrhythmias.

NON-SELECTIVE CHANNELS

Pacemaker Current I_f

I_f was so named because it was a "funny" current, which activated slowly upon hyper-polarization, in contrast to previously described cation currents activated by depolarization (DiFrancesco, 1981a,b, 1982, 1985, 1986, 1995). It is similar to the hyperpolarization-activated current I_h in neurons. I_f is not selective between Na and K, but other monovalent cations (Li, Cs, Rb) are almost impermeant. The reversal potential is typically about –15 mV and unitary conductance is small (~1 pS). Thus at negative E_m net inward current is carried by Na and contributes to diastolic depolarization. The time constant of I_f activation at –90 mV in SA node cells is ~500 ms (and ≥2 sec at –70 mV). Thus I_f activates gradually at negative E_m, and it does not inactivate.

The protein responsible for I_f has recently been cloned (HCN1, 2 & 4; Ludwig *et al.*, 1998, 1999; Gauss *et al.*, 1998; Santoro *et al.*, 1998; Shi *et al.*, 1999) and is related to a class of cyclic nucleotide gated cation channels. HCN stands for **H**yperpolarization-activated **C**yclic **N**ucleotide-gated. These 700-900 amino acid channels appear to be homologous to the E_m-dependent K channels (Fig 38B) including 6 transmembrane domains, positive charges on every third amino acid in the S_4 domain and the GYG signature sequence in the P-loop. Differences in amino acids neighboring GYG may result in lower selectivity for K over Na (P_K/P_{Na} = 3-4; Clapham, 1998). With these similarities it is not clear why this channel activates upon hyperpolarization, rather than depolarization (as for E_m-dependent K channels). One possibility is that these channels have activation and inactivation like I_{to}, but are fully activated at all relevant E_m values. Then hyperpolarization may allow E_m-dependent recovery from inactivation (as for E_m-dependent K, Na & Ca channels) such that I_f is really like a window current (see Miller & Aldrich, 1996).

I_f is present in SA & AV node cells, Purkinje fibers, and also atrial & ventricular myocytes, although myocytes do not readily display prominent pacemaker activity (DiFrancesco, 1995). The E_m-dependence of activation differs dramatically in different tissues (Fig 42). In SA node cells the E_m-dependent activation range overlaps with the range of E_m during pacemaker activity (–40 to –60 mV) and the same is true for Purkinje fibers (–80 to –100 mV). While I_f exists in ventricular myocytes (Yu *et al.*, 1993, 1995) it is probably non-functional due to the very negative E_m range of activation (Fig 42). An exception could be if the E_m-dependence becomes more positive as a result of cAMP or some other potentially pathophysiological modulatory effect. There also remains some controversy about the role of I_f in SA node cells (see pg 94-97), based on relatively negative activation E_m in some reports. This would certainly be the case if one assumed that the E_m-dependence of I_f in Purkinje fibers also was relevant to SA node. Shi *et al.* reported that rabbit SA nodal cells expressed mainly HCN4, Purkinje fibers express HCN1 & 4 equally and ventricular myocytes express only HCN2. Thus there may be a molecular correlate to the different E_m-dependence of I_f in different cardiac tissues.

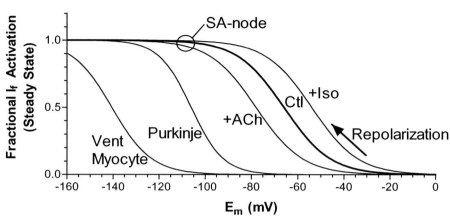

Figure 42. E_m-dependence of I_f activation during hyperpolarization. The rightmost 3 Boltzmann curves are for SA node and have half-maximal E_m ($E_{0.5}$) at -78, -66 and -54 mV for acetylcholine (ACh), control (Ctl) and isoproterenol (Iso) respectively (slope values are 10 mV/e-fold change). Values for Purkinje fibers and ventricular myocytes are taken from Yu *et al.* (1995; $E_{0.5} = -106$ & -140 and slopes are 7 & 8.7 mV respectively).

Sympathetic stimulation or β-adrenergic agonists (e.g. isoproterenol) and also para-sympathetic stimulation by acetylcholine (ACh) release alter the E_m-dependence of I_f, but not the maximal current available (see Fig 42). The positive shift with isoproterenol means that at any E_m there will be more depolarizing inward current via I_f, and this would increase the rate of depolarization and thereby the heart rate. ACh has the opposite effect, reducing I_f at any E_m and thereby slowing the rate of depolarization and heart rate. Thus, I_f and $I_{K(ACh)}$ contribute significantly to the slowing of heart rate induced by parasympathetic stimulation of the heart. Elevated $[Ca]_i$ also increases I_f (Hagiwara & Irisawa, 1989) and this would also tend to increase heart rate.

The mechanism of sympathetic activation of I_f is mediated by the β-adrenergic receptor and production of cAMP by adenylyl cyclase. However, transduction does not depend upon activation of PKA, but is due to a direct affect of cAMP on the I_f channel (DiFrancesco & Tortora, 1991). This makes sense now that we know that this channel is related to a class of cyclic nucleotide gated channels. Parasympathetic regulation is mediated via muscarinic receptor and pertussis-sensitive G-protein (DiFrancesco & Tromba, 1988).

Ca-activated nonselective monovalent cation current $I_{ns(Ca)}$.

$I_{ns(Ca)}$ was first described in heart by Colquhoun *et al.* (1981) and also characterized by Ehara *et al.* (1988) in guinea-pig ventricular myocytes. Unitary currents (conductance =15 pS) did not show any rectification and the channels were not selective among K, Na or Cs. $I_{ns(Ca)}$ was half-maximally activated by 1.2 μM Ca with a Hill coefficient of 3 in excised patches. This channel has the potential to contribute inward current upon spontaneous SR Ca release and contribute to DADs along with $I_{Cl(Ca)}$ and $I_{Na/Ca}$. The relative contribution of $I_{ns(Ca)}$ however is small and it is not clear how functionally important this current is in ventricular myocytes.

Na/Ca EXCHANGE

Na/Ca exchange will be discussed in detail in Chapter 6, so I will only mention a few salient characteristics here which are most relevant to Na/Ca exchange current ($I_{Na/Ca}$) during the AP (Fig 45). The accepted stoichiometry of this reversible countertransport system is 3Na to 1Ca such that 1 positive charge is moved in the direction of Na transport. Thus Ca influx via Na/Ca exchange produces outward $I_{Na/Ca}$ and Ca extrusion causes inward $I_{Na/Ca}$ (Fig 43). The direction and amplitude of $I_{Na/Ca}$ flow depends on E_m as well as the intra- and extracellular Na and Ca concentrations. $I_{Na/Ca}$ has a reversal potential ($E_{Na/Ca}$) analogous to that of ion channels. Under normal diastolic conditions $E_{Na/Ca}$ is typically about –40 mV, and inward $I_{Na/Ca}$ occurs (Ca extrusion) at resting E_m –80 mV (A in Fig 43). However, since resting $[Ca]_i$ is low the amplitude of diastolic inward $I_{Na/Ca}$ is small (i.e. substrate concentration is limited). Upon depolarization to the AP peak E_m passes through the $E_{Na/Ca}$ and $I_{Na/Ca}$ reverses and becomes outward (Ca influx, B in Fig 43). Since $[Ca]_i$ rises rapidly due to I_{Ca} and SR Ca release, the $E_{Na/Ca}$ rapidly shifts to much more positive potentials (note the shift in x-intercept in Fig 43, of the 1 µM *vs.* 150 nM curve). This favors more inward $I_{Na/Ca}$ (Ca extrusion, 1 µM curve in Fig 43). The net $I_{Na/Ca}$ current as the AP proceeds through the plateau phase depends on both the time course of the Ca transient and trajectory of the AP. As AP repolarization proceeds and $[Ca]_i$ remains elevated, $I_{Na/Ca}$ becomes strongly inward, as Na/Ca exchange extrudes Ca (from C to D to A in Fig 43). As $[Ca]_i$ declines at diastolic E_m, inward $I_{Na/Ca}$ gradually declines (for more detail see pg 147-151).

When $[Ca]_i$ is elevated at resting E_m during a spontaneous SR Ca release (E in Fig 43) a large inward $I_{Na/Ca}$ can be generated and this contributes to both a transient inward current (I_{ti}) as well as the genesis of DADs. The relative contribution of $I_{Na/Ca}$, $I_{Cl(Ca)}$ and $I_{ns(Ca)}$ to DADs will be discussed below (pg 97-99). Whatever Ca enters the cell via I_{Ca} at each beat, must be extruded from the cell via Na/Ca exchange. Thus if 10 µM Ca enters via I_{Ca} 30 µM Na must enter to extrude it. Interestingly, this Na influx is likely to be 2-3 times as much as enters via I_{Na} during the AP. The Na ions which enter must in turn be extruded from the cell via the sarcolemmal Na/K-ATPase.

NA/K-ATPase

The Na/K-ATPase transports 3 Na ions out and 2 K ions into the cell using the energy of one ATP molecule, and thus moves one net charge out per cycle. This is the key transporter that sets up the sarcolemmal ionic gradients for Na, K and Ca and consequently allows ion channels to function. As indicated in Table 13 (pg 62) the Na/K-ATPase can generate a $[Na]_o/[Na]_i$ gradient of about 14 and a $[K]_i/[K]_o$ gradient of ~25 (based on ΔG_{ATP}). ATP is normally not rate limiting for Na/K-ATPase, and local glycolysis may regenerate ATP, making the pump less directly dependent on oxidative phosphorylation (Glitsch & Tappe, 1993). The main regulators of Na/K-ATPase are the substrates $[Na]_i$ and $[K]_o$. The activating K_m for $[Na]_i$ is ~10 mM and for $[K]_o$ is ~1.5 mM, so the pump is almost 80% saturated with respect to $[K]_o$ at normal $[K]_o$ of 5 mM. Normal $[Na]_i$ of ~10 mM is right at the K_m for $[Na]_i$, assuring responsiveness to altered $[Na]_i$ under physiological conditions. The precise K_m for $[Na]_i$ may vary with different Na/K-ATPase isoforms and could cause resting $[Na]_i$ differences among species or regions (e.g. higher $[Na]_i$ in rat than rabbit or guinea-pig ventricle; Shattock & Bers, 1989; Harrison *et al.*, 1992a).

Na/Ca Exchange Current ($I_{Na/Ca}$)

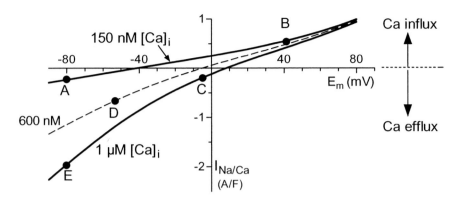

Figure 43. E_m-dependence of $I_{Na/Ca}$ at different $[Ca]_i$. $I_{Na/Ca}$ was calculated using the equation and constants in Luo & Rudy (1994a) for $[Na]_i = 10$ mM and $[Ca]_o = 2$ mM. Inward currents ($I_{Na/Ca} < 0$) reflect Ca efflux. As $[Ca]_i$ rises the reversal E_m for $I_{Na/Ca}$ ($E_{Na/Ca}$) becomes more positive. Abruptly increasing $[Ca]_i$ at −80 mV as with caffeine increases inward $I_{Na/Ca}$ greatly (A to E). During the AP upstroke $I_{Na/Ca}$ reverses and becomes outward (A to B). As repolarization and $[Ca]_i$ decline $I_{Na/Ca}$ becomes inward again (C & D).

Like the Na/Ca exchanger, transport by Na/K-ATPase has a functional reversal potential which depends on both intracellular and extracellular [Na] and [K] as well as the ΔG_{ATP}. Under normal conditions this has been estimated to be about −180 mV (Glitsch & Tappe, 1995), such that Na/K-ATPase current (and Na transport) is outward over the whole physiological range. However, this can change as ΔG_{ATP} declines during ischemia or energetic compromise, limiting the Na/K-ATPase at negative E_m (e.g. E_{rev} shifts to −60 mV when ΔG_{ATP} falls from −58 to −39 kJ/mol). It is worth noting that at −80 mV almost all (95%) of the energy used by the Na/K-ATPase goes into pumping Na out of the cell, because the electrochemical gradient for Na is so much steeper than for K (150 mV *vs.* 8 mV). That is, at resting E_m (close to E_K) it takes little energy to pump K in, but a great amount to pump Na out. Aside from this thermodynamic effect Na/K-ATPase current is also weakly dependent on E_m with a broad peak between −80 and 0 mV (Gadsby *et al.*, 1993; Bielen *et al.*, 1993). The result of these characteristics is that the Na/K-ATPase contributes a relatively small outward (repolarizing) current throughout the AP (Fig 45). The sustained outward Na/K-ATPase current thus also contributes slightly to the negative diastolic E_m. Abrupt block of the Na/K-ATPase normally only causes 2-4 mV depolarization acutely (due to block of outward current), but of course in the long term would completely dissipate E_m and render cells inexcitable as the ion gradients run down.

Under typical experimental conditions the mean Na/K-ATPase current is 0.3 A/F over the cardiac cycle (Fig 45). Since the Na/K-ATPase must extrude Na which enters the cell via I_{Na} and Na/Ca exchange, it would be useful to know how well this current accounts for the known Na influx. For 15 μM Na entry via I_{Na} plus 36 μM Na entry via $I_{Na/Ca}$ (to extrude 12 μM Ca entry via I_{Ca}) per beat at 1 Hz would require extrusion of 17 μM charge per second, or 0.27 A/F of required Na/K-ATPase current. Thus there is good quantitative agreement between flux estimates and Na/K-ATPase current measurements and >2/3 of Na entry is via Na/Ca exchange.

The Na/K-ATPase is a member of the P-type ATPase pumps (like the SR and sarcolemmal Ca-ATPases) and was first cloned by Shull *et al.* (1985) and Kawakami *et al.*, 1985). Three Na/K-ATPase isoforms exist in rat and human heart (α_1, α_2 & α_3, each ~1000 amino acids or 110 kDa; Lucchesi & Sweadner, 1991; Wang *et al.*, 1996c). These α subunits exhibit all of the ion transport, ATPase activity and digitalis glycoside binding sites. The associated β subunits (β_1 & β_2; 35 kDa) may play a role in ensuring appropriate processing and insertion of the pump in the membrane, but only β_1 is appreciable in human heart (McDonough *et al.*, 1990; Wang *et al.*, 1996c). Expression of Na/K-ATPase is higher in ventricle than atrium. McDonough *et al.* (1996) demonstrated that in rat ventricular myocytes the α_1 isoform (lower ouabain affinity) is preferentially in T-tubules, whereas α_2 was homogeneously distributed. Conversely, in rat vascular smooth muscle the α_2 & α_3 isoforms (high ouabain affinity) were preferentially localized to junctions between SR and sarcolemma, while α_1 was ubiquitous (Juhaszova & Blaustein, 1997). This could reflect functionally important spatial compartmentalization. The α subunit has 10 transmembrane domains (with amino and carboxy tails intracellular) and the 5th and 6th domains seem to be most important in ion binding and may form the pore through which Na and K flow (Lingrel *et al.*, 1997). External sites between domains 1-2, 5-6 and 6-7 appear to be most important for specific binding of ouabain and other cardiac glycosides. These compounds are specific inhibitors of Na/K-ATPase and have been used to enhance cardiac contractility in the treatment of congestive heart failure for more than 200 years. The inotropic mechanism of cardiac glycosides will be discussed in depth in Chapter 10. Suffice it to say here that Na/K-ATPase inhibition would cause [Na]$_i$ to rise and this would shift the balance of fluxes on the Na/Ca exchange to favor more Ca influx and less Ca efflux.

Figure 44 shows the accepted Na/K-ATPase transport mechanism as sequential in the following sense (Läuger, 1991; Rakowski *et al.*, 1997). In the E_1-ATP state of the enzyme the cation binding sites face the cytosol, ready to bind Na. When 3 Na ions bind this causes ATP hydrolysis and phosphorylation of the enzyme in a state where the Na ions are occluded (inaccessible from either side). Then the pump shifts to the E_2 conformation where the Na ions are released to the outside and are replaced by 2 K ions. Binding of K ions stimulates dephosphorylation and K occlusion. Finally, intracellular ATP binds to the pump causing reversion to the E_1 state where K is released to the cytosol and the pump is ready for another cycle. The turnover rate is 75-100/sec (Nakao & Gadsby, 1986), ~4 orders of magnitude slower than the flux rate through a Na channel. The number of sarcolemmal Na/K-ATPase sites is much higher than for Na channels (1200 *vs.* 3/μm^2).

Na/K-ATPase in guinea-pig ventricle can be inhibited by β-adrenergic agonists via a cAMP/PKA pathway (Gao *et al.*, 1996, 1998a) and stimulated by α-adrenergic activation (Wang *et al.*, 1998a). The β-adrenergic-induced depression of Na/K-ATPase is still somewhat controversial, since Ishizuka & Berlin (1993) found no effect on Na/K-ATPase current in rat myocytes and increases in Na/K-ATPase were reported in rabbit, guinea-pig and sheep ventricle (Désilets & Baumgarten, 1986; Glitsch *et al.*, 1989; Kockskämper *et al.*, 2000). While there may be some species-dependent differences, technical issues may also obscure the depressant effect of β-adrenergic agonists (Gao *et al.*, 1997c). The depressant effect also agrees with data in renal cells, and there may also be isoform-specific differences (Blanco & Mercer, 1998). Reduction of

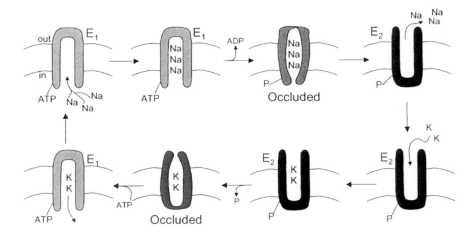

Figure 44. Post-Albers scheme of Na/K-ATPase mechanism (see text; based on Läuger, 1991).

Na/K-ATPase upon sympathetic stimulation could exacerbate the rise in [Na]$_i$ which occurs with increased heart rate.

Different Na/K-ATPase isoforms have differing glycoside and [Na]$_i$ sensitivity (Blanco & Mercer, 1998). Thus, alteration in the balance of isoform expression or cellular localization could be important in determining function and [Na]$_i$. In failing human heart there is decreased expression of the 2 main human Na pump isoforms (α_1 and α_3; Schwinger *et al.*, 1999b). This could cause [Na]$_i$ to rise in heart failure and contribute to altered Ca homeostasis.

CURRENTS DURING VENTRICULAR ACTION POTENTIAL

Figure 45 shows a rabbit ventricular myocyte AP and the ionic currents which occur. One practical way to evaluate the complex interacting currents during the AP is the following. First one measures the E_m- and time-dependence (& [Ca]$_i$-dependence where relevant) of each current, under well controlled voltage clamp conditions.   Then the time-, E_m- and [Ca]$_i$-dependence of each current can be calculated at each point in time and used to calculate how the integrated currents affect E_m and [Ca]$_i$ during the next instant.   These sort of numerical integration models can be quite complicated, but some excellent versions have been developed (e.g. Noble's Oxsoft Heart, Luo & Rudy, 1991, 1994a, Zeng *et al.*, 1995; Jaffri *et al.*, 1998; Winslow *et al.*, 1999; Nordin, 1993, Demir *et al.*, 1994; Lindblad *et al.*, 1996). Figure 45 uses the system of equations in the Luo-Rudy guinea-pig ventricular myocyte AP model (Luo & Rudy, 1991, 1994a; Zeng *et al.*, 1995) with some adjustments to make it more appropriate for rabbit ventricular myocytes (e.g. I_{to} is included and I_{Kr} & I_{Ks} are adjusted; Salata *et al.*, 1996). Dr. J.L. Puglisi and I have mounted this on a user friendly platform (LabHeart) and we plan to make it available in 2000. These models are certainly imperfect, but are being continually improved and can be valuable adjuncts to guide appropriate experimental tests. One of the imperfections is simply that the model can be no better than the precision and completeness of the data concerning channel behavior, and one must always compromise with results from different species and obtained under differing experimental conditions. An additional key issue is how to deal with specialized spaces (SR-T-tubule junctions and subsarcolemmal space), where ions and/or regulators may accumulate or deplete. With these caveats in mind let's consider which currents contribute to each phase of the ventricular AP.

Rapid Upstroke of AP (Phase 0)

Myocyte depolarization is normally initiated by passive current spread from a neighboring active region (Fig 37), which can bring the cell to the threshold point where a sufficient number of Na channels are activated that inward I_{Na} exceeds outward I_K. The rapid upstroke of the AP in atrial and ventricular myocytes is primarily due to the regenerative activation of I_{Na}. That is, once threshold depolarization is reached for an AP, the opening of Na channels leads to further depolarization, which activates additional Na channels and depolarization etc. This positive feedback creates a very rapid depolarization (200 V/sec) toward E_{Na}. Since there is always some finite K permeability, the E_m never reaches E_{Na} (+70 mV), but in ventricular myocytes often reaches +35-50 mV. Depolarization also rapidly shuts off the inwardly rectifying I_{K1}, limiting outward current during the AP upstroke (and later phases). Depolarization stops, in part because Na channels inactivate, and this constitutes a built-in negative feedback or brake on I_{Na}. Strictly speaking, the AP peak is where inward current ($I_{Na} + I_{Ca}$) exactly equals outward current (carried mostly by K). With depolarization the driving force for I_{Na} ($E_m - E_{Na}$) gets smaller, while for K currents the driving force ($E_m - E_K$) increases. In addition, the K conductance increase, rapidly for I_{to} & I_{Kur} (more slowly for I_{Kr} & I_{Ks}). By the peak of the AP I_{Na} is back down to ~1% of its peak value and I_{Ca} is already at 43% of maximum (see inset in Fig 45). Coincidentally, the absolute value of $I_{Ca,L}$ and I_{Na} are both ~4 A/F at this point. Again, at the AP peak total inward and outward current are exactly balanced.

Early Repolarization (Phase 1)

Several factors contribute to the early repolarization phase, including additional I_{Na} inactivation and activation of outward I_{to} and $I_{Cl(Ca)}$ (although the latter is not in the Fig 45 model). The same SR Ca release which contributes to the activation of $I_{Cl(Ca)}$ also inactivates I_{Ca} and that is responsible for the initial rapid decrease in $I_{Ca,L}$ in Fig 45. I_{Kur} also activates very rapidly and may contribute to early repolarization. Probably I_{to} is the most dominant contributor to the AP notch, and the decrease in the AP notch seen from epi- to endocardium follows that of I_{to} expression (see pg 78-79). Nevertheless, inhibition of SR Ca release can also diminish the notch (due to effects on $I_{Cl(Ca)}$ and I_{Ca}). Atrial myocytes and rat and mouse ventricular myocytes have much more I_{to}, and consequently greater early repolarization. Moreover, in rat and mouse ventricular myocytes there is almost no plateau phase, because early repolarization is so great. $I_{Ca,T}$ is not normally observed in rabbit ventricular myocytes, and was not included in the model calculations. It is shown in Fig 45 simply to indicate the expected timecourse for an AP like this.

Plateau (Phase 2)

The long plateau phase of the AP can be relatively flat, domed, gradually declining or some combination thereof. Its key characteristic is that E_m does not change rapidly. This is because inward and outward current are nearly balanced. During this time the inward current is mostly carried by $I_{Ca,L}$ and the outward current by delayed rectifier K currents (I_{Kur}, I_{Kr} & I_{Ks}). I_{Kur} follows roughly the shape of the AP because its gating responds so rapidly to E_m. The shape is distorted with respect to the AP, mainly because currents are much larger at positive E_m due to

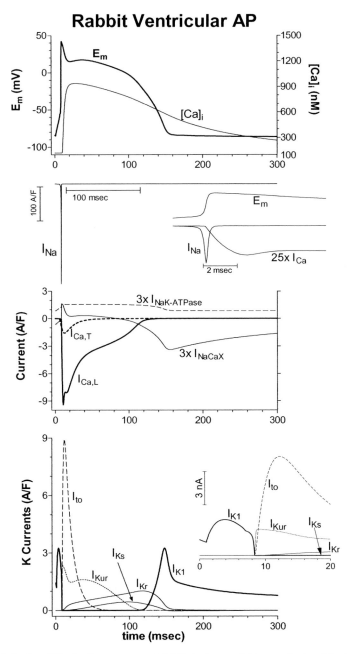

Rabbit Ventricular AP

Figure 45. Calculated E_m, ionic currents and $[Ca]_i$ during a rabbit ventricular AP. Calculations were done using the LabHeart program (J.L. Puglisi & D.M. Bers) and the Luo & Rudy (1991, 1994a; Zeng *et al.*, 1995) equations and parameters for guinea-pig ventricle with some adjustments to better represent rabbit ventricle (e.g. inclusion of I_{to}, altered I_{Kr} and I_{Ks}; Salata *et al.*, 1996). $I_{Ca,T}$ was also not included, but it is shown for general information. $I_{Na/Ca}$ and Na/K-ATPase current are scaled up by a factor of 3 to make them clearer. The time-expanded insets illustrate the temporal relationship of E_m, I_{Na} and $I_{Ca,L}$ in the first 9 msec (upper) and K currents near the rapid AP upstroke at ~8 msec (lower).

the higher driving force on K ($E_m - E_K$). I_{Ks} activates more slowly and I_{Kr} increases as repolarization progresses (Fig 41) and these two outward current sustain the latter plateau. There is a delicate balance of currents during the plateau phase so rather modest differences in any of the currents can alter plateau duration. For example, there is less I_{Ks} in midmyocardial cells and this contributes to a very long APD in these cells and the U-wave on the ECG (Liu & Antzelevitch, 1995). PKA-dependent phosphorylation also alters I_{Ks} and $I_{Ca(cAMP)}$ to shorten the plateau. Moreover, mutations in HERG and KvLQT1, the genes which code for the channels which carry I_{Kr} and I_{Ks} cause congenital long QT syndrome in humans (Sanguinetti *et al.*, 1995, 1996a,b) in which ventricular APD is abnormally long. Alterations in other ionic currents can also perturb the delicate balance and plateau duration.

Late Repolarization (Phase 3)

At some point repolarization accelerates greatly and E_m goes from the plateau level near 0 mV back toward the diastolic E_m. There is a negative slope in the current-voltage relationship of I_{Kr} and I_{K1} (Fig 41B,C), which means that as repolarization proceeds outward current increases (causing further repolarization). This sort of positive feedback results in progressive acceleration of repolarization. Since this occurs at more positive E_m for I_{Kr}, that current is particularly important in the early part of this accelerating phase of late repolarization. As repolarization proceeds I_{Kr} deactivates at more negative E_m. At E_m below -30 mV I_{K1} increases with repolarization, again accelerating repolarization. During repolarization inward $I_{Na/Ca}$ (Ca extrusion) becomes more prominent because [Ca]$_i$ is still relatively high and the more negative E_m causes a stronger driving force favoring inward $I_{Na/Ca}$ (see Chapter 6).

PACEMAKERS (AP PHASE 4)

Many cells in the heart exhibit spontaneous pacemaker activity, e.g. SA node, AV node and Purkinje fibers. Many different currents are involved in pacemaker activity and the relative amounts vary in different regions and under different conditions (Irisawa *et al.*, 1993; Anumonwo & Jalife, 1995; Noma, 1996). This also depends on the E_m range, [Ca]$_i$ and the history. Figure 46 shows APs typical of SA node cells with some of the key players implicated in pacemaker activity. Figure 47 is from the rabbit SA node model of Demir *et al.* (1994, 1999) and includes more details and quantitative estimates. Notably, these cells have little or no I_{K1}, and this is largely responsible for their relatively positive diastolic potential. As repolarization proceeds in these cells delayed rectifier K currents are decreasing ($\tau \sim 300$ msec, Fig 47) and a loss of outward current (even with an unchanging inward background current) will tend to move the E_m in a depolarizing direction. Thus turning off of K currents contributes to pacemaker activity in a permissive sense (Noma, 1996). I_f is an inward current activated by hyperpolarization and is often referred to as the pacemaker current. While there is little doubt that I_f contributes substantially to pacemaker activity (especially in Purkinje fibers), there is significant controversy about the predominance of I_f in SA node cells (DiFrancesco, 1995; Vassale, 1995; Noma, 1996). The key aspects of debate are whether the I_f activation only occurs appreciably at E_m more negative than the pacemaker range, and also whether the activation is sufficiently fast (especially at the positive end of their activation range). While I_f may be minor in true primary pacemaker cells at the core of the SA node (with most negative $E_m = -60$), it may be more

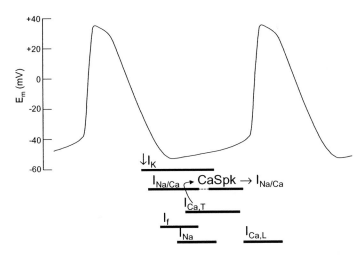

Figure 46. Currents contributing to pacemaker activity in nodal cells (SA or AV). The schematic shows that declining outward I_K and inward I_f, $I_{Na/Ca}$, $I_{Ca,T}$, $I_{Ca,L}$, and I_{Na} can all make contributions. Background inward current and a sustained inward current activated by depolarization may also be involved (see text).

important in peripheral nodal cells and/or with the normal degree of sympathetic tone that the SA node receives *in vivo*. I_f is also more generally accepted to play an important role in Purkinje fiber pacemaking. Note that these subsidiary (slower) pacemakers are normally suppressed (or overdriven) by the SA node. They only become the functional cardiac pacemaker when the more primary pacemakers are non-functional (e.g. sinus block, AV block).

Nodal cells and Purkinje fibers also have much higher $I_{Ca,T}$ density than do most ventricular myocytes and the activation E_m range for this channel is in the pacemaker range (Fig 40C). Thus $I_{Ca,T}$ contributes inward current toward the pacemaker depolarization, and 40 μM [Ni] which blocks $I_{Ca,T}$ rather selectively can slow pacemaker activity (Hagiwara *et al.*, 1988; Zhou & Lipsius, 1994). $I_{Ca,L}$ may also participate in pacemaker activity, but with the relatively positive E_m for activation this is probably only relevant in the latter part of pacemaking. On the other hand, the regenerative activation of $I_{Ca,L}$ is responsible for the upstroke of the AP in nodal cells (just as I_{Na} is in myocytes and Purkinje cells). The slower activation of $I_{Ca,L}$ and the lower overall current density compared to myocyte I_{Na} are responsible for the much slower rate of rise of nodal compared to ventricular AP (~5 *vs.* 200 V/sec).

As E_m declines faster than $[Ca]_i$, there is also an inward $I_{Na/Ca}$ component which may contribute to early pacemaking. In subsidiary pacemaker cells Zhou & Lipsius (1993) showed that there is a late component of diastolic depolarization which depends on both SR Ca release and $I_{Na/Ca}$. Hüser *et al.*(2000) provided evidence consistent with an intriguing local $[Ca]_i$ signaling model (Fig 46). The activation of $I_{Ca,T}$ may raise local $[Ca]_i$ sufficiently to trigger local SR Ca release events (Ca sparks, see Chapters 7 & 8). This local amplification of $[Ca]_i$ increases inward $I_{Na/Ca}$ (Ca efflux). This may occur late in diastolic depolarization because of recovery times required for either $I_{Ca,T}$ or the SR Ca release channel (see Chapters 5-9).

In nodal cells which show slowly rising APs, I_{Ca} (rather than I_{Na}) is the primary current responsible for the upstroke of the AP. These cells do have Na channels (Muramatsu *et al.*,

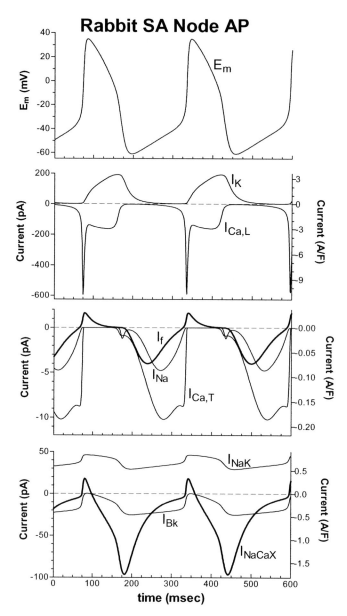

Figure 47. Calculated E_m and ionic currents during rabbit SA node APs, done using the Demir *et al.* (1994, 1999) model. I_{Bk} is a composite background current, corresponding to Ca, Na & K leak currents.

1996), but since E_m never gets very negative, they are mostly inactivated. The few Na channels available, can contribute to the inward currents associated with diastolic depolarization (Fig 47). However, based on pacemaker TTX sensitivity this may only be in perinodal cells with relatively negative E_m (Li *et al.*, 1997a; Kodama *et al.*, 1997). Figures 45 and 47 show that in SA nodal cells I_{Na} density is >1000 times less than in ventricular myocytes and >50 times less than $I_{Ca,L}$.

Guo *et al.* (1995) also reported a sustained inward current which is activated by depolarization in the range of the pacemaker potential. This may be distinct from I_{Ca} or the background inward current (I_{Bk} in Fig 47) which reverses at –21 mV (Hagiwara *et al.*, 1992; Noma, 1996). This I_{Bk} may be a relatively non-selective Na, Ca, K conductance (Demir *et al.*, 1994). It is not entirely clear yet how these inward currents contribute to pacemaker activity.

In conclusion there are multiple, overlapping and redundant currents involved in cardiac pacemaker activity. There is a hierarchy where the SA node is normally the primary or fastest pacemaker, but if the SA node fails to activate the rest of the heart, there are other normally slower pacemakers which can take over this role. These latent or subsidiary pacemakers exist in regions near the SA node, in the atria, AV node (and valves) and in the His-Purkinje system. Even ventricular myocytes can exhibit spontaneous pacemaker activity under unusual circumstances (particularly when sympathetic activity is very high). The differing balances of pacemaker mechanisms in different regions also provides a different sort of fail-safe, because agents which abolish SA node function may have little impact on other pacemakers.

EARLY AND DELAYED AFTERDEPOLARIZATIONS

Two AP aberrations that can be pro-arrhythmic are EADs and DADs (Cranefield & Aronson, 1988). These are usually categorized by the take-off potential (see Fig 48). If E_m has already returned to the diastolic E_m prior to the depolarization it is a DAD, whereas if it takes off (net depolarization) from somewhere on the plateau or late repolarization phase it is an EAD. These are also called triggered activities, because they depend on prior stimulation.

Early Afterdepolarizations (EADs)

EADs are more prone to occur with prolonged APDs. This can happen with bradycardia or partial inhibition of K channels. The latter can happen as a consequence of hypokalemia (which reduces outward I_{K1} and I_{Kr}), pharmacological action (e.g. K channel blocker) or congenital channel defects (long QT linked mutations which alter I_{Na}, I_{Kr} and I_{Ks}). Midmyocardial (or M) cells are particularly prone to EADs because of their long APD (Nuss *et al.*, 1999). EADs can occur at either the plateau range of E_m or in late repolarization. It is likely that those that occur at plateau E_m are attributable to reactivation of Ca channels, which can partially recover during very long APs, especially as [Ca]$_i$ declines (January & Riddle, 1989; Shorofsky & January, 1992; Luo & Rudy, 1994b; Sipido *et al.*, 1995a). That is, as E_m falls into the range of I_{Ca} window current, Ca channels recover such that they can cause depolarization.

EADs which occur late in repolarization (e.g. below –40 mV) are not due to reactivation of I_{Ca} because the Ca channels which recovered from inactivation during the AP would not be activated at this negative E_m (Fig 40C). EADs occurring in this E_m range may be due to Ca-activated currents, and as such have more in common mechanistically with DADs discussed below. Nuss *et al.* (1999) also reported spontaneous depolarizations (especially in heart failure) which were [Ca]$_i$-independent, but of unknown basis.

Delayed Afterdepolarizations (DADs)

DADs are most frequently observed under conditions that increase cellular and SR Ca loading. The high SR Ca load and [Ca]$_i$ cause apparently spontaneous SR Ca release events

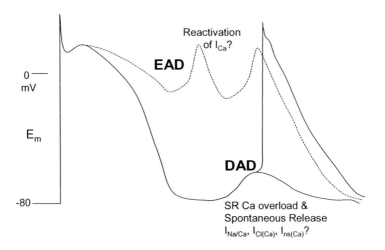

Figure 48. Afterdepolarizations in cardiac myocytes. This schematic shows fundamental differences in early- and delayed afterdepolarizations (EADs & DADs) and the likely underlying mechanisms.

which elevate $[Ca]_i$ and activate $[Ca]_i$-dependent currents. I say "apparently spontaneous" because the events are probably stochastic (making them seem random or spontaneous), but we now know that elevated $[Ca]_i$ and SR Ca load increase their probability. There is also a delay in the availability of SR Ca release events after prior activation (Satoh *et al.*, 1997), explaining why DADs typically occur after a finite time of repolarization. Digitalis glycosides, which block Na/K-ATPase and cause cellular Na and thus Ca loading, are a common mode of induction of DADs (Rosen *et al.*, 1973a; Ferrier & Moe, 1973). β-adrenergic agonists which stimulate both I_{Ca} and SR Ca uptake can also increase the probability of DADs (Belardinelli & Isenberg, 1983a).

The elevation of $[Ca]_i$ activates a transient inward current (I_{ti}) in voltage clamp studies (Lederer & Tsien, 1976; Kass *et al.*, 1978). Without voltage clamp this inward current would depolarize the membrane transiently, causing a DAD. There are three potential candidates for the Ca-activated inward I_{ti}, namely $I_{Na/Ca}$, $I_{Cl(Ca)}$ and $I_{ns(Ca)}$. Most investigators find no evidence for significant contribution of $I_{ns(Ca)}$ to I_{ti} or DADs in ventricular myocytes, but there is evidence for $I_{Cl(Ca)}$ and extensive data supporting a major role of $I_{Na/Ca}$ (Fedida *et al.*, 1987b; Laflamme & Becker, 1996; Zygmunt *et al.*, 1998; Schlotthauer & Bers, 2000). Kimura (1988) concluded that 85% of the I_{ti} was attributable to $I_{Na/Ca}$ (at -80 mV and $[Ca]_i = 0.5$ μM). Zygmunt *et al.* (1998) attributed 60% of I_{ti} to $I_{Na/Ca}$ and 40% to $I_{Cl(Ca)}$ in dog ventricular myocytes, but in rabbit we find I_{ti} to be almost exclusively $I_{Na/Ca}$ (Schlotthauer & Bers, 2000; Schlotthauer *et al.*, 2000).

It is important to consider not only the I_{ti}, but the amount of depolarization that it produces. E_{Cl} is typically -50 or -55 mV. Thus, while $I_{Cl(Ca)}$ is inward at -80 mV, it will become smaller as depolarization occurs, because the driving force would be reduced by 50% by a 12 mV depolarization. This will limit the ability of $I_{Cl(Ca)}$ to produce robust DADs. At high $[Ca]_i$ the value of $E_{Na/Ca}$ is positive (Fig 43) so this argument is not as relevant for $I_{Na/Ca}$. In addition, we find that the depolarization induced by rapid caffeine-induced SR Ca release can trigger an AP, even when $I_{Cl(Ca)}$ is blocked by niflumate (Schlotthauer & Bers, 2000). Moreover, blocking

Na/Ca exchange by replacing Na with Li completely blocks depolarization (although $I_{Cl(Ca)}$ and $I_{ns(Ca)}$ could still function). In conclusion, ventricular DADs are primarily due to $I_{Na/Ca}$, with $I_{Cl(Ca)}$ contributing somewhat less (especially near threshold) and $I_{ns(Ca)}$ is probably unimportant.

In heart failure the Na/Ca exchanger is upregulated and I_{K1} is decreased (Studer *et al.*, 1994; Beuckelmann *et al.*, 1993; Kääb *et al.*, 1996; Pogwizd *et al.*, 1999). The greater Na/Ca exchange increases the inward $I_{Na/Ca}$ for any given SR Ca release. The reduced I_{K1} destabilizes the resting E_m and allows a given inward current to more readily trigger an AP. This is the likely basis for increased triggered arrhythmias in heart failure (see pg 299 & 322). Indeed, in the human, triggered arrhythmias above (plus possibly abnormal automaticity) are responsible for initiation of almost all arrhythmias in non-ischemic heart failure and ~50% of those in ischemic heart failure (Pogwizd *et al.*, 1992, 1997, 1998). Thus nonreentrant mechanisms are likely to account for initiation of most arrhythmias in patients with heart failure.

REENTRY OF EXCITATION

While reentry may only initiate a minority of arrhythmias, it is the main mechanism responsible for the subsequent faulty propagation of the cardiac impulse leading to ventricular tachycardia and fibrillation. I will not discuss the complexities of this issue in any detail here, but simply indicate the classic picture of reentry and of spiral waves in the genesis and propagation of reentrant arrhythmias.

Figure 49A shows a multicellular conduction pathway around an anatomical obstruction (e.g. a blood vessel). The impulse goes around the ring in both directions. When the wavefronts meet head-on, they annihilate each other because the previously activated tissue (well behind both fronts) is refractory. This is a benefit of the long cardiac AP. This prevents propagation from jumping ahead to re-excite tissue behind the opposing wavefront. Several pathophysiological conditions set the scene for reentry in this situation (Fig 49B). There must be unidirectional conduction block, often due to decremental conduction approaching an inexcitable core from one side. Reduced or heterogeneous refractory period (due to short APD) and slowed conduction can also facilitate the appearance of reentry. Now as the same impulse approaches it can travel down one branch but dies out going down the other (decremental conduction and inexcitable core). One can think of this as a progressive decrease in space constant (λ) such that propagation is extremely weak near the inexcitable core. This time when the normal impulse reaches the annihilation point (from Fig 49A) the impulse proceeds through. Now it can reach the damaged region from the other side and can jump the inexcitable gap (unidirectional block) and re-excite the tissue on the other side. Here one can consider that λ is much longer when it gets to the inexcitable gap from this side, and so can bring cells on the other side to threshold for an AP. Since conduction to that point has been slowed (and especially if refractory periods are short) the impulse may propagate retrograde, and go around the ring again. This can produce a continuing propagation around the ring (circus movement) and also branch off in other directions.

Spiral waves can be initiated by either a break in a propagating wavefront or crossing of fronts in cells and multicellular tissues (Lechleiter *et al.*, 1991; Davidenko *et al.*, 1992; Lipp & Niggli, 1993). Indeed, this is a general property of excitable media (Winfree, 1973). The break creates an edge of very high convex curvature which slows conduction due to the relatively large current sink to source ratio. This causes the wavefront to bend around this tip forming the

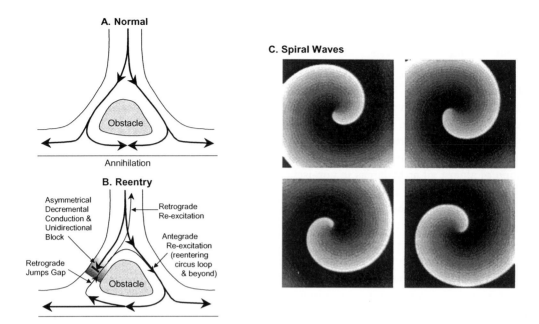

Figure 49. Reentrant excitation in heart. **A-B**. Classical model of reentry around an anatomical region. Unidirectional conduction block, decremental conduction and reduced refractory period in a damaged region contribute to increased probability of re-excitation. **C**. Spiral waves simulated in 2D cardiac tissue (3×3 cm) using a modified Luo-Rudy AP model at 4 successive 12 ms intervals. White is depolarized and the spiral period is 50 ms (B was generaously supplied by J.N. Weiss).

curved arm of a spiral wave (Fig 49C). Further out along the arm the current sink-source mismatch is less severe and the curvature decreases progressively, forming the increasing spiral pattern. The exact form of this spiral, its stability and how it moves in the tissue depends on the electrophysiological characteristics of the substrate, mass and geometry of the tissue (Weiss *et al.*, 1999). Indeed, the spirals can meander, break, up and form multiple spirals.

Thus alterations in myocyte properties as well as anatomical obstacles or architectural features (which can change with cardiac ischemia and remodeling) can contribute to the genesis and propagation of cardiac arrhythmias. It is important to extend the kind of understanding we are developing for electrophysiological properties of ion channels and single cells to increasingly complex tissues in approaching the real physiological situation. The focus in this chapter has been more on the understanding of normal properties of cardiac ion channels and fundamental electrophysiological properties of cardiac myocytes. It is important to keep in mind that the balance of currents during the AP is delicate, and that any increase in inward current will tend to prolong the APD and any increase in outward current will tend to shorten AP. Moreover, in different regions of the heart the AP is probably tuned for optimal physiological function and the AP characteristics are determined by the ion channels expressed, the cell characteristics and also the cells with which it is electrically connected. The information here sets the scene for more detailed discussion of Ca channels and transporters in the next few chapters.

D.M. Bers.
Excitation-Contraction Coupling and Cardiac Contractile Force.
2nd Ed., Kluwer Academic Publishers, Dordrecht, 2001

101

CHAPTER 5

Ca INFLUX VIA
SARCOLEMMAL Ca CHANNELS

Since the time of Ringer (1883) it has been known that extracellular [Ca] is important in cardiac muscle contraction. Cardiac Ca currents were first characterized as "slow inward current" or I_{si}, since several tens of msec were required for peak current to be achieved (e.g. Rougier *et al.*, 1969; Mascher & Peper, 1969; Beeler & Reuter, 1970; Ochi, 1970). Since the advent of the patch-clamp and isolated myocyte techniques it is now clear that Ca current (I_{Ca}) can reach a peak value in ~2-3 msec after a depolarization (e.g. see Fig 50). Thus the moniker of slow inward current seems inappropriate, although I_{Ca} could be considered secondary, in deference to I_{Na} which activates still faster than I_{Ca} (Fig 45). The inward I_{Ca} during the normal cardiac action potential contributes to the AP plateau and is also involved in the activation of contraction (directly and/or indirectly).

Ca CHANNEL TYPES

Hagiwara *et al.* (1975) were probably the first to demonstrate two classes of Ca channels in a single cell type. Nowycky *et al.* (1985) characterized three types of Ca channels in dorsal root ganglion cells, giving them names which have been adopted generally in the present nomenclature. L-type Ca channels are characterized by a **L**arge conductance (~25 pS in 110 mM Ba), **L**ong lasting openings (with Ba as the charge carrier), sensitivity to 1,4-dihydropyridines (DHPs) and activation at **L**arger depolarizations (i.e. at more positive E_m). T-type channels are characterized by a **T**iny conductance (~8 pS in 110 mM Ba), **T**ransient openings, insensitivity to DHPs, and activation at more negative E_m. N-type Ca channels are **N**either T nor L, are predominantly found in **N**eurons, and are intermediate in conductance and voltage dependence.

There are also other Ca current types distinguished by electrophysiological and pharmacological phenotype (e.g. P/Q & R), which are more prominent in neurons and neuroendocrine cells. The T-type Ca channels are the only low-voltage-activated (LVA) type, while all of the other types are referred to as high-voltage-activated (HVA), although the E_m-dependence is not always as distinct as one would like. The ten different E_m-dependent Ca channel genes are indicated in Table 15, along with alternate names and properties.

This L, T, N classification is an oversimplification because there are large differences even among L-type channels. For example, ω-conotoxin can strongly inhibit neuronal L-type Ca channels, but not cardiac or skeletal muscle L-type channels (McCleskey *et al.*, 1987). In addition the activation and inactivation kinetics in skeletal muscle L-type channels are ~10-fold slower than in cardiac muscle (Bean, 1989). Discussion here will focus on the Ca channel types in heart, mainly L- and T-type (due to α_{1C}, α_{1D}, α_{1G} and α_{1H}).

Table 15

Ca channel Types

Isoform	Gene name	Type	Blockers	Tissue
α_{1A}	CACNA1A	P/Q	ω-agatoxin-IVA (<100 nM) ω-conotoxin-MVIIC (>100 nM)	Neurons
α_{1B}	CACNA1B	N	ω- conotoxin-GVIA (<100 nM)	Neurons
α_{1C}	CACNA1C	L	DHP, ΦAA, BTZ	Heart, brain, lung smooth muscle, endocrine
α_{1D}	CACNA1D	L	DHP, ΦAA, BTZ	Neurons, heart
α_{1E}	CACNA1E	R	100 μM Ni	Neurons, heart?
α_{1F}	CACNA1F	L?		?
α_{1S}	CACNA1S	L	DHP, ΦAA, BTZ	skeletal muscle
T-Type (LVA)				
α_{1G}	CACNA1G	T	Mibefradil, Ni (K_i =250 μM)	Neurons, cardiac Purkinje
α_{1H}	CACNA1H	T	Mibefradil, Ni (K_i =12 μM)	Heart, kidney, liver
α_{1I}	CACNA1I	T	Mibefradil, Ni (K_i =216 μM)	Neurons

DHP is dihydropyridine, ΦAA is phenylalkylamine (e.g. D600) and BTZ is benzothiazepine (e.g. diltiazem). Information in table is from various sources (e.g. Varadi *et al.*, 1999; Lee *et al.*, 1999b).

Cardiac muscle contains both L- and T-type Ca channels (e.g. see Fig 50 & Table 16), but not N-type channels (Bean, 1985, 1989; Nilius *et al.*, 1985). $I_{Ca,L}$ is ubiquitous in cardiac myocytes, whereas cardiac $I_{Ca,T}$ was first described in atrial cells (Fig 50A, Bean, 1985). In canine cardiac Purkinje cells there is robust $I_{Ca,T}$ (Fig 50B, Hirano *et al.*, 1989). For a test E_m of –20 mV $I_{Ca,L}$ and $I_{Ca,T}$ in Fig 50B are about equal, whereas at 0 mV peak $I_{Ca,L}$ is 3 times larger than $I_{Ca,T}$. L-type I_{Ca} appears to be prominent in all cardiac myocytes, whereas T-type I_{Ca} is much more variable. Figure 50C shows total I_{Ca} current-voltage relationships in four different cell types. The extent of the hump at negative E_m (about –40 mV) reflects the relative amount of $I_{Ca,T}$. Purkinje cells seem to have the most, while pacemaker and some atrial myocytes also have significant amounts (Hagiwara *et al.*, 1988; Bean, 1989), but the amount of $I_{Ca,T}$ in ventricular myocytes is either modest in guinea-pig (Mitra & Morad, 1986) or undetectable in bullfrog, calf, cat, rabbit, rat and ferret (Bean, 1989; Nuss and Houser, 1993; Yuan and Bers, 1994; Yuan *et al.*, 1996). Neonatal rat ventricular myocytes exhibit $I_{Ca,T}$ (Wetzel *et al.*, 1993; Gaughan *et al.*, 1998) and significant $I_{Ca,T}$ may reappear in ventricular myocytes during the development of ventricular hypertrophy in cat (Nuss and Houser, 1993) and rat (Martinez *et al.*, 1999).

Thus T-type current is typically small or absent in ventricular myocytes, but may be more prominent during development and hypertrophy. The relative prominence of $I_{Ca,T}$ in pacemaker and conducting cells, and its activation at E_m in the pacemaker range has led to suggestions and evidence for a role of $I_{Ca,T}$ in atrial pacemaking (see pg 94-96 and Hagiwara, 1988; Wu & Lipsius, 1990). Because $I_{Ca,T}$ is relatively small and inactivates very rapidly the total amount of Ca flux via $I_{Ca,T}$ is small compared to that via $I_{Ca,L}$ and negligible in most ventricular myocytes. This may reflect different functional roles, where $I_{Ca,L}$ is more involved in triggering SR Ca release and refilling SR Ca stores (see below), rather than pacemaking.

Since $I_{Ca,L}$ inactivation is Ca dependent (Kokubun & Irisawa, 1984; Lee et al.,1985; see pg 116-119) $I_{Ca,L}$ is transient and the kinetics can be confused with T type I_{Ca}. Therefore, L-type

A. Dog Atrium (115 mM Ba; Bean, 1985)

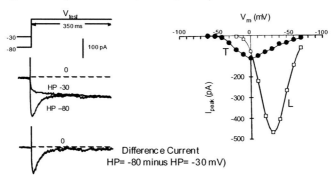

B. Dog Purkinje Fiber (2 mM Ca; Hirano et al., 1989)

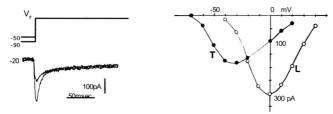

C. Several Species (Total I_Ca)

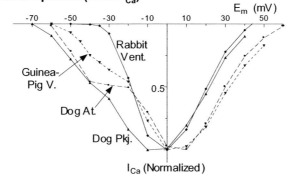

Figure 50. Voltage-dependence of whole cell L- and T-type Ca channel currents. **A.** Ba currents (with 115 mM Ba) induced by E_m steps to test potentials from holding potentials (HP) of –80 or –30 mV. The E_m protocol is shown in the top trace, currents in the middle trace, and the difference between these currents in the bottom panel. The peak I_{Ba} activated from –30 mV is attributed to L-type Ca channels (o) and the additional transient difference current activated from –80 mV (•) is attributed to T-type Ca channels (from Bean, 1985, with permission). **B.** Similar protocol to A, but in dog Purkinje cells and with 2 mM Ca as charge carrier (from Hirano *et al.*, 1989, with permission). The shifts in E_m between A and B are due to surface potential differences in 2 mM Ca *vs.* 115 mM Ba (see Fig 55, pg 115). **C.** Total I_{Ca} from several sources (HP = –80 to –100 mV), where the hump at –40 mV is due to T-type current and differs among the tissues and species studied. Dog Purkinje (from Hirano *et al.*, 1989) and rabbit ventricle (GM Briggs & DM Bers, unpublished) are in 2 mM Ca and dog atrium (from Bean, 1985) and guinea-pig ventricle (from Mitra & Morad, 1986) are in 5 mM Ca, but are shifted –10 mV to compensate for surface potential.

and T-type channels can be best distinguished when Ba is the charge carrier since L-channel inactivation is then rather slow (e.g. Fig 50A). Where T-type current is prominent, it can also be resolved by the difference in E_m-dependence (Fig 50). In cells which have substantial $I_{Ca,T}$ the current-voltage relationship (from holding E_m of –80 or –90 mV) also shows a prominent "shoulder" at negative E_m. While only T and L-type I_{Ca} is apparent in cardiac myocytes, N-, P/Q- or R currents can be seen in intracardiac neurons (Jeong & Wurster, 1997).

The cardiac cell types in which $I_{Ca,T}$ is more prominent also happen to be the cells which have less extensive T-tubules (see Table 1). It is not known explicitly whether T-type Ca channels are excluded from T-tubules, but L-type Ca channels in cardiac and skeletal muscle may be concentrated there (see Chapter 1). In general, unless otherwise specified below, Ca channels and I_{Ca} will refer to L-type Ca channels or $I_{Ca,L}$ for cardiac myocytes.

MOLECULAR CHARACTERIZATION OF Ca CHANNELS

L type Ca channels are characteristically sensitive to dihydropyridines (DHPs). Most DHPs act as Ca channel blockers or antagonists (e.g. nifedipine, nisoldipine and nitrendipine, isradipine), while some DHPs act as Ca channel agonists (e.g. Bay K 8644, but only the (-) enantiomer). The agonist agents appear to greatly prolong the open time of the channel (see Fig 61). The DHP-sensitivity of L-type Ca channels and high density of DHP receptors in skeletal muscle T-tubules were crucial to the initial extensive biochemical characterization and isolation of the L-type channel proteins from skeletal muscle (Curtis & Catterall, 1984; Borsotto *et al.*, 1984; Flockerzi *et al.*, 1986). Five protein subunits were found to constitute the skeletal muscle Ca channel (α_1, α_2, β, γ and δ) and all have been sequenced (Tanabe *et al.*, 1987; Ellis *et al.*, 1988; Ruth *et al.*, 1989; Jay *et al.*, 1990; Bosse *et al.*, 1990). The α_1 subunit of skeletal muscle (α_{1S}) is distinct from the cardiac channel clone (α_{1C} Mikami *et al.*, 1989). The α_1 subunit appears to bear the main known functional characteristics of these Ca channels. That is, the α_1 subunit bears the channel, the DHP, phenylalkylamine and benzothiazepine receptors (Galizzi *et al.*, 1986; Sharp *et al.*, 1987; Sieber *et al.*, 1987; Vaghy *et al.*, 1987; Striessnig *et al.*, 1990a,b) and may contain the sites phosphorylated by protein kinases A, CaMKII (Curtis & Catterall, 1985; Hosey *et al.*, 1986, 1987; Imagawa *et al.*, 1987a; Nastainczyk *et al.*, 1987) and protein kinase C (O'Callahan *et al.*, 1988). Transfection of DNA coding for the α_{1C} subunit into a cell line lacking the other subunits was sufficient to produce E_m-dependent I_{Ca} (Perez-Reyes *et al.*, 1989). Moreover, the α_1 subunit structure is very much like the E_m-dependent Na channel and tetrameric K channels in Fig 38. That is, α_{1C} has 4 homologous domains (I-IV), each of which has 6 transmembrane spans (S_1-S_6, with charged S_4) and pore loops between S_5 and S_6, and has a long carboxy tail (Fig 51). There are alternate splice variants of α_{1C} (reviewed in Bers & Perez-Reyes, 1999). There is also α_{1D} expressed in the heart (Takimoto *et al.*, 1997; Wyatt *et al.*, 1997), but it is not clear if there is functional consequence to α_{1D} *vs.* α_{1C} expression.

As for the E_m-dependent channels discussed in Chapter 4, Ca channels have the same repeating positive charge at every third amino acid for a stretch of 10-15 amino acids in each S_4 span. This is undoubtedly involved in the E_m-dependent gating of the Ca channels. There are differences in activation among different types of Ca channels, e.g. the skeletal muscle Ca channel (α_{1S}) activates very slowly in comparison to the cardiac α_{1C}. In studies with chimeric Ca channels Tanabe *et al.* (1991) found that differences in domain I between α_{1S} and α_{1C} could

Table 16
Properties of Cardiac L- and T-type Ca Channels

	L-type	T-type
Activation range		
5 mM Ca	Positive to −30 mV	Positive to −60 mV
110 mM Ba	Positive to −10 mV	Positive to −50 mV
Inactivation		
Range	Positive to −40 mV	−90 to −60 mV
Ca dependent	Yes	No
Voltage dependent	Slow	Fast
Tail deactivation	Fast	Slow
Conductance		
110 Ba	25 pS	8 pS
110 Ca	8 pS	8 pS
150 Na, EDTA	80 pS	50 pS
Mean open time	Typically <1 ms	Short, 1-2 ms
Kinetics (Ba)	Multiple bursts/pulse	1 burst per pulse, (inactivation)
Pharmacological sensitivity:		
Dihydropyridines	Yes	No
Cd	High	Low
Ni	Low	High
Isoproterenol	Yes	No
Excised patch	Loses activity	Retains activity

This tabulation is from Hess (1988) with values mostly obtained at room temperature.

explain this activation difference, while Spaetgens & Zamponi (1999) found domains II and III (& maybe IV) confer the more positive E_m-dependent inactivation of α_{1C} *vs.* α_{1E}.

Ellis *et al.* (1988) cloned and expressed the α_2 subunit and it is now clear that the α_2 and δ subunit are from the same $\alpha_2\delta$ gene (Jay *et al.*, 1991). However, the $\alpha_2\delta$ protein gets cleaved so that 2 different proteins were expected based on biochemical work. Normally the $\alpha_2\delta$ connection is by one or more disulfide links and the δ portion anchors the complex in the membrane (Fig 51). So far most work has been on one gene known to code $\alpha_2\delta$, but alternative splicing in different tissues gives rise to splice variants (Williams *et al.*, 1992; Kim *et al.*, 1992; Angelotti & Hofmann, 1996). The α_{2a} is predominant in skeletal muscle and α_{2b} in brain, whereas the α_{2c} and α_{2d} variants are most common in heart (and are slightly shorter). Klugbauer *et al.* (1999) recently found 2 more $\alpha_2\delta$ isoforms that are expressed primarily in brain.

When $\alpha_2\delta$ is coexpressed with α_{1C} there is a ~2-fold increase in expression of DHPR binding sites, gating currents, and ionic currents (Wei *et al.*, 1995; Singer *et al.*, 1991; Bangalore *et al.*, 1996). This may indicate that $\alpha_2\delta$ plays a role in the formation of functional channels at the plasma membrane surface. However, coexpression of $\alpha_2\delta$ also increases the apparent affinity of those channels for DHPs by 4-fold (Wei *et al.*, 1995) and accelerates channel opening and closing (Bangalore *et al.*, 1996; see review by Felix, 1999). The $\alpha_2\delta$ subunit may also directly bind drugs, such as the anticonvulsant, gabapentin (Gee *et al.*, 1996), but the therapeutic impact is unclear. Most of the δ component seems merely to anchor the $\alpha_2\delta$ subunit in the membrane (since other transmembrane spanning domains can substitute), whereas the heavily glycosylated extracellular α_2 domain seems to interact with the α_1 subunit, at least in domain III (Gurnett *et al.*, 1997; Felix *et al.*, 1997).

The γ subunit appears to be restricted to the skeletal muscle Ca channel (Ruth *et al.*, 1989; Jay *et al.*, 1990), but coexpression with α_{1S} can also increase DHP binding, and alter allosteric action of phenylalkylamines (Suh-Kim *et al.*, 1996). Although there is no evidence for a cardiac γ subunit, additional γ genes may be expressed in brain (Letts *et al.*, 1998).

There are four β subunit genes (β_1-β_4), but the main cardiac isoform is β_2. There is alternative splicing of β_2 exons near the amino terminus and in a central region near the α_1 interaction domain (Perez-Reyes & Schneider, 1995; De Waard *et al.*, 1994). Recent data suggests that the β_{2a} isoform is only expressed in brain (Qin *et al.*, 1998). β_3 and β_1 variants have also been detected in heart (Collin *et al.*, 1993; Hullin *et al.*, 1992). Northern analysis of rat and rabbit tissues indicates that β_2 mRNA is the most abundant β in heart, while β_3 is the most abundant in lung. A β_2 specific antibody also was able to immunoprecipitate 80% of the DHP binding sites from rabbit heart. Therefore β_2 is the predominant cardiac β.

Coexpression of β_2 with α_{1C} causes a 10-fold increase in current, accelerates activation and inactivation kinetics, shifts steady-state inactivation and greatly increases the number of high affinity DHP binding sites (Perez-Reyes *et al.*, 1992; Neely *et al.*, 1993; Mitterdorfer *et al.*, 1994). Phosphorylation of the β_2 subunit may also be involved in the β-adrenergic-induced increased in I_{Ca} (Haase *et al.*, 1993; Bünemann *et al.*, 1999). The β subunit may act in part like a molecular chaperone, helping nascent α_{1C} molecules to fold properly and reach the plasma membrane (Gao *et al.*, 1999). However, the β subunit may also facilitate pore opening (Costantin *et al.*, 1998; Yamaguchi *et al.*, 1998; Gerster *et al.*, 1999) and stabilize a state of the α_{1C} which has intrinsically higher DHP affinity (Mitterdorfer *et al.*, 1994, 1998).

Specific interaction domains between α_1 and β subunits have been elucidated (AID and BID in Fig 51; De Waard *et al.*, 1994; Pragnell *et al.*, 1994). The site on α_1 that interacts with β (AID) is in the loop between domain I and II. Splice variants of this loop may allow β's to interact differentially with the α_1 variants. The site on β which interacts with α_1 (BID) occurs just after a region in β_2 that is highly spliced, again, indicating functional variations in α_1-β subunit interactions. Indeed, splice variants of both this site and the amino terminus (β_{2a} *vs.* β_{2b}) can alter channel kinetics when co-expressed with α_{1E} (Olcese *et al.*, 1994; Qin *et al.*, 1996). One major difference between β_{2a} and β_{2b} is that only β_{2a} is palmitoylated. Mutation of the palmitoylated residues alters its interaction with the α subunit (Qin *et al.*, 1998; Chien *et al.*, 1996).

Neuronal N- and P-type Ca channels are also strongly modulated by G-proteins binding to the AID region of α_{1A} and α_{1B}, where they interact with β subunits (see Dolphin, 1998; Ikeda & Dunlap, 1999 for more detailed discussion and references). Stimulation of various 7 transmembrane spanning receptors activates heterotrimeric G-proteins which release their $\beta\gamma$ subunit. This $G_{\beta\gamma}$ binds to the I-II loop of these Ca channel α_1 subunits (at least partly displacing the bound Ca channel β subunit) and causes depression of I_{Ca} activation rate and amplitude. This depressant effect on I_{Ca} (which may be tonic) can be relieved by strong depolarization, resulting in an E_m-dependent facilitation of neuronal I_{Ca}. This may enhance Ca influx in neurons firing at higher frequencies. Large depolarizations appear to cause dissociation of $G_{\beta\gamma}$ from the Ca channel α_1 subunit, relieving the inhibition. G-protein dependent inhibition (and E_m-dependent

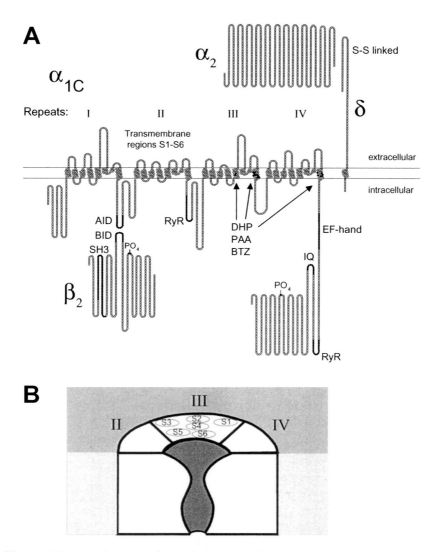

Figure 51. **A.** Schematic diagram and subunit structure of the cardiac L-type Ca channel. **A.** Each ball represents one amino acid. The main α_1 subunit has the four domains (I-IV), each with 6 transmembrane spans (S_1-S_6) and a pore loop (as in Fig 38). Ca channel antagonists dihydropyridines, phenylalkylamines and benzothiazapines (DHP, PAA & BTZ) bind to the $IIIS_5$, $IIIS_6$ & IVS_6 regions. Possible interaction sites between the α_1 subunit and the ryanodine receptor (RyR) are indicated, as well as a potentially important phosphorylation site (PO_4), an EF-hand region and an IQ motif where calmodulin binds. The β_2 subunit is cytosolic, can be phosphorylated (PO_4), has an apparent SH3 domain and interacts with α_1 at the α- and β-interaction domains (AID, BID). The $\alpha_2\delta$ subunit is coded by one gene, but then cleaved, but still interconnected by sulfhydryl bridges. **B.** A cutaway view of how the α_1 subunits may encircle a central pore (see also Fig 38 & 39; drawings kindly supplied by E. Perez-Reyes).

relief) does not occur appreciably in cardiac I_{Ca}, but this effect emphasizes the potential modulatory roles for Ca channel subunits.

Other sites on the α_{1C} subunit shown in Fig 51 (to be discussed in greater detail later) are possible interacting sites for the cardiac ryanodine receptor (II-III loop and carboxy tail), phosphorylation sites on the carboxy tail (Ser-1928), EF-hand and IQ motifs (involved in Ca-dependent inactivation) and sites where the 3 main classes of Ca channel blockers (DHPs, phenylalkylamines and benzothiazepine) bind ($IIIS_5$, $IIIS_6$ and IVS_6). In heart the α_{1C}, $\alpha_2\delta$ and β_2 subunits are about 200, 175 and 60 kDa respectively (with the α_2-δ split at about 150 α_2, 30 δ).

The three T-type Ca channels α_{1G}, α_{1H} and α_{1I} have recently been cloned and expressed (Perez-Reyes *et al.*, 1998; Cribbs *et al.*, 1998; Lee *et al.*, 1999a,b). These channels are structurally very similar to L-type Ca channels (e.g. I-IV domains, S_1-S_6 transmembrane spans and pore loop). The sequence is most highly conserved in the S_4 and pore loop regions. However, the overall sequence identity between T-type and any high voltage activated Ca channel is low (<15%). Notably, the pore loop in domain III has an aspartate rather than the glutamate which is in all four domains of all other Ca channels forming the EEEE locus which is critical for permeation (see pg 117) and all 3 T-type Ca channels have SKD in this spot rather than TFE in α_{1C}). Two motifs present in α_{1C} that are not found in α_{1H} are the β subunit interaction region (I-II loop) and the putative EF hand which might be involved in Ca-dependent inactivation (below). The latter is not surprising because $I_{Ca,T}$ does not exhibit Ca-dependent inactivation. Mibefradil is a somewhat selective $I_{Ca,T}$ inhibitor, with a K_i ~1 µM for all three $I_{Ca,T}$ types (about ten times lower than for $I_{Ca,L}$ block, Cribbs *et al.*, 1998). Ni also blocks $I_{Ca,T}$, but α_{1H} is particularly sensitive (Table 15), whereas α_{1G} and α_{1I} have Ni-sensitivity that is not much different from that of $I_{Ca,L}$ (Lee *et al.*, 1999b). Since the $I_{Ca,T}$ in cardiac pacemaker cells is highly Ni-sensitive, it seems likely to be mediated by α_{1H}. On the other hand, $I_{Ca,T}$ in Purkinje cells in the heart is less Ni-sensitive, and may reflect α_{1G}.

Messenger RNA for both α_{1G} and α_{1H} are found in human heart. Although α_{1H} was cloned from an adult human heart library, much more mRNA is expressed in kidney and liver (Cribbs *et al.*, 1998). Future studies are required to determine which of these T channel subtypes is expressed in pacemaker tissue and which is expressed in vascular smooth muscle. While $I_{Ca,T}$ seems to be recapitulated by expression of the α_1 subunit alone, it is not yet known whether auxiliary subunits contribute to $I_{Ca,T}$ function (as seen for other Ca channels). While a small amount of α_{1E} may be expressed in atria and contribute to $I_{Ca,T}$ (Piedras-Rentería *et al.*, 1997), the significance of this contribution to I_{Ca} in heart remains to be clarified.

Ca CHANNEL SELECTIVITY AND PERMEATION

McCleskey and Almers (1985) determined the narrowest point in the Ca channel pore to be ~6 Å diameter since tetramethylammonium can permeate. Thus, the Ca channel must exert selectivity by means other than exclusion by size. Hagiwara *et al.* (1974) observed that Ba current through Ca channels was greater than Ca current, but that the Ba current was more susceptible to block by Co. They concluded that this was due to competition at a binding site within the channel, with a weaker affinity for Ba than for Ca, such that Co would prevent Ba current more effectively. This also explains the higher control Ba *vs.* Ca current. Since Ba doesn't "stick" as well in the channel, it can go through more quickly.

Hess *et al.* (1986) measured cardiac Ca channel selectivity based on current reversal potentials in asymmetric salt solutions (see Table 17). They also reported single channel conductances for several permeant ions. In the absence of divalent cations Ca channels carry very large nonspecific monovalent cation current (I_{NS}, typically inward Na current). Na does not

Table 17
Selectivity of Cardiac L-type Ca Channel

Ion	P_{ion}/P_{Cs}	Single-channel Conductance (pS)[†]	Unhydrated Radius (Å)
Ca	4200	9	0.99
Sr	2800	9	1.13
Ba	1700	25	1.35
Li	9.9	45	0.60
Na	3.6	85	0.95
K	1.4	-	1.33
Cs	1.0	-	1.69
Mg	~0	-	0.65

*Selectivities as permeability ratios based on reversal potential measurements by Hess *et al.*, 1986, with values from Tsien *et al.*, 1987. [†]From Hess *et al.*, 1986 with 110 mM divalent and 150 mM monovalent (the latter is at pH 9.0 to limit proton block of the channel, Prod'hom *et al.*, 1987).

compete very well for the Ca-selective site in the pore. Indeed, as $[Ca]_o$ is increased Na current through cardiac and skeletal Ca channels is blocked by Ca with a K_d ~1 µM [Ca] (see Fig 52A; Almers & McCleskey, 1984; Almers *et al.*, 1984, Hess & Tsien, 1984). Mg also blocks I_{NS} (K_i ~50 µM) and it may be noted that one must chelate both extracellular Ca and Mg to measure unblocked I_{NS} (e.g. with EDTA, rather than EGTA). As $[Ca]_o$ rises further in Fig 52A, I_{Ca} is not measurable until nearly mM $[Ca]_o$ and saturates with a K_d ~14 mM (Hess *et al.*, 1986). This disparity is consistent with more than one Ca binding site is in the Ca channel.

The anomalous mole fraction effect is a related phenomenon which is also consistent with more than one site in the channel (Yue & Marbán, 1987; Friel & Tsien, 1989). This effect is where the current through a Ca channel is paradoxically smaller in mixtures of Ca and Ba (at constant total [Ca]+[Ba]) than in either ion alone (Hess & Tsien, 1984).

These types of experiments led Almers & McCleskey (1984) and Hess & Tsien (1984) to propose a model for Ca channel permeation which includes 2 Ca selective sites in the permeation pathway (Fig 52C). The potential energy ($\Delta G/RT$) for a Ca or Na ion as it goes through an unoccupied Ca channel are indicated by the solid (Ca) and dashed curves (Na). The two energy wells correspond to 2 Ca binding sites. Ca can enter one site and change the energy profile (due to its two positive charges). Ca can also move between these sites more easily than it can escape the pore. When a Na ion enters the open site, it will not dwell long due to electrostatic repulsion and lower affinity. Thus, Na current is blocked by µM [Ca]. Single occupancy by Ca would also decrease the affinity for Ca at the other site from K_d ~0.5 µM to ~10 mM. If another Ca ion does enter the other site, the repulsive forces are very strong, so there is a 50% chance that the first Ca ion will rapidly leave the pore (even at E_m=0). With the usual strong inwardly directed electrochemical driving force for Ca entry (E_{Ca} ~ +120 mV), this will result in a rapid inward Ca current. In this way the strong repulsion of double occupancy overcomes the anticipated slow off-rate expected of a high affinity site and allows both rapid ion flux through the channel and high divalent cation selectivity. Indeed, the high Ca flux rates do not occur until mM [Ca], where double occupancy of the channel is expected with this model (see Fig 52B). More than 2 binding sites in the pore might even help to explain some results (Yue & Marbán, 1990).

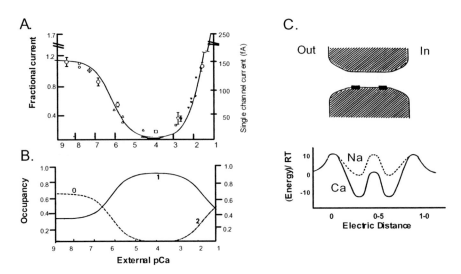

Figure 52. Ca channel permeation. **A.** Increasing [Ca]$_o$ blocks Na current through the Ca channel at K$_d$ ~1 μM. At higher [Ca]$_o$ (mM) the current is carried by Ca ions. **B.** fractional occupancy of the Ca channel by none (0), 1 or 2 ions. Ca current increases when the channel is occupied by 2 Ca ions. **C.** Schematic diagram of the Ca channel, showing two binding sites and the energy profile for a single Ca or Na ion as they traverse the channel where the abscissa is the electrical distance across the membrane (from Almers & McCleskey, 1984, with permission).

This strict sequential site model is heuristic, but similar characteristics can also be obtained with a single selective site and repulsive interactions with an incoming Ca ion (Armstrong & Neyton, 1992; Dang & McCleskey, 1998). Indeed, the key molecular site in the selectivity filter is a ring of glutamate residues, one from each pore loop known as the EEEE locus (EI, EII, EIII & EIV, Yang *et al.*, 1993) . The carboxyl groups of these glutamates could wrap around Ca in a similar manner to the 4 carboxyl groups of EGTA. These glutamates were individually changed to glutamines in heterologously expressed α$_{1C}$, neutralizing the negative charges (Yang *et al.*, 1993; Ellinor *et al.*, 1995). This resulted in different shifts in the [Ca]$_o$ required to half-block I$_{NS}$ carried by Li (Fig 53A). These 4 glutamates were not equivalent and mutating two simultaneously resulted in an even more dramatic shifts in Ca block (nearly 1000-fold). Since single point mutations alter K$_d$(Ca) there cannot be 2 discrete independent sites. Additional mutagenesis studies of the EEEE locus (Ellinor *et al.*, 1995; Chen *et al.*, 1996a; Chen & Tsien, 1997) have provided much additional detailed information and insight. Figure 53B shows how the EEEE locus might provide coordinated Ca ion binding in the pore (Varadi *et al.*, 1999). These 4 glutamates probably do not form two discrete binding sites, but rather a more complex domain that can bind one Ca with high affinity (K$_d$ ~1 μM) or two Ca ions with low affinity (K$_d$ ~10 mM; Yang *et al.*, 1993; McCleskey, 1999). While the molecular details may be getting a bit clearer, the functional behavior is not grossly different from that envisioned in the two-site models. That is, a negatively charged region creates high affinity Ca binding, and approach of another Ca ion (favored by other negative charges) stimulates the first Ca to move

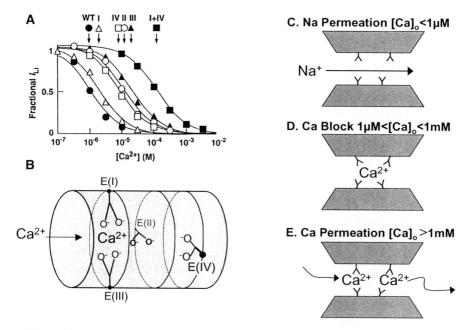

Figure 53. Critical pore glutamates and Ca channel permeation. **A.** Shifts in the [Ca]$_o$-dependence of block of Li current (I$_{Li}$) through wild type (WT) rabbit α_{1C} Ca channel expressed in *Xenopus* oocytes. Mutant channels were also expressed in which each of the P-loop glutamates in the EEEE locus (I, II, III, IV) were substituted by glutamine as well as a simultaneous swap in I & IV (data from Yang *et al.*, 1993, with permission). **B.** Depiction of how the EEEE locus may coordinately bind Ca in the pore (based on Yang *et al.*, 1993 and Varadi *et al.*, 1999). **C-E.** Schematic of Na permeation at low [Ca]$_o$, block by 1-500 μM [Ca]$_o$ (one Ca in channel) and high Ca flux at mM [Ca]$_o$ when the channel is doubly occupied.

on down the channel (Fig 53C-E). Moreover, Ca will be much more effective than Na in driving off Ca (or blocking Na flux).

Nonner & Eisenberg (1998) proposed a continuous Poisson-Nernst-Planck (PNP) model of Ca channel permeation, using a rigid electronegative tube, rather than the localized binding sites and discrete steps of the other models above. Remarkably, this channel exhibited Ca-selectivity and Ca block of Na current. While it could not readily explain the non-equivalent effects of different glutamates in the EEEE locus (McCleskey, 1999), it is wise to consider these challenging problems from multiple perspectives.

There is flickering block of Ca channels by protons (Prod'hom *et al.*, 1987) and certain multivalent cations (Lansman *et al.*, 1986). If the blocking events are fast the single channel conductance simply looks reduced, because the individual blocking events are not resolvable. This is true at neutral pH for I$_{NS}$, and raising pH to 9 can allow the full 85 pS conductance to be observed. This flickering block may reflect transient binding of these competing ions to the sites in the pore and has allowed estimates of on- and off-rates in some of the studies cited above. The block of Ca channels by other multivalent ions can also indicate the selectivity of the sites in the channel. Certain ions may also block the channel, but still pass through. The voltage dependence for the relief of block can indicate whether the ion can be "forced" through the channel (e.g. at large negative E$_m$), or must exit from the same side it entered (Lansman *et al.*, 1986). It is interesting that Mg can readily permeate skeletal muscle Ca channels, but is almost impermeant in the cardiac channel (Almers & Palade, 1981; Hess *et al.*, 1986). This permeation difference is particularly striking because the 4 P-loop cores are identical between α_{1S}, α_{1C} and α_{1D}. There may also be more subtle species differences in cardiac Ca channel permeation which cannot be attributed to P-loop differences (Yuan *et al.*, 1996). Thus, there are likely to be more factors involved in permeation than just the core P-loop regions. In symmetrical solutions the Ca channel exhibits a very linear current-voltage relationship (Rosenberg *et al.*, 1986) indicating that the permeation pathway is functionally symmetrical.

It is worth considering what the single Ca channel current and conductance are under physiological conditions. We often consider ion channel conductance to be a relatively linear function of permeant ion concentration. In the limit this is not the case for any channel, partly due to limitations created by ion binding in the pore. However, it can also be due to access resistance; i.e. as the current increases there is depletion of ions at one mouth of the channel and accumulation at the other (Peskoff & Bers, 1988; Bers & Peskoff, 1991). This effect is slightly mitigated by the local potentials created by the ion depletion and accumulation and any fixed negative charges on or near the channel (or an applied field). That is, a local depletion of $[Ca]_o$ outside a Ca channel will create a local negative potential which helps draw Ca toward the channel mouth from the medium. The maximal flux through a channel would be $2\pi rD[X]_o$, where X is the permeant ion, r is the channel radius (e.g. 0.3 nm) and D is the diffusion coefficient ($\sim 10^{-5}$ and $\sim 3 \times 10^{-6}$ cm^2/s for Na and Ca respectively). For a narrow Na or K channel (at 140 mM) maximal theoretical current would be ~ 50 pA. For a Ca channel at 2 and 110 mM $[Ca]_o$ maximal current would be 0.4 and 24 pA respectively (Peskoff & Bers, 1988). Since single channel I_{Ca} of 0.2 pA occur physiologically in cardiac Ca channels, significant Ca depletion occurs at the outer channel mouth and accumulation at the inner mouth (Bers & Peskoff, 1991; see also Chapter 8, Fig 118, pg 222).

Having said this, Ca depletion/accumulation is not the normal limiting factor for I_{Ca}, especially at high $[Ca]_o$. Single channel I_{Ca} is normally measured at various E_m to measure the channel conductance (the slope in Fig 54A; Yue & Marbán, 1990). Conductance measurements at various $[Ba]_o$ indicate that the conductance saturates at high $[Ba]_o$ (although depletion would be less severe). Figure 54B-C shows mean Ba and Ca conductance compiled by McDonald *et al.* (1994) from 24 different studies of this sort (13 in cardiac and 11 in smooth muscle). Maximal Ca and Ba conductance are 10 and 27 pS, with half-maximal values at 4 mM $[Ca]_o$ and 10 mM $[Ba]_o$. These K_m values may be related to the affinity of the binding site in the channel in the doubly occupied state (Fig 53E). Notably, conductance for Na (which does not bind strongly) is 10 times higher than for Ca (or 20 times if we count ions rather than charge). Thus, the key feature in limiting Ca (or Ba) flux through the channel is binding in the channel, or more accurately the rate of Ca dissociation from the binding site(s) in the channel.

In discussing Ca fluxes it is common to infer Ca flux by integrating the Ca current. In general this is reasonable when one has taken the care to block all other currents. The implicit assumption is that all of the I_{Ca} is carried by Ca ions. For much of the voltage range this is not a bad assumption, especially as P_{Ca}/P_{Cs} is >1000. Figure 54D shows currents carried by Ca and Cs according to the Goldman-Hodgkin-Katz (GHK) current equation

A. Unitary Ba Currents

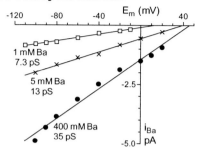

B. Ca Channel Conductance

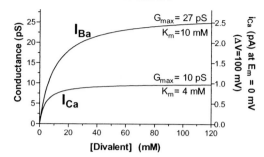

C. Ca Channel Conductance

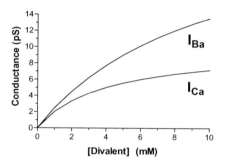

D. Ca Channel Current (GHK)

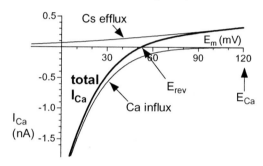

Figure 54. Ca channel conductance and I_{Ca} near E_{rev}. **A**. Single channel Ba currents at different E_m values and $[Ba]_o$ (redrawn from Yue & Marbán, 1990), where linear regressions yield the indicated conductances. **B**. Single channel Ca and Ba conductance as a function of $[Ca]_o$ and $[Ba]_o$. The curves are fits to data compiled by McDonald *et al.* (1994) from 24 different studies (using $G=G_{max}/(1+K_m/[X])$, where X is Ca or Ba). The right ordinate assumes ohmic conductance and a driving force of 100 mV (as would be the case for E_m =0 mV and E_{Ca} = 100 mV). **C**. Same data as B, expanded to emphasize the physiological range. **D**. Whole myocyte I_{Ca} calculated from the GHK equation (see text) with $P_{Ca} = 4\times10^{-5}$ cm/s and $P_{Ca}/P_{Cs} = 1000$ for a 150 pF cell. Ca influx and Cs efflux are shown separately along with total Ca channel current.

$$I_{Ca} = FkE_m \left\{ \frac{4P_{Ca}([Ca]_o - [Ca]_i \exp(-2kE_m))}{1 - \exp(2kE_m)} + \frac{P_{Cs}([Cs]_i - [Cs]_o \exp(-kE_m))}{1 - \exp(-kE_m)} \right\} \quad (1)$$

where $k = 1/(25.7 \text{ mV})$ and $P_{Ca}/P_{Cs} = 1000$. The left term is the Ca flux and the right term is the Cs flux. There will be little error in assuming that I_{Ca} at +10 mV is all Ca influx (Ca influx would be underestimated by only 4%). However, at the I_{Ca} reversal potential ($E_{rev} = +52$ mV) one would assume zero Ca influx, whereas the actual Ca influx is 11% of the value which occurs at +10 mV. E_{rev} is the E_m where Ca influx is exactly balanced by Cs efflux through the channel. This is distinct from the Ca equilibrium potential ($E_{Ca} = +125$ mV) where there would be no net Ca influx. Zhou & Bers (2000) demonstrated just this sort of Ca entry via I_{Ca} at E_m above E_{rev} (by measuring Ca channel influx with a fluorescent indicator while measuring I_{Ca} by voltage clamp). While this was an expected finding based on GHK theory, it should also be noted that the Ca channel does not truly behave ideally with respect to GHK assumptions. This is due in part to the binding sites in the pore and the ion-ion interactions which are known to exist. Ca influx above the E_{rev} for I_{Ca} is important to keep in mind experimentally, since some investigators have depolarized to E_{rev} with the intention of stopping Ca influx (e.g. in E-C coupling studies).

NUMBERS OF Ca CHANNELS

Schwartz *et al.* (1985) estimated that there are 30-50 times as many specific DHP receptors in frog skeletal muscle as functional L-type Ca channels. In isolated mammalian ventricular myocytes, the density of L-type Ca channels has been estimated from single channel and whole cell I_{Ca} measurements to be 3-5/μm^2 (McDonald *et al.*, 1986; Tsien *et al.*, 1983). Bers & Stiffel (1993) measured specific DHP binding to isolated adult rabbit, rat, guinea-pig and ferret ventricular myocytes to be ~150 fmol/mg protein (as did Green *et al.*, 1985 and Kokubun *et al.*, 1986 in rat myocytes). In rabbit ventricular homogenate the receptor density is somewhat lower (~90 fmol/mg homogenate protein), due to dilution with other proteins. Assuming 120 mg protein/cm^3, 25% extracellular space and a surface to volume ratio of 0.6/μm (including T-tubules, Table 1), this would correspond to ~20 DHP receptors/μm^2. This is in the same range as estimates of Ca channel density based on non-linear charge movement in cardiac myocytes thought to represent gating of the Ca channel (3.7-5.5 nC/μF, Field *et al.*, 1988; Bean & Ríos, 1989; Hadley & Lederer, 1989). Assuming that 6 elementary charges cross the membrane field when a channel opens, these "gating currents" would correspond to 37-57 channels/μm^2.

Ca channel density (N) can also be estimated based on whole cell and the single channel current (I_{Ca} & i_{Ca}) using the relationship $N = I_{Ca}/(i_{Ca} \times p_o)$. The calculated channel density depends critically on the open channel probability (p_o). The value of p_o assumed from single channel records must represent the true mean open probability of all functional Ca channels. The relatively high p_o (~0.8) used for the whole cell I_{Ca} by McDonald *et al.* (1986) was probably far too high, since whole cell I_{Ca} can be increased several-fold in the presence of Bay K 8644 which is known to increase p_o (Hess *et al.*, 1984a; Bean & Rios, 1989). Lew *et al.* (1991) found mean overall $p_o = 0.03$ at peak current (including those in relatively inactive modes) and with the measured i_{Ca} and I_{Ca} the calculated N is 18 channels/μm^2, equal to the density of DHP receptors in the same rabbit ventricular myocytes (13-15/μm^2). Thus, the number of Ca channels and DHP receptors are the same (~15/μm^2 or ~300,000/cell) and only ~3% of the Ca channels are open at peak I_{Ca}. Thus, there is no discrepancy between the density of cardiac DHP receptors and L-type Ca channels. This may also be true for skeletal muscle Ca channels if the average p_o at the peak of the whole cell I_{Ca} is on the order of 0.03, rather than the value of 1.0 assumed by Schwartz *et al.* (1985). Of course the Ca channels are not uniformly distributed, but clustered near SR junctions (see Chapter 1).

Ca CHANNEL GATING

Surface Potential and Activation

Cardiac I_{Ca} is rapidly activated by depolarization, reaching a peak in ~2-7 msec, depending on the temperature and E_m (see Figs 45 & 50). Ca channel activation seems to depend primarily on E_m, but as for most voltage sensitive channels, is also sensitive to changes in surface

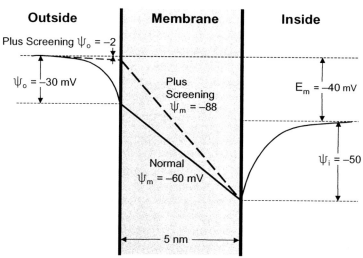

Figure 55. Surface potential and channel gating. At higher extracellular divalent ion concentration, external surface charge is screened thereby decreasing ψ_o and making trans-bilayer potential (ψ_m) more negative for the same E_m. Thus greater E_m depolarization is required to reach the same activating ψ_m.

potential (e.g. Wilson *et al.*, 1983; Hille, 1992). The surface potential arises from fixed negative charges on the membrane surface (McLaughlin, 1977, 1989). Figure 55 illustrates the effect that changing surface potential (ψ_o and ψ_i) can have on the electric field within the membrane (ψ_m), which may be what the voltage sensors of the channel respond to. I have selected to consider the situation near the threshold of I_{Ca} activation ($E_m = -40$) in a physiological medium (2 mM Ca and ~150 mM ionic strength) and used the Gouy-Chapman theory of the diffuse double layer (Grahame, 1947). The values for the surface potentials are somewhat arbitrarily chosen, but would correspond to surface charge densities of ~1 elementary charge/ 100-300 Å^2 (which roughly corresponds to expected surface densities of acidic phospholipids and sugars). This is also similar to the value estimated by Kass & Krafte (1987) from divalent cation-induced shifts of Ca channel gating in cardiac Purkinje fibers (i.e. 1/250 Å^2). The ψ_i was assumed to be larger, since negatively charged phospholipids are preferentially on the inner sarcolemmal leaflet in cardiac muscle (Post *et al.*, 1988) and the divalent cation concentration is lower inside the cell than out. Divalent cations are especially effective in screening surface charge since they are concentrated by the negatively charged surface and also bind to the negatively charged sites to neutralize them (McLaughlin *et al.*, 1981; Bers *et al.*, 1985). Indeed, at 1 mM [Ca]$_o$ we estimate surface [Ca]$_o$ and [Na]$_o$ to be 25 mM and 700 mM respectively (and surface [Cl] is also reduced).

Given these conditions, the "normal" state at $E_m = -40$ mV in Fig 55 would correspond to a trans-bilayer potential of $\psi_m = -60$ mV. If extracellular divalent cation concentration is increased such that the external surface potential (ψ_o) is nearly abolished then the trans-bilayer potential is considerably more polarized ($\psi_m = -88$ mV) for the same $E_m = -40$. Thus a greater E_m depolarization will be required for the channel to "see" the same trans-bilayer field and hence threshold for activation. This is why the current-voltage relationship with 115 mM Ba in Fig 50A is shifted to more depolarized E_m compared with 2 mM Ca in Fig 50B (and I_{NS} activation in divalent-free solution is shifted −20 mV compared to I_{Ca}). Ba does not shift activation as much as Ca does, probably because it does not bind as avidly to negative membrane surface sites (the pure charge screening effect should be the same for all divalents). This effect applies to all E_m-dependent channels and applies equally to the E_m-dependence of inactivation. It readily explains the increased excitability of cells in low divalent cation concentrations. That is, low $[Ca]_o$ shifts the activation and inactivation of channels to more negative E_m (closer to the resting E_m).

The effect of the surface potential decays exponentially over a few Debye lengths (one Debye length ~1 nm). Surface potential clearly effects channel gating, but might also alter Ca channel conductance, because of the surface Ca concentrating effect of the negative potential. However, Coronado & Affolter (1986) demonstrated single channel conductance was relatively insensitive to the surface potential. Thus, in contrast to the gating sensor, the opening into the permeation pathway may be relatively shielded from ψ_o effects (due to elevation above the bilayer surface and/or a charge-free disc around the pore of about 2 nm).

As discussed in Chapter 4, most of the E_m-dependence in Ca channel activation is between closed states, with the final closed to open transition being relatively E_m-independent. Analogous to Fig 40B, the E_m-dependence of Ca channel gating charge movement occurs at more negative E_m than that of I_{Ca} (Bean & Ríos, 1989).

I_{Ca} Inactivation

Inactivation of Ca channels is time-, E_m- and $[Ca]_i$-dependent (Lee *et al.*, 1985; Kass & Sanguinetti, 1984; Hadley & Hume, 1987). Figure 56A shows that inactivation of I_{NS} is very slow ($t_{1/2} > 500$ ms) and probably reflects purely E_m-dependent inactivation which is very slow at this test E_m (–30 mV). As an aside, $E_m = -30$ mV in the absence of divalent cations produces a membrane field and ψ_m comparable to that at $E_m = -10$ or 0 mV with normal $[Ca]_o$ (due to surface charge screening by Ca, see above). The divalent cation currents were recorded during pulses to 0 mV. I should note that when E_m is 40-50 mV more positive to this range the inactivation of I_{NS} increases (i.e. E_m-dependent inactivation is more prominent, but still incomplete even at large positive E_m). The Ba current (I_{Ba}) in Fig 56A inactivates more rapidly ($t_{1/2} = 161$ ms) than I_{NS}, and this may reflect a modest ability of Ba to mimic Ca-dependent inactivation (Ferreira *et al.*, 1997). When Ca is the charge carrier, with 10 mM EGTA in the pipette to abolish cellular Ca transients (and in this case SR Ca release), inactivation is faster still ($t_{1/2} = 37$ ms). This probably reflects Ca-dependent inactivation due to Ca entering via the channel itself. EGTA is a slow Ca buffer and thus cannot prevent a rise in local $[Ca]_i$ near the mouth of the Ca channel. High concentrations of faster Ca buffers (like BAPTA) can slow this Ca-dependent inactivation. During normal E-C coupling there is also Ca released from the SR and this can further elevate local $[Ca]_i$ near the L-type Ca channel. The top I_{Ca} trace in Fig 56A is under conditions where a normal Ca transient occurs in the cell (clamped using perforated patch mode). I_{Ca} inactivates much faster ($t_{1/2} = 17$ ms) and this emphasizes that SR Ca release also plays a major role in I_{Ca} inactivation in a physiological setting. Indeed, in action potential clamp experiments (Fig 60), normal SR Ca release reduces the integrated Ca influx via $I_{Ca,L}$ by 50% (Puglisi *et al.*, 1999).

Figure 56B shows the E_m-dependence of inactivation at the end of a 500 ms pulse to the indicated E_m (Hadley & Hume, 1987). It can be seen that I_{NS} inactivation was incomplete after 500 ms, even at +60 mV. At strong positive E_m (where little Ca enters), there is little difference between I_{Ca} and I_{NS} inactivation (i.e. it is more purely E_m-dependent). The additional I_{Ca} inacti-

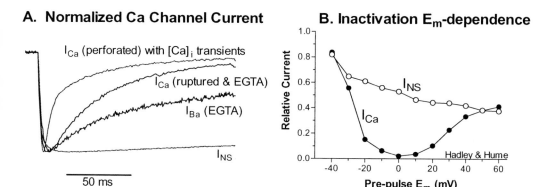

A. Normalized Ca Channel Current

B. Inactivation E_m-dependence

Figure 56. Cardiac Ca channel inactivation. **A.** Normalized Ca, Ba and Na currents (I_{Ca}, I_{Ba} & I_{NS}) meas-ured at 0 mV (except I_{NS} at –30 mV to obtain comparable activation state). I_{Ca} was recorded under both perforated patch conditions (where normal SR Ca release and Ca transients occur) and in ruptured patch with cells dialyzed with 10 mM EGTA (to prevent global Ca transients). I_{Ba} was also recorded with ruptured patch (with 10 mM EGTA in the pipette). Extracellular [Ca] and [Ba] were both 2 mM and I_{NS} was measured in divalent-free conditions (10 mM EDTA inside and out) with $[Na]_o$ at 20 mM and $[Na]_i$ at 10 mM. Peak currents were 1370, 808, 780 and 5200 pA and were attained at 5, 7, 10 and 14 ms for I_{Ca} (perforated), I_{Ca} (ruptured), I_{Ba} and I_{NS} respectively, with $t_{1/2}$ of current decline of 17, 37, 161 and >500 ms respectively. **B.** Amplitude of I_{NS} and I_{Ca} through Ca channels (at –10 mV) after 500 msec pulses to the indicated E_m in guinea-pig ventricular myocytes. I_{NS} inactivation is E_m-dependent, and the additional inactivation with Ca is attributed to Ca-dependent inactivation (redrawn from Hadley & Hume, 1987).

vation at intermediate E_m has the same E_m-dependence as inward I_{Ca} amplitude (e.g. maximal at ~0mV, see Fig 50C). This fast Ca-dependent inactivation is the overwhelmingly dominant inactivation on the time scale of an AP (or voltage clamp pulse in Fig 56A).

The Ca-dependent inactivation of I_{Ca} appears to depend on $[Ca]_i$ and as such may provide a sort of feedback control to limit further Ca entry. A remarkable feature of the Ca_i-dependent inactivation is that it is still readily apparent even when $[Ca]_i$ is fairly heavily buffered by EGTA or BAPTA, which abolishes contraction. This suggested that Ca entering via I_{Ca} must exert the inactivating effect locally, and perhaps directly at the channel, prior to mixing with bulk $[Ca]_i$. Höfer *et al.* (1997) estimated a K_i for $[Ca]_i$ of 4 µM based on single Ca channel currents.

Novel insight into the molecular mechanism was provided by de Leon *et al.* (1995) in studies of a putative Ca-binding EF-hand region present in the cardiac α_{1C} (Fig 51) that is not in α_{1E} (a neuronal Ca channel which does not show Ca-dependent inactivation). By donating this EF-hand region of α_{1C} into α_{1E} in chimeric Ca channels they could confer Ca-dependent inacti-vation upon α_{1E}. However, a study disrupting the Ca binding site by mutagenesis did not confirm this (Zhou *et al.*, 1997). More recently three independent groups have demonstrated that calmodulin may mediate Ca-dependent inactivation of α_{1C}, converging on the following model (Zulkhe & Reuter, 1998; Peterson *et al.*, 1999; Qin *et al.*, 1999; Zulkhe *et al.*, 1999). Calmodulin may already be bound to the Ca channel at rest. This may require 1 Ca bound to calmodulin-α_{1C} with relatively high affinity (K_d =29 nM) in the carboxy terminal of α_{1C} near the IQ motif (amino acids 1624-5 in Fig 51) prior to Ca channel activation. When the channel opens and local [Ca] rises, more Ca binds to calmodulin (which has 4 Ca binding sites) causing a stronger interaction with the IQ motif of the Ca channel and consequent inactivation. Some aspects of this model

A. Activation & Availability

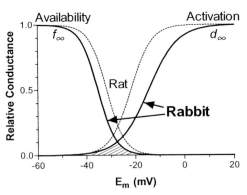

B. Recovery from Inactivation

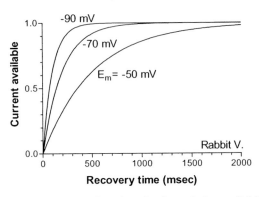

Figure 57. Cardiac Ca channel activation, availability and recovery from inactivation. **A.** I_{Ca} availability is measured by depolarizing from –90 mV to the indicated E_m for 2 sec and then testing the remaining available I_{Ca} at $E_m = 0$ mV ([Ca]$_o$=2 mM). The result is referred to as a steady state inactivation curve. Activation is measured by dividing the peak current by the apparent driving force ($E_m - E_{rev}$) according to Ohm's law (G=I/ΔV). Both curves are described by a Boltzmann relation (pg 70). Thick curves are for rabbit and broken curves for rat (data from Yuan *et al.*, 1996). **B.** Time and E_m dependence of recovery from inactivation of rabbit ventricular I_{Ca}. After a 2 sec pulse to +10 mV to induce complete inactivation, E_m is held at the values indicated for different times before testing I_{Ca} available with a pulse to 0 mV. Data are composite from several studies in our lab at 2 mM [Ca]$_o$ and 23°C.

require further clarification, including whether the Ca-calmodulin-IQ region functions like a "ball and chain" as in N-type inactivation (pg 72).

If voltage clamp pulses (or presumably action potentials) are very long, I_{Ca} can be largely inactivated during the cytosolic Ca transient, but then partly recover as [Ca]$_i$ declines (Sipido *et al.*, 1995a). This sort of reactivation of L-type Ca channels during long action potentials may contribute to arrhythmogenic early afterdepolarizations (EADs; January & Riddle, 1989).

Figure 57A shows typical steady state activation and availability (or inactivation) curves for I_{Ca} in rat and rabbit ventricular myocytes, where SR Ca load and transients were prevented by high intracellular EGTA (from Yuan *et al.*, 1996). The Ca channel activation variable (d_∞) starts increasing at –40 mV and is maximal by 0 mV. The inactivation variable (f_∞) begins decreasing at –45 and is nearly 0 at –15 mV. Rat *vs.* rabbit I_{Ca} activates at more negative E_m, inactivates at more positive E_m, has slower Ca-dependent inactivation and shows a larger window current. In both cases the maximal steady state window I_{Ca} occurs at about –28 mV and the conductance at that point is 1% of maximum for rabbit, but 5% for rat ($d_\infty \times f_\infty$). This could provide significant sustained Ca influx at E_m from –45 to –15 mV. Josephson *et al.* (1984) reported that guinea-pig ventricle shows a larger window current than rat. Cohen & Lederer (1988) showed a develop-mental decrease in window I_{Ca} after birth in rats, but in their case there was SR Ca release and they attributed this difference to maturation of SR Ca release and cross-signaling.

Once the Ca channel is inactivated, recovery from inactivation is also [Ca]$_i$- and E_m-dependent. Figure 57B shows that recovery is much slower at $E_m = -50$ than at –90 mV. This means that Ca channel recovery only becomes very fast as AP repolarization is nearly complete. At –50 mV one can appreciate that frequency-dependent accumulation of inactivated channels may occur (e.g. at 1 Hz). Moreover, drugs like the protein kinase inhibitors H-89, KN-62 and

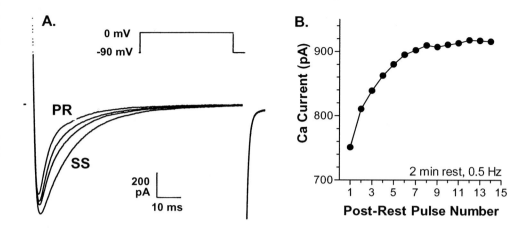

Figure 58. Ca-dependent facilitation of I_{Ca} or I_{Ca} staircase. I_{Ca} at 0.5 Hz (from -90 to 0 mV) after a 2 min rest period in a ferret ventricular myocyte. The first post-rest pulse (PR) and the second, third and steady state (SS) pulses are shown in **A** and the whole post-rest I_{Ca} "staircase" in **B**. It may be noted that when the holding E_m is -40 mV a declining I_{Ca} "staircase" is seen (redrawn from Hryshko & Bers, 1990).

KN-93 can slow recovery at -90 mV, so that it resembles that seen at $E_m = -50$ mV (Yuan & Bers, 1994; Li *et al.*, 1997b). Clearly, this can reduce apparent I_{Ca} in a protocol dependent way.

Ca-dependent I_{Ca} Facilitation or I_{Ca} Staircase

        Increasing the frequency of voltage clamp pulses from a holding potential of about -40 mV typically results in a progressive decline in I_{Ca} amplitude (Tseng, 1988; Hryshko & Bers, 1990). This negative I_{Ca} staircase probably reflects insufficient time for Ca channels to recover from the inactivated state between pulses (at -40 mV). In contrast at suitably physiological holding potentials (-80 mV), Fig 58 shows that there is a pulse-dependent progressive increase in I_{Ca} amplitude and a prominent slowing of inactivation (Mitra & Morad, 1986; Lee, 1987; Argibay *et al.*, 1988; Boyett, & Fedida, 1988; Fedida *et al.*,1988a,b; Gurney *et al.*,1989; Hryshko & Bers, 1990; Tseng, 1988; Zygmunt, & Maylie, 1990). This positive I_{Ca} staircase is Ca-dependent (not apparent with Ba as the charge carrier), still occurs in the absence of SR Ca release, and three groups independently demonstrated that Ca-dependent I_{Ca} facilitation is mediated by CaMKII-dependent phosphorylation (Yuan & Bers, 1994; Anderson *et al.*, 1994a; Xiao *et al.*, 1994a; Dzhura *et al.*, 2000). Of course SR Ca release (a much larger local Ca flux than I_{Ca}) can amplify the effect, explaining some disparate results (Delgado *et al.*, 1999). Since this Ca-dependent facilitation is still observed when cells are dialyzed with 10 mM EGTA (but is abrogated by 20 mM BAPTA), the Ca-dependent activation of CaMKII must be highly localized near the L-type Ca channel (Hryshko & Bers, 1990). This facilitatory effect of Ca entry on subsequent I_{Ca} is distinct from, but coexists with the Ca_i-dependent inactivation described above. Indeed, biphasic effects of $[Ca]_i$ on unitary I_{Ca} have been reported (Hirano & Hiraoki, 1994).

        Zuhlke *et al.* (1999) found that point mutations in the isoleucine in the IQ domain which abolish Ca-calmodulin dependent inactivation could either enhance (Ile to Ala) or abolish (Ile to

Glu) Ca-dependent I_{Ca} facilitation. Thus the calmodulin involved in activating CaMKII and I_{Ca} may be the same tethered calmodulin which is involved in Ca-dependent inactivation. I further speculate that the slowing of I_{Ca} inactivation during this positive I_{Ca} staircase (Fig 58) might result from some degree of functional shift of calmodulin from the "inactivation target" to CaMKII as a target. The physiological impact of this Ca-dependent facilitation is not entirely clear. However, it may partly offset direct Ca-dependent inactivation and create an additional Ca channel memory that has a time scale of at least a few seconds.

A voltage-dependent facilitation of I_{Ca} has also been described in chromaffin cells (Artelejo *et al.*, 1990, 1992), skeletal (Sculptoreanu *et al.*, 1993a) and cardiac Ca channels (Pietrobon & Hess, 1990; Sculptoreanu *et al.*, 1993b; Xiao *et al.*, 1994a; Kamp *et al.*, 2000). In cardiac Ca channels this effect seems to be mediated by cAMP dependent protein kinase and may require coexpression of Ca channel β subunits (but is distinct from the G-protein mediated modulation of neuronal Ca channels discussed on pg 106). This facilitation occurs with pulses to very positive potentials (e.g. >+100 mV) and also dissipates extremely rapidly upon repolarization to physiological membrane potentials in ventricular myocytes. For example, if one repolarizes from +100 to −60 mV for more than ~10 ms the facilitation is almost abolished (and even faster at more negative, diastolic E_m). Thus this voltage-mediated I_{Ca} facilitation is probably not physiologically important in the normal cardiac myocyte.

AMOUNT OF Ca ENTRY VIA Ca CHANNELS

The amount of Ca entry via I_{Ca} is functionally important with respect to the Ca requirements for myofilament activation. During a square voltage clamp pulse to 0 mV the I_{Ca} waveform can be integrated to infer a Ca influx of ~10 μmol/L cytosol (see pg 55; this is equivalent to peak I_{Ca} = 1 nA, triangular shape 120 ms long for 30 pL myocyte cytosol). However, Ca influx during the AP may differ significantly from the usual square pulse. Figure 59 compares square pulses and AP waveforms used as command potentials in voltage clamp (i.e. AP clamp; Doerr *et al.*, 1990; Arreola *et al.*, 1991; Yuan *et al.*, 1996; Grantham & Cannell, 1996; Linz & Meyer, 1998). Peak I_{Ca} during the AP clamp is lower and occurs later than for the square pulse. This is because at the AP peak (+50 mV) Ca channels activate rapidly, but the driving force for Ca is initially low because E_m is close to the reversal potential for I_{Ca} (~+60 mV). As E_m falls the driving force apparently increases faster than the channels inactivate, producing a larger current at later times during the AP. In rabbit ventricle I_{Ca} is also more sustained during the AP than a square pulse. The bottom panels in Fig 59 show running integrals of Ca influx. In rat ventricular myocytes the amount of Ca influx for the same 200 ms square pulse is higher than in rabbit (Yuan *et al.*, 1996). This is due to the difference in I_{Ca} activation and inactivation. However, the rat ventricular AP is very brief and with species-appropriate AP waveforms the Ca influx is much higher in rabbit *vs.* rat ventricular myocyte (21 *vs.* 14 μmol/L cytosol).

The data shown in Fig 59 overestimate physiological Ca influx because these measurements were in cells dialyzed with EGTA (such that there was less Ca-dependent inactivation of I_{Ca}). We also recently measured integrated I_{Ca} during AP clamp in rabbit ventricular myocyte at 25 and 35°C where normal SR Ca release occurred, but all other currents, including $I_{Na/Ca}$ and $I_{Cl(Ca)}$ were blocked (Puglisi *et al.*, 1999). Figure 60A shows that for steady state AP clamps (and contractions) I_{Ca} peaks earlier and higher at 35°C than at 25°C, but the integrated Ca influx is

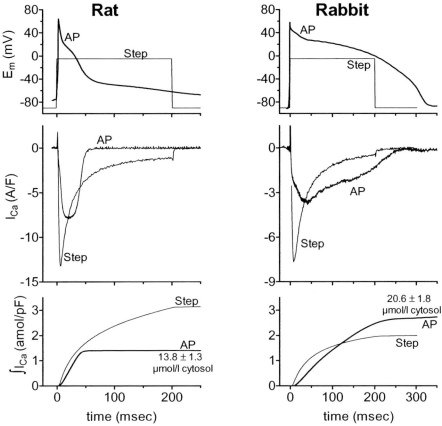

Figure 59. I_{Ca} during square pulse and AP-clamp. Rat and rabbit ventricular myocytes (25°C) were voltage clamped with either a square voltage step or an AP waveform (measured from 5 other cells under physiological conditions). All other currents were blocked e.g. by replacement of K with Cs and Na with TEA (inside and out) and cells were dialyzed with 10 mM EGTA to prevent Ca transients. Running integrals of Ca influx during AP-clamp are shown along with mean values (data from Yuan *et al.*, 1996).

almost the same. Figure 60B shows how I_{Ca} changes during APs as the SR is refilled (after prior depletion) and contractions recover to steady state (at 25°C). As the contractions and SR Ca release get larger I_{Ca} inactivates more rapidly and completely during the AP. This is an obvious consequence of more profound Ca-dependent inactivation of I_{Ca}. Considering that there is no SR Ca at the first pulse (and peak I_{Ca} hardly changes), the decline in integrated I_{Ca} from pulse 1 to steady state (pulse 10) indicates how SR Ca release limits Ca influx. Figure 60C shows that at both 25 and 35°C integrated I_{Ca} decreases from 12 to 6 µmol/L cytosol. This indicates that I_{Ca} inactivation due to SR Ca release decreases net Ca influx by ~50% at both temperatures. Quantitatively similar conclusions were found in square voltage clamp pulse experiments in rat, ferret and guinea-pig myocytes (Adachi-Akahani *et al.*, 1996; Sham *et al.*, 1995a; Trafford *et al.*, 1997; Terraciano & MacLeod, 1997; Linz & Meyer, 1998).

The kinetics of this SR Ca release-induced I_{Ca} inactivation can also provide information about the timing of SR Ca release (Puglisi *et al.*, 1999; Linz & Meyer, 1998). We took the

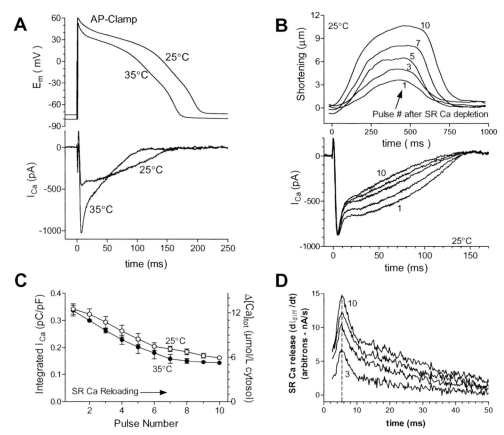

Figure 60. Ca influx during AP at 25 and 35°C in rabbit ventricular myocyte. I_{Ca} during AP-clamp. **A**.
AP waveforms and I_{Ca} during steady state AP-clamps. The AP waveform was recorded under physiological
ionic conditions (another cell) and used as the command E_m in this cell, where all other ionic currents were
blocked (Cs and TEA replacing K and Na). **B**. After SR Ca was depleted by a brief caffeine-application
(with Na), a series of AP-clamps were given, and the SR and contraction recover to steady state over 10
sequential pulses. **C**. Integrated I_{Ca} for each pulse during SR Ca reloading in experiments like panel B at 25
and 35°C. **D**. The difference current between pulse 1 in panel B and pulses 3, 5, 7 & 10 (I_{diff} taken as an
index of local [Ca] due to SR Ca release) was differentiated (dI_{diff}/dt) to provide an index of SR Ca release
rate as sensed by the L-type Ca channel (data are from Puglisi *et al.*, 1999).

difference in I_{Ca} traces between pulse #1 and the other pulses in Fig 60B (I_{Diff}) as an index of the
local $[Ca]_i$ produced by SR Ca release, as sensed by the L-type Ca channel. The rate at which
this local $[Ca]_i$ changes (dI_{Diff}/dt) may thus be the locally sensed rate of SR Ca release. Figure
60D shows that the local SR Ca release flux sensed by the Ca channel reaches a peak in 5 ms,
regardless of the amplitude of release (or 2.5 ms at 35°C). This is much faster than the rate of
rise of the global cellular Ca transient, but is not surprising given our expectation that Ca release
via ryanodine receptors occurs very near the L-type Ca channel. It also emphasizes that Ca-
sensitive ionic currents can be excellent sensors of local $[Ca]_i$ in the cell.

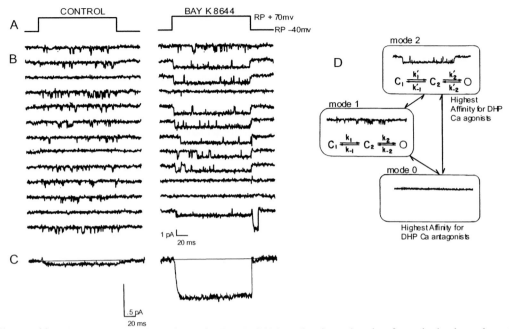

Figure 61. Effect of the Ca channel agonist Bay K 8644 on Ca channel gating from single channel patch clamp recordings. **A.** Voltage clamp protocol referenced to the resting potential (RP) of about –60 mV. **B.** Single sweeps in the absence (left) and presence (right) of 5 µM Bay K 8644. **C.** Average current from all single sweeps. **D.** Model of Ca channel gating modes proposed by Hess *et al.* (1984). The transitions between modes is slow compared to the gating within a mode (indicated as C_1, C_2 and O for two closed and one open state). (All panels are from Hess *et al.*, 1984, with permission).

MODULATION OF I_{Ca} BY AGONISTS AND ANTAGONISTS

A hallmark of L-type Ca channels is their sensitivity to DHPs (e.g. nifedipine, nitrendipine, nimodipine, nisoldipine, isradipine or PN200-110, Bay K 8644, azidopine and iodipine). Indeed, the specific binding of DHPs to the α_1 subunit of the L-type Ca channel was important in the isolation of the protein. Most of these DHPs decrease I_{Ca} and are known as Ca channel blockers or Ca channel antagonists. Some DHPs, notably (–) Bay K 8644, (+) S-202-791 and CGP 28392 (known as Ca channel agonists), greatly increase I_{Ca} by increasing the duration of single Ca channel openings, without appreciably altering single channel conductance (Brown *et al.*, 1984; Hess *et al.*, 1984a; Kokubun & Reuter, 1984; Kokubun *et al.*, 1986). Bay K 8644 can increase channel open times from ~0.6 msec to ~20 msec and Hess *et al.* (1984a) suggested that Bay K 8644 binding to the Ca channel stabilized a state of the channel, called "mode 2" in which long stable openings occur (see Fig 61). In the presence of Bay K 8644 the channel can still switch to the normal state (mode 1) where the openings are shorter and indistinguishable from the control conditions. The mode 2 type openings can also be seen under control conditions, but they are quite rare (Hess *et al.*, 1984a; Yue *et al.*, 1990). Thus, Ca agonists can greatly increase the likelihood of these long lasting mode 2 openings. Ca antagonist DHPs, on the other hand, inhibit I_{Ca} apparently by favoring a mode of channel gating (mode 0) characterized by the channel being unavailable to open. Switching between modes occurs on a slower time scale than bursts of activity (several seconds). Indeed, normal Ca channels can be quiescent for many seconds of depolarizing pulses (mode 0), can then have very infrequent and brief opening of 0.15 ms (mode 0_a; Yue *et al.*, 1990), switch to a mode where occasional bursts of 0.5-1 ms occur (mode 1) and rarely make excursions to mode 2 (where openings of 10-20 ms are observed). While this modal model of Ca channel gating is widely used, its applicability has also been challenged (Lacerda & Brown, 1989).

The long openings induced by Bay K 8644 would be expected to lead to slower I_{Ca} inactivation during a voltage clamp pulse. This is not usually observed for I_{Ca} because the larger Ca influx also produces greater Ca-dependent inactivation. Interestingly, when Bay K 8644 and β-adrenergic agonists (which also enhance mode 2) are applied together there is a dramatic slowing of I_{Ca} inactivation (Tsien *et al.*, 1986; Tiaho *et al.*, 1990). A prominent feature of I_{Ca} in the presence of Bay K 8644 is large, long-lasting "tail" currents. Tail currents are due to the rapid increase in Ca driving force when repolarization occurs with Ca channels still open (before they deactivate at negative E_m). The last sweep in Fig 61B with Bay K 8644 shows a single channel tail Ca current. Bay K 8644 also shifts activation and inactivation to more negative E_m (by 10 to 20 mV). The non-DHP Ca channel agonist FPL-64176 also shifts activation and inactivation E_m negative and produces even more dramatic tail I_{Ca} than Bay K 8644, but it does not compete with DHPs at their binding site (Rampe & Lacerda, 1991; Kunze & Rampe, 1992). Bay Y 5959 is a new DHP Ca channel agonist (Bechem *et al.*, 1997) which also produces very prolonged tail I_{Ca} and slows I_{Ca} activation (both like FPL-64176).

Early experiments indicated that the affinity of cardiac microsomes for nitrendipine was 1000 times higher than the concentrations required to block I_{Ca} (Bellemann *et al.*, 1981; Lee & Tsien, 1983). This was explained by the voltage dependence of DHP binding to Ca channels. For example, Bean (1984) showed that depolarization of E_m from −80 to −10 mV in ventricular myocytes decreased the apparent K_d for I_{Ca} inhibition by nitrendipine by >1000×, from ~500 nM to 0.36 nM (Fig 62). Similar results were found by Sanguinetti & Kass (1984) and they concluded that DHPs bind preferentially to the inactivated state of the channel. This conclusion was supported by ^{3}H-DHP binding experiments in isolated sarcolemmal vesicles (Schilling & Drewe, 1986) and myocytes (Green *et al.*, 1985; Kokubun *et al.*, 1986). These results fit well with the modulated receptor hypothesis described by Hondeghem & Katzung (1977) and Hille (1977) to explain the voltage- and use-dependent block of Na channels by local anesthetics.

Sanguinetti & Kass (1984) also compared DHPs (and verapamil) which are neutral at physiological pH (nitrendipine and nisoldipine) with ones that bear a net charge at pH = 7.4 (verapamil and to an intermediate degree, nicardipine). The charged ligands appeared to block the channel only when it was in the open state (i.e. requiring voltage pulses) and as such are strictly *use-dependent*. These charged ligands may need for the channel to open to gain access to the receptor site. The neutral ligands, on the other hand appear able to block I_{Ca} whether the channel is in the open or inactivated state (i.e. at depolarized holding potentials without requiring pulses) and as such are more strictly *voltage-dependent* than use-dependent.   The more hydrophobic nature of these ligands may allow them to gain access to the receptor site even when the channel is inactivated. It is also possible that uncharged lipophilic DHPs act by first partitioning into the membrane bilayer and approaching DHP receptors by lateral diffusion (Herbette *et al.*, 1989; Valdivia & Coronado, 1988). There is good evidence to support the idea

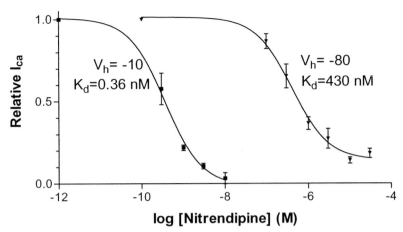

log [Nitrendipine] (M)

Figure 62. Different I_{Ca} blocking effectiveness of nifedipine in canine cardiac myocytes depends on holding potential (V_h). The apparent K_d for I_{Ca} block decreased by 1200-fold when V_h was depolarized from -80 to -10 mV (curves are fit to original data taken from Bean, 1984). Incomplete I_{Ca} block occurred when $V_h = -80$ may be due to a fraction of I_{Ca} which is not through L-type Ca channels.

that DHPs gain access to the receptor from the external side of the membrane (and external protons can get access whether the channel is open or not; Kass & Arena, 1989; Kass *et al.*, 1991; Strubing *et al.*, 1993). This would be consistent with the receptor being at the external end of the channel. Benzothiazepine Ca channel blockers (e.g. diltiazem) also appear to gain access from the extracellular side (Hering *et al.*, 1993a,b). Access for phenylalkylamines (another class of Ca channel blockers, e.g. verapamil) appears to be at the inner sarcolemmal surface since impermeant ligands are relatively ineffective from the outside (Hescheler *et al.*, 1982; LeBlanc & Hume, 1989).

The voltage-dependence of the DHPs compared to the use-dependence of verapamil may explain the greater efficacy of the DHPs as vasodilators and the relative lack of effect on cardiac muscle at therapeutic levels. That is, since resting vascular smooth muscle is usually at more depolarized levels of E_m and can undergo long further depolarizations, DHPs will interact preferentially with these smooth muscle Ca channels rather than cardiac Ca channels which do not spend long enough times at depolarized enough potentials to be blocked by therapeutic concentrations of DHPs. Of course this also explains why the cardiac effects observed with Ca antagonists are more pronounced in pacemaker cells which have relatively depolarized diastolic E_m level. This effect also contributes to the antiarrhythmic effect of Ca channel blockers.

At least three classes of drugs interact specifically with the L-type Ca channel: 1) DHPs (above), 2) phenylalkylamines (ΦAAs, such as verapamil, D600, D888 and D890) and 3) benzothiazepines (BTZs e.g. diltiazem), and these sites in turn interact allosterically (Fig 63A, Glossmann *et al.*, 1984, 1985). DHP and benzothiazepine binding reciprocally stimulate binding at the other site and ΦAA binding reciprocally inhibits DHP binding and benzothiazepine binding. Ca and other divalent cations stimulate DHP binding, but depresses ΦAA and benzothiazepine binding. It has also been argued that there are two distinct DHP receptors, one

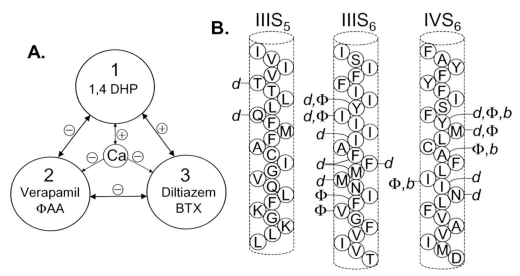

Figure 63. Ca antagonist binding to Ca channel. **A.** Functional interrelationship between dihydropyridine (1,4 DHP), phenylalkylamine (ΦAA) and benzothiazepine (BTX) receptor sites on the L-type Ca channel (e.g. DHP occupancy increases BTX and Ca binding, but inhibits ΦAA binding; after Glossmann *et al.*, 1984, 1985). **B.** Sites on the α_{1C} channel IIIS$_5$, IIIS$_6$ and IVS$_6$ transmembrane domains which are thought to be critical in binding DHP (*d*), ΦAA (Φ) and BTZ (*b*) (based on review by Mitterdorfer *et al.*, 1998).

for Ca antagonists and one for Ca agonists (Kokubun *et al.*, 1986; Brown *et al.*, 1986), but in general these DHPs exhibit competitive binding. The stereoisomers of two well known Ca agonists appear to act as pure Ca antagonists ((−)-R-202-791 and (+) Bay K 8644; Williams *et al.*, 1985; Franckowiak *et al.*, 1985; Kokubun *et al.*, 1986) A further complication is that one stereoisomer which is a Ca agonist ((+)-S-202-791), switches from an I_{Ca} agonist at negative test potentials to an I_{Ca} antagonist at E_m ~0 mV (along with a change from allosteric enhancement of PN200-110 binding to competitive inhibition; Kokubun *et al.*, 1986; Kamp *et al.*, 1989). Even nitrendipine, a DHP known as a Ca antagonist, can increase I_{Ca} activated from negative holding potentials (Brown *et al.*, 1986). Thus, while the precise nature of the DHP receptor(s) is not entirely clear, these compounds are extremely valuable tools in understanding and modulating Ca channels. Diphenylbutylpiperidine neuroleptics (e.g. fluspiriline and pimozide) and the benzoyl-pyrrole Ca agonist FPL-64176 may also bind to the Ca channel at an independent receptor (Gould *et al.*, 1983; Galizzi *et al.*, 1986; Kunze & Rampe, 1992).

Substantial information has been obtained about the sites of interaction of DHPs, ΦAAs and benzothiazepines with the Ca channel α_{1C} subunit (reviewed in Hockerman *et al.*, 1997; Mitterdorfer *et al.*, 1998). Studies using photoaffinity labeling with reactive ligands such as ^{3}H-azidopine indicated that sites in IIIS$_6$ and IVS$_6$ interact with DHPs and BTZs (Striessnig *et al.*, 1990a, 1991; Nakayama *et al.*, 1991; Kraus *et al.*, 1996). Similar studies with ΦAAs only identified sites on IVS$_6$ (Striessnig *et al.*, 1990b). Mutational "gain of function" analysis has identified α_{1C} amino acids that when substituted into non-DHP-sensitive channels (e.g. α_{1A}) can endow them with DHP sensitivity (Grabner *et al.*, 1996). Sinnegger *et al.* (1997) found 9 non-conserved amino acids on α_{1C} (in IIIS$_5$, IIIS$_6$ and IVS$_6$) which could confer full DHP sensitivity

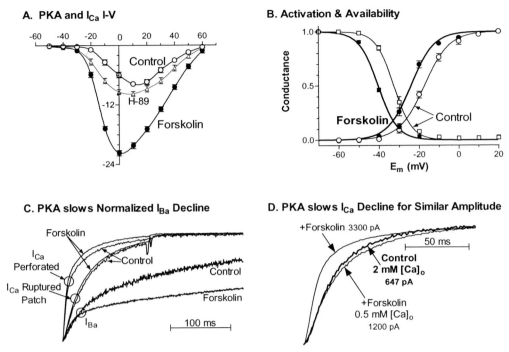

Figure 64. β-adrenergic agonist effects on I_{Ca}. Forskolin (1 μM, a direct activator of adenylyl cyclase) was applied for 5-10 min to increase cAMP and activate PKA (see Fig 65). **A.** Forskolin increases I_{Ca} at all E_m values, but especially at negative E_m (200 ms pulses from $E_m = -90$ mV to indicated E_m). **B.** Activation and inactivation curves after forskolin are both shifted to more negative E_m values (methods as in Fig 57). **C-D.** Effect of forskolin on normalized I_{Ca} and I_{Ba} decline measured in perforated patch mode and I_{Ca} in ruptured patch with 10 mM EGTA in the pipette. I_{Ca} and I_{Ba} were recorded by Yuan & Bers (1995) in ferret ventricular myocytes at 23°C in perforated (A, C & D) and ruptured patch modes (B & C) with all other ionic currents blocked.

to $α_{1A}$ (Figs 51A and 63B). The converse "loss-of-function" approach substituting $α_{1C}$ residues with either alanine or $α_{1E/B}$ residues provided complementary data about 13 sites which contribute to DHP binding on $α_{1C}$ (2 on IIIS$_5$, 7 on IIIS$_6$ and 4 on IVS$_6$; Peterson *et al.*, 1996, 1997; Schuster *et al.*, 1996). Similar studies with ΦAAs and BTZs identified key sites on IIIS$_6$ and IVS$_6$ only (Fig 63B; Hockerman *et al.*, 1997; Hering *et al.*, 1996). Notably, there is significant overlap of the sites involved in antagonist binding, despite a lack of classical competition among these drug classes. Additionally, this S$_5$-S$_6$ region is likely to form part of the pore lining and activation gate regions of these channels though not the selectivity filter (see Figs 38 & 39).

β-ADRENERGIC MODULATION OF CARDIAC Ca CURRENT

The activation of I_{Ca} by β-adrenergic agonists in cardiac muscle is a classic observation (e.g. Reuter, 1967). This occurs mainly through PKA, causes a 2-4 fold increase in basal I_{Ca} in ventricular myocyte and shifts the voltage-dependence of activation and inactivation to more negative E_m (Fig 64A-B; Tsien *et al.*1986; Hartzell, 1988; McDonald *et al.*, 1994). The shift in activation gating causes the I_{Ca} increase to be most prominent at negative E_m and maximal I_{Ca} to be at more negative E_m. At the single channel level PKA has no effect on unitary conductance, but there are fewer blank sweeps (without any openings) and an apparent increase in open times which may reflect a shift toward mode 2 gating (Cachelin, 1983; Yue *et al.*, 1990).

The β-adrenergic cascade also interacts with other signaling pathways in modulating I_{Ca}. For example, acetylcholine (ACh) has no effect on basal I_{Ca} in ventricular myocytes, but strongly antagonizes the catecholamine- or forskolin-stimulated I_{Ca} (Fischmeister & Hartzell, 1986; Hescheler *et al.*, 1986). Part of this effect of ACh may be mediated by the muscarinic receptor-mediated activation of G_i which inhibits adenylyl cyclase and thus net cAMP production (Lindeman & Watanabe, 1989). In addition, ACh increases cGMP which can either decrease cAMP by stimulating a cGMP-activated phosphodiesterase (PDE-II) in frog (Fischmeister & Hartzell, 1987) or increase cAMP in mammalian heart by a cGMP-inhibited PDE-III (Ono & Trautwein, 1991; McDonald *et al.*, 1994). Indeed, in atrial latent pacemaker cells, where ACh depresses basal I_{Ca} (due to higher basal cAMP than in ventricular myocytes), withdrawal of ACh causes a dramatic overshoot of I_{Ca} amplitude above control (Wang & Lipsius, 1996). They attributed this to further elevation of cAMP, and concluded that this rebound increase in I_{Ca} was responsible for transient post-vagal tachycardia. Increased cGMP can also activate cGMP-dependent protein kinase (PKG), which does not appear to alter basal I_{Ca}, but can (like ACh and cGMP) antagonize cAMP-mediated increases in I_{Ca} (Ono & Trautwein, 1991). Nitric oxide also stimulates cGMP production in cardiac myocytes (Balligand *et al.*, 1993) and this can mediate I_{Ca} regulation as above (Mery *et al.*, 1993; Kirstein *et al.*, 1995; Han *et al.*, 1994a). Indeed, there is evidence to suggest that nitric oxide is required for the ACh-mediated antagonism of cAMP-activated I_{Ca} in cardiac myocytes (Han *et al.*, 1994a; Wang & Lipsius, 1995b). ACh has also been shown to stimulate protein phosphatase activity, which would also reverse PKA mediated phosphorylation (Herzig *et al.*, 1995).

Figure 65 indicates the β-adrenergic agonist pathway. Occupation of the β-adrenergic receptor by an agonist activates a GTP binding protein (G_s) and the α subunit ($G_{s\alpha}$) dissociates and activates adenylyl cyclase, producing cAMP. The increase in cAMP leads to the dissociation of the regulatory and catalytic subunits of the cyclic AMP-dependent protein kinase (PKA). The PKA catalytic subunit phosphorylates several proteins including the L-type Ca channel and also the ryanodine receptor, phospholamban and troponin I.

Support for this β-adrenergic pathway for I_{Ca} comes from experiments showing that the effect can be mimicked by intracellular cAMP, cAMP analogs and phosphodiesterase inhibitors (Tsien *et al.*, 1972; Tsien, 1973; Vogel & Sperelakis, 1981; Cachelin *et al.*, 1983; Nargeot *et al.*, 1983; Kameyama *et al.*, 1985), direct activation of adenylyl cyclase by forskolin (Wahler & Sperelakis, 1985; Hescheler *et al.*, 1986) or non-hydrolyzable GTP analogs (Josephson & Sperelakis, 1978) and intracellular application of PKA catalytic subunit (Osterrieder *et al.*, 1982; Brum *et al.*, 1983). Dephosphorylation of the Ca channel by protein phosphatases (1 and 2A) also abolishes the increase in I_{Ca} seen with isoprenaline (Hescheler *et al.*, 1987a), but does not decrease basal I_{Ca}. The latter finding also indicates that phosphorylation of the Ca channel is not **required** for channel activity in ventricular myocytes.

PKA is probably anchored in the vicinity of the Ca channel by an "A kinase anchoring protein" AKAP-79 (Gao *et al.*, 1997a; Fraser *et al.*, 1998). This crucial localization may have caused difficulties in demonstrating PKA-dependent activation of I_{Ca} in heterologous expression

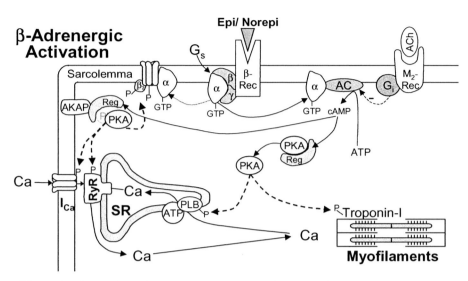

Figure 65. Dual pathways for activation of Ca channels by β-adrenergic stimulation. The classic pathway is via stimulation of adenylyl cyclase (AC, via activation of the GTP binding protein G_s), increased [cAMP] and phosphorylation of the Ca channel by the catalytic subunit of the cAMP-dependent protein kinase (PKA, where Reg is the regulatory subunit of PKA). Another minor pathway is via a direct effect of the activated α subunit of G_s on the Ca channel (β-Rec= β adrenergic receptor, Epi= epinephrine, Norepi= norepinephrine, M_2-Rec= M_2-muscarinic receptor, AKAP=PKA anchoring protein, PLB= phospholamban, ACh = acetylcholine.

systems (Zong *et al.*, 1995). Forskolin, which increases cAMP (by stimulating adenylyl cyclase) activates PKA and strongly activates I_{Ca} in heart cells (Fig 64), fails to effect the heterologously expressed α_{1C}, although the PKA inhibitor H-89 could decrease I_{Ba} (Perez-Reyes *et al.*, 1994). Despite this issue, the cloned α_{1C} and β_{2A} subunits have been shown to be substrates for PKA and PKC (Haase *et al.*, 1993; Puri *et al.*, 1997). The phosphorylation site on α_{1C} (Ser-1928) can increase I_{Ca} in an AKAP-dependent manner, but in heart cells Ser-1928 and the distal part of the C-terminus might be cleaved off in some fraction of Ca channels (Gao *et al.*, 1997b). Two non-consensus PKA sites on the β_{2A} subunit (Ser-478 & 479) can be phosphorylated by PKA and increase I_{Ca} (Bünemann *et al.*, 1999).

A more rapid direct activation of I_{Ca} by $G_{S\alpha}$ was suggested to be physiologically important (Yatani *et al.*, 1987; Yatani & Brown, 1989), but this effect (when observed) is a very small fraction of the overall β-adrenergic response (Pelzer *et al.*, 1990; MacDonald *et al.*, 1994).

How is Ca channel gating modified by β-agonists? Here let us consider the relationship between whole cell I_{Ca} (I) and single channel current (i): $I = N_f \times p_o \times i$, where N_f is the number of functional channels in the cell and p_o is the probability that the channel will be open. Since single channel conductance is unaltered, i is not changed (Reuter *et al.*, 1982). Single channel recording indicated that p_o was increased by β-agonists or dibutyryl-cAMP (Cachelin *et al.*, 1983; Brum *et al.*, 1984). There may also be some increase in N_f, but truly "new" channels do not appear in membrane patches with β-stimulation (as would be expected if dormant channels become functional; Bean *et al.*, 1984). The apparent increase in N_f could also be due to an apparent shift toward greater mode 1 and mode 2 gating (*vs.* mode 0, 0_a and mode 1; Yue *et al.*, 1990; Cachelin *et al.*, 1983; Brum *et al.*, 1984). Thus, the increase in I_{Ca} induced by β-adrenergic stimulation (and channel phosphorylation) is probably entirely due to an increase in p_o of the channel. This increased p_o is mediated either by a change in the E_m dependence of activation or a shift toward modes of channel gating where longer openings are favored.

As shown in Fig 64, PKA causes greater increase of I_{Ca} at more negative potentials and this is due to negative shifts in the E_m dependence of both activation and inactivation. This shift brings the E_m-dependence of I_{Ca} activation closer to the E_m-dependence of Ca channel gating current (which is not much shifted by β-stimulation; Bean, 1990). Bean suggested that β-stimulation may increase I_{Ca} by making the coupling between the charge movement and opening of the Ca channel more efficient. It is of interest to note that the negative E_m shift in gating is the opposite direction that one would expect for simple surface potential effects of adding negative PO_4 groups to the membrane or channel surface (see Fig 55). Thus the phosphorylation must change the channel sufficiently to overcome this effect.

PKA typically accelerates I_{Ca} inactivation, but this is probably due in large part to the greater Ca-dependent inactivation secondary to larger I_{Ca} amplitude. Figure 64C-D shows that I_{Ba} inactivation is slowed by PKA-dependent phosphorylation, and that if $[Ca]_o$ is lowered in the presence of forskolin (to limit the increase in I_{Ca}) I_{Ca} inactivation is also slowed by PKA. Thus Ca channel phosphorylation slows both Ca- and E_m-dependent inactivation, but higher Ca influx and SR Ca release may functionally reverse this effect in the normal cellular environment.

Both $β_1$ and $β_2$-adrenergic agonists couple to G_s and can produce inotropic effects in heart, but they may couple differentially to L-type Ca channels *vs.* other cellular targets (Xiao & Lakatta, 1993; Xiao *et al.*, 1994b; Hool & Harvey, 1997). Additionally the $β_2$-adrenergic receptor may also couple to a G_i transduction system (Zhou *et al.*, 1999), complicating the resulting effects and interpretations. Intracellular Mg can block I_{Ca}, but Mg-ATP also stimulates I_{Ca} independent of phosphorylation (O'Rourke *et al.*, 1992). At physiological intracellular Mg-ATP this regulatory effect is probably maximal.

OTHER MODULATORS OF Ca CURRENT

Other hormones are known to modify cardiac Ca currents, although for many of these results are conflicting or the effects are relatively small (McDonald *et al.*, 1994). For example, most results with α-adrenergic agonists indicate no affect on I_{Ca} (Hescheler *et al.*, 1988; Hartmann *et al.*, 1988; Ertl *et al.*, 1991). However, phenylephrine induced a small transient decrease followed by a substantial increase in I_{Ca} only when using perforated patch recording (Zhang *et al.*, 1998; Liu & Kennedy, 1998). This variation of whole cell voltage clamp limits rundown of I_{Ca} and prevents the washout of normal intracellular constituents which occur in conventional ruptured-patch recording and can alter cellular responses. Histamine, acting at H_2 receptors, can also increase cardiac I_{Ca} by activating adenylyl cyclase and the cAMP cascade (Hescheler *et al.*, 1987b; Levi & Alloatti, 1988). Atrial natriuretic peptide (ANP) can reduce I_{Ca}, but this may depend on intracellular GTP and cAMP levels (Anand-Srivastava & Cantin, 1986; Cramb *et al.*, 1987, Gisbert & Fischmeister, 1988; LeGrand *et al.*, 1992). ANP may activate G_i and prevent cAMP dependent enhancement of cardiac I_{Ca} in a similar manner to acetylcholine.

ANP may also activate guanylyl cyclase and cGMP production, which can modulate I_{Ca} via PKG as well as stimulate breakdown of cAMP by phosphodiesterase type II. As mentioned earlier, cGMP is not generally found to alter basal I_{Ca} (Ono & Trautwein, 1991), but some investigators contend that PKG can directly decrease cardiac I_{Ca} (Wahler *et al.,* 1990; Sperelakis *et al.,* 1996). Endothelin increases I_{Ca} in smooth muscle (Inoue *et al.,* 1990), but in cardiac myocytes it either produces a small reduction of I_{Ca}, particularly without pipette GTP, but could enhance I_{Ca} with GTP in the pipette (Tohse *et al.,* 1990; Lauer *et al.,* 1992). In perforated patch measurements endothelin had no effect on basal I_{Ca}, but reversed β-adrenergic agonist stimulation of I_{Ca} via the ET_A receptor and pertussis toxin-sensitive G_i (Thomas *et al.,* 1997).

Adenosine, acting at P_1-purinergic receptors can activate G_i and prevent I_{Ca} activation by β-adrenergic agonists, but does not alter basal I_{Ca}, analogous to ACh above (Belardinelli & Isenberg, 1983b; West *et al.,* 1986). Activation of P_2-purinergic receptors by adenosine can increase I_{Ca} via stimulation of G_s (Scamps *et al.,* 1992), but inhibitory effects have also been reported (e.g. Qu *et al.,* 1993). Angiotensin II can increase I_{Ca}, possibly via stimulation of protein kinase C (PKC) rather than PKA (Allen *et al.,* 1988; Dösemeci *et al.,* 1988; LeGrand *et al.,* 1991). Phorbol esters directly stimulate protein kinase C (PKC) and in cardiac myocytes were shown to increase (Dösemeci *et al.,* 1988; Lacerda *et al.,* 1988), decrease (Tseng & Boyden, 1991; Scamps *et al.,* 1992; Zhang *et al.,* 1997a), have biphasic effects (Lacerda *et al.,* 1988) or not change I_{Ca} (Walsh & Kass, 1988). While this leaves the issue somewhat unclear, Zhang *et al.* (1997a) have shown that the inhibitory effect of the phorbol ester PMA that they observe is attributable to a C2-containing PKC isoform (PKC-α, -β or -γ).

Protein tyrosine kinase (PTK) inhibitors (e.g. genestein) decrease I_{Ca} in ruptured patch experiments (Katsube *et al.,* 1998; Hool *et al.,* 1998; Ogura *et al.,* 1999), but also have a coexistent larger and slower stimulatory effect that is apparent in perforated patch experiments (Wang & Lipsius, 1998). This may mean that a membrane associated PTK stimulates basal I_{Ca}, while a cytosolic PTK is normally inhibitory. Blocking PTKs with genestein also increases the sensitivity to β-adrenergic agonists with respect to stimulation of I_{Ca} and I_K (Hool *et al.,* 1998). Thus tyrosine kinases may depress responsiveness to adrenergic signaling and reflects a cross-talk between these kinase cascades. Arachadonic acid and some of its metabolites (epoxy-eicosatrienoic acids, EETs) can also inhibit cardiac I_{Ca} (Petit-Jaques & Hartzell, 1996; Chen *et al.,* 1999a). While arachadonate may act by stimulating a phosphatase, EETs seem to directly accelerate inactivation and decrease single channel p_o and conductance.

Regulation of I_{Ca} by these other pathways is indeed potentially confusing given the number of conflicting results. However, most of these seem to work via G_s, G_i (and possibly other G-proteins) and modulation of cyclic nucleotides (cAMP & cGMP) and protein kinases (PKA, PKC, PTK and PKG). Clearly additional work will be required to clarify the details of these intermingling pathways for many of these important modulatory mechanisms.

In conclusion, I would like to emphasize that L-type I_{Ca} is the main route of Ca entry into the cell (*vs.* leak, Na/Ca exchange or $I_{Ca,T}$) and that I_{Ca} plays a central role in cardiac E-C coupling and overall Ca regulation and contraction. The kinetics and amplitude of the I_{Ca} during the action potential are critical factors in controlling the amount of Ca released by the SR (see Chapter 8). Ca which enters as I_{Ca} may also contribute directly to the activation of the myofilaments as well as to the replenishment of SR Ca stores (see Chapter 9). The amount of Ca influx via I_{Ca} must be extruded from the cell during the same cardiac cycle (e.g. via Na/Ca exchange) for a steady state to exist. Any uncompensated Ca influx could constitute a progressive Ca load for the cell. Due to the high conductance of these ion channels, a relatively small number of Ca channels which fail to inactivate could lead to substantial Ca gain (e.g. during a window I_{Ca}, especially at depolarized E_m). This, of course, can compromise relaxation and contraction and even be arrhythmogenic (see Chapters 4, 6 & 10).

D.M. Bers.
Excitation-Contraction Coupling and Cardiac Contractile Force.
2nd Ed., Kluwer Academic Publishers, Dordrecht, 2001

CHAPTER 6

Na/Ca EXCHANGE AND THE SARCOLEMMAL Ca-PUMP

THE SARCOLEMMAL Ca-PUMP

The two known mechanisms responsible for extrusion of Ca from cardiac myocytes are the sarcolemmal Ca-ATPase pump and Na/Ca exchange. A plasma membrane Ca-pump was first reported in erythrocytes (Schatzmann, 1966), but is ubiquitous (Schatzmann, 1982, 1989; Carafoli & Stauffer, 1993; Guerini et al., 1998). The red cell plasma membrane Ca-pump has been most extensively characterized and appears closely related to that in other tissues. Two key features of the Ca-pump are its stimulation by Ca-calmodulin and by PKA-dependent phosphorylation. The plasma membrane Ca-pump is a P-type ATPase (like the Na/K-ATPase, H/K-ATPase and the SR Ca-ATPase). That is, it transfers the energy of ATP to a high energy phosphorylated intermediate (aspartyl residue), energy which is then used in the ion transport step (e.g. Figs 44 & 83). The purified protein (138 kDa) is no more similar to the SR Ca-pump protein than it is to the Na/K-ATPase or H/K-ATPase (Niggli et al., 1981a; Verma et al., 1988). The plasma membrane Ca-ATPase was first cloned by Shull & Greeb (1988) and there are four human isogenes (PMCA1-4) and also numerous splice variants (Carafoli, 1994). A central stretch of ~80 kDa is all that is required for Ca transport (James et al., 1988). The overall structure is similar to the related, and better characterized SR/ER Ca-ATPase (SERCA; see Chapter 7, Fig 81-82). There are probably 10 transmembrane domains (TM1-10) which make up ~20% of the protein, while the cytosolic domains make up ~80%. The data are much more compelling for the SR Ca-ATPase, but TM4, 5 and 6 may be involved in Ca translocation. The TM2-3 loop is analogous to the *hinge* domain of SERCA which is thought to couple ATP hydrolysis to Ca transport. The even larger TM4-5 loop contains the site which binds ATP (and fluorescein isothiocyanate or FITC) and also the aspartate which is phosphorylated at the active site of the enzyme. A third important cytosolic domain is the carboxy terminal tail where a 30 amino acid stretch contains the regulatory calmodulin binding domain and also has regulatory sites which are phosphorylated by PKA and PKC (James et al., 1988, 1989; Wang et al., 1991). This carboxy terminal is thought to interact with the other 2 cytosolic domains in an autoinhibitory manner, such that Ca-calmodulin binding and phosphorylation relieve this inhibition (Carafoli, 1994). One Ca ion seems to be transported per ATP hydrolyzed (Rega & Garrahan, 1986) and Ca extrusion by this pump appears coupled to proton influx (1Ca:1H, Kuwayama, 1988). The turnover rate of plasma membrane Ca-pumps may approach ~20/sec with $K_m(Ca)$ ~1 μM (Schatzmann, 1989).

The cardiac sarcolemmal Ca-pump was first described in vesicle studies by Caroni & Carafoli (1980). They also demonstrated a stimulatory effect of cAMP-dependent phosphorylation (~3-fold) and calmodulin on the pump (Caroni & Carafoli 1981a,b). They found a $K_m(ATP)$~30 µM, $K_m(Ca)=0.3$ µM and $V_{max}=31$ nmol/mg protein/min in the presence of endogenous calmodulin *vs.* $K_m(Ca)=11$ µM and $V_{max}=10$ nmol/mg protein/min in calmodulin depleted preparations. Dixon & Haynes (1989) measured the cardiac sarcolemma Ca-ATPase activity stimulation by calmodulin, cAMP-dependent protein kinase or both (Table 18). Calmodulin profoundly effects $K_m(Ca)$ and V_{max}, while smaller effects were observed with PKA.

Table 18

Kinetic Properties of the Cardiac Sarcolemmal Ca-Pump

	V_{max} nmol/mg pn/min	$V_{max}*$ µmol/L cytosol/sec	$K_m(Ca)$ nM	n (Hill)
Basal	1.7 ± 0.3	0.28	1800 ± 100	1.6 ± 0.1
+PKA	3.1 ± 0.5	0.50	1100 ± 100	1.7 ± 0.1
+Calmodulin	15.0 ± 2.5	2.43	64 ± 1.4	3.7 ± 0.2
+PKA+calmodulin	36.0 ± 6.5	5.83	63 ± 1.7	3.7 ± 0.1

Data are taken from Dixon & Haynes (1989). *assuming 30-fold enrichment of sarcolemma, 120 mg protein/g wet wt and 2.43 g wet wt/ml cytosol (see Table 9, pg 42).

The maximum rate of Ca extrusion via the sarcolemmal Ca-pump from cardiac myocytes based on these V_{max} values is ~5.8 µmol/L cytosol/sec. Bassani *et al.* (1995a) found a very similar V_{max} in intact ventricular myocytes (2 µmol/L cytosol/sec in rabbit and 10 µM/sec in ferret), but the apparent $K_m(Ca) = 0.3$ µM was intermediate and closer to the Caroni & Carafoli value above. This might reflect a partial calmodulin activated state in the intact cell. The affinity of the sarcolemmal Ca-pump for Ca-calmodulin is high (K_m ~1 nM; Graf & Penniston, 1981), but direct information about dynamic regulation in myocytes is lacking. The activating effect of calmodulin on the Ca-ATPase can also be mimicked by acidic phospholipids, and in the normal cellular environment this may produce 50% maximal activity (Niggli *et al.*, 1981b).

There are no highly selective inhibitors of the sarcolemmal Ca-ATPase. However, eosin and other fluorescein analogues can potently inhibit plasma membrane Ca-ATPase (Gatto & Milanick, 1993). Eosin and carboxyeosin inhibit the pump with K_i values of 50 and 20 nM respectively, without altering Na/Ca exchange (Gatto *et al.*, 1995). In ventricular myocytes 15 µM carboxyeosin blocked sarcolemmal Ca-ATPase function, but may also inhibit the SR Ca-ATPase by ~20% (Bassani *et al.*, 1995a).

During normal cellular Ca transients in rabbit ventricular myocytes the transport rate by the sarcolemmal Ca-ATPase is probably <1 µM/sec and also it would take ~60 sec to produce relaxation by itself (see Fig 30, pg 53) . This rate of Ca transport is quite slow compared to that by sarcolemmal Ca channels (300 µM/sec), SR Ca release (1000 µM/sec), SR Ca-ATPase (200 µM/sec) or Na/Ca exchange (30 µM/sec); see Figs 29 and 45. Thus, while the sarcolemmal Ca-pump can have a high affinity for $[Ca]_i$, the transport rate is too slow for it to be a major contributor to Ca fluxes during the cardiac cycle. The sarcolemmal Ca-ATPase appears to be nearly 5 times stronger in ferret than in rabbit or rat ventricular myocytes (Bassani *et al.,* 1994b, 1995a). Even in the absence of SR Ca uptake, Choi & Eisner (1999) showed that Ca removal by this system in Wistar rats is only ~25% of that by the Na/Ca exchange, whereas our estimates are <13%, 6% and 14% in in Sprague Dawley rats, rabbits and ferrets, respectively (Bassani *et al.,*

1994a, 1995a). Thus, even with species differences the sarcolemmal Ca-ATPase is only a minor Ca transporter on a beat-to-beat basis. It might, however be more important in slow longer term extrusion of Ca by the cell (but see Lamont & Eisner, 1996, and the end of this chapter).

Na/Ca EXCHANGE

Von Wilbrandt & Koller (1948) proposed that the site of action of Ca on the heart was likely to be at the cell membrane and that contractions depended on the ratio $[Ca]_o/[Na]_o$. Lüttgau & Niedergerke (1958) suggested that Na and Ca compete for an anionic site (R^{2-}) responsible for bringing Ca into the cell, consistent with a Ca/Na^2 model. Repke (1964) and Langer (1964) suggested that intracellular Na might be linked to Ca influx in some way. This helped explain the basis of digitalis inotropy and the "staircase" or positive force-frequency relationship in cardiac muscle (where increasing frequency leads to increased contractile force). Reuter & Seitz (1968) in heart and Baker *et al.* (1969) in squid giant axon were the first to document the presence of a Na/Ca exchange countertransport system. In the ensuing 30 years Na/Ca exchange has been characterized and its role in cardiac Ca regulation clarified (see reviews by Khananshvili, 1998; Reeves, 1998; Blaustein & Lederer, 1999; Egger & Niggli, 1999; Philipson & Nicoll, 2000; Hryshko, 2001).

Early Characterizations in Sarcolemmal Vesicles

Much important seminal work on sarcolemmal Na/Ca exchange came from studies of isolated cardiac sarcolemmal vesicles (**SLV**). The general strategy for studying Na/Ca exchange in SLV is illustrated in Figure 66. Reeves & Sutko (1979) were the first to demonstrate Na/Ca exchange in SLV by measuring ^{45}Ca uptake into a relatively crude preparation of SLV preloaded passively with Na and diluted into a Na-free medium. Pitts (1979) made early estimates that the Na/Ca exchange stoichiometry was 3:1 (Na:Ca). Studies showed that Na/Ca exchange is both sensitive to E_m (since more positive intravesicular potential increased Ca uptake) and can generate a voltage gradient (Bers *et al.*, 1980; Reeves & Sutko, 1980; Philipson & Nishimoto, 1980; Caroni *et al.*, 1980). These results were consistent with an electrogenic Na/Ca exchange (i.e. >2Na:1Ca), but the stoichiometry was most clearly demonstrated by Reeves & Hale (1984) using a thermodynamic approach. Their measurements of the [Na] gradient required to prevent net Ca transport at various membrane potentials indicated a stoichiometry of 3Na:1Ca. This stoichiometry is completely consistent with a wide array of other studies and is now generally accepted as *the* true stoichiometry of Na/Ca exchange in cardiac muscle (e.g. Philipson & Nicoll, 2000). Some intriguing new data indicate a higher stoichiometry of ~4:1 (Fujioka *et al.*, 2000) or a loss of electrogenicity at very acidic external pH (Egger & Niggli, 2000). It is probably premature to dismiss the enormous body of work consistent with the 3:1 stoichiometry, but it may not be quite as rigidly fixed as we have thought for the past 15 years. Thus, in most of the ensuing discussion I will retain the 3:1 stoichiometry, unless otherwise noted.

It was surprisingly difficult to separate inside-out and right-side out sarcolemmal vesicles to study the symmetry of the Na/Ca exchange. Philipson & Nishimoto (1982a) and Philipson (1985) circumvented this limitation by comparing Na/Ca exchange in vesicles which were loaded with Na only by the action of the sarcolemmal Na/K-ATPase pump (i.e. inside-out vesicles) with that in the whole population of SLV. They found a similar $K_m(Ca)$ (~25 µM) and Na-dependence

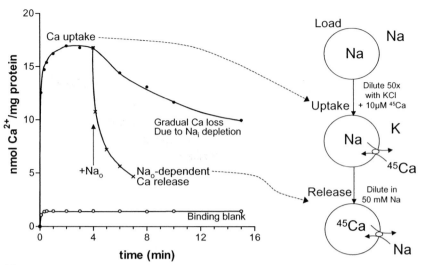

Figure 66. Na/Ca exchange in isolated cardiac sarcolemmal vesicles. Vesicles are pre-equilibrated with 140 mM Na and then diluted 50× into a solution with ^{45}Ca and 140 mM KCl or, in the case at left, 280 mM sucrose + 50 μM CaCl$_2$. Parallel samples diluted without changing [Na] serve as binding blanks. Samples are filtered or quenched with a La containing solution. After uptake has occurred, addition of 50 mM NaCl induced a rapid efflux of Ca, indicative of the reversibility of the Na/Ca exchange system (left panel is reproduced from Bers *et al.*, 1980, with permission).

of Ca efflux (K$_m$~30 mM) in both populations, suggesting a relatively symmetrical exchanger, although their later work clearly showed asymmetry (see below; Li *et al.*, 1991). In SLV the K$_m$(Na) is generally 20-30 mM, while values for K$_m$(Ca) vary widely (2-200 μM), although most reports give 20-40 μM (Reeves & Philipson, 1989). Electrophysiological measurement described below, where the siddedness is more clearly defined, have provided more direct concentration dependence and symmetry information.

Isolation, Cloning and Structure

Philipson *et al.* (1988) identified 70 and 120 kDa proteins as the Na/Ca exchanger and suggested that the smaller protein may be a proteolytic fragment of the larger. Nicoll *et al.* (1990) cloned the cardiac Na/Ca exchange (NCX1) and found it to consists of 970 amino acids (MW = 108 kDa) including 12 putative transmembrane domains and one very large cytoplasmic hydrophilic domain. The first 32 amino acids and first transmembrane span constitute a signal peptide which is cleaved off during processing (Durkin *et al.*, 1991; Hryshko *et al.*, 1993), such that the mature protein is 938 amino acids long and the amino terminal is glycosylated and extracellular. Earlier models suggested 11 transmembrane domains. However, new topological data indicate only 9 transmembrane spans (Fig 67) based on access of epitope-specific antibodies and of sulfhydryl reagents to substituted cysteine residues (Nicoll *et al.*, 1999; Iwamoto *et al.*, 1999; Doering *et al.*, 1998). In the current model there are 5 transmembrane domains on the amino part of the molecule, a large cytoplasmic or f-loop (550 amino acids or 59% of the whole protein) and 4 additional transmembrane domains on the carboxy end plus a putative P-loop like domain. Deletion of the large intracellular f-loop (Matsuoka *et al.*, 1993) showed that the loop is not essential for transport of Na or Ca, but it does abolish allosteric regulation by [Ca]$_i$ and [Na]$_i$

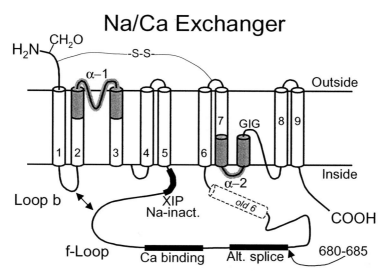

Figure 67. Working model of the Na/Ca exchanger based on the work of Nicoll *et al.* (1999) indicating 9 membrane spanning segments, glycosylation (CH_2O), α-repeats and alternative splicing domain (Alt. splice). The original 1st transmembrane domain (TM) is cleaved during maturation and not shown. Former TM6 (old-TM6) is now thought to be in the cytosolic f-loop. Former TM9 is now modeled as a P-like loop (as in ion channels) between TM7 & TM8. The figure is based on Philipson & Nicoll (2000).

(see below). Similarly, chymotrypsin treatment of the intracellular side of Na/Ca exchange in excised membrane patches also abolishes these modes of regulation (Hilgemann, 1989). There are also two 23 amino acid regions of intramolecular homology (α repeats α-1 & α-2) which face opposite sides of the membrane. There is also a region that is somewhat similar to a region of the Na/K-ATPase and SR Ca-ATPase that is thought to be involved in Ca transport (Clarke *et al.*, 1989b; Nicoll *et al.*, 1996). The second transmembrane domain and the α-repeats may contribute to the ion translocation pathway (Nicoll *et al.*, 1996), but additional clarification is required. There is also a charged segment of 20 residues (219-238) at the amino end of the f-loop (XIP) which resembled a calmodulin binding domain, and may be autoinhibitory. Exogenous XIP (exchange inhibitory peptide) can inhibit Na/Ca exchange from the cytosolic side in SLV, excised sarcolemmal patches and when dialyzed into whole myocytes (Li *et al.*, 1991; Chin *et al.*, 1993).

In addition to the gene which generates the cardiac Na/Ca exchanger (NCX1) there are two other genes (NCX2 & NCX3) which are mainly found in brain and skeletal muscle (Li *et al.*, 1994; Nicoll *et al.*, 1996). All 3 isoforms have similar, but not identical functional properties (Linck *et al.*, 1998). NCX1 is present in heart (one of the richest sources of Na/Ca exchange) and the gene is subject to alternative splicing in the f-loop. Six exons (A-F) participate and all NCX1 splice variants have either exon A or B, but not both. Exon A is more common in excitable cells (e.g. heart, neurons and skeletal muscle) while exon B is more commonly found in kidney, liver, lungs and astrocytes (Quednau *et al.*, 1997; He *et al.*, 1998). Na/Ca exchange activity in cardiac muscle is >10-fold higher than in smooth and skeletal muscle and neuronal tissue (Slaughter *et al.*, 1989; Donoso & Hidalgo, 1989; Blaustein, 1989; Barzilai *et al.*, 1984, 1987). Cardiac NCX1.1 expresses exons ACDEF (Philipson & Nicoll, 2000; Kim *et al.*, 1998).

Another Na/Ca exchanger family (NCKX) which exchanges 4Na for 1 Ca plus 1K is prominent and functionally important in rod cells in the retina (Schnetkamp *et al.*, 1989; Reïlander *et al.*, 1992). Further discussion will concentrate on cardiac NCX1.

The Na/Ca exchanger is reversible and carries out ion transport in a consecutive or "ping-pong" reaction mechanism (Khananshvili, 1990; Hilgemann *et al.*, 1991) similar to the Na/K-ATPase in Fig 44 (pg 91). For example, 3 Na ions bind with the exchanger open toward the outside and are then transported by a conformational change allowing dissociation of 3Na inside and binding of an intracellular Ca ion. The conformation then switches back to face outside and the Ca can be released to the extracellular space, completing a cycle. This would result in movement of one net charge inward per cycle and thus Ca extrusion constitutes an inward $I_{Na/Ca}$. This electrogenicity also indicates that Na/Ca exchange is sensitive to E_m as well as intracellular and extracellular [Ca] and [Na]. The Na/Ca exchanger can also operate in Na/Na exchange or Ca/Ca exchange modes (Reeves & Sutko, 1979; Philipson & Nishimoto, 1981; Slaughter *et al.*, 1983). These modes are most evident in the absence of Ca or Na respectively, but do not produce net ion movement. Thus, these fluxes are not functionally important.

Na/Ca Exchange Current in Myocytes and Excised Patches

Cardiac ionic currents attributed to Na/Ca exchange were first reported by Horackova & Vassort (1979), but acceptance was slow because of voltage clamp limitations in multicellular preparations and lack of clear expectations for the measured current. The developments of whole cell voltage clamp, ventricular myocyte isolation techniques and SLV data on Na/Ca exchange allowed faster progress. Na_o-dependent inward currents were observed in single myocytes during caffeine-induced or spontaneous SR Ca release (Clusin *et al.*, 1983; Mechmann & Pott, 1986) and were attributed to Na/Ca exchange. These currents are likely responsible for the transient inward currents ($I_{ti}s$) and delayed afterdepolarizations (DADs) discussed on page 98. Another manifestation of $I_{Na/Ca}$ is the so called "creep" currents described by Eisner & Lederer (1979) and Hume & Uehara (1986a,b). Depolarizing voltage clamp pulses in Na_i loaded cells are associated with a declining outward "creep" current (likely due to declining Ca entry via Na/Ca exchange). Repolarization also produces an inward tail current which slowly declines as Ca is extruded via Na/Ca exchange current. These creep currents were [Na] and [Ca]-dependent and could be suppressed by La and dichlorobenzamil (Bielefeld *et al.*, 1986; Hume, 1987).

Kimura *et al.* (1986, 1987; Miura & Kimura, 1989) provided key compelling electro-physiological characterizations of Na/Ca exchange in intact ventricular myocytes. They blocked all other known ionic currents (including Na/K-ATPase) and dialyzed the cell with known [Na] and [Ca] solutions. Figure 68 shows that with [Ca]$_i$ near zero, there was no current activated by 140 mM Na_o. However, when [Ca]$_i$ was raised to 430 nM, application of 140 mM Na_o activated an E_m-dependent current (Fig 68B-D) which was inward at $E_m = -90$ mV. Thus this inward current was dependent on [Na]$_o$, [Ca]$_i$ and E_m. They also demonstrated an E_m-dependent outward current which depended on [Na]$_i$ and [Ca]$_o$. The outward $I_{Na/Ca}$ (Na efflux and Ca influx) also appeared to require a certain amount of [Ca]$_i$ acting as an allosteric regulator ($K_{1/2}$ ~22 nM [Ca]$_i$, Miura & Kimura, 1989). Stimulation by Ca$_i$ was also suggested in sarcolemmal vesicle studies (Reeves & Poronnik, 1987).

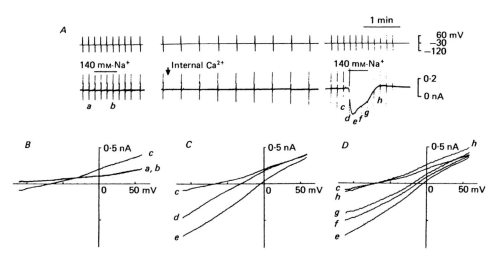

Figure 68. Na/Ca exchange current recording in a dialyzed and voltage-clamped guinea-pig ventricular myocyte. A) Slow recording of E_m (top) and $I_{Na/Ca}$ where the spikes are from ramp depolarizations used to generate the current voltage relationships in **B**, **C** and **D** at the times indicated (a-h). The bars in A refer to changing the extracellular solution from 140 mM LiCl to 140 mM NaCl ([Ca]$_o$ was 1 mM throughout). At the arrow [Ca]$_i$ was increased from nominally Ca free to 430 nM with 42 mM EGTA and 140 CsCl throughout. Ouabain, Ba, Cs, D600 and tetraethylammonium were used to inhibit other ionic currents. Application of Na$_o$ stimulated $I_{Na/Ca}$ only after [Ca]$_i$ was raised. The gradual decline in $I_{Na/Ca}$ (d-g) was supposed to be due to local Ca depletions (from Kimura *et al.*, 1987, with permission).

Hilgemann (1990) developed the giant excised patch technique to study cardiac Na/Ca exchange under more controlled conditions in patches detached from the cell. By dialyzing patch pipettes and rapidly changing bath solution around the intracellular surface of the Na/Ca exchanger (Fig 69A), Hilgemann and colleagues comprehensively characterized cardiac Na/Ca exchange (Hilgemann, 1990; Hilgemann *et al.*, 1992a,b; Matsuoka and Hilgemann, 1992; Hilgemann & Collins, 1992; Collins *et al.*, 1992). Figure 69 shows the method and some characteristics of $I_{Na/Ca}$ measured this way. Regulatory [Ca]$_i$ is required ($K_m \sim 0.3$ μM) for $I_{Na/Ca}$ activity, even when Na$_i$ is the transport substrate on the inside. With high [Ca] in the pipette ([Ca]$_o$) application of 100 mM Na to the inside surface activates outward $I_{Na/Ca}$ (Fig 69B). Sustained exposure to high [Na]$_i$ results in a Na-dependent inactivation of $I_{Na/Ca}$. Notably this Na$_i$-dependent inactivation is prominent only at high [Na]$_i$ (e.g. >30 mM), levels which may not be attained under normal physiological conditions. In addition, Fig 69C shows that when [Ca]$_i$ is high, Na$_i$-dependent inactivation does not occur. However, removal of [Ca]$_i$ still deactivates outward $I_{Na/Ca}$. Reported kinetics of Ca$_i$-dependent activation and deactivation vary (Fig 69C, Hilgemann *et al.*, 1992a; Kappl & Hartung, 1996; Weber *et al.*, 2001). We find that outward $I_{Na/Ca}$ in intact ventricular myocytes is activated during SR Ca release just as fast as [Ca]$_i$ rises (~50 ms), and that $I_{Na/Ca}$ Ca$_i$-activation state can vary dynamically during Ca transients over the physiological range with K_m=125 nM, Weber *et al.*, 2001). Thus, Ca$_i$-dependent activation may have a short-term memory of [Ca]$_i$.

Levitsky *et al.* (1994) found high affinity Ca binding to two neighboring acidic regions in NCX1 (446-454 & 498-509). Mutations of the three sequential aspartate residues in these regions disrupt both Ca binding and allosteric regulation of $I_{Na/Ca}$ by [Ca]$_i$ (Matsuoka *et al.*,

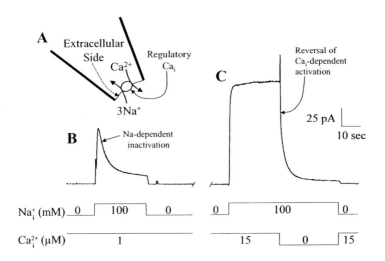

Figure 69. Na/Ca exchange current in giant excised patch showing secondary regulation by Ca_i and Na_i.
A) inside-out patch conditions (~10 μm diameter tip) with external surface bathed in high [Ca], but without
Na. **B**. Application of 100 mM Na_i (at 1 μM Ca) causes activation and then inactivation of $I_{Na/Ca}$. **C**. when
bath [Ca] is elevated to 15 μM application of 100 mM Na_i activates outward $I_{Na/Ca}$, but inactivation is not
seen. Deactivation is observed upon removal of regulatory $[Ca]_i$. The patch here is from a *Xenopus* oocyte
expressing NCX1. (modified from Philipson & Nicoll, 2000, with permission).

1995). In the *Drosophila* Na/Ca exchanger (Calx), Ca binding to the analogous region decreases
$I_{Na/Ca}$ and this effect is prevented by similar mutations (Hryshko *et al.*, 1996; Dyck *et al.*, 1998).
This raises the intriguing possibility that Ca binding to the same site produces opposite effects in
NCX1 *vs.* Calx. A deletion mutation (Δ680-685; see Fig 67) in the NCX1 f-loop abolishes
allosteric regulation by both Ca_i and Na_i (Maxwell *et al.*, 1999: Weber *et al.*, 2001), so this
region is also crucial in regulation. The XIP region of NCX1 is involved in Na_i-dependent
inactivation since mutations in this region alter the process (Matsuoka *et al.*, 1997).

The physical functions of the Ca_i-dependent activation and Na_i-dependent
inactivation in intact cells are still not clear. However, the Ca_i-dependent activation could
stimulate Ca extrusion by $I_{Na/Ca}$ when $[Ca]_i$ is relatively high and turn the exchanger off as $[Ca]_i$
falls to diastolic levels (thereby limiting how low $[Ca]_i$ goes). This Ca_i-dependent activation
could also stimulate greater Ca influx via Na/Ca exchange when conditions favor this direction
of Ca flux. The Na_i-dependent inactivation could prevent excess Ca influx and cellular Ca
overload under conditions of high $[Na]_i$ where net Ca influx might be strongly favored.
However, the very high $[Na]_i$ required to observe Na-dependent inactivation of $I_{Na/Ca}$ may render
this regulatory mechanism physiologically unimportant.

Figure 70 shows the E_m- and $[Na]_i$-dependence of $I_{Na/Ca}$ at two $[Ca]_i$ which reflect resting
and peak systolic $[Ca]_i$ (Matsuoka & Hilgemann, 1992). These data were obtained at
physiological $[Na]_o$ (140 mM) and $[Ca]_o$ (2 mM) and after treatment with chymotrypsin to
remove allosteric regulation by Na_i and Ca_i. The complex dependence of the $I_{Na/Ca}$ on Na, Ca and
E_m can be seen and is further addressed below (see *Thermodynamics*, pg 147).

Ca and Na affinities as substrates for ion transport have also been measured by several
groups under a variety of conditions and there is functional competition between Ca and Na at

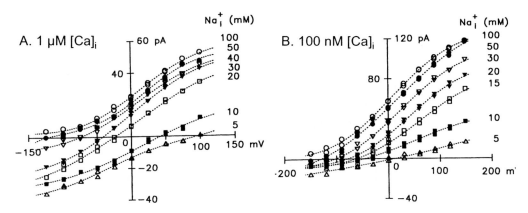

Figure 70. $I_{Na/Ca}$ Current-voltage relationships from excised giant patches from guinea-pig ventricular myocytes. Patches were treated with chymotrypsin to remove secondary regulation and all other known currents were blocked. **A.** With constant $[Ca]_o$ (2 mM), $[Na]_o$ (150 mM) and $[Ca]_i$ (1 μM), $[Na]_i$ was varied from 5 to 100 mM. The lower 3-4 curves probably reflect the $I_{Na/Ca}$ expected in intact cells when $[Ca]_i$ is high (e.g. peak systole). **B.** The same conditions as A, except $[Ca]_i$ is reduced to 100 nM, comparable to diastolic $[Ca]_i$ (from Matsuoka & Hilgemann, 1992, with permission).

both sides. There is general agreement that the $K_m(Na_i)$ of the Na/Ca exchanger is 20-30 mM, with a somewhat higher value of $K_m(Na_o)$ 50-70 mM. Moreover, the [Na]-dependence exhibits a Hill coefficient of 2-3, consistent with the stoichiometry of 3Na per transport cycle (Miura & Kimura, 1989). Miura & Kimura (1989) estimated $K_m(Ca_i)$ to be 0.6 μM, while values of 1-4 μM were found by Hilgemann *et al.* (1991; Hilgemann, 1996). Some $K_m(Ca_i)$ estimates may also be complicated by the coexistence of Ca_i-dependent allosteric regulation. Values for $K_m(Ca_o)$ have ranged from 0.1 to 1.5 mM, but most estimates are near the 1.2 mM value reported by Kimura *et al.* (1987). It should be borne in mind that the experimentally measured $K_m(Ca)$ can also be affected by other conditions such as [Na], E_m and pH.

Figure 71 shows simultaneous measurement of $I_{Na/Ca}$ and Ca transients in a guinea-pig ventricular myocyte where other channels and transporters including SR were blocked (Barcenas-Ruiz *et al.*, 1987). During long depolarizing voltage clamp steps the Na/Ca exchanger can bring in enough Ca to produce high $[Ca]_i$ (>1 μM). Then on repolarization $I_{Na/Ca}$ also produces an inward tail $I_{Na/Ca}$ (lower traces in Fig 71A) as well as $[Ca]_i$ decline. The plot of $I_{Na/Ca}$ as a function of $[Ca]_i$ is fairly linear, suggesting that Ca extrusion via Na/Ca exchange is not saturated even at relatively high physiological $[Ca]_i$. This result suggests that the functional $K_m(Ca_i)$ for the Na/Ca exchange is probably higher than 1 μM.

Many di- and trivalent cations block Na/Ca exchange activity (e.g. $Cd^{2+} > La^{3+} > Y^{3+} > Mn^{2+} > Co^{2+} > Mg^{2+}$; Bers *et al.*, 1980). Trosper & Philipson (1983) found that trivalent cations were more effective than divalents and that Ba^{2+} and Sr^{2+} also inhibited Na/Ca exchange (Table 19). Tibbits & Philipson (1985) also showed that Sr^{2+} and to a lesser extent Ba^{2+} could also substitute for Ca^{2+} and be transported in exchange for Na. Egger *et al.* (1999) also showed that Ni can be transported weakly by Na/Ca exchange, probably by an electroneutral Ni/Ca exchange, thus explaining the abolition of $I_{Na/Ca}$ typically observed with mM Ni.

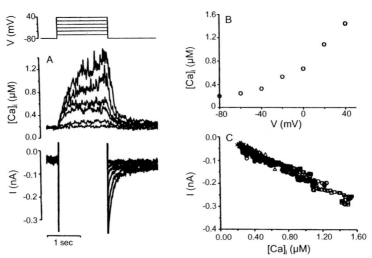

Figure 71. Ca influx and extrusion by $I_{Na/Ca}$ in a guinea-pig ventricular myocyte. **A**. Pipette [Na] was 7.5 mM. Outward currents during depolarization were off-scale. **B** and **C** show the E_m dependence of the Ca_i transient and the $[Ca]_i$-dependence of the "tail" current observed upon repolarization to –80 mV. Other ionic currents were blocked by Cs, tetraethylammonium, verapamil and ryanodine and $[Ca]_i$ was assessed by fura-2 fluorescence (from Barcenas-Ruiz *et al.*, 1987, with permission).

Charge movements by the Na/Ca exchanger have been used to measure "half-reaction cycles" (Hilgemann *et al.*, 1991; Niggli & Lipp, 1994). The idea is to start with all of the exchangers facing inside (e.g. due to high $[Na]_o$ without Ca anywhere) and then suddenly apply substrate (e.g. $[Na]_i$) to the inside such that neither the full Na/Ca exchange cycle nor net ion movement can occur. In this case the added $[Na]_i$ will bind and be translocated through a half-reaction such that the exchanger will move to face outside. Hilgemann *et al.* (1991) found that charge moved across the membrane when Na was carried, but not when Ca was carried. Furthermore, their results suggested that one positive charge moves per Na-half cycle and that this occurs near the extracellular end of the ion pathway. This would be consistent with the "unloaded" exchanger having two negative charges. The number of charges moved then provided an estimate of the surface density of Na/Ca exchanger in the membrane ($400/\mu m^2$) and with a V_{max} for $I_{Na/Ca}$ (20-30 A/F) they calculated a maximal molecular turnover rate (5000/sec). Niggli & Lipp (1994) used flash photolysis to rapidly raise $[Ca]_i$ and found that some charge moves with both the Na and Ca transporting half reaction. Interestingly, Hilgemann's group found that squid Na/Ca exchanger (NCX-SQ1) gave the opposite result from canine or guinea-pig heart NCX1, in that all of the charge moved in the Ca translocation step and none in the Na translocation step (He *et al.*, 1998).

Modulation of Na/Ca exchange

Table 19 lists some factors which alter cardiac sarcolemmal Na/Ca exchange. Early evidence, partly from SLV, suggested stimulatory effects of ATP on Na/Ca exchange and Ca affinity (Caroni & Carafoli, 1983; DiPolo & Beaugé, 1988; Hilgemann, 1990). MgATP can reactivate inactivated $I_{Na/Ca}$ in giant excised patches (K_m ~3 mM) and it was suggested that this might be due to activation of phospholipid translocase or flippase reorienting phosphatidylserine to the inner surface (Collins *et al.*, 1992; Hilgemann & Collins, 1992), consistent with activation by acidic phospholipids (Philipson, 1984). Further studies showed that ATP could activate a lipid kinase causing phosphorylation of phosphatidylinositol (PI) to form PIP_2 (Hilgemann & Ball, 1996). Apparently PIP_2 stimulates $I_{Na/Ca}$ by preventing Na_i-dependent inactivation and might interact with the positively charged XIP domain (He *et al.*, 2000; Philipson & Nicoll, 2000). Under physiological conditions ($[ATP]_i > 5$ mM) it would be expected that this PIP_2 pathway would always be fully active. This would again imply that Na_i-dependent inactivation does not occur, except under pathophysiological conditions where $[ATP]_i$ falls appreciably.

Na/Ca exchange is remarkably sensitive to alteration of the lipid bilayer. Exchange is increased by a) reconstitution with acidic phospholipids, b) addition of exogenous negatively charged amphiphiles or c) phospholipase cleavage of native phospholipids to yield negatively charged membrane lipids. Certain anionic head groups are more stimulatory for Na/Ca exchange than others and several cationic amphiphiles are inhibitory (Philipson, 1984). The effects of charged amphiphiles and phospholipids does not appear to be simply due to surface charge effects (e.g. concentrating Ca near the exchanger). Indeed, Na/Ca exchange is virtually unaffected by changes in surface charge or surface [Ca] (Bers *et al.*, 1985). The organic divalent cation dimethonium screens surface charge and thereby reduces surface [Ca] and Ca binding. But even when dimethonium strongly decreased Ca binding to SLV, it did not affect Na/Ca exchange. Thus, the negatively charged amphiphiles may enhance Na/Ca exchange via a more specific interaction with a site on the Na/Ca exchanger.

The stimulatory effect of negatively charged amphiphiles on exchange activity is enhanced if the lipophilic portion of the molecule also disorders the bilayer, especially toward the center of the bilayer (e.g. by unsaturated bonds or inclusion of doxyl- groups; Philipson & Ward, 1987). Optimal reconstitution of exchange activity requires acidic phospholipids and ~20% cholesterol with other related sterols unable to substitute (Vemuri & Philipson, 1988a).

Low pH inhibits Na/Ca exchange in SLV, while alkalosis enhances exchange (Philipson *et al.,* 1982). Giant patch recordings of outward $I_{Na/Ca}$ confirmed this, but also showed that chymotrypsin almost abolished pH_i-dependence (Doering & Lederer, 1993, 1994). Possibly the pH regulation (like that of regulation by Ca_i and Na_i) is mediated by the large cytosolic loop f. Egger & Niggli (2000) evaluated the effect the effect of extracellular pH (pH_o) on cardiac $I_{Na/Ca}$. They found maximal $I_{Na/Ca}$ at $pH_o = 7.6$ and 50% of that value at pH_o of 10 and 5.5. At very low pH_o (<6) inward $I_{Na/Ca}$ declined much more than Ca transported by Na/Ca exchange, suggesting a progressive reduction of the electrogenic nature of Ca transported by Na/Ca exchange.

The pathophysiological consequences of the pH and lipid effects above are not yet clear. However, during cardiac ischemia, the declining pH would be expected to decrease Na/Ca exchange, production of fatty acids (e.g. arachidonate, see Chien *et al.*, 1984; Philipson & Ward, 1985) would increase Na/Ca exchange and redox stimulation might also stimulate Na/Ca exchange. These latter effects might limit the depression of Na/Ca exchange during ischemia and help minimize cardiac Ca overload. On the other hand SLV from ischemic myocardium exhibit reduced Na/Ca exchange (Bersohn *et al.*, 1982) and fatty acids also increase passive Ca permeability in SLV (Philipson & Ward, 1985) so that the net result in ischemia is still unclear.

Ca chelators, such as EGTA stimulate Na/Ca exchange at a given [Ca], by reducing $K_m(Ca)$ (e.g. from ~20 to ~1 μM, Trosper & Philipson, 1984) and similar effects have been reported for the plasma membrane Ca-pump (Schatzmann, 1973; Sarkadi et al., 1979). This might partly account for the lower $K_m(Ca)$ estimated in intact cells perfused with EGTA buffers than in SLV where $K_m(Ca)$ determinations were often made without Ca chelators. It is not yet known whether the Ca affinity of the exchanger is also increased by the related Ca chelators which are used as fluorescent Ca indicators in intact cells (e.g. indo-1 and fura-2). This could complicate the use of these indicators in the study of Na/Ca exchange.

The Na/Ca exchanger can be inhibited by a number of drugs (Table 19), but most of these agents are neither very potent nor very selective. That is, they inhibit other ion transport systems and channels at even lower concentrations than those required to inhibit Na/Ca exchange (Kaczorowski et al., 1989). For example, dichlorobenzamil inhibits sarcolemmal Ca channels, and related amiloride derivatives are potent inhibitors of Na/H exchange, Na-coupled sugar and amino acid transport, Na, K & Ca channels, and cholinergic and adrenergic receptors This lack of a specific inhibitor (ligand) of Na/Ca exchange has been a serious limitation, both to the isolation of the protein and characterization of the physiological action of the Na/Ca exchanger.

XIP inhibits Na/Ca exchange non-competitively at low μM concentrations. However, it is of quite limited use in physiological experiments because the peptide must be applied intracellularly and because XIP also potently inhibits both the sarcolemmal and SR Ca-ATPase (Enyedi & Penniston, 1993). Side effects are not entirely surprising since XIP resembles a calmodulin binding domain and 8 of the 20 amino acids are positively charged. Thus while XIP may be useful in studying isolated $I_{Na/Ca}$ in excised patches, it is less help in clarifying the role of Na/Ca exchange in the complex cellular environment. FMRF-amide is a tetrapeptide which can inhibit Na/Ca exchange non-competitively with a K_i ~1 μM (DiPolo & Beaugé, 1994; Khananshvili et al., 1993). An analogous cyclic hexapeptide (FRCRCF-amide) was also a potent Na/Ca exchange inhibitor with K_i between 2-10 μM in SLV (Khananshvili et al., 1995, 1996) and in patch clamped myocytes an apparent K_i of ~20 nM (Hobai et al., 1997a).

KB-R7943, an isothiourea derivative, has been reported to be a relatively selective inhibitor of Na/Ca exchange (Watano et al., 1996; Iwamoto et al., 1996a; Watano & Kimura, 1998; Iwamoto & Shigekawa, 1998). KB-R7943 blocked outward $I_{Na/Ca}$ in myocytes with a $K_i =$ 0.32 μM, while much higher concentrations were required to block inward $I_{Na/Ca}$ ($K_i = 17$ μM; Watano et al., 1996). This apparently selective block of outward $I_{Na/Ca}$ (Ca influx) with low [KB-R7943] has been confirmed in cellular [Ca]$_i$ measurements (Satoh et al., 2000), where 5 μM KB-R7943 blocked Ca influx via Na/Ca exchange upon abrupt [Na]$_o$ removal, but had no effect on [Ca]$_i$ decline during relaxation when the SR Ca-pump was not functional. They also showed that KB-R7943 could prevent Ca overload and spontaneous arrhythmias induced by strophanthidin-induced block of the Na/K-ATPase, without preventing the inotropic effects. While this intriguing compound may be useful, it also inhibits I_{Na} ($K_i = 14$ μM), I_{Ca} ($K_i = 8$ μM) and inward rectifying I_K ($K_i = 7$ μM; Watano et al., 1996). It is also unclear from a mechanistic standpoint how it seems to produce relatively direction-specific block (Kimura et al., 1999). Thus, KB-R7943 should be used cautiously and with appropriate controls.

Table 19

Factors That Alter Cardiac Sarcolemmal Na/Ca Exchange

Enhancers of Na/Ca Exchange

		Reference
E_m	Depolarization $\rightarrow\uparrow$ Ca entry	a
pH	Alkalosis	b
ATP	mM ATP ($\downarrow K_m(Ca)$)	c,d
PIP_2	via ATP-stimulated lipid kinase	e
$[Ca]_i$	40-125 nM $\rightarrow\uparrow I_{Na/Ca}$ (regulatory)	d,f
Proteinase	Trypsin, Chymotrypsin, Pronase, Papain, Ficin	g
Phospholipase	Phospholipase C & D $\rightarrow\uparrow$ Exchange	h
Anionic Amphiphiles	SDS, Lauric acid $\rightarrow\uparrow$ Exchange ($\downarrow K_m$)	i,j
Redox Modification	$FeSO_4$ & DTT, Glutathione	k
Ca Chelator	EGTA, EDTA, CDTA ($\downarrow K_m$)	l
Lipids	Cholesterol, Unsaturated/doxyl lipids	m

Inhibitors of Na/Ca Exchange

		Reference
pH	$\downarrow$ pH $\rightarrow\downarrow$ Exchange	b
Inorganic Cations	$La^{3+}>Nd^{3+}>Tm^{3+}\sim Y^{3+}>Cd^{2+}>$ $Sr^{2+}>Ba^{2+}\sim Mn^{2+}>Mg^{2+}$	n,a
Cd^{2+}, Ni^{2+}	$K_i(Cd)$= 320 μM; $K_m(Ni)$ = 200 μM	o
XIP	K_i = 0.1-1 μM	p
FMRF-amide	K_i = 1.5 μM	q
Cationic Amphiphiles	Dodecylamine $\rightarrow\downarrow$ Exchange ($\downarrow V_{max}$)	j
Adriamycin (doxorubicin)		r
Chlorpromazine		r
Tetracaine, Dibucaine, Ethanol		s
Verapamil, D600	K_i(Verapamil)= 50-200 μM; K_i(D600)= 22 μM	t
Quinidine		u
Polymyxin B		g
Quinacrine	K_i = 10-50 μM	v,w
Bepridil	K_i = 30 μM	x
Dichlorobenzamil	K_i = 4 - 17 μM	y,w
Harmaline	K_i = 250 μM	z
Methylation		α
KB-R7943	$K_i(I_{Na/Ca})$= 17 μM inward, 0.3 μM outward	β

a) Bers *et al.*, 1980; Caroni *et al.*, 1980, Philipson & Nishimoto, 1980, **b)** Philipson *et al.*, 1982, **c)** Caroni & Carafoli, 1983; DiPolo & Beaugé, 1987, **d)** DiPolo & Beaugé, 1988, Hilgemann, 1990, **e)** Hilgemann & Ball, 1996, **f)** Miura & Kimura, 1989; Weber *et al.*, 2001, **g)** Philipson & Nishimoto, 1982b, **h)** Philipson & Nishimoto, 1984, **i)** Philipson, 1984, **j)** Philipson *et al.*, 1985, **k)** Reeves *et al.*, 1986, **l)** Trosper & Philipson, 1984; **m)** Philipson & Ward. 1985; Philipson & Ward, 1987; Vemuri & Philipson, 1987, **n)** Trosper & Philipson, 1983, **o)** Hobai *et al.*, 1997a, **p)** Li *et al.*, 1991, **q)** DiPolo & Beaugé, 1994; Khananshvili *et al.*, 1993, **r)** Caroni *et al.*, 1981, **s)** Michaelis *et al.*, 1987; Michaelis & Michaelis, 1983, **t)** Van Amsterdam & Zaagzma, 1986; Kosnev *et al.*, 1989; Kimura *et al.*, 1987, **u)** Ledvora & Hegvary, 1983; Mentrard *et al.*, 1984, **v)** De la Peña & Reeves, 1987, **w)** Bielefeld *et al.*, 1986, **x)** Garcia *et al.*, 1988, **y)** Kaczarowski *et al.* 1985, **z)** Suleiman & Reeves, 1987, **α)** Vemuri & Philipson, 1988b, **β)** Watano *et al.* 1996.

Phosphorylation

Evidence that Na/Ca exchange can be stimulated by phosphorylation in squid giant axon (see DiPolo & Beaugé, 1991) has generally not extended to cardiac Na/Ca exchange despite attempts to evaluate this sort of effect (Philipson & Nicoll, 2000). There are a couple of exceptions to the predominantly negative results with respect to phosphorylation. Iwamoto *et al.* (1995, 1996b, 1998) detected effects of PKC on cardiac and smooth muscle Na/Ca exchange that were initially attributed to phosphorylation, but the functional effects were modest and the latter work indicated that NCX1 phosphorylation was not required. Stimulatory effects reported for Phenylephrine, angiotensin II and endothelin-1 may be via PKC (Ballard & Schaffer, 1996). Fan *et al.* (1996) found that PKA activation can inhibit Na/Ca exchange activity in frog heart, an effect which might be due to a unique exon present in the frog, but not mammalian Na/Ca exchanger (Shuba *et al.*, 1998).

V_{max} vs. Ca Requirements, Site Density and Localization

To appreciate the contribution of Na/Ca exchange to cellular Ca fluxes, let us consider the rate at which this system transports Ca. In SLV, Ca transport rates of ~25 nmol/mg protein/sec are typically observed (Reeves & Philipson, 1989). Assuming 30-fold purification of SLV and 120 mg tissue protein/g wet wt tissue this would be ~240 μmol/L cytosol/sec. $I_{Na/Ca}$ of ~300 pA (or 3 A/F) are also typical in mammalian ventricular myocytes (e.g. Miura & Kimura, 1989), corresponding to 200 μmol/L cytosol/sec. Based on the rate of Ca extrusion during caffeine-induced contractures maximal physiological Ca efflux is ~50 μmol/L cytosol/sec (Bassani *et al.,* 1994a). Thus Ca transport rates under physiological conditions probably are <100 μmol/L cytosol (1 A/F).   However, when outward $I_{Na/Ca}$ is driven by saturating concentrations of substrate (100 mM [Na]$_i$ & >10 mM [Ca]$_o$) and large positive E_m the maximal $I_{Na/Ca}$ can be 30 A/F or 10-20 times higher (Li & Kimura, 1990; Hilgemann, 1990). It is under these real V_{max} conditions that the turnover rate of 5000/sec was estimated (Hilgemann *et al.*, 1991). This is much higher than most membrane transporters such as Na/K-ATPase, which has a maximum turnover rate of 60-200/sec (Freidrich *et al.*, 1996).   The site density for Na/Ca exchangers is 200-400/μm^2 (Hilgemann *et al.*, 1991). This is lower than the value of 1000/μm^2 which can be inferred for the Na/K-ATPase (Colvin *et al.*, 1985), but 10-20 times higher than the density of DHPR and functional Ca channels (see pg 114). There is some controversy about the spatial distribution of Na/Ca exchange molecules in the ventricular sarcolemma. Frank *et al.* (1992) indicated that Na/Ca exchangers are located preferentially in T-tubules, while Kieval *et al.* (1992) found a more uniform sarcolemmal distribution.

Under physiological conditions the Na/Ca exchanger probably only reaches a turnover rate of ~300-500/sec (because of non-V_{max} conditions). While this is still fast flux for an ion pump, it is more than 1000 times smaller than an L-type Ca channel (or RyR). A single Ca channel current of 0.3 pA at 2 mM [Ca]$_o$ corresponds to 10^6 Ca ions/sec (~3000 times larger). Thus, while the normal cellular peak I_{Ca} (6 A/F) and $I_{Na/Ca}$ (1 A/F) may differ by only a factor of 6 (and for Ca flux by only a factor of 3), it will take ~1000 times as many Na/Ca exchange molecules to carry out this Ca transport. This has important implications with respect to spatial aspects of Ca signaling which are important in E-C coupling. For example, the opening of a single Ca channel in the junctional cleft will bring in 1000 Ca ions/ms in a membrane area of 0.0003 μm^2, whereas ~3000 Na/Ca exchange molecules would be required to produce the same Ca influx. These Na/Ca exchange molecules (even at 400/μm^2) would occupy ~8 μm^2 of membrane or a disc of 2.5 μm diameter, which is more than 10 times larger that the whole junctional region and more on the scale of an entire sarcomere. Thus, Ca entry via I_{Ca} is 25,000 times more "focused" than $I_{Na/Ca}$, making it a much more effective way to elevate local [Ca]$_i$ to relatively high levels. Na/Ca exchange is still an important quantitative mode of Ca transport during the cardiac cycle, it is simply less capable of producing local $[Ca]_i$ spikes than is I_{Ca}.

The ability of Na/Ca exchange to extrude Ca in ventricular myocytes varies in different species. Sham *et al.* (1995b) found the amount of inward $I_{Na/Ca}$ to vary with hamster >guinea-pig > rat ventricle. I would extend this provisionally based on our data on Na/Ca exchange-dependent $[Ca]_i$ decline of caffeine-induced contractures in several papers to be hamster>guinea-pig >rabbit >ferret >cat >dog >mouse ~ rat. Su *et al.* (1999) found an almost inverted sequence when measuring outward $I_{Na/Ca}$ induced by abrupt Na_o withdrawal (mouse >rat > rabbit >dog > human). It is not clear why these observations differ, but the former data are for forward mode (Ca extrusion) whereas the latter are for Ca-influx mode. It is possible that this discrepancy is partially attributable to higher $[Na]_i$ in rat and mouse, which favors outward $I_{Na/Ca}$.

Ca Entry via Na/Ca Exchange and Contraction

Rapid reduction of $[Na]_o$ around intact cardiac muscle cells causes large contractions attributed to Ca influx via Na/Ca exchange (e.g. Chapman & Tunstall, 1980). However, this doesn't address whether Ca entry via Na/Ca exchange can contribute appreciably to force development under more physiological conditions. Many results indicate that Ca entry via Na/Ca exchange *can* contribute quantitatively to the direct activation of the myofilaments, since contractions and Ca transients can be activated by action potentials and long depolarizing voltage clamp pulses even when both sarcolemmal Ca channels and SR Ca release are inhibited (e.g. Eisner *et al.*, 1983; Cannell *et al.*, 1986; Hume & Uehara, 1986b; Barcenas-Ruiz *et al.*, 1987; Bers *et al.*, 1988). However, with $[Na]_i$ of only ~7 mM very large or very long depolarizations are required (Fig 71).

In intact rabbit ventricular muscle, we showed that action potential activated contractions can be nearly abolished by blocking Ca channels with nifedipine (Bers *et al.*, 1988). However, if $[Na]_i$ is elevated (e.g. to 15-20 mM), large twitch contractions can still be elicited in the presence of nifedipine (see Fig 124). We concluded that Ca entry via Na/Ca exchange does not normally contribute significantly to the activation of contraction, but can if $[Na]_i$ is elevated by inhibition of the Na-pump. There was also indirect evidence to suggest that, with elevated $[Na]_i$, Ca entry via Na/Ca exchange could trigger Ca release from the SR. While Cannell *et al.* (1987) indicated that this may not occur when $[Na]_i$ is only ~7 mM, Leblanc & Hume (1990) showed that Ca entry via Na/Ca exchange may induce SR Ca release. In the latter case, they suggest that tetrodotoxin-sensitive Na entry may increase the local subsarcolemmal $[Na]_i$ thereby activating Ca entry and SR Ca release. The possible role of Na/Ca exchange in SR Ca release will be discussed further in Chapters 8 & 10, but this is probably only relevant when $[Na]_i$ is high.

Thermodynamic Considerations

Before further discussion of cellular Ca flux via Na/Ca exchange it is worth considering the thermodynamic basis that governs net transport. If there is more energy in the inwardly directed electrochemical gradient for 3 Na ions than for one Ca ion, Ca extrusion via this coupled transporter is thermodynamically favored (Mullins, 1979). That is

$$n(E_{Na} - E_m) > 2(E_{Ca} - E_m) \qquad (6.1)$$

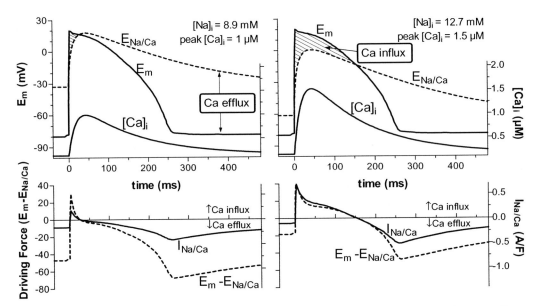

Figure 72. Changes in $E_{Na/Ca}$ and $I_{Na/Ca}$ during an action potential in rabbit ventricle. When $E_m > E_{Na/Ca}$, Ca influx via the Na/Ca exchanger is thermodynamically favored (shaded areas). When $E_m < E_{Na/Ca}$, Ca extrusion is favored. Resting $[Ca]_i=150$ nM, $[Ca]_o=2$ mM and $[Na]_o=140$ mM for all traces, with peak $[Ca]_i$ (at 40 ms) indicated. Na activity coefficient of 0.786 is assumed (i.e. $[Na]_i$ of 8.9 & 12.7 implies aNa_i of 7 & 10 mM). $E_{Na/Ca}$ is from Eq 6.2 and current uses the Luo & Rudy (1991) equation:
$$I_{Na/Ca}= k_{Na/Ca}\{e^{\eta Vk}[Na]_i^3[Ca]_o - e^{(\eta-1)Vk}[Na]_o^3[Ca]_i\}\}/\{(K_{mNa}^3 + [Na]_o^3)(K_{mCa}+[Ca]_o)(1+k_{sat}e^{(\eta-1)Vk})\},$$
with $k_{Na/Ca}= 2000$ A/F, $K_{m,Na}=87.5$ mM, $K_{m,Ca}=1.38$ mM, $k_{sat}= 0.25$, $\eta=0.35$ and $k=F/RT=1/(26$ mV).

where n is the coupling ratio and E_{Ca} and E_{Na} are the equilibrium potentials for Ca and Na ($E_x = (RT/zF) \log ([X]_o/[X]_i)$). Then for $n=3$, the potential at which the gradients are equal ($E_{Na/Ca}$) is the $I_{Na/Ca}$ reversal potential or the E_m at which the $I_{Na/Ca}$ is zero (exactly analogous to the reversal potential of an ion channel). Hence,

$$E_{Na/Ca} = 3E_{Na} - 2E_{Ca} \tag{6.2}$$

Thus, whenever E_m is more positive than $E_{Na/Ca}$ Ca entry via the exchanger is favored and when E_m is negative to $E_{Na/Ca}$ Ca extrusion is favored.

Figure 72 illustrates how $E_{Na/Ca}$ may be expected to change during the action potential in ventricular muscle under normal conditions. The shape of the $E_{Na/Ca}$ curve is dictated here by the $[Ca]_i$ transient (which alters E_{Ca}). For typical diastolic values of $[Na]_o$ and $[Na]_i$ (140 and 8.9 mM respectively; $E_{Na} = +73$ mV) and $[Ca]_o$ and $[Ca]_i$ (2 mM and 150 nM, respectively; $E_{Ca} = +125.8$ mV) $E_{Na/Ca}$ would be -32.6 mV. Thus at a resting E_m of -80 mV Ca extrusion and inward $I_{Na/Ca}$ would be thermodynamically favored ($E_{Na/Ca} > E_m$). During the action potential, there is a very brief period where Ca influx via the exchanger is favored ($E_m > E_{Na/Ca}$, shading in Fig 72). It can be appreciated that the precise length of this period is rather sensitive to changes in peak $[Ca]_i$, the time course of the Ca transient, $[Na]_i$ and the shape of the action potential. The lower panels show how the thermodynamic driving force ($E_m - E_{Na/Ca}$) and $I_{Na/Ca}$ changes during the AP. This illustrates the dynamic, yet delicate balance of Ca fluxes mediated by the Na/Ca exchanger.

Indeed, increasing intracellular Na activity from 7 to 10 mM (8.9 to 12.7 mM [Na]$_i$) in the right panel prolongs the time when Ca influx would be favored, even though peak [Ca]$_i$ is much higher (which by itself would favor Ca efflux).

While the simple thermodynamic consideration above can be sufficient to predict the direction of Ca transport by Na/Ca exchange and the driving force, the I$_{Na/Ca}$ amplitude is also subject to kinetic limitations (depending on substrate concentrations). Indeed, as [Ca]$_i$ declines, the inward I$_{Na/Ca}$ in Fig 72 is not as large as might be expected from the driving force. That is, the driving force for Ca extrusion via Na/Ca exchange during diastole is large, but the net Ca extrusion is limited by the low diastolic [Ca]$_i$. Several quantitative models of I$_{Na/Ca}$ have included these considerations (e.g. DiFrancesco & Noble, 1985; Hilgemann, 1989; Beuckelmann & Wier, 1989; Matsuoka & Hilgemann, 1992; Luo & Rudy, 1994a). Figure 72 uses the equation of Luo & Rudy (1994a), but I now prefer a more complete version:

$$I_{Na/Ca} = \frac{(V_{max}/(1+\{K_{mAllo}/[Ca]_i\}^2))\ ([Na]_i^3[Ca]_o e^{\eta Vk} - [Na]_o^3[Ca]_i\ e^{(\eta-1)Vk})}{\left[\begin{array}{l} K_{mCao}[Na]_i^3 + K_{mNao}^3[Ca]_i + K_{mNai}^3[Ca]_o(1+[Ca]_i/K_{mCai}) + \\ K_{mCai}[Na]_o^3(1 + \{[Na]_i/K_{mNai}\}^3) + [Na]_i^3[Ca]_o + [Na]_o^3[Ca]_i) \end{array}\right]\left[1 + k_{sat}e^{(\eta-1)Vk}\right]} \tag{6.3}$$

where K$_{mAllo}$ is the K$_m$ for allosteric Ca$_i$-activation (125 nM). Other constants are transport K$_m$s for Na & Ca inside and out (in mM): K$_{mCao}$ (1.4), K$_{mCai}$ (0.0036), K$_{mNao}$ (88), K$_{mNai}$ (12). The k$_{sat}$ (0.27) assures saturation at very negative E$_m$, η (0.35) is the energy barrier position controlling E$_m$-dependence of I$_{Na/Ca}$ and k=F/RT (V$_{max}$ ~10-20 A/F). We developed this equation during studies of allosteric regulation (first factor in numerator) of I$_{Na/Ca}$ by [Ca]$_i$ (Weber *et al.*, 2000).

The I$_{Na/Ca}$ analysis in Fig 72 is simplified because it assumes that [Ca]$_i$ is uniform during the Ca transient. However, during the twitch there are likely to be spatial gradients of [Ca] near the membrane and sites of SR Ca release (Langer & Peskoff, 1996). Trafford *et al.* (1995) used I$_{Na/Ca}$ to demonstrate that the local subsarcolemmal [Ca]$_i$ ([Ca]$_{sm}$) sensed by the Na/Ca exchanger differed from the global [Ca]$_i$ during caffeine-induced Ca transients. Figure 73 shows this type of experimental analysis. Figure 73B shows [Ca]$_i$ and I$_{Na/Ca}$ plotted against each other for each time point in Fig 73A. During the rising phase of the Ca transient (Activation) I$_{Na/Ca}$ amplitude is much larger than for the same [Ca]$_i$ during relaxation. Using I$_{Na/Ca}$ as a bioassay for local [Ca]$_i$ and assuming that [Ca]$_i$ = [Ca]$_{sm}$ during the latter part of [Ca]$_i$ decline (regression line), we can infer [Ca]$_{sm}$ from I$_{Na/Ca}$ for any point. Figure 73C shows that [Ca]$_{sm}$ rises earlier and to a much higher peak value than [Ca]$_i$ sensed by the bulk cytosolic Ca indicator. This emphasizes the utility of electrophysiological indicators of local [Ca]. It also indicates that large spatial gradients of [Ca]$_i$ exist during what appear to be relatively homogeneous signals from fluorescent Ca indicators (see also Fig 60, pg 122, where I$_{Ca}$ was used in a similar manner).

During a normal twitch these gradients could be even faster and steeper due to the rapid and highly synchronized twitch SR Ca release compared to that induced by caffeine. Indeed, Egan *et al.* (1989) interrupted the action potential by repolarization and used tail I$_{Na/Ca}$ to predict the twitch Ca transient sensed by the Na/Ca exchanger. Figure 74 combines these considerations into the context of Fig 72 concerning I$_{Na/Ca}$ during the cardiac action potential. The Ca transient in Fig 74A produces a change in E$_{Na/Ca}$ that is between the two cases shown in Fig 72, and the

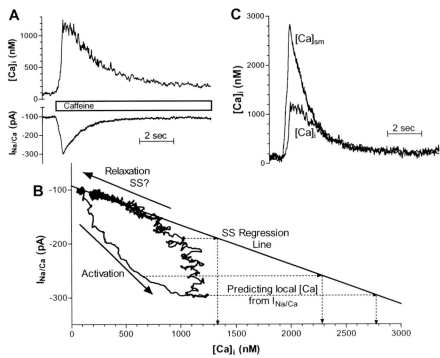

Figure 73. Submembrane [Ca] predicted from $I_{Na/Ca}$. **A.** caffeine-induced Ca transient and $I_{Na/Ca}$ in a rabbit ventricular myocyte. **B.** $I_{Na/Ca}$ plotted as a function of global [Ca]$_i$ for the traces in A (note that during activation $I_{Na/Ca}$ is larger in amplitude than for the same [Ca]$_i$ during [Ca]$_i$ decline). During [Ca]$_i$ decline the [Ca]$_i$ is assumed to directly control $I_{Na/Ca}$, such that a linear regression (between resting [Ca]$_i$ and [Ca]$_i$ decline below 800 nM) predicts local submembrane [Ca]$_i$ ([Ca]$_{sm}$). Dotted lines indicate [Ca]$_{sm}$ sensed by the Na/Ca exchanger at 3 different points before the steady state (SS) relation is assumed. **C.** Complete plot of [Ca]$_{sm}$ and [Ca]$_i$ for this caffeine-induced Ca transient (data acquired by K.S. Ginsburg).

$I_{Na/Ca}$ in Fig 74C (driven by global [Ca]$_i$ and [Na]$_i$) is similar to that in Fig 72. However, if we instead allow the [Ca]$_{sm}$ in Fig 74B to drive $I_{Na/Ca}$ the initial outward current only lasts 0.3 ms instead of 75 ms (and reduces total Ca influx from 0.3 to 0.01 µmol/L cytosol). Thus the high local [Ca]$_i$ in the junctional cleft (produced by I_{Ca} and SR Ca release) can shift Na/Ca exchange rapidly into the Ca efflux mode. Thus high local [Ca]$_i$ may limit any net Ca entry via Na/Ca exchange during the AP. On the other hand, there may also be a transient increase in subsarcolemmal [Na]$_i$ ([Na]$_{sm}$, Fig 74B; Leblanc & Hume, 1990). The high [Na]$_{sm}$ favors more outward $I_{Na/Ca}$ and in the example in Fig 74C this increases the peak and prolongs the outward $I_{Na/Ca}$ duration to 3 ms (with total integrated Ca influx of 0.08 µmol/L cytosol). While this by itself does not preclude a potential triggering role for outward $I_{Na/Ca}$, the total Ca influx via Na/Ca exchange is negligible with respect to total cellular Ca fluxes.

It seems probable that under normal conditions the Na/Ca exchanger serves mainly as a means of Ca extrusion and that Ca current is the main means of Ca entry into cardiac myocytes. Figure 75 shows the quantitative functional relationship of I_{Ca} and $I_{Na/Ca}$ when SR function was suppressed by 10 mM caffeine (Bridge *et al.,* 1990). A guinea-pig ventricular myocyte was voltage clamped using a dialyzing pipette containing Na-free, 130 mM CsCl solution to prevent Ca entry via Na/Ca exchange and K currents, respectively. Depolarization in the absence of Na$_o$-

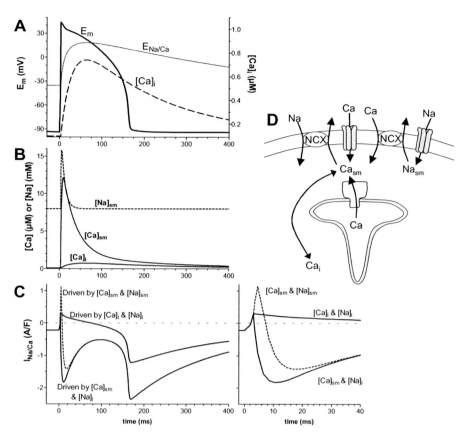

Figure 74. Local $[Ca]_i$ and $[Na]_i$ effects $I_{Na/Ca}$ during cardiac action potential (AP). **A.** Bulk $[Ca]_i$ and $E_{Na/Ca}$ during a normal AP in rabbit ventricular myocyte. **B.** Submembrane $[Ca]_i$ ($[Ca]_{sm}$) and $[Na]_i$ ($[Na]_{sm}$) predicted using exponential time constants of rise (2 and 1 ms respectively) and fall (30 and 8 ms, respectively) where the $[Ca]_{sm}$ was added to the global $[Ca]_i$ (which rises and falls with time constants of 30 and 200 ms respectively). **C.** $I_{Na/Ca}$ calculated from Eq 6.3 using the different $[Ca]$ & $[Na]$ values as indicated and the same parameters as Fig 72, except $E_{Na/Ca}$ =700 A/F and k_{sat} = 0.1 (expanded time scale at right). **D.** Cartoon showing how local $[Ca]$ and $[Na]$ in the junctional region are interdependent.

activated inward I_{Ca} and cell contraction. Repolarization by itself did not induce relaxation until Na_o was added using a quick solution switch. This relaxation was associated with an inward $I_{Na/Ca}$ producing Ca extrusion and relaxation. Integration of the nifedipine-sensitive I_{Ca} and the $I_{Na/Ca}$ (Fig 75B) showed twice as much I_{Ca} as $I_{Na/Ca}$, consistent with all Ca entry via I_{Ca} (2 charges/ Ca) and all extrusion via a 3Na:1Ca Na/Ca exchange (1 charge/Ca). This demonstrates the ability of Ca influx via I_{Ca} to support contraction and $I_{Na/Ca}$ to extrude Ca and produce relaxation. Keep in mind that under normal twitch conditions (with functional SR) the Na/Ca exchanger removes only 8-30% of the total activator Ca during relaxation. As stressed in Chapter 3 the amount of Ca extrusion from the cell must be matched by the Ca influx per beat for the cell to remain in steady state Ca balance. Since Ca influx via Na/Ca exchange is likely to be very small (Fig 74), I_{Ca} provides almost all of the Ca influx.

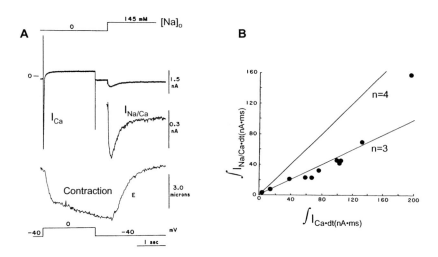

Figure 75. Ca entry via I_{Ca} and Ca efflux via $I_{Na/Ca}$. **A.** A voltage clamped guinea-pig ventricular myocyte was equilibrated with 10 mM caffeine to prevent SR Ca uptake and release. The I_{Ca} associated with the 2 sec depolarizing pulse in Na-free 2.7 mM Ca solution activated a contraction. Relaxion was induced when $[Na]_o$ was rapidly returned, activating Ca extrusion via $I_{Na/Ca}$. **B.** The integral of $I_{Na/Ca}$ is plotted as a function of the integrated I_{Ca}. The $\int I_{Ca}$ is roughly twice the $\int I_{Na/Ca}$ as would be expected for a Na/Ca exchange coupling ratio of n=3. (from Bridge *et al.*, 1990, with permission).

COMPETITION AMONG Na/Ca EXCHANGE, SARCOLEMMAL Ca-PUMP AND SR Ca-PUMP DURING RELAXATION AND AT REST

As discussed in Chapter 3 (pg 52-54), during relaxation there is dynamic competition among Na/Ca exchange and the SR Ca-pump, sarcolemmal Ca-pump and mitochondrial Ca uniporter. During relaxation the SR Ca-pump is generally dominant over the Na/Ca exchanger in mammalian ventricle, but this dominance varies between 2-3:1 in rabbit and guinea-pig to >10:1 in rat and mouse. Table 20 lists estimates of the quantitative contribution of Na/Ca exchange *vs.* other Ca transporters to relaxation and $[Ca]_i$ decline during twitches and also during caffeine-induced contractures (where net SR Ca uptake is blocked). During a twitch, the Na/Ca exchange contributes a variable amount toward relaxation or $[Ca]_i$ decline (3 - 47%) depending on species and condition. Almost all of the remaining Ca removal is due to the SR Ca-pump (50-96%), with the combined action of the sarcolemmal Ca-pump plus mitochondrial uniport never being as much as 10%. During caffeine-induced contractures or twitches when the SR Ca-pump is blocked with thapsigargin the Na/Ca exchange is by far dominant (75-93%). This suggests that Na/Ca exchange is several times more effective in mediating Ca efflux from the cell than is the sarcolemmal Ca-ATPase (see also below).

Figure 76 shows paired rapid cooling contractures (RCCs), a complementary approach to that shown in Fig 30 for evaluating the competition between the SR Ca-pump and Na/Ca exchange during relaxation (Hryshko *et al.*, 1989c; Bers *et al.*, 1989). Rapid cooling of cardiac

Table 20

Ca Transport During Ventricular Myocyte and Muscle Relaxation

Species	ref	Temp (°C)	—Twitch— NCX	SR	Slow	—Caffeine/Thapsigargin— NCX	SL-pump	Mito
Rabbit [Ca]$_i$	a	22	28	70	2	93	3	3
	b	35	27	70	3			
	b	25	23	74	3			
	g	22				91	6	3
Rat [Ca]$_i$	a	22	7	92	1	87	— 13 —	
	c	27	9	87	4	68	— 32 —	
	d	23	8	87	5	80	20	0
Mouse [Ca]$_i$	e	23	9	90	1			
(PLB-KO)	e	23	3	96	<1			
Rat neonate [Ca]$_i$	f	22	46	50	4			
Ferret [Ca]$_i$	g	22	29	65	6	75-85	14-20	4
Rabbit Relax	b	25	28	70	2			
	b	35	21	76	3			
Ferret Relax	b	25	30	63	7			
	b	35	28	67	5			
Cat Relax	b	25	47	51	2			
	b	35	32	66	2			
Dog [Ca]$_i$	l	37	27	73	-			
Failing [Ca]$_i$	l	37	56	44	-			
Paired RCCs								
Rabbit Relax	h	29	23	76	1			
Rabbit Relax	h	29	27	73	-			
Guinea-pig [Ca]$_i$	i	30	36	64	-			
Guinea-pig [Ca]$_i$	j	22	30	67	3			
Human Normal	k	37	37	63	-			
Human Failing	k	37	42	58	-			

PLB-KO, phospholamban knock out, NCX=Na/Ca exchange, SR=SR Ca-pump. Slow=combined sarco-lemmal Ca-ATPase (SL-pump)+mitochondrial uniporter (Mito). Caffeine/thapsigargin=relaxation with non-functional SR. In some cases, the Slow sytems were not assessed, so all is assumed to be SR+NCX. **a)** Bassani *et al.* 1992, 1994a, **b)** Puglisi *et al.* 1996, **c)** Negretti *et al.* 1993, **d)** Choi & Eisner, 1999, **e)** Li *et al.* 1998, **f)** Bassani *et al.*, 1994c, **g)** Bassani *et al.* 1994b, 1995a, **h)** Hryshko *et al.* 1989, **i)** Bers *et al.* 1989, **j)** Terracciano & MacLeod, 1994, 1997, **k)** Pieske *et al.* 1999. **l)** O'Rourke *et al.*, 1999.

muscle to ~0-1°C in <1 sec causes release of all SR Ca while simultaneously inhibiting Ca transport mechanisms (see also details in Chapter 7).   This [Ca]$_i$ results in slowly activating contractures at this temperature and the RCC amplitude is a useful index of the amount of Ca which was in the SR at the time of cooling.   Rewarming the muscle re-activates Ca transport systems (e.g. SR and sarcolemmal Ca pumps and Na/Ca exchange) allowing relaxation to occur.

In Fig 76 we used paired RCCs such that the second RCC (RCC$_2$) is used to assess the fraction of Ca released at the first RCC (RCC$_1$) which was resequestered by the SR during relaxation of RCC$_1$.   For example, if all of the Ca released from the SR at RCC$_1$ were resequestered during relaxation, RCC$_2$ should be the same amplitude as RCC$_1$ (RCC$_2$/RCC$_1$ =100%). This is essentially the case in Fig 76B where the rabbit myocyte was bathed in Na-free,

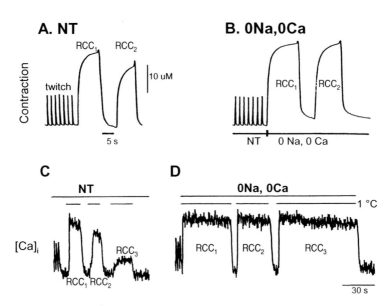

Figure 76. Paired rapid cooling contractures (RCCs) used to assess the resequestration of Ca by the SR. **A)** Paired RCCs induced after a train of electrically evoked twitches in a rabbit ventricular myocyte. RCC_2 is smaller because some of the Ca released during RCC_1 is extruded by Na/Ca exchange during relaxation. **B)** When Na/Ca exchange is prevented during rewarming (by Na-free, Ca-free solution), the SR can resequester all of the Ca released at RCC_1 (so RCC_2/RCC_1 is 1). **C** and **D**) A similar protocol in a guinea-pig ventricular myocyte except that $[Ca]_i$ was measured (using indo-1) and three RCCs were used instead of two (from Hryshko *et al.*, 1989c (top) and Bers *et al.*, 1989 (bottom), with permission).

Ca-free solution during cooling and rewarming (to prevent Na/Ca exchange). However if Na/Ca exchange was allowed to compete with the SR (Fig 76A), $RCC_2/RCC_1 \sim 75\%$. This again implies that Na/Ca exchange extrudes an amount of Ca responsible for $\sim 25\%$ of developed tension in the presence of an intact SR. Fig 76C-D show similar data for $[Ca]_i$ during triple RCCs in guinea-pig ventricular myocytes. In this case Na/Ca exchange reduced the amplitude of the second and third Ca_i transients by 36% and 51% (with respect to the preceding RCC).

Figure 77 shows the voltage-dependence of relaxation mediated by the SR and Na/Ca exchange (Bers & Bridge, 1989). When relaxation was mediated by Na/Ca exchange (in the presence of caffeine) relaxation was highly voltage-dependent (voltage clamp data are also shown from Bridge *et al.*, 1988). This is expected on thermodynamic grounds, since Ca extrusion via Na/Ca exchange is favored by more negative E_m (see above). A slight acceleration of relaxation by nifedipine at depolarized E_m raises the possibility of a small window I_{Ca} at these potentials which could slow relaxation. In contrast to the results with Na/Ca exchange, relaxation mediated by the SR (in Na-free, Ca-free solution) was entirely independent of voltage. Crespo *et al.* (1990) reached similar conclusions, by comparing the slow phase of $[Ca]_i$ decline in ryanodine-treated guinea-pig ventricular myocytes (attributed to Na/Ca exchange) with the rapid $[Ca]_i$ decline in rat ventricular myocytes (attributed primarily to SR Ca uptake).

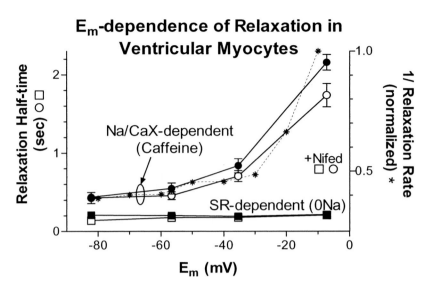

***Figure* 77**. Voltage dependence of relaxation when Na/Ca exchange is prevented. RCCs and rewarming of rabbit ventricular muscle were done in solution which either prevented SR Ca reuptake by 10 mM caffeine (●○) or blocked Na/Ca exchange by 0Na,0Ca solution (■□, E_m was varied by altering $[K]_o$ during the RCC and rewarming). Parallel data were obtained with 10 μM nifedipine to block I_{Ca} (○ □, data from Bers & Bridge, 1989). Also shown are voltage clamp data (* from Bridge *et al.*, 1988) from guinea-pig ventricular myocytes where relaxation rate was measured in the steady presence of 10 mM caffeine.

Figure 78 shows an experiment in which the Na_o-dependent component of relaxation was examined in a voltage clamped rat ventricular myocyte where $[Ca]_i$ was measured using indo-1 (Bers *et al.*, 1990). The cell was depolarized from −50 to +15 mV for 50 msec (top) or 1 sec (bottom) in the presence (left) or absence (right) of 145 mM Na_o. After repolarization to −50 mV the decline of $[Ca]_i$ for both short and long pulses was monoexponential and the time constant (τ) was slowed by ~20% by blocking Na/Ca exchange ($0[Na]_o$). During the long pulses at +15 mV $[Ca]_i$ also declined along a monoexponential, but was relatively insensitive to $[Na]_o$. This is consistent with the voltage dependence expected of Na/Ca exchange, where Ca extrusion is less favored at more positive E_m (such that Ca is preferentially pumped into the SR).

Figures 76-78 demonstrate that the Na/Ca exchange can compete with the SR Ca-pump during the relaxation of cardiac contraction with the Na/Ca exchanger being responsible for ~20 - 30% of the decline in $[Ca]_i$ or force during cardiac relaxation. Despite the general similarity of the numbers it should also be appreciated that this fraction will vary depending on certain variables such as the action potential configuration, the resting $[Ca]_i$ and $[Na]_i$, peak $[Ca]_i$, the timecourse of the Ca_i transient and the state of the SR and the Na/Ca exchanger itself. For example, the long depolarization at +15 mV in Fig 78 (bottom left) biases the competition between the SR Ca-pump and the Na/Ca exchange in favor of the SR. Indeed, the next contraction and Ca transient after that pulse was larger, reflecting the enhanced SR Ca load. On the other hand, if the cell and SR are already heavily Ca loaded, the decline of $[Ca]_i$ can still be accelerated by Na_o at +15 mV (see Fig 10 in Bers *et al.*, 1990).

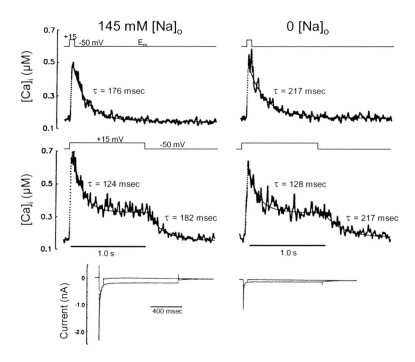

Figure 78. The effect of Na_o on the decline of $[Ca]_i$ in a rat ventricular myocyte with depolarizing pulses from –50 mV to +15 mV for 50 msec (top) or 1 sec (bottom). The dialyzing patch-clamp pipette contained <0.5 mM Na to prevent Ca influx via Na/Ca exchange and 70 μM indo-1 to assess $[Ca]_i$. During the long pulses and after repolarization, the $[Ca]_i$ was fit with a monoexponential decline (curves superimposed and time constants τ indicated). During the long depolarizations there may be a small residual Ca influx via Ca channels (see current records at bottom). (from Bers *et al.*, 1990, with permission).

Resting Ca efflux from Cells

Finally, let us consider the relative roles of Na/Ca exchange and sarcolemmal Ca-pump in diastolic efflux of Ca. Indeed, without energy-dependent Ca extrusion the resting E_m would drive $[Ca]_i$ to nearly 1 M at equilibrium! This is emphasized by the work of Choi & Eisner (1999). They showed that when Na/Ca exchange and sarcolemmal Ca-pump are both blocked (by $0Na_o$ and carboxyeosin) raising $[Ca]_o$ from 0 to 0.1 mM caused large $[Ca]_i$ increases. Moreover the rate of diastolic Ca influx into cells has been estimated to be 0.5-3 μmol/L cytosol/sec (Díaz *et al.*, 1997a; Trafford *et al.*, 1997). This would rapidly load the cell if the Ca extrusion mechanisms were not able to counterbalance this Ca influx at resting $[Ca]_i$.

Philipson & Ward (1986) extrapolated SLV results and concluded that Na/Ca exchange and the sarcolemmal Ca-ATPase pump were likely to extrude Ca from the cell at comparable rates. Barry and Smith (1984) suggested that a Na_o-independent mechanism was responsible for the major fraction of ^{45}Ca efflux from cultured chick heart cells. These initial studies were complicated by undetermined Ca-Ca exchange and Barry *et al.* (1986) later concluded that this Na_o-independent component of ^{45}Ca efflux was only ~20% of the Ca efflux via Na/Ca exchange.

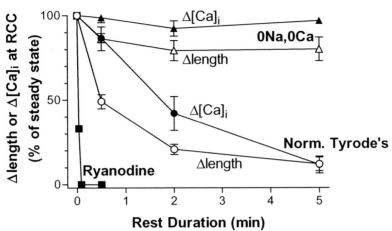

Figure 79. Rest decay of SR Ca relies on Na/Ca exchange. After steady state 0.5 Hz stimulation guinea-pig ventricular myocytes were rested in either normal Tyrode's or 0Na, 0Ca solution (to block Na/Ca exchange). RCCs were used to assess SR Ca content as either $\Delta[Ca]_i$ (indo-1) or cell shortening (Δlength). Ryanodine (1 μM, 20 min,■) did not abolish RCCs, but greatly accelerated the rate of rest decay (see Chapter 7) (data from Bers *et al.*, 1989).

We have generally found that blocking either Na/Ca exchange or the sarcolemmal Ca-ATPase does not produce a significant rise in resting $[Ca]_i$, although blocking either one may slow the decline in $[Ca]_i$ during repetitive stimulation (since Ca enters with each pulse). Most would concede that the Na/Ca exchange is dominant over the sarcolemmal Ca-pump during $[Ca]_i$ decline. However, some posit that the sarcolemmal Ca-pump may be especially important in governing diastolic Ca efflux because it can have a higher affinity ($K_m(Ca)\sim60$ nM, see Table 18) than the Na/Ca exchange ($K_m(Ca) \geq 1$ μM).

We have examined which Ca transport system functions during prolonged rest, when $[Ca]_i$ remains low (Bers *et al.*, 1989; Bassani *et al.*, 1994b; Bassani & Bers, 1994). During rest there is some finite rate of Ca leak from the SR lumen to the cytoplasm. Ca in the cytoplasm is then subject to either extrusion from the cell (via Na/Ca exchange or the sarcolemmal Ca-pump) or resequestration by the SR (for the moment ignoring mitochondrial uptake). If all of this Ca is resequestered by the SR, then the Ca content of the SR would stay constant at rest. If some of this Ca is extruded from the cell, then the SR Ca content would progressively decline during rest. Thus the rate of decline of SR Ca content during rest provides an index of how well the trans-sarcolemmal Ca transporters compete with the SR Ca-ATPase (reflecting cellular Ca efflux by the Na/Ca exchange or sarcolemmal Ca-pump).

Figure 79 illustrates the process of rest decay in guinea-pig ventricular myocytes. RCCs were induced at various times after the last stimulated twitch and Ca transients and myocyte contraction were recorded (Bers *et al.*, 1989). With longer rest intervals in normal Tyrode's (NT) the amplitude of the RCC and accompanying Ca transient are progressively smaller. When the rest period is in Na-free, Ca-free solution (0Na,0Ca) there is almost no decline in the amplitude

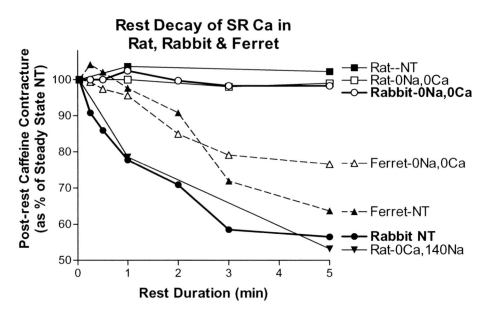

Figure 80. Rest decay of SR Ca in rabbit, rat and ferret. After steady state stimulation myocytes were rested in either normal Tyrode's (NT ■▲ ●), 0Na,0Ca solution (to block Na/Ca exchange □○△) or 0Na, 140 mM Na_o (after depleting Na_i, to enhance Ca extrusion by Na/Ca exchange, ▼). Caffeine-induced contractures were used to assess SR Ca content. (data from Bassani *et al.*, 1994b, Bassani & Bers, 1994).

of the post-rest RCCs and Ca transients even after 5 min of rest. This is consistent with Na/Ca exchange being the main means by which Ca is extruded from the resting cell. Indeed, the Na-free solution which is used to prevent Na/Ca exchange is also Ca-free to prevent Ca gain via Na/Ca exchange in the absence of Na_o. Under these conditions the sarcolemmal Ca-pump should be even better able to extrude Ca into the Ca-free solution. Even so, there is practically no rest decay in the absence of Na/Ca exchange. This result demonstrates that in intact guinea-pig ventricular myocytes, Ca efflux during rest (as well as during relaxation) is mainly via Na/Ca exchange with the sarcolemmal Ca-pump making at most a very small contribution.

Figure 80 shows that the same results are obtained in rabbit ventricular myocytes (in this case using caffeine-induced contractures to assess SR Ca content after rest. That is, 0Na, 0Ca during rest completely abolishes resting loss of SR Ca in rabbit (○ *vs.* ●). In rat ventricular myocytes SR Ca content is stable during rest and usually does not decline (■, Bassani & Bers, 1994). This may be due to the relatively high $[Na]_i$ reported in rat (16 mM or aNa_i =12.7 mM) which would place $E_{Na/Ca}$ at or below resting E_m (–80 mV), such that Ca extrusion via Na/Ca exchange is not thermodynamically favored (Shattock & Bers, 1989; see also Chapter 9, Fig 140). In this case blocking Na/Ca exchange in rat by 0Na,0Ca solution (□) does not change things much, despite the fact that the sarcolemmal Ca-pump should be unimpeded. On the other hand, if rat myocytes are pre-depleted of Na_i (by exposure to 0Na,0Ca) and Ca extrusion by Na/Ca exchange is stimulated in $0Ca_o$, 140 mM Na_o solution (▼) rat myocyte SR loses Ca during rest as fast as rabbit. So again it seems that the Ca transport across the sarcolemma is dictated by the Na/Ca exchanger, not the sarcolemmal Ca-ATPase. Finally, we turn to ferret ventricular myocytes, where rest decay of SR Ca content occurs in NT as well as in 0Na, 0Ca solution. The inability of 0Na, 0Ca to completely block resting SR Ca loss suggests that the sarcolemmal Ca-ATPase does indeed contribute to resting cellular Ca efflux (perhaps about equally with the Na/Ca exchanger). This is completely consistent with the relatively powerful sarcolemmal Ca-ATPase reported in ferret ventricular myocytes (i.e. 5 fold higher V_{max} than in rabbit; Bassani *et al.*, 1994a,b, 1995a). Indeed, in ferret *vs.* rabbit we find that the sarcolemmal Ca-ATPase contributes more significantly to twitch relaxation (6 *vs.* 0.5%) and to [Ca]$_i$ decline during caffeine exposure (14-20% *vs.* 3% see Table 20). Thus, one should be careful about generalizations and there are significant species differences in how Na/Ca exchange and sarcolemmal Ca-ATPase interact.

Transgenic Mice and Antisense Knock-down of Na/Ca exchange

Philipson's group generated transgenic mice overexpressing canine NCX1 and myocytes from these mice have been studied (Adachi-Akahane *et al.*, 1997; Yao *et al.*, 1998; Terraciano *et al.*, 1998; Weber *et al.*, 2001). Exchanger activity was increased 2-3 fold based on $I_{Na/Ca}$ or [Ca]$_i$ decline during caffeine exposure, whereas other Ca transport systems (e.g. I_{Ca} and SR Ca-ATPase) appeared unaltered. One could imagine that higher Na/Ca exchanger expression might reduce SR Ca content, based on the foregoing discussion about the dominant role of this system in Ca extrusion from the cell and its minor role in Ca influx. The first two groups above found no change in either twitch amplitude or SR Ca content (based on caffeine-induced Δ[Ca]$_i$ and integrated $I_{Na/Ca}$). This could be explicable if (as described above for the rat) $E_{Na/Ca}$ is poised right at the resting E_m. Indeed, Yao *et al.* (1998) found [Na]$_i$ to be ~16 mM in both wild type and transgenic mice, giving an $E_{Na/Ca}$ = –85 mV for [Ca]$_i$ = 125 nM or –80 for [Ca]$_i$ = 150 nM. Thus, it is plausible that the Na/Ca exchange reaches equilibrium during diastole and doesn't then support substantial diastolic Ca flux. Terraciano *et al.* (1998) found a large increase in SR Ca content and consequently larger twitch size in the mice overexpressing NCX1. The difference is unexplained, but even a small systematic difference in myocyte [Na]$_i$ could have a large impact. Moreover, Yao *et al.* (1998) claimed the additional Na/Ca exchanger could provide triggering for Ca-induced SR Ca-release (based on lower sensitivity to nifedipine block of twitches), while Adachi-Akahane *et al.* (1997) found no evidence for Na/Ca exchange-mediated Ca-induced Ca-release in the transgenic mice. Clearly more work is needed to clarify some of these points.

In the absence of highly selective blockers of Na/Ca exchange some groups have used an antisense mRNA approach to knock-down Na/Ca exchanger expression in myocytes (Lipp *et al.*, 1995; Slodzinski & Blaustein, 1998a,b). While the technique looks promising, it has not yet been applied to new mechanistic questions.

In conclusion, it is evident that the Na/Ca exchange system is very important in myocardial Ca regulation. Key fundamental characteristics of this system and its function are becoming increasingly clear. Na/Ca exchange is the main means by which Ca is extruded from the cell, during both relaxation and diastole. By comparison, the sarcolemmal Ca-pump seems relatively unimportant in cardiac muscle (particularly because net Ca movement in either direction via Na/Ca exchange would normally appear able to overwhelm this pump). Indeed, Na/Ca exchange can even compete with the powerful SR Ca-pump for cytoplasmic Ca and thereby contribute to relaxation. The Na/Ca exchange can also mediate Ca influx sufficient to activate contraction, but this probably does not occur under normal physiological conditions (where the main role of the Na/Ca exchange seems to be to extrude Ca from the cell). In fact, Na/Ca exchange must extrude as much Ca as enters the cell via Ca current in each cardiac cycle, in order for a steady state to be achieved. Finally, since the Na/Ca exchange is the main means by which the cell extrudes Ca, anything which prevents this Ca extrusion will increase cellular Ca loading and can lead to Ca overload. These issues will be addressed further in Chapter 10.

D.M. Bers.
Excitation-Contraction Coupling and Cardiac Contractile Force.
2nd Ed., Kluwer Academic Publishers, Dordrecht, 2001

CHAPTER 7

SARCOPLASMIC RETICULUM
Ca UPTAKE, CONTENT AND RELEASE

SR Ca-PUMP

Kielley & Meyerhoff (1948) first described a Mg-activated ATPase in a microsomal fraction from muscle. Ebashi (1961; Ebashi & Lipmann, 1962) and Hasselbach & Makinose (1961) later identified this as the membrane associated Ca-ATPase or "relaxing factor" in muscle responsible for lowering cytoplasmic [Ca]. This Ca-pump has been the subject of intensive study since that time (see reviews by Inesi, 1985, 1987; Fleischer & Tonomura, 1985; Entman & Van Winkle, 1986; Schatzmann, 1989; Mintz & Guillain, 1997; MacLennan et al., 1997; Anderson & Vilsen, 1998; Tada, 2001).

Skeletal and cardiac muscle SR vesicles isolated on sucrose density gradients can be separated into two types (Meissner, 1975; Campbell et al., 1980; Jones & Cala, 1981; Saito et al., 1984). A heavy SR fraction is obtained at higher density and contains terminal cisternae and the Ca-release channel (or ryanodine receptor) as well as the Ca-pump. At lower density, a light SR fraction is obtained in which most of the protein (~90%) is the Ca-pump (Meissner, 1975; Campbell, 1986; Fleischer & Inui, 1989). The light SR fraction probably originates from the longitudinal SR. Thus, Ca is pumped into the SR along the longitudinal tubules (and terminal cisternae) and is released from the terminal cisternae, where the SR "foot" processes span the gap from the SR to the sarcolemma (see Chapter 1). I will focus initially on the SR Ca-pump, while the release process will be discussed below (pg 186). However, it should be noted that many characteristics of the Ca-pump have been studied in mixed populations of SR vesicles (heavy plus light). In heavy SR vesicles Ca uptake can be "short circuited" by open Ca-release channels (which seems to be the usual state of cardiac SR release channels in isolated vesicles). Ca uptake in cardiac heavy SR vesicles can be dramatically increased by inclusion of agents which block the Ca release channel (e.g. ruthenium red or Mg;, Meissner & Henderson, 1987).

The sarco(endo)plasmic reticulum Ca-ATPase (SERCA) is a member of the P-type ion transporting ATPase family (as are Na/K-ATPase, sarcolemmal Ca-ATPase and H/K-ATPase). Two striated muscle SERCA proteins have been sequenced and cloned and exhibit 84% amino acid identity (MacLennan et al., 1985; Brandl et al., 1986). One of these is from fast twitch muscle (SERCA1, MW =110,331 Da) and the other from slow twitch skeletal and cardiac muscle (SERCA2a, which has 4 less amino acids; Brandl et al., 1986, 1987; MacLennan et al., 1987). In fast twitch skeletal muscle the SERCA1a isoform predominates in adult, whereas SERCA1b is present in fetal and neonatal stages. SERCA2b and a third isoform (SERCA3; Dode et al., 1996) are ubiquitous in the endoplasmic reticulum of non-muscle cells. While SERCA1 and SERCA2a have very similar properties, SERCA2b has a two-fold higher Ca affinity with slower V_{max} and

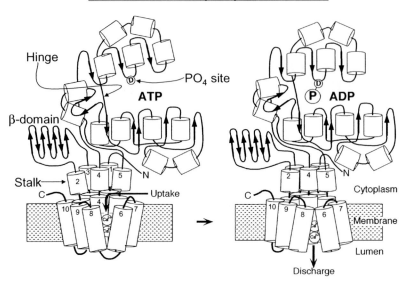

Figure 81. Schematic of SR Ca-ATPase structure. Most of the protein (70%) is on the cytoplasmic side of the SR membrane including β-strand, phosphorylation (D351, P), nucleotide binding, stalk domains and a Hinge. Ten transmembrane spans (M_1- M_{10}) are shown as 1-10. Amino acids on M_4-M_6 and M_8 are important in Ca-binding and transport (Glu-309 in M_4, Glu-771 in M_5, Asn-796, Thr-799 & Asp-800 in M_6 and Glu-908 in M_8). Left shows Ca entry from cytosol and right shows Ca release into the SR lumen (From MacLennan *et al.*, 1992, with permission).

SERCA3 has a comparable turnover rate, but much lower Ca affinity (Lytton *et al.*, 1992; Verboomen *et al.*, 1994; Anderson & Vilsen, 1998). Figure 81 shows an early proposed secondary structure of SERCA by MacLennan's group, indicating where ATP binds (nucleotide binding domain), phosphorylation site (Asp-351), a β-strand domain and a hinge region. The protein has 10 membrane spanning regions (M_1-M_{10}), where M_1-M_5 each have an additional α-helical "stalk" region on the cytoplasmic side (S_1-S_5). Crucial high affinity Ca binding sites initially proposed to reside in the anionic stalk region (Brandl *et al.*, 1986), have now been localized in the transmembrane domains (M_4-M_6 and M_8, Clarke *et al.*, 1989a,b). Figure 82 shows a newer look, based on crystal structure from X-ray diffraction (Toyoshima *et al.*, 2000) greatly extending prior electron microscopic reconstructions (e.g. Stokes & Green, 2000).

The transport reaction starts with two Ca ions and one ATP molecule binding to high affinity binding sites on the cytoplasmic side of the pump (see Figs 81 & 83). The terminal phosphate of ATP is then transferred to Asp-351 on the Ca-pump inducing Ca ion "occlusion" (which means that Ca cannot be readily released to either side). Based on the results of Clarke *et al.* (1989a,b), Ca binds to sites in transmembrane regions M_4-M_6 & M_8 which may form a channel, and phosphorylation alters the structure such that Ca cannot return to the cytoplasmic side from which it came (occlusion). The phosphorylation causes a transition from the E_1P to E_2P state, thereby reducing Ca affinity such that Ca can be released to the lumen of the SR via the channel. This reduction in affinity is important for the rapid release of Ca into the SR lumen

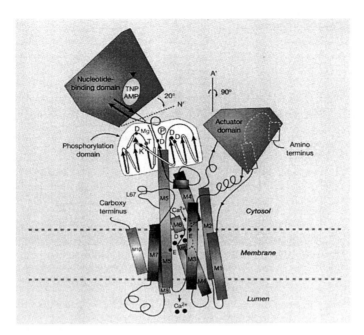

Figure 82. Structure of the skeletal muscle SR Ca-pump. Diagram by MacLennan & Green (2000) based on the crystal structure by Toyoshima *et al.* (2000). M_5 seems to provide a central axis, Ca sites in M_4-M_6 and M_8 are formed in part by disruption of the M_4 and M_6 helices. The nucleotide binding domain is above and must tilt to bring ATP to the phosphorylation site, which lies in a region of 7 stranded parallel β-sheets (arrows). The actuator domain (was β domain) may rotate 90° toward the phosphorylation domain. The cytosolic phospholamban interaction site is at the bottom of the nucleotide binding domain.

where ambient [Ca] is higher. The catalytic site for ATP is at least 4 nm away from the pore, requiring long range functional linkages to couple the ATPase to channel reorientation.

Two Ca ions are transported by the Ca-pump for each ATP molecule consumed in both skeletal and cardiac SR (Tada *et al.*, 1982; Reddy *et al.*, 1996). The lower stoichiometries often reported for the *in vitro* cardiac Ca-pump probably reflect Ca-pump-independent leak of Ca from the vesicles or contaminating ATPases. The lipid environment is also important for this enzyme and removal of the ~30 lipid molecules associated with the SR Ca-pump decreases Ca-dependent ATPase activity (Hidalgo *et al.*, 1976; Hesketh *et al.*, 1976) .

The number of SR Ca-pumps estimated from phosphoenzyme formation in guinea-pig and dog ventricle was 14 and 47 μmol/L cytosol respectively (Levitsky *et al.*, 1981; Feher & Briggs, 1982). Hove-Madsen & Bers (1993b) used thapsigargin titration to estimate the number of pump sites in permeabilized myocytes from rat *vs.* rabbit ventricle. We estimated 19 μmol/L cytosol in rabbit and several fold higher in rat (perhaps as high as 100 μmol/L cytosol) . While these are only estimates and I used 47 μM in Chapter 3, I consider that the likely range is 15-75 μmol/L cytosol and species-dependent (e.g. guinea-pig < rabbit< dog < rat ~ mouse). The maximum turnover rate for the cardiac SR Ca-pump has been estimated to be 10-15 Ca ions/ pump/sec in dog and guinea-pig (Shigekawa *et al.*, 1976; Levitsky *et al.*, 1981). This is similar to the turnover rate of the skeletal muscle SR Ca-pump and Shigekawa *et al.* (1976) attributed the

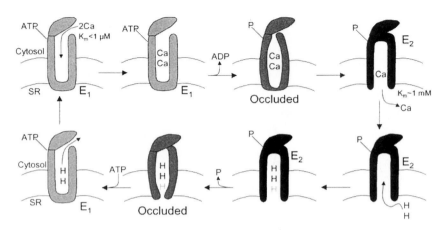

Figure 83. SR Ca-pump transport scheme. Starting from top left, 2 Ca ions bind with high affinity, then bound ATP is used to phosphorylate aspartate-351 and modify the conformation of the protein so that the Ca ions are occluded. The Ca_2E-P undergoes a conformational change (to E_2) and the Ca ions are released to the interior of the SR (due to a lower Ca affinity). Protons are carried during the lower part of the cycle to return from E_2 to E_1 state where Ca can be reloaded.

slower cardiac Ca-pumping rate to ~4-fold lower pump site density and lower Ca affinity in heart. These values mean that for the cardiac SR to take up 50 µmol Ca/L cytosol during relaxation each SR Ca-pump would only need to cycle only about once!

Regulation of the Cardiac SR Ca-pump by Phospholamban

A major difference between the cardiac and skeletal muscle Ca-pumps is that cardiac muscle contains the regulatory protein phospholamban (PLB; Tada & Katz, 1982; see reviews by Koss & Kranias, 1996; Simmerman & Jones, 1998; Tada & Toyofuku, 1998; MacLennan *et al.*, 1997). PLB exists as a homopentamer (apparent total MW ~22,000 Da) and the amino acid sequence has been deduced from cDNA (Fujii *et al.*, 1987). The monomer is 6080 Da (52 amino acids) and it exhibits one hydrophobic and one hydrophilic domain. Simmerman *et al.* (1986) proposed a structural model of the pentamer which could have a hydrophilic pore through the SR membrane with phosphorylation sites on the cytoplasmic surface (Fig 84A). Provocative initial observations suggesting that dephosphorylated PLB might form Ca-selective channels in lipid bilayers (Kovacs *et al.*, 1988) are still not widely accepted. Figure 84 shows the pentameric structure of PLB in the membrane, and that transmembrane α-helices may form a leucine zipper to stabilize this complex (Simmerman *et al.*, 1996; Kimura *et al.*, 1996, 1997). That is, a series of leucines and isoleucines at the *a* and *d* positions of the helical wheel plot (Fig 84B) can interdigitate to stabilize the interaction throughout the membrane (Fig 84C). Moreover, these authors showed that mutations along this leucine zipper could prevent pentamerization.

PLB is an endogenous inhibitor of SERCA (Hicks *et al.*, 1979; Inui *et al.*, 1986) and decreases Ca transport and ATPase activity, especially at low [Ca] because it increases $K_m(Ca)$ without altering V_{max} (see Fig 85; WT with PLB *vs.* PLB knockout or PLB (-/-)). PLB inhibits both SERCA1a and SERCA2a, but not SERCA3 (Toyofuku *et al.*, 1993). PLB is present at high concentration in ventricular myocytes, probably comparable to the concentration of the SR Ca-

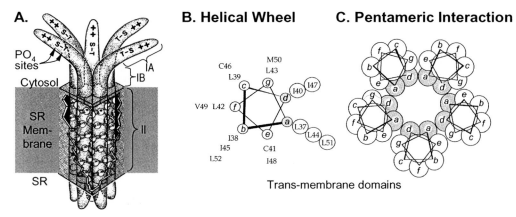

Figure 84. Phospholamban structure and pentamerization. **A**. Domain I of PLB extends above the SR membrane surface and includes phosphorylation sites Ser-16 and Thr-17 (Domain IA is residues 1-20 and IB is 21-29). The transmembrane domain II (residues 30-52) interacts with neighboring monomers to stabilize a pentameric structure (based on Simmerman *et al.*, 1986). **B**. Helical wheel plot of the transmembrane residues (i.e. 7 residues /2 full turns) in a monomer where the *a* and *d* positions are occupied by either leucine (L) or isoleucine (I). **C**. The *a* domain of one PLB monomer may interdigitate with the *d* domain of another forming leucine zippers stabilizing the pentameric array (B and C are based on Simmerman *et al.*, 1996, with images generously provided by L.R. Jones).

ATPase (Tada *et al.*, 1983; Louis *et al.*, 1987). Colyer & Wang (1991) estimated that ventricular SR has 0.4 mol PLB pentamer per SR Ca-ATPase (or 2 PLB monomers/ per pump molecule). This would imply that there is ~100 μmol PLB/L cytosol (also comparable to [TnC]). There is ~10 times less PLB in atrial muscle and lower concentrations are also present in slow skeletal and smooth muscle (Briggs *et al.*, 1992). However, even in ventricle PLB overexpression in transgenic mice (doubling PLB protein with respect to the SR Ca-ATPase) produces a proportional shift to lower Ca affinity (Fig 85), suggesting that the Ca-pumps are not nearly saturated with PLB *in situ* (Kadambi *et al.*, 1996; Chu *et al.*, 1997). In heterologous coexpression studies Reddy *et al.* (1995) found maximal inhibition with 3 PLB monomers per SR Ca-ATPase. Titration of PLB overexpression in transgenic mice indicated that ~40% of the SR Ca-pumps are normally regulated by PLB, and that maximal pump inhibition took place at 2.6-fold overexpression of PLB (Brittsan *et al.*, 2000).

Figure 85 shows the [Ca] dependence of forward SR Ca-pumping. With endogenous PLB in ventricular SR (WT) the $K_m(Ca)$ is typically ~300 nM. The maximal Ca-pump rate is shown in the usual cellular units and typical of that in rat ventricular myocytes (Bassani *et al.*, 1994a; Balke *et al.*, 1994). Recent values for K_m in the literature vary considerably (e.g. from 234 nM to >1 μM; Sasaki *et al.*, 1992; Toyofuku *et al.*, 1993; Hove-Madsen & Bers, 1993b; Kiss *et al.*, 1994; Bassani *et al.*, 1994a; Balke *et al.*, 1994; Mattiazzi *et al.*, 1994; Lu & Kirchberger, 1994; Reddy *et al.*, 1996; Luo *et al.*, 1994; Odermatt *et al.*, 1996). Part of the variation may be the difficulty in making precisely calibrated Ca-EGTA buffers. Thus a K_m value of 300 nM is an educated guess.

PLB can be phosphorylated by cAMP-dependent protein kinase (PKA) at serine-16 (Kirchberger *et al.*, 1974; Tada *et al.*, 1974; Simmerman *et al.*, 1986). This largely reverses the

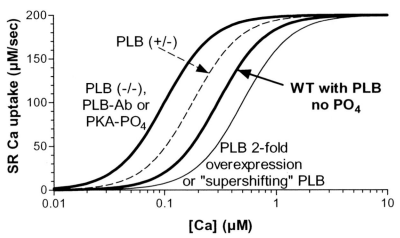

Figure 85. Influence of phospholamban on SR Ca transport. Curves of Ca uptake $(200/(1+\{K_m/[Ca]\}^2))$ in μmol/L cytosol/sec using K_m values from various sources (see text). For wild type (WT) SR Ca-pump $K_m= 300$ nM. Either PLB phosphorylation (PKA-PO$_4$), gene knockout (-/-) or application of an antibody that prevents the PLB-SERCA interaction (PLB-Ab) reduce K_m to 100 nM. SR with half the normal amount of PLB (+/–) has an intermediate K_m (178 nM) and two-fold overexpression of WT PLB or certain "supershifting" mutant PLBs (which don't form homopentamers) can increase K_m to higher values (500 nM). Note the different Ca transport rates expected at 0.1-0.3 μM [Ca]$_i$.

PLB-induced Ca affinity shift, increasing the Ca affinity of the SR Ca-pump by 2-3 fold (e.g. changing K_m from 300 to 100 nM in Fig 85). Thus for most relevant [Ca]$_i$ values (0.1 -1 μM) there is a substantial increase in Ca-pump rate. Application of a PLB antibody which interferes with the interaction between PLB and the SR Ca-ATPase produces similar effects (PLB-Ab in Fig 85; Sham *et al.*, 1991; Suzuki and Wang, 1986). Furthermore when either the cardiac or skeletal muscle SR Ca-pump (SERCA2A or SERCA1) is expressed without PLB the Ca pumping and ATPase activity properties are like the endogenous PKA phosphorylated Ca-pump (e.g. Toyofuku *et al.*, 1993; Reddy *et al.*, 1996).

PKA-dependent phosphorylation of PLB at Ser16 has been observed in intact perfused hearts in response to catecholamines (Le Peuch *et al.*, 1980; Kranias & Solaro, 1982; Lindeman *et al.*, 1983). This stimulation of Ca uptake rate by catecholamines appears to be the main means by which β-adrenergic agonists accelerate relaxation in the heart (*vs.* TnI phosphorylation; see pg 277-278; McIvor *et al.*, 1988; Li *et al.*, 2000). Moreover, the activation and washout of the lusitropic effect (acceleration of relaxation) of catecholamines in heart occurs in parallel to the phosphorylation and dephosphorylation of PLB at Ser-16, while dephosphorylation of Thr-17 (site of CamKII phosphorylation, see below) or TnI occur more slowly (Wegener *et al.*, 1989; Talosi *et al.*, 1993). Catecholamines would also bias the competition between the SR Ca-pump and the sarcolemmal Na/Ca exchange in favor of the former, increasing SR Ca load and limiting Ca extrusion from the cell via Na/Ca exchange (see Chapters 3, 6 & 10). In combination with the potent stimulation of sarcolemmal Ca current by β-adrenergic agonists (see Chapter 5), this increase in SR Ca-pumping normally results in a substantial increase in SR Ca content available for release.

PLB is also phosphorylated by CaMKII at Thr-17 (Le Peuch *et al.*, 1979; Simmerman *et al.*, 1986) which produces a similar lowering of $K_m(Ca)$ as PKA phosphorylation of Ser-16 (Kranias, 1985; Sasaki *et al.*, 1992; Odermatt *et al.*, 1996). While less generally accepted there are also reports that suggest an increase of V_{max} due to CaMKII phosphorylation of PLB with less effect on K_m (*vs.* PKA; Mattiazzi *et al.*, 1994; Antipenko *et al.*, 1997a,b). Bassani *et al.* (1995c) showed that CaMKII phosphorylation might be responsible for a frequency-dependent acceleration of SR Ca uptake and relaxation in intact cells (see pg 270). However, this effect is still observed in mice in which the PLB gene has been knocked out (Luo *et al.*, 1994; Li *et al.*, 1998). In intact hearts, β-adrenergic agonists produce phosphorylation at Ser16, but also more gradually at Thr-17 (Wegener *et al.*, 1989; Talosi *et al.*, 1993; Kuschel *et al.*, 1999a). This may be partly due to adrenergic enhancement of Ca transients. However, it may also be due to cAMP-dependent inhibition of phosphatase 1 and also PKA-dependent stimulation of a phosphatase inhibitor (Ahmad *et al.*, 1989; Neumann *et al.*, 1991). Indeed, elevation of Ca transients alone (by high $[Ca]_o$ or Bay K 8644) does not normally result in Thr-17 phosphorylation (Lindemann & Watanabe, 1985b; Napolitano *et al.*, 1992; Vittone *et al.*, 1993) except when low concentrations of the phosphatase inhibitor okadaic acid is included or the pH is acidic (Mundiña-Weilenmann *et al.*, 1996; Vittone *et al.*, 1998). On the other hand, Hagemann *et al.* (2000) recently showed a frequency-dependent increase in PLB Thr-17 phosphorylation in rat myocytes in the absence of Ser-16 phosphorylation.

PLB can also be phosphorylated by PKC at serine 10 *in vitro* (Iwasa & Hosey, 1984; Movesian *et al.*, 1984). While Rogers *et al.* (1990) found that PKC decreased SR Ca uptake in permeabilized myocytes, it is not clear whether PKC-dependent PLB phosphorylation actually occurs *in vivo* or has any functional impact. PLB can also be phosphorylated at Ser-16 by cGMP-dependent protein kinase, but whether this occurs physiologically is not clear (Huggins *et al.*, 1989; Bartel *et al.*, 1995).

Some reports suggest that CaMKII can directly phosphorylate cardiac (but not skeletal) SR Ca-ATPase increasing the V_{max} for Ca transport (Xu *et al.*, 1993; Toyofuku *et al.*, 1994c). However, this result is controversial and two major studies have directly contradicted it (Reddy *et al.*, 1996; Odermatt *et al.*, 1996). Thus, PLB (and its phosphorylation state) seems to be the main endogenous regulator of SR Ca-pump function. Of course, the Ca-ATPase is also sensitive to the concentrations of substrates (Ca and ATP) as well as pH and other small molecules (see pg 169; Tada, 2001).

James *et al.* (1989) crosslinked Lys-3 on PLB to either Lys-397 or 401 on the Ca-pump, but this only worked when PLB was dephosphorylated. Toyofuku *et al.* (1993, 1994a) showed that residues 397-402 of SERCA2a (KDDKPV) were essential for PLB interaction, by measuring Ca transport function with SERCA2a/ SERCA3 chimeras. An elegant series of functional mutational analyses of PLB coexpressed with SERCA has resulted in unique insights and the hypothetical model in Fig 86 (Toyofuku *et al.*, 1994b; Kimura *et al.*, 1996, 1997; Autry & Jones, 1997; Cornea *et al.*, 1997). This intriguing working hypothesis considers PLB monomers to be the active inhibitors of the pump, whereas the pentamers constitute a PLB reservoir. Some loss of PLB function occurs with alanine substitutions for cytosolic residues 2,4,7,9,12 and 14. It was suggested that the cytoplasmic domain of PLB is not intrinsically inhibitory, but based on charge and hydrophobicity this region can interact with SERCA and modulate the inhibitory effects,

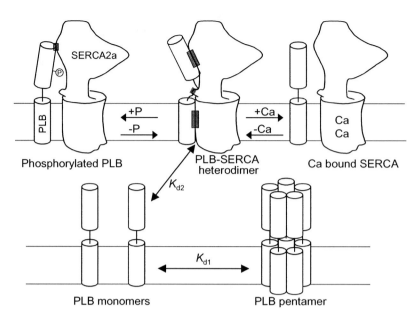

Figure 86. Model of phospholamban (PLB)-SERCA2 interaction. PLB can be either mono- or pentameric with a dissociation constant (K_{d1}). PLB mutations which disturb the leucine zipper (Fig 84) shift K_{d1} toward more monomers without altering the intrinsic affinity of monomeric PLB for the SR Ca-ATPase (K_{d2}), which causes greater pump inhibition. Other PLB mutations can increase or decrease K_{d2} without altering K_{d1}. Heterodimeric PLB-SERCA inhibits SR Ca-ATPase (Fig 85), but either phosphorylation of PLB or Ca binding to the pump can reduce PLB binding and relieve inhibition. Based on diagram in Kimura *et al.* (1997), modified and kindly provided by D.H. MacLennan.

which are caused mainly by interactions in the transmembrane regions. Interestingly, PLB and SERCA2a still co-immuno–precipitate when the inhibitory effect is reversed by either PLB phosphorylation or antibody, but they are dissociated at high [Ca] (Asahi *et al.*, 2000). Thus elevation of [Ca]$_i$ could reduce the fraction of SR Ca-pumps inhibited by PLB and this might contribute to frequency-dependent acceleration of relaxation by speeding SR Ca transport (when time-averaged [Ca]$_i$ is high).

Mutations in the PLB transmembrane domain which disturb the leucine zipper in Fig 84 (e.g. residues 37,40,44,47) result in de-pentamerization and greater Ca-pump inhibition. These monomeric mutants or "supershifters" (Fig 85) were suggested to be more effective simply because they were not in pentameric complexes, and so were free to interact with SERCA2a (i.e. a leftward shift along the K_{d1} balance in Fig 86, resulting in more PLB-SERCA heterodimers). Conversely, mutations on the opposite side of the PLB helix lost inhibitory function (without pentamer changes). This was attributed to reduced inhibitory interaction of PLB monomers with SERCA2a (a downward shift along K_{d2} in Fig 86). Phosphorylation drives the PLB equilibrium in favor of pentamers and reduces the inhibitory effect of PLB on the Ca-pump. This might simply be a downward shift along K_{d2} in Fig 86, resulting in more pentamers (or phosphorylated PLB may cause the K_{d1} to shift in favor of pentamers). A remarkable gain of PLB inhibitory function was seen when Arg-27 was mutated to alanine (N27A). This resulted in a 10-fold reduction in Ca affinity, without any loss of pentamers. Moreover, transgenic mice expressing this pentameric N27A mutant PLB exhibit decrease of SR Ca transport, cellular contraction and relaxation, and prolongation of isovolumic relaxation of the ventricle *in vivo* (Zhai *et al.*, 2000).

There is also evidence to suggest that PLB may decrease the energetic efficiency of the SR Ca-ATPase (Frank *et al.*, 2000; Shannon *et al.*, 2001) and the effect can be reversed by PKA phosphorylation. This would mean that in the presence of unphosphorylated PLB the SR Ca-ATPase would not be able to establish as large a [Ca] gradient (see *Thermodynamics*, pg 173).

Thus PLB is an extremely important physiological regulator of cardiac contraction. The remarkable enhancement of cardiac function in the PLB knockout mouse (Luo *et al.*, 1994) without any striking down-sides may indicate that selective inhibition of PLB expression or PLB-SERCA2a interaction could be a powerful cardiac inotropic strategy. Indeed, an advantage of this explicit PLB target is that one can increase SR Ca transport and Ca transients, without the physiological concomitant effects of PKA activation. That is, one could avoid PKA-dependent: a) reduction of myofilament Ca sensitivity (which would limit inotropy), b) increased I_{Ca} (which could lead to Ca overload), c) activation of the ryanodine receptor (which could increase spontaneous SR Ca release) and d) reduced energetic efficiency of contraction and metabolism.

SR Ca-ATPase inhibitors

While there are many modulators of SR Ca-ATPase, there is a group of three key agents which are widely used and potent inhibitors. These are thapsigargin (TG; Thastrup *et al.*, 1990; Sagara & Inesi, 1991), cyclopiazonic acid (CPA, Goeger *et al.*, 1988; Seidler *et al.*, 1989) and 2,5-di(*tert*-butyl)-1,4-benzohydroquinone (TBQ, Nakamura *et al.*, 1992). TG is the highest affinity and most selective of these tools (K_d < 2 pM, Davidson & Varhol, 1995). This extremely high affinity allows TG to be used very selectively to inhibit SERCA pumps. However, one must keep in mind that the concentration of SR Ca-ATPase molecules in myocytes is ~50 µM, so higher [TG] than 1-10 nM are often used as a practical matter to obtain rapid and complete block of SR Ca-ATPase. It is often better to consider [TG] in terms of nmol/mg protein to avoid not having enough TG molecules to bind to all of the SR Ca-pumps. In permeabilized myocytes in a cuvette ~1 nmol/ mg protein is sufficient for complete block, and at 5 nmol/mg it takes less than 5 sec for >95% block (Hove-Madsen & Bers, 1993b). In superfused intact myocytes, exposure to 5 µM TG blocks SR Ca-ATPase by ~95% in 60 sec and completely in <90 sec (Bassani *et al.*, 1993b). Curiously, when TG (or CPA) are superfused around thin multicellular preparations, it is almost impossible to completely block the SR Ca-ATPase (Baudet *et al.*, 1993). The high affinity of TG for the SR Ca-ATPase makes TG exposure essentially irreversible. CPA and TBQ can be used as more reversible SR Ca-pump inhibitors. CPA also has submicromolar affinity and ~10 µM is typically used to inhibit SR Ca-ATPase. TBQ inhibits the SR Ca-ATPase with a K_m~1.5 µM (Nakamura *et al.*, 1992) and 10 µM is typically used experimentally. While these agents are quite selective for SERCA pumps (as opposed to other P-type pumps) they may not be without complicating effects (e.g. Dettbarn & Palade, 1998).

Regulation of the SR Ca-pump by Ca, pH, ATP and Mg

SERCA has a high affinity ATP site (K_d ~1 µM) which is the substrate site and a second lower ATP affinity site (K_d ~200 µM) which serves a regulatory role (deMeis & Vianna, 1979; DuPont, 1977; Verjovski-Almeida & Inesi, 1979). Generally [ATP] is in excess for the SR Ca-

ATPase and $[Ca]_i$ is the limiting substrate. When cellular ATP levels fall during ischemia, there may be some decline in SR Ca-pumping and slowing of relaxation due to the allosteric effect, but [ATP] would have to be extremely low to prevent ATP binding to the substrate site (but see also *Thermodynamics* below). The actual substrate for the Ca-pump is probably MgATP, but other nucleotides can also be used (Tada *et al.*, 1978). However, the GTPase activity of the cardiac Ca-pump has different characteristics (e.g. very low Ca sensitivity; Tate *et al.,* 1985, 1989).

The SR Ca-pump is also pH-sensitive. Shigekawa *et al.* (1976) found a broad pH optimum around 8, which was more alkaline than that observed for skeletal muscle. Fabiato & Fabiato (1978a; Fabiato, 1985e) found that the Ca uptake by cardiac SR in mechanically skinned cell was progressively reduced as pH was decreased from 7.4. Thus, acidosis associated with ischemia may be expected to depress the rate of SR Ca-pumping and thus slow relaxation as is observed during acidosis. Of course acidosis can also reduce the Ca sensitivity of the myofilaments, Ca current, Na/Ca exchange etc. (see Chapter 10).

It should also be noted that there is a broad range of values reported for the optimum pH and this may depend on the assay conditions (e.g. [Ca], oxalate, [Mg], temperature, [ATP], phosphorylation state, the type of SR vesicles etc.). Indeed, this consideration is valid for the [Ca] and [ATP] dependence as well and it is a constant challenge to mimic accurately the intracellular physiological conditions for *in vitro* experiments aimed at determining the *in vivo* Ca-pump dependence on [Ca], [Mg], [ATP], etc. The situation is further complicated by the Ca release channel which alters **net** Ca transport by the Ca-pump and the gating of this channel is also affected by [Ca], ATP, Mg and pH (see below). For example, Fabiato & Fabiato (1978a) reported that at pH 7.4 the Ca uptake by the SR was optimal at [Ca]=18 nM, since under their particular conditions higher [Ca] induced Ca release. Indeed, Wimsatt *et al.* (1990) found maximal SR Ca uptake rate in permeabilized rat myocytes at ~500 nM Ca and lower uptake at 1-100 μM Ca. They attributed this decrease to Ca-induced Ca-release, because addition of SR Ca release channel blockers (procaine or ruthenium red) converted this to a monotonically increasing function (with much higher Ca uptake at 10 μM than at 500 nM Ca).

Figure 87 shows an on-line approach we have used to measure SR Ca uptake rate in both digitonin-permeabilized and intact ventricular myocytes (Hove-Madsen & Bers, 1993b; Bassani *et al.*, 1994a). The free Ca transient is converted to a total cytoplasmic transient ($\Delta[Ca]_{tot}$ in Fig 87A) using the Ca buffering characteristics measured in cells (as in Chapter 3) or in permeabilized cells (after pump blockade). The derivative with respect to time of the $\Delta[Ca]_{tot}$ signal is a Ca transport rate and under our conditions this Ca transport was entirely due to the SR Ca-ATPase. Plotting $d[Ca]_{tot}/dt$ as a function of $[Ca]_i$ for each individual point during $[Ca]_i$ decline (Fig 87B) gives the $[Ca]_i$ dependence of SR Ca transport rate (with K_m values ~200-300 nM and Hill coefficients of 2-4). The maximal SR Ca uptake rate in rat is ~2.4 times higher than in rabbit myocytes, and this is true for both intact and permeabilized cells. The extrapolated Ca transport rate in permeabilized cells was ~50% lower than that obtained in intact myocytes. It is not clear whether this difference is due to decreased function of some permeabilized cells in the cuvette (*vs.* intact cells) or other systematic differences in analysis.

Oxalate is frequently used as a precipitating anion in studies of SR Ca uptake. The principle is that oxalate is rapidly transported across the SR membrane (by an anion transporter)

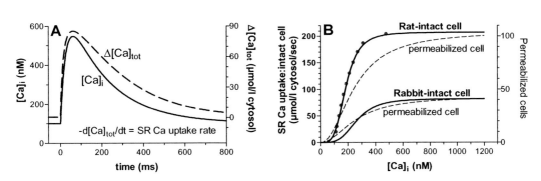

Figure 87. SR Ca transport measured in intact and permeabilized ventricular myocytes. **A.** Ca transient ($[Ca]_i$) from a rat ventricular myocyte where the Na/Ca exchange is prevented by complete Na depletion (as in Bassani *et al.,* 1994a). The $[Ca]_i$ is converted to total cytosolic Ca ($[Ca]_{tot}$) using buffering data as in Fig 26, pg 43: $[Ca]_{tot} = (236 \ \mu M / \{1+(498 \ nM/[Ca]_i)\}) -39 \ \mu M)$. **B.** The $d[Ca]_{tot}/dt$ is plotted as a function of $[Ca]_i$ for each point in time during $[Ca]_i$ decline (a few example points are shown). These curves are then fit by a Hill equation $V = V_{max}/(1+ \{K_m/[Ca]_i\}^n)$. The same analysis was used for intact rabbit myocytes and a similar approach was used for digitonin-permeabilized myocytes. Intact cell data are from Bassani *et al.* (1994a) and permeabilized cell data are from Hove-Madsen & Bers (1993b).

and as intra-SR free [Ca] ($[Ca]_{SR}$) increases it binds to oxalate and then precipitates, thereby limiting further rise in $[Ca]_{SR}$ which would prevent net uptake (see pg 175). This allows SR Ca uptake to continue almost linearly as a function of time at a given [Ca]. This greatly simplifies measurement of the [Ca]-dependence of SR Ca transport. Otherwise one would be restricted to an initial uptake rate at very short times (before $[Ca]_{SR}$ changes appreciably). However, the oxalate method is not physiological and the precipitated SR Ca is not readily releasable.

Calsequestrin

Physiologically intra-SR [Ca] is buffered in large part by calsequestrin, which was first described in skeletal muscle SR by MacLennan & Wong (1971). Meissner (1975) suggested that calsequestrin was primarily localized in the terminal cisternae of the SR. Calsequestrin in cardiac muscle was first identified and purified by Campbell *et al.* (1983) and Jorgensen & Campbell (1984) provided evidence that cardiac calsequestrin is localized to junctional SR (and corbular SR). The primary structure of cardiac calsequestrin has been deduced by cDNA cloning (MW = 45,269; Scott *et al.,* 1988) and is only 63% homologous with the fast twitch skeletal muscle calsequestrin (MW = 42,435; Fliegel *et al.,* 1987). As with the SR Ca-pump and PLB, "cardiac" calsequestrin is also expressed in slow twitch skeletal muscle (Scott *et al.,* 1988). The crystal structure of skeletal calsequestrin has been elucidated (Wang *et al.,* 1998b) and it has 3 thioredoxin folds which condense upon binding Ca. Ca binding seems to be by bridging of negatively charged surfaces between domains, rather than in EF-hand type loops as seen in TnC and calmodulin.

Cardiac calsequestrin is highly acidic and each molecule binds ~35-40 Ca ions (or ~900 nmol Ca/mg protein, Mitchell *et al.,* 1988) with an apparent $K_m(Ca) \sim 500 \ \mu M$. Assuming the maximum yield of isolated cardiac calsequestrin reported by Campbell (1986, 40 mg/kg wet wt) represents a true yield of 25-50% of whole heart calsequestrin, and the extrapolation conventions from Chapter 3, this corresponds to 175- 350 µmol of Ca binding sites per liter cytosol (3.2-6.4

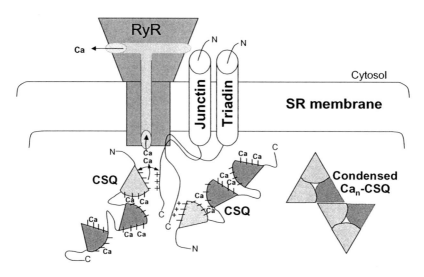

Figure 88. Association of calsequestrin (CSQ) with junctional SR proteins. These include the ryanodine receptor (RyR), triadin and junctin. Ca binds to negative charges (−) on CSQ, bridging the domains and limiting association with triadin and junctin. Higher $[Ca]_{SR}$ may lead to tighter CSQ condensation and multimerization (Ca_n-CSQ). Based on diagrams by Zhang *et al.* (1997b) and Wang *et al.* (1998b).

mM of Ca binding sites in the SR). Thus, these sites could buffer a substantial fraction of the Ca taken up by the SR with an appropriately low affinity. Shannon & Bers (1997) measured intra-SR free [Ca] and also total SR Ca content in rat ventricular myocytes. From these measurements we determined that the B_{max} for intra-SR Ca was ~14 mM with a K_d of 0.63 mM. This K_d is very close to the *in vitro* value above and the B_{max} for Ca is a bit higher than expected. Related recent results in intact myocytes give a B_{max} of ~3 mM intra-SR Ca sites (Shannon *et al.*, 2000a).

Calsequestrin appears to be attached to the junctional face membrane in the terminal cisternae of the SR (e.g. Franzini-Armstrong *et al.*, 1987) and when Ca binds to calsequestrin the shape of the molecule changes (Ikemoto *et al.*, 1972, 1974; Cozens & Reithmeier, 1984). Ikemoto *et al.* (1989, 1991) have even proposed that calsequestrin is involved in the regulation of the SR Ca release channel, but more work will be needed to clarify this possibility. Triadin and the structurally related protein junctin (Caswell *et al.*, 1991; Knudson *et al.*, 1993a,b; Jones *et al.*, 1995; Zhang *et al.*, 1997b) are also co-localized to the junctional region and interact with each other, calsequestrin and the ryanodine receptor. Thus there may be a physical interaction among these proteins as illustrated in the schematic in Fig 88. Three cardiac triadins exist (MW 35, 40 & 92 kDa for type 1, 2 & 3) with triadin-1 being dominant in heart. Skeletal muscle expresses a 95 kDa triadin, and junctin (26 kDa) is expressed in both cardiac and skeletal muscle. While functional information is limited, Zhang *et al.* (1997b) suggested that triadin and junctin may physically couple calsequestrin to the RyR as a junctional complex (Fig 88). They also showed that interactions between these proteins and calsequestrin are Ca-sensitive. Thus, as $[Ca]_{SR}$ falls during SR Ca release, calsequestrin may bind more strongly to triadin and/or junctin. This cooperative "zipping up" of this association could, in principle, facilitate Ca unloading of calsequestrin and thereby facilitate SR Ca release. This schematic model is speculative, but could help to explain the intriguing results of Ikemoto *et al.* (1989, 1991).

Calsequestrin has been overexpressed >10-fold in mouse heart (Jones *et al.*, 1998; Sato *et al.*, 1998b) and the mice develop cardiac hypertrophy. In myocytes there is a massive increase in SR Ca content (assessed by caffeine application) as expected for a greater amount of intra-SR Ca buffer. There was also a marked reduction in twitch Ca transients and contractions. One possible explanation for this somewhat unexpected result is that the free $[Ca]_{SR}$ may be low due to exceptionally heavy Ca buffering, and low $[Ca]_{SR}$ can strongly depress fractional SR Ca release (Bassani *et al.*, 1995b; Shannon *et al.*, 2000b).

Several other Ca binding proteins are in the SR. A 53 kDa SR glycoprotein appears to be the C-terminal half of sarcalumenin, which is 160 kDa in skeletal muscle and ~130 kDa in heart (Leberer *et al.*, 1989a,b, 1990). Sarcalumenin does not alter Ca-pump function in cotransfection studies, but the amino-terminal half is highly acidic, and like calsequestrin binds ~35 mol Ca/mol protein. The carboxy end (i.e. the 53 kDa glycoprotein) does not bind Ca appreciably. A histidine rich Ca-binding protein (~140 kDa) also exists in the SR lumen, but is a minor protein (Hoffman *et al.* 1989). Another minor luminal Ca binding SR protein calreticulin (MW = 46,567, Fliegel *et al.*, 1989b) binds 1 Ca with high affinity and ~25 Ca with low affinity (MacLennan *et al.*, 1972; Ostwald & MacLennan, 1974) and is present in both muscle and non-muscle cells (Fliegel *et al.*, 1989a,b). Indeed, calreticulin terminates with the ER retention signal peptide KDEL, whereas the muscle-specific proteins calsequestrin, sarcalumenin and histidine rich Ca-binding protein lack this sequence (Milner *et al.*, 1992). Calreticulin and the analogous (and ubiquitous) calnexin may both function primarily as molecular chaperones, assisting in protein folding and stabilization (John *et al.*, 1998; Danilczyk *et al.*, 2000). Thus, there are other SR Ca binding proteins, but from a quantitative standpoint calsequestrin is overwhelmingly dominant.

Thermodynamics and Ca-pump backflux

The SR Ca-pump can work in both directions. That is, it is a reversible enzymatic reaction and Ca can move out of the SR and even make ATP in doing so (Takenaka *et al.*, 1982; Feher, 1984). As such, the net direction of Ca-pump movement is dictated by thermodynamics (as was the case for Na/Ca exchange, Chapter 6). The free energy from ATP required to build the [Ca] gradient is $\Delta G_{SR\text{-}CaP} = 2RT \bullet \ln([Ca]_{SR}/[Ca]_i)$ and provided that $\Delta G_{ATP} + \Delta G_{SR\text{-}CaP}$ is negative, net Ca uptake occurs. Shannon & Bers (1997) measured $[Ca]_{SR}$ and thus the [Ca] gradient that could be generated by the cardiac SR Ca-pump. We found that $[Ca]_{SR}/[Ca]_i$ was constant at ~7000 over the whole range where measurements could be made (10-300 nM $[Ca]_i$). Thus, for $[Ca]_i = 150$ nM, $[Ca]_{SR}$ would be 1 mM. Chen *et al.* (1996b) also measured $[Ca]_{SR}$ using a low affinity Ca-binding NMR probe (TF-BAPTA) and found $[Ca]_{SR}$ in the intact beating heart to be ~1.5 mM. Figure 89 shows that the [Ca] gradient of 7000 corresponds to $\Delta G_{SR\text{-}CaP}$ of 44 kJ/mol, which is 74% of the energy available from ATP (for ΔG_{ATP}=59 kJ/mol, Allen *et al.*, 1985a). This is a fairly high energetic efficiency, but seems to be typical of ion transport pumps (see Table 13, page 62).

Net reverse Ca-pump flux is not expected physiologically, because the [Ca] gradient would have to exceed that required to make ΔG_{ATP} (and of course it is ΔG_{ATP} that builds the [Ca] gradient in the first place). Nevertheless it is important to consider the backwards flux through

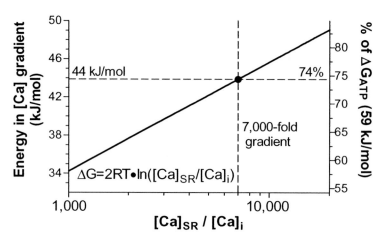

Figure 89. Energy in the trans-SR [Ca] gradient. Energy to transport 2 Ca ions/ATP is a logarithmic function of $[Ca]_{SR}/[Ca]_i$ (inset equation) and measurements indicate the pump can achieve a gradient of 7,000, equivalent to 44 kJ/mol, requiring 74% of the energy of ΔG_{ATP} (Based on Shannon & Bers., 1997).

the SR Ca-pump, as emphasized by Fig 90. Based on the forward Ca-pump rate (V_{For}) one would expect Ca influx into the SR at 100 nM $[Ca]_i$ to be 21 µmol/L cytosol/sec. If this unidirectional influx were balanced only by a leak flux, the leak flux rate (V_{Leak}) would also have to be 21 µmol/L cytosol/sec for the SR Ca content to be at a steady state. Indeed, this sort of V_{Leak} has been required to analyze SR Ca fluxes in cardiac myocytes (e.g. Balke *et al.*, 1994; Bassani *et al.*, 1994a). However, this is almost 100 times higher than the measured unidirectional Ca leak rate with the SR Ca-pump blocked in intact cells (0.3 µmol/L cytosol/sec; Bassani & Bers, 1995). With this V_{For} of 21 and V_{Leak} of 0.3, the reverse Ca-pump rate (V_{Rev}) would need to be 20.7 µmol/L cytosol/sec for the SR to be in Ca balance (Fig 90B). The implication of this is that the SR Ca-ATPase may approach thermodynamic equilibrium at physiological $[Ca]_i$ (i.e. with forward and reverse rates nearly balanced). Is it reasonable that V_{Rev} is this high? This requires a bit more quantitative consideration. Ca-pump flux can be written as

$$V_{net} = \frac{V_{mFor}([Ca]_i/K_{mFor})^2 - V_{mRev}([Ca]_{SR}/K_{mRev})^2}{1 + ([Ca]_i/K_{mFor})^2 + ([Ca]_{SR}/K_{mRev})^2} \tag{7.1}$$

where V_{mFor} and V_{mRev} are the forward and reverse maximum rates, and K_{mFor} and K_{mRev} are the forward and reverse dissociation constants. Hill coefficients were assumed to be 2 for flux in both directions. With $[Ca]_{SR} = 0$, the last term in both numerator and denominator drop out and Eq 7.1 reduces to the standard Hill equation ($V=V_{max}/(1+\{K_m/[Ca]_i\}^n)$), but as $[Ca]_{SR}$ rises reverse flux becomes more important and limits net Ca-pump flux. Indeed, at steady state ($V_{net} = 0$), the numerator of Eq 7.1 is 0. If we assume that maximal pump velocity is the same forward and reverse (Takenaka *et al.*, 1982), then $V_{mFor} = V_{mRev} = V_{max}$ and it follows that $K_{mRev}/K_{mFor} = [Ca]_{SR}/[Ca]_i$. Thus for a [Ca] gradient of 7000 and K_{mFor} of 300 nM, K_{mRev} would be 2 mM. Moreover, if $[Ca]_{SR}$ is 1 mM the V_{Rev} value in Fig 90B is predicted and this low affinity K_{mRev} is consistent with kinetic analysis of the SR Ca-pump transport cycle (e.g. see Fig 83).

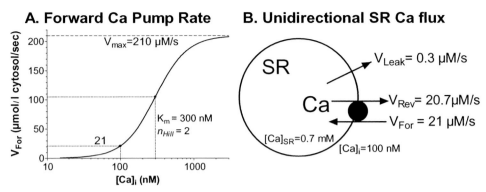

Figure 90. Unidirectional SR Ca-pump flux. **A**. Forward pump rate based on simple Hill relations as in Fig 85 ($V_{For} = V_{max}/(1+\{K_m/[Ca]_i\}^n)$). **B**. For $[Ca]_i = 100$ nM and $[Ca]_{SR} =700$ μM, values indicate expected forward and reverse Ca-pump flux rates and also SR Ca leak rate.

We tested the impact of SR Ca leak on the maximum steady state SR Ca load by measuring maximal SR Ca load in intact voltage clamped ventricular myocytes (Ginsburg *et al.*, 1998). If the leak does limit SR Ca load, then accelerating the SR Ca-pump (with isoproterenol) or slowing the pump (with submaximal thapsigargin exposure) should alter maximal SR Ca load accordingly. On the other hand, if the leak is inconsequential, then the Ca-pump should approach the thermodynamically limiting gradient, even when the pump is significantly slowed (it just takes more time). Essentially, the same maximal SR Ca load was reached when the SR Ca-pump was activated by isoproterenol, partially blocked by thapsigargin or untreated. Of course a different number of pulses were needed with isoproterenol or thapsigargin. The implication is that the normal resting SR Ca leak does not appreciably limit the SR Ca load.

This can also be appreciated on quantitative theoretical grounds. Figure 91 shows that the SR Ca load is not expected to be greatly decreased by the Ca leak until V_{Leak} approaches the forward rate of the pump (42 μmol/L cytosol/sec at 150 nM $[Ca]_i$). Furthermore, at physiological leak rates (0.3 μmol/L cytosol/s) slowing or accelerating the Ca-pump does not affect the steady state SR Ca load, although the time required to attain that load is altered accordingly. For pump inhibition by thapsigargin V_{max} was decreased by 50% and for Ca-pump stimulation by isoproterenol, K_m was reduced by 50%. Even a V_{Leak} ten times higher than measured would reduce SR Ca by less than 10%. This is consistent with observed results of Ginsburg *et al.* (1998) and re-emphasizes the importance of considering this backward pump flux in realistic models of SR Ca regulation in intact cells.

Not all results agree with this interpretation. Indeed, blocking leak via the ryanodine receptor with tetracaine can dramatically increase SR Ca content (Györke *et al.*, 1997; Overend *et al.*, 1998), an effect that would not be expected if leak were very small. More work is needed to clarify this discrepancy. However, a possible explanation may be that V_{Leak} increases very steeply as both $[Ca]_{SR}$ and $[Ca]_i$ rise (see *Regulation of SR Ca release*, pg 192-195 and Chapters 8-9). Thus, at relatively high SR Ca loads (and $[Ca]_i$) leak may be much higher and may more strongly affect SR Ca load.

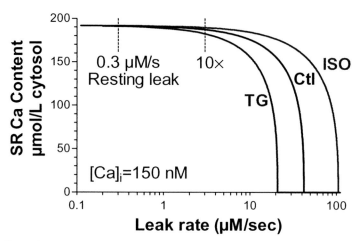

Figure 91. Effect of SR Ca leak rate on SR Ca content. Curves are based on Eq 7.1 in the steady state ($V_{net} = V_{For} - V_{Rev}$) and consideration that V_{net} is balanced by V_{Leak}. Then $[Ca]_{SR}$ is a function of V_{Leak} and $[Ca]_i$: $[Ca]_{SR} = 7000\{([Ca]_i^2 \, (V_{max}/V_{Leak} - 1) - (K_{mFor})^2)/ (V_{max}/V_{Leak} + 1))\}^{1/2}$ and total SR Ca ($[Ca]_{SRtot}$) is related to $[Ca]_{SR}$: $[Ca]_{SRtot} = [Ca]_{SR} + (B_{maxSR}/(1+\{K_{dSR}/[Ca]_{SR}\})$, where B_{maxSR} is the intra-SR binding capacity and K_{dSR} is the dissociation constant. Thus $[Ca]_{SR}$ and $[Ca]_{SRtot}$ can be predicted as a function of $[Ca]_i$, V_{max}, V_L and K_{mFor}. The control values used are $V_{max} = 210$ µmol/L cytosol/s, $K_{mFor} = 300$ nM, $B_{maxSR} = 3.95$ mM and $K_{dSR} = 600$ µM. For $[Ca]_i = 150$ nM at low leak levels $[Ca]_{SR} = 1$ mM and $[Ca]_{SRtot}$ of 191 µmol/L cytosol corresponds to 3.5 mM intra-SR Ca (see Ginsburg et al., 1998).

Figure 92 shows incorporation of Eq 7.1 into detailed quantitative analysis of real cellular Ca transients (Shannon et al., 2000a). Associated with SR Ca release there is a decline in SR Ca content (and $[Ca]_{SR}$) and consequently reverse Ca-pump flux is decreased, while forward Ca-pump flux is stimulated by high $[Ca]_i$. Thus there is an increase in net SR Ca uptake by the pump. As $[Ca]_i$ declines and $[Ca]_{SR}$ rises the forward Ca-pump rate falls and reverse Ca-pump rate increases, until the net pump flux is almost zero (only balancing the small leak). At that point the SR Ca content has returned, and in this case the amount of Ca which entered via I_{Ca} was also accumulated by the SR because these experiments were done in Na-free conditions to avoid complicating Na/Ca exchange fluxes.

The functional consequence of this thermodynamic consideration is that Ca uptake by the SR (especially during late relaxation and diastole) will be sensitive to energetic limitations that may occur under pathophysiological conditions. For example, if [ATP] declines or [ADP] or [PO$_4$] rise, the ΔG_{ATP} available to the Ca-pump will be reduced. While this may not alter V_{max} or initial rates of $[Ca]_i$ decline, it will reduce the [Ca] gradient that the SR Ca-pump can generate. This will have preferential effects on the latter phase of $[Ca]_i$ decline and on diastolic $[Ca]_i$ as the pump approaches a different thermodynamic equilibrium (at lower $[Ca]_{SR}$ and higher $[Ca]_i$). A lower SR Ca content may also have a disproportionately depressant impact on Ca transients by reducing both the amount of SR Ca available and also the fraction released (see pg 224-225).

As a protective mechanism with respect to changes in ΔG_{ATP}, many glycolytic enzymes appear to be closely associated with the SR Ca-pump (Xu et al., 1995; Xu & Becker, 1998). These enzymes can produce ATP locally (and consume local ADP) and this ATP appears to have preferential access to the SR Ca-pump. This may ensure optimal ΔG_{ATP} availability for Ca

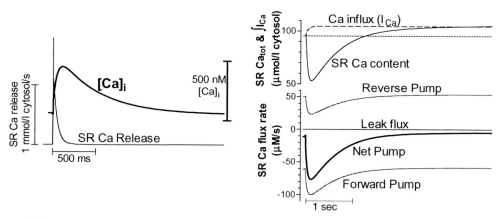

Figure 92. SR Ca-pump fluxes during a cellular Ca transient. Left panel shows a Ca transient and SR Ca release flux in a voltage clamped rabbit ventricular myocyte in Na-free conditions to block Na/Ca exchange (data from Shannon *et al.*, 2000b). Data were analyzed to provide running information about forward and reverse SR Ca-pump rate (using Eq 7.1) and SR Ca leak ($k([Ca]_{SR} -[Ca]_i)$. During this twitch SR Ca content fell by ~45% during SR Ca release, but was higher at the end of the trace by the amount of integrated Ca entry via I_{Ca} (i.e. this cell was being progressively Ca loaded).

transport. On the other hand, Chen *et al.* (1998) showed that $[Ca]_{SR}/[Ca]_i$ varies in parallel to ΔG_{ATP} and Tian *et al.* (1998) found that inhibition of creatine kinase (which phosphorylates ADP to ATP) limits SR Ca handling and thereby limits contractile reserve in the intact heart.

This raises the issue of energetic requirements for Ca transport (see also pg 62). In guinea-pig ventricle Schramm *et al.* (1994) determined that 15% of cardiac energy expenditure is due to the SR Ca-ATPase *vs.* 76% for myofilament ATPase and 9% for Na/K-ATPase (remember that ~75% of the Na extruded was that used to extrude Ca via Na/Ca exchange). This ~20% of total energy expenditure for Ca transport is a major energetic investment. Two Ca ions can be pumped into the SR per molecule of ATP, while only one Ca ion per ATP can be extruded via Na/Ca exchange (indirectly, since 3 Na are moved per cycle by Na/Ca exchange and Na/K-ATPase). Thus, any shifts from SR Ca transport to greater transsarcolemmal fluxes, as may occur in heart failure, will also carry an extra energetic cost.

It is clear from the foregoing that the rate of Ca transport by the SR Ca-ATPase is sufficient to drive cardiac relaxation, even if there is also a variable parallel contribution from the Na/Ca exchange (as discussed in Chapter 6). The amount of Ca stored in the SR is obviously a crucial parameter in understanding SR function and that will be discussed here.

SR Ca CONTENT: ASSESSMENT IN
INTACT CARDIAC MUSCLE AND MYOCYTES

A number of different experimental approaches have been used to measure the SR Ca content in ventricular muscle. These have included ^{45}Ca fluxes in intact cells and tissue as well as in homogenates and SR vesicles. Some of the more recent measurements in intact cells have come from the amplitude of caffeine-induced Ca transients as well as integration of $I_{Na/Ca}$ during caffeine-induced contractures. Table 21 shows a compilation of some measurements, with all converted to the units μmol/L cytosol. The top group are relatively high and are generally at an ambient [Ca] higher than the diastolic $[Ca]_i$ of 100-150 nM. Most of the values in the lower section of Table 21 are at physiological [Ca] and many are from intact cells. Most of these values range from 32-58 μmol/L cytosol in guinea-pig ventricular myocytes to 210-260 μmol/L cytosol in rat or ferret ventricle. This provides a realistic consensus range despite the variety of experimental approaches, conditions and laboratories. For now, 50-150 μmol/L cytosol is a likely range of steady state SR Ca content in intact ventricular myocytes at typical stimulation frequencies. For an SR volume of 3.5% of the cell this would correspond to 1.5-3 mM total SR Ca (with about half bound to calsequestrin). Let's consider how SR Ca content is measured.

Electron Probe Microanalysis

Electron probe microanalysis (EPMA) can directly assess Ca in junctional SR (jSR) in electron microscopic specimens, using emitted X-ray spectra (Wheeler-Clark & Tormey, 1987; Jorgensen *et al.*, 1988; Wendt-Gallitelli & Isenberg, 1989; Moravec & Bond, 1990). These studies have indicated jSR Ca contents (under non-Ca-depleting conditions) of ~15 mmol/kg dry wt. Under conditions expected to deplete the SR of Ca (e.g. long rest periods, ryanodine or freeze clamping during the rising phase of a contraction) values of 3-7 mmol/kg dry wt were reported. Extrapolation of these values to either mmol Ca/L jSR (or μmol/L cytosol) must take technical limitations into account (e.g. dispersion of the X-ray beam into non-jSR regions and geometry of jSR within the depth of section, ~200 nm). At the simplest level, assuming 4 kg wet jSR/kg dry jSR, a jSR density of 1.1 g/cm^3 and 0.3% of cell volume as jSR or terminal cisternae (see Table 3, page 7), 15 mmol/kg dry jSR would correspond to ~4 mM total [Ca] in the jSR or ~20 μmol/L cytosol. The jSR is only ~10% of the SR volume, but may have 5-10 times more total Ca/L than network SR, due to the localization of calsequestrin. This may imply that there is about the same amount of total Ca in network and jSR. This would make total SR Ca load ~40 μmol/L cytosol, which is about 50% of the SR Ca content estimated by biochemical or physiological approaches. It is also similar to the Ca required to activate a normal contraction (see page 47). Therefore, while electron probe microanalysis is probably the most direct and absolute method of measurement of SR Ca content, it may slightly underestimate SR Ca and it is technically difficult, tissue destructive and challenging to extrapolate to the intact cell.

Caffeine-Induced Contractures, $\Delta[Ca]_i$ and $\int I_{Na/Ca}$

Two of the most useful means to assess SR Ca "on line," with intact, contracting cardiac muscle or myocytes are rapid application of caffeine or cold solution (~1°C). Caffeine and cooling induce SR Ca release at a desired time and the amplitude of the resulting contracture or Ca transient can be used as an index of the SR that is Ca available for release at that time. With these indirect approaches the actual amount of Ca released (in μmol/L cytosol) is inferred, but this limitation can be modest and may not outweigh the great advantages of these approaches (on-line, reproducible, sensitive and non-destructive).

Caffeine-induced contractures were first described by Endo (1975b) in mechanically skinned skeletal muscle fibers and by Fabiato (1985b; Fabiato & Fabiato, 1975a,1978a) in mechanically skinned cardiac myocytes. Early uses of this approach in intact cardiac muscle and

TABLE 21

SR Ca Content Measurements

Reference	Species	Prep	SR Ca Load μmol/L cytosol	Conditions
Solaro & Briggs, 1974	dog	V homog	427	1 μM [Ca], ^{45}Ca
Dani *et. al.*, 1979	rabbit	perm V myo	171-512	< 1 μM [Ca], ^{45}Ca
Levitsky *et. al.*, 1981	g-p	V homog	376	24 μM [Ca], ^{45}Ca
Bridge, 1986	rabbit	papillary	645	2.7 mM [Ca]$_o$, aa, resting Ca loss
H-M & Bers, 1993a	rabbit	perm V myo	884	> 7.5 μM [Ca]
Shannon & Bers, 1997	rat	perm V myo	880	~1 μM [Ca]$_i$ ^{45}Ca
Kawai & Konishi, 1994	ferret	perm papillary	372	1 μM [Ca], fl
Solaro & Briggs, 1974	dog	V homog	68	100 nM [Ca], ^{45}Ca
Hunter *et. al.*, 1981	rat	perfused heart	119	2.5 mM [Ca]$_o$, rest-dep ^{45}Ca loss
Fabiato, 1983	rat	skinned fiber	142	~100 nM [Ca]
Moravec & Bond, 1990	hamster	papillary	40	0.2 Hz, 1.9 mM [Ca]$_o$, EPMA
Callewaert *et al.*, 1989	rat	isol V myo	90	66 nM [Ca]$_c$, caff, $I_{Na/Ca}$
	g-p		32	~70 nM [Ca]$_c$, caff, $I_{Na/Ca}$
H-M & Bers, 1993a	rabbit	perm V myo	~100	~100 nM [Ca]$_c$
Shannon & Bers 1997	rat	perm V myo	415	100 nM [Ca]$_i$ ^{45}Ca
Varro, *et. al.*, 1993	rat	isol V myo	185	1 mM [Ca]$_o$, caff, $I_{Na/Ca}$
Trafford *et al.*, 1997	ferret	isol V myo	118	0.33 Hz, 2 mM [Ca]$_o$, caff, $I_{Na/Ca}$
Pytkowski 1989	rabbit	papillary	408*	1 Hz, 1.8 mM [Ca]$_o$, ^{45}Ca
Langer & Rich 1993	rat	isol V myo	210*	1 mM [Ca]$_o$, ^{45}Ca flux, caff
Kawai & Konishi, 1994	ferret	perm papillary	260	100 nM [Ca]$_c$, fl
Bassani *et. al.*, 1995a	ferret	isol V myo	141	0.5 Hz, 2 mM [Ca]$_o$, caff, fl
Bassani & Bers, 1995	rat	isol V myo	114	0.5 Hz, 1 mM [Ca]$_o$, caff, fl
	rabbit	isol V myo	106	0.5 Hz, 2 mM [Ca]$_o$, caff, fl
Terracciano *et al.*, 1995	g-p	isol V myo	58	0.5 Hz, 2 mM [Ca]$_o$, caff, $I_{Na/Ca}$
Terr. & MacLeod, 1997	g-p	isol V myo	38	0.5 Hz, 1 mM [Ca]$_o$, caff, $I_{Na/Ca}$
	rat	isol V myo	73	0.5 Hz, 1 mM [Ca]$_o$, caff, $I_{Na/Ca}$
Delbridge *et. al.*, 1996	rabbit	isol V myo	87	0.5 Hz, 2 mM [Ca]$_o$, caff, fl, $I_{Na/Ca}$
Ginsburg *et al.*, 1998	ferret	isol V myo	149-190	0.5 Hz, 2 mM [Ca]$_o$, caff, fl, $I_{Na/Ca}$

The line separates measurements of maximum SR Ca content (above) from those under more normal cellular conditions. All values are converted to μmol/L cytosol. H-M is Hove-Madsen, Terr. is Terracciano, g-p is guinea-pig. *represents caffeine and ryanodine sensitive component of kinetically defined ^{45}Ca washout (~20% of total component). aa= atomic absorption spectroscopy, caff = caffeine-induced release, fl = Ca-sensitive fluorescence, isol V myo. = isolated ventricular myocytes, $I_{Na/Ca}$ = Ca efflux measured via Na/Ca exchange current, EPMA=electron probe microanalysis, perm = sarcolemma permeabilized by digitonin or saponin. Table prepared with help from T.R. Shannon.

myocytes were by Chapman & Léoty (1976), Bers (1987a), Smith *et al.* (1988) and O'Neill *et al.* (1990a). One can use the myofilaments as a Ca bioassay, measuring the caffeine-induced contracture, and these have been widely useful. Of course whenever tension is being measured to assess SR Ca load, one must be careful that an intervention under study does not alter myofilament Ca sensitivity (e.g. as is the case for β-adrenergic agonists). Caffeine itself increases myofilament Ca sensitivity (Fabiato, 1981b; Wendt & Stephenson, 1983; Eisner & Valdeolmillos, 1985), which means that force (or cell shortening) in the presence of caffeine cannot be directly related to the force in its absence (e.g. during a twitch). More robust quantitative versions of this approach include measurement of [Ca]$_i$ and $I_{Na/Ca}$.

Figure 93A shows caffeine-induced Ca transients and $I_{Na/Ca}$, which can both be used independently to assess SR Ca load. The amplitude of the Ca transient (Δ[Ca]$_i$) can be used as a

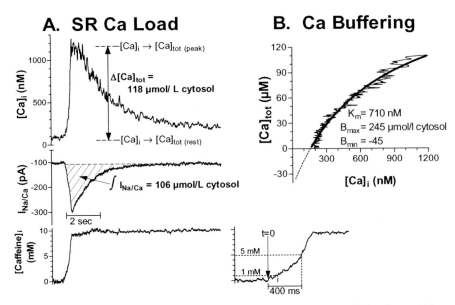

Figure 93. Caffeine-induced Ca transient, SR Ca content and cytosolic buffering in a rabbit ventricular myocyte under voltage clamp. **A.** Caffeine (10 mM) was rapidly applied and the Ca-independent indo-1 fluorescence signal was used to infer [caffeine]$_i$ (bottom; O'Niell *et al.*, 1990a). Amplitude of the Ca transient (top) is used to calculate total SR Ca released after conversion to total cytosolic Ca (using buffering curve #1, pg 43). SR Ca content is also obtained from the integral of I$_{Na/Ca}$ (×6.44 pF/pL cytosol, ÷96,490 C/mol and 0.93 to account for non-I$_{Na/Ca}$ mediated Ca transport). **B.** Ca buffering curve is obtained by backward integration of I$_{Na/Ca}$, conversion to [Ca]$_{tot}$ and fitting as a function of [Ca]$_i$ ([Ca]$_{tot}$ ={B$_{max}$/(1+K$_m$/[Ca]$_i$)}+B$_{min}$, Trafford *et al.*, 1999). Data here were recorded by K.S. Ginsburg.

crude index of SR Ca content, but can be made more quantitative by using cytosolic Ca buffering values (see pages 42-46) to translate [Ca]$_i$ to total cytosolic [Ca] ([Ca]$_{tot}$). Then the difference between resting and peak [Ca]$_{tot}$ provides the SR Ca content (in this case 118 μmol/L cytosol). This method, as shown, can underestimate peak [Ca]$_i$ because Ca extrusion by I$_{Na/Ca}$ begins as [Ca]$_i$ rises and hence can curtail the peak [Ca]$_i$ (by up to ~25%, Bassani *et al.*, 1994a). This limitation can be circumvented by applying caffeine in 0Na, 0Ca solution.

Indo-1 fluorescence is strongly quenched by caffeine, but in a wavelength-independent manner. Thus, fluorescence ratios used to infer [Ca]$_i$ are unaffected (if background fluorescences are appropriately subtracted). O'Neill *et al.* (1990a) turned this potential problem into an advantage by using indo-1 quench to indicate intracellular [caffeine]. The two usual indo-1 fluorescence signals can be combined to provide a Ca-independent signal that indicates the time course of quench. That signal can then be translated to the intracellular [caffeine] as in the lower panel of Fig 93A. In this case [caffeine]$_i$ rose to 1 mM (sufficient to trigger SR Ca release) in less than 60 ms. Caffeine must be applied very rapidly. Otherwise contractions can be biphasic, because myofilament Ca sensitization occurs progressively after SR Ca release. Slow caffeine application also causes asynchronous cellular SR Ca release, which damps the global Ca transient (lower & slower) as cellular release and extrusion progress as in propagating Ca waves.

During a caffeine-induced Ca transient the [Ca]$_i$ decline is almost entirely due to Ca extrusion from the cell via Na/Ca exchange (93% in rabbit, Table 20). Varro *et al.* (1993) first used integrated $I_{Na/Ca}$ to measure SR Ca content. The Ca-activated inward current in rabbit cells (Fig 93A) is entirely $I_{Na/Ca}$, because it is abolished in 0Na, 0Ca solution, whereas other candidate Ca-activated currents ($I_{Cl(Ca)}$ & $I_{ns(Ca)}$) should still have functioned (Delbridge *et al.*, 1996). Thus, caffeine-induced $I_{Na/Ca}$ can be integrated to measure the number of Ca ions released and extruded (and divided by 0.68-0.93 to correct for the non-$I_{Na/Ca}$ Ca removal, depending on species). In this rabbit myocyte we find 106 µmol/L cytosol, in close agreement with that based on $\Delta[Ca]_i$ (especially considering that the two methods have very different assumptions and limitations).

In addition, since we know the rate of total Ca removal (measured by $I_{Na/Ca}$) and the $[Ca]_i$ at each point in time, this data can also be used as an on-line cytosolic Ca buffering titration (Fig 93B). This method, devised by Trafford *et al.* (1999), integrates $I_{Na/Ca}$ from the end of the caffeine-induced contracture backward in time for the falling phase of the Ca transient. The analysis in Fig 93B yielded buffering values almost identical to curve #1 in Fig 26 (which were used to calculate $\Delta[Ca]_{tot}$ in Fig 93A), so it would produce the same resultant $\Delta[Ca]_{tot}$.

Caffeine-induced SR Ca release is thus a very powerful and useful approach, especially in isolated myocytes where diffusional limitations are minimal. Other effects of caffeine such as myofilament Ca sensitization (above) and phosphodiesterase inhibition (Butcher & Sutherland, 1962) which can increase cAMP and activate protein kinase A, can complicate interpretations (but are generally not problematic during the few sec of caffeine exposure). The fact that the Ca released is immediately subject to transport systems such as Na/Ca exchange (above) is also a limitation. Finally, due to the transient nature of the $[Ca]_i$ rise diffusional barriers in multicellular preparations mean that the $[Ca]_i$ transient will occur at different times throughout the preparation. This lack of synchrony can prevent measurable overall muscle contraction or global $\Delta[Ca]_i$ from being observed. Indeed, we find that caffeine-induced contracture amplitude is inversely related to the diameter of the multicellular preparation. For multicellular preparations rapid cooling contractures are far more useful because heat diffuses much faster than caffeine and the cold also greatly inhibits Ca transport rates.

Rapid Cooling Contractures (RCCs)

Rapidly cooling cardiac muscle (to ~1°C) induces contractures attributable to SR Ca release. Rapid cooling contractures (RCCs) were first described in skeletal muscle fibers (Sakai, 1965), but required pretreatment with 0.3-1 mM caffeine. This contrasts with mammalian cardiac muscle, where RCCs are induced normally in the absence of caffeine (Kurihara & Sakai, 1985; Bridge, 1986) and prior caffeine exposure only inhibits RCCs (K_m ~1 mM, with abolition at 5-10 mM caffeine, Bers *et al.*, 1987; Bers & Bridge, 1988).

Figures 94 and 95A show typical RCCs in rabbit ventricular muscle and guinea-pig ventricular myocytes after stimulation was terminated. Rapid cooling from 29°C to 0-1°C induces a rapid release of the available SR Ca to the cytoplasm. This Ca then activates a contracture (slowly at 1°C), the amplitude of which indicates the SR Ca available for release at the time of cooling. During the time at 0-1°C, ion transport mechanisms (e.g. Na/Ca exchange and Ca-pumps) are strongly inhibited so $[Ca]_i$ declines slowly. Upon rewarming, a "rewarming spike" is observed on the tension record, but not on the $[Ca]_i$ trace. This rewarming spike is due to the rapid increase in myofilament Ca sensitivity induced by rewarming, before $[Ca]_i$ declines (as expected from page 29; Harrison & Bers, 1989a). Rewarming also reactivates the ion

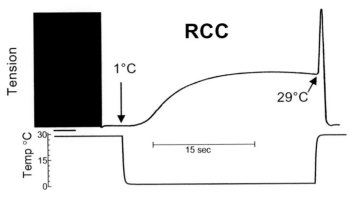

Figure 94. Rapid cooling contracture (RCC) in rabbit ventricular muscle. Steady state field stimulation (0.5 Hz) was terminated and 2 sec later (↓) superfusate was switched from 29°C to 1°C. The surface temperature of the muscle decreased rapidly. After the RCC reached a maximum solution was switched back to 29°C, inducing a rewarming spike (due to increased myofilament sensitivity) and rapid relaxation.

transport mechanisms which had been inhibited by the cold (e.g. SR Ca-pump and Na/Ca exchange). Reactivation of these processes causes rapid relaxation, and by changing solution composition during the cold and rewarming one can evaluate the Ca transport mechanisms responsible for relaxation (Bers & Bridge, 1989, see pg 52 & 152-4).

The muscle surface in Fig 94 was cooled below 5°C in < 300 msec, reaching a stable value of ~1°C in about 1.5 sec. We estimate the core of a 400 µm diameter muscle to be cooled to <5°C in <2 sec (very much faster than caffeine would equilibrate in this muscle). Additionally, because Ca transport systems are largely inhibited at 1°C, the $[Ca]_i$ rise during an RCC is less transient than with caffeine. This makes RCCs of greater practical utility in multicellular preparations. While RCCs are not as quantitative (in absolute Ca terms) as caffeine-induced Ca transients (above), RCCs can be repeated to assess changes in SR Ca load on-line.

$[Ca]_i$ can rise very rapidly during an RCC (see Figs 76 & 95). This Ca comes from the SR, since RCCs can be abolished by depleting the SR with caffeine, ryanodine and long rest periods (Bers *et al.*, 1987). RCCs also do not depend on Ca influx since their amplitude is unaffected by the absence of $[Ca]_o$ (Bers *et al.*, 1989; Fig 95A *vs.* D), even after long times (Fig 95D-F). Sitsapesan *et al.* (1991) showed that cooling single cardiac Ca-release channels (in bilayers) to 5°C dramatically increases the channel open probability (from $p_o = 0.004$ to 0.35 at 100 nM Ca), mainly by tremendous increase in open time. Much evidence also suggests that RCCs can release all of the available SR Ca (e.g. Bers *et al.*, 1989).

RCCs measured as isometric force are generally smaller than twitch contractions, despite the high $[Ca]_i$. This is due to decreased myofilament Ca sensitivity and maximal force at 1°C (pg 29). When RCCs are measured as unloaded shortening in isolated myocytes or muscle they can greatly exceed twitch amplitude (Fig 95; Hryshko *et al.*, 1989c). The explanation is that prolonged $[Ca]_i$ elevation in the RCC allows the cell to progressively shorten (since force needs only overcome passive restoring force). Fig 95A-C shows that increasing rest duration results in gradual decreases in RCC amplitude (rest decay, see pg 157 & Chapter 9). When Ca extrusion via Na/Ca exchange is prevented during the rest (0Na,0Ca solution) then this loss of SR Ca is

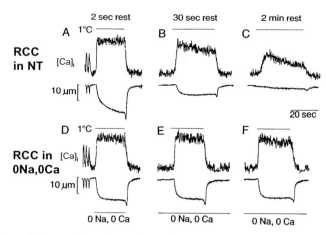

Figure 95. RCCs and Ca transients in a guinea-pig ventricular myocyte. Shortening (in μm) and [Ca]$_i$ during the last stimulated twitches (at 0.5 Hz in **A** and **D**) and during RCCs induced 2 sec after the last twitch (**A** and **D**), 30 sec after termination of another train of pulses (**B** and **E**) and after a similar 2 min rest (**C** and **F**). In **A-C** the superfusate during rest and RCCs was NT. In **D-F** the superfusate during rest and RCCs was Na-free and Ca-free, with 500 μM EGTA). The horizontal bar indicates the time during which the superfusate was at 1°C (from Bers *et al.*, 1989, with permission).

also prevented (Fig 95D-F). [Ca]$_i$ does slowly decline during long RCCs, reflecting incomplete inhibition of Ca transport systems (and RCCs relax faster at 3-5°C than at 0-1°C).

Ryanodine effects on SR Ca were extensively probed using RCCs (Bers *et al.*, 1987, 1989; Bers & Bridge, 1989; Hryshko *et al.*, 1989c). After equilibration with 100-500 nM ryanodine, RCCs of similar amplitude could still be measured in rabbit ventricular muscle, but only immediately after a series of contractions (see Fig 96). With ryanodine, RCC amplitude declined as a function of rest with a t½=0.73 sec, which is ~100 times faster than control (t½=81 sec). These results indicated that ryanodine did not stop the SR from accumulating Ca when [Ca]$_i$ was high, but that it greatly accelerated the leak of Ca back to the cytoplasm. This agrees with observations that ryanodine preferentially slows relaxation at low [Ca]$_i$ and depresses post-rest contractions at lower [ryanodine] than that required to depress steady state twitches (Bers & Bridge, 1989; Malécot & Katzung, 1987). This relates to the pump-leak considerations above. That is, when [Ca]$_i$ is high (and SR [Ca] is low) the Ca-pumping rate exceeds the rate of ryanodine-induced Ca leak. However as [Ca]$_i$ declines (and [Ca]$_{SR}$ rises) the leak becomes greater and the SR loses Ca. These results agree with the action of ryanodine to "lock" the SR Ca release channel in a submaximal open state (see pg 187,;Rousseau *et al.*, 1987).

Cumulative Extracellular Ca Depletions

A surprisingly useful tool to study changes in SR Ca is extracellular Ca microelectrodes used to monitor net Ca gain or loss (as local [Ca]$_o$ depletions or accumulations, Bers, 1983, 1985, 1987; Bers & MacLeod, 1986; MacLeod & Bers, 1987). In the steady state Ca entry at one beat must be extruded prior to the next beat; otherwise progressive Ca loading will occur (note steady initial [Ca]$_o$ traces in Fig 97). However, under non-steady state conditions, such as termination of stimulation, the cell may lose Ca (rest decay), observable as a rise in [Ca]$_o$. With a long

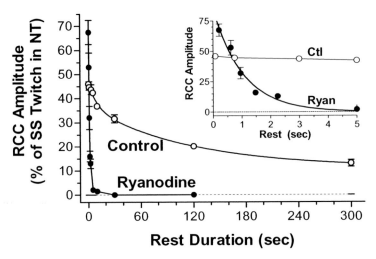

Figure 96. Ryanodine (100 nM) accelerates rest decay of SR Ca content in rabbit ventricular muscle. Stimulation at 0.5 Hz was terminated and the muscle cooled after rest time indicated on the abscissa. Inset shows an expanded time scale (redrawn from data in Bers *et al.*, 1987).

enough rest interstitial $[Ca]_o$ gradually returns to steady state. Resumption of stimulation results in net Ca cellular uptake as the SR refills toward steady state (see $[Ca]_o$ depletions in Fig 97). These cumulative cellular Ca losses and gains are due mainly to changes in SR Ca. They are inhibited by caffeine and require transsarcolemmal Ca flux, since they can be blocked by Co and nifedipine (Bers & MacLeod, 1986). Furthermore, larger Ca_o depletions are observed after long rest intervals where the SR has lost its Ca (MacLeod & Bers, 1987). Since the SR is then empty, a larger net Ca uptake is required to return it to steady state (hence the larger Ca_o depletion).

With ryanodine (Fig 97B) termination of stimulation results in a large and rapid Ca extrusion from the cell ($[Ca]_o$ rise). This is because all of the SR Ca is rapidly extruded from the cell by Na/Ca exchange (due to the rapid Ca leak from the SR). This fits with the above mechanism of ryanodine action based on RCCs. That is, during trains of pulses the SR may accumulate large amounts of Ca, because Ca_o depletions (& RCCs) in the presence of ryanodine are as large as control, and are caffeine sensitive (MacLeod & Bers, 1987; Bers & MacLeod, 1986). During SR Ca leak and efflux $[Ca]_i$ remains low, because resting force is not elevated.

Reduction of the transsarcolemmal [Na] gradient inhibits Ca_o accumulations and depletions (Fig 165B; Bers & MacLeod, 1986; Bers, 1987b). This is because the lower [Na] gradient limits Ca extrusion by Na/Ca exchange. If Na/Ca exchange is unable to extrude Ca from the cell during rest, the SR stays full of Ca (see pp 156-9), there will be no Ca_o accumulation during rest and no Ca_o depletion with resumption of stimulation (i.e. the SR doesn't lose Ca during rest, so it doesn't need more to be reloaded to reach steady state).

It may seem surprising that measuring $[Ca]_o$ is useful as an on-line monitor of changing SR Ca content, but this emphasizes that Ca can shift from SR to interstitium and back (depending on SR Ca-pump/Na/Ca exchange competition) without much change in diastolic $[Ca]_i$. One

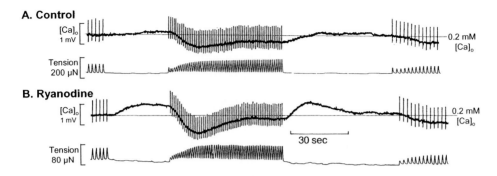

Figure 97. Extracellular Ca depletions in rabbit ventricular muscle. Local $[Ca]_o$ (upper traces) and tension before (**A**, bath $[Ca]_o$ =0.2 mM) and after equilibration with 1 µM ryanodine (**B**). Both panels begin with steady state stimulation (0.5 Hz), 30 sec rest, 1 Hz for ~ 1 min and 0.5 Hz again after a 1 min rest period. The spikes on the $[Ca]_o$ trace are stimulus artifacts. Extracellular [Ca] was measured with a double-barreled Ca-selective microelectrode (from Bers & MacLeod, 1986, with permission).

limitation of this approach is that Ca_o depletions are difficult to extrapolate in absolute units of µmol/L cytosol. A lower limit estimate of Ca uptake into the SR from this approach is 64 µmol/L cytosol (MacLeod & Bers, 1987), but this does not account for interstitial Ca binding sites. Hilgemann *et al.* (1983, Hilgemann & Langer, 1984) also studied cumulative cardiac Ca_o depletions using extracellular Ca indicator dyes. These 2 types of $[Ca]_o$ measurements also sense net sarcolemmal Ca fluxes during single contractions (Bers, 1983, 1985, 1987b; Dresdner & Kline, 1985; Pizarro *et al.*, 1985; Hilgemann, 1986a,b; Shattock & Bers, 1989).

Direct Chemical and Radiotracer Techniques

Classical chemical measurements (e.g. atomic absorption spectrometry and [45]Ca flux) can provide values that are easily extrapolated in units of µmol/L cytosol. However, the precise intracellular location of the Ca and temporal resolution of these approaches is limited. Long rest periods (after rest decay) were associated with Ca losses of >400 µmol/L cytosol in rabbit and guinea-pig ventricle (Pytkowski *et al.*, 1983; Lewartowski *et al.*, 1984; Bridge, 1986; Lewartowski & Pytkowski, 1987; Pierce *et al.*, 1987; Pytkowski, 1989). These values are high and may include Ca from compartments other than the SR. Pytkowski (1989) also measured the caffeine-induced decrease in [45]Ca content in rabbit heart (408 µmol/L cytosol), which was only 44% of the rest dependent loss of [45]Ca. Langer *et al.* (1990; Langer & Rich, 1993) also estimated a caffeine-sensitive fraction of cellular Ca content in rat ventricle (210-240 µmol/L cytosol) which accounted for 21% of the Ca in an "intermediate compartment" of [45]Ca washout ($t_{1/2}$ = 3-19 sec). Unfortunately, interpretations using this general approach are complicated by contributions of non-SR compartments and the observation that caffeine did not decrease the [45]Ca content in guinea-pig ventricle (Lewartowski & Pytkowski, 1987). On the other hand, radiotracer approaches have the unique advantage that one can measure unidirectional (as opposed to net) fluxes. That is because one can have [45]Ca on one side and [40]Ca on the other and we assume that the membrane does not distinguish between these isotopes.

In conclusion, the absolute SR Ca content varies in different species and under different conditions. On the other hand, we are approaching a consensus where SR Ca content is probably in the general range of 50-150 μmol/L cytosol. For an SR Ca content of 100 μmol/L cytosol we would require about 50% of this amount to be released in terms of the Ca requirements for activation of contraction (see Chapter 3). That conveniently matches estimates of fractional SR Ca release during the twitch (Bassani *et al.*, 1993b, 1995b).

SR Ca RELEASE CHANNEL OR RYANODINE RECEPTOR

Isolation and molecular identification of the SR Ca-release channel was greatly accelerated by the recognition that the neutral plant alkaloid ryanodine is a selective and specific ligand for the channel (also called the ryanodine receptor, RyR). Ryanodine produces irreversible contracture of skeletal muscle, but progressive decline in cardiac muscle twitches (Jenden & Fairhurst, 1969; Hajdu & Leonard, 1961; Sutko & Willerson, 1980). Ryanodine opens the SR Ca release channel in both skeletal and cardiac muscle (see below). In cardiac muscle the Ca lost from the SR is extruded by Na/Ca exchange, thereby unloading the SR and cell of Ca, and depressing contractions. In skeletal muscle with much weaker Na/Ca exchange and higher SR Ca content, much of the SR Ca remains cytosolic, activating a contracture which consumes cellular ATP before the [Ca]$_i$ declines (making contracture irreversible). Some useful RyR reviews are by Coronado *et al.* (1994), Meissner (1994), Sutko & Airey (1996), Xu *et al.*, (1998a), Zucchi & Ronca-Testoni (1997), Shoshan-Barmatz & Ashley (1998) and Sitsapesan & Williams (1998).

Ryanodine, at low concentrations (1-1000 nM), accelerates Ca loss from heavy SR vesicles, but at very high concentrations (>100 μM) it slows Ca efflux (Fig 98D; Nayler *et al.*, 1970; Fairhurst & Hasselbach, 1970; Jones *et al.*, 1979; Jones & Cala, 1981; Fabiato, 1985d; Meissner, 1986a). Smith *et al.* (1985a, 1986) demonstrated that the Ca release from these heavy SR vesicles from skeletal muscle could be attributed to a high conductance Ca channel which they incorporated into lipid bilayers (i.e. the channel was similarly modulated by [Ca], ATP, ruthenium red and Mg). Rousseau *et al.* (1986, 1987) demonstrated similar channels in heart and also showed that ryanodine induced a long lived subconducting state of the SR Ca-release channel (Fig 98C). That is, ryanodine (at least up to 10 μM) appears to lock the Ca release channel into an open, but lower than normal conducting state. Williams and coworkers have shown that different ryanoids produce a different fraction of maximal conductance and also alter the dwell time in the open state (Tanna *et al.*, 1998, 2000). These studies have provided unique insights into the kinetics of ryanoid binding to the channel and also into conductance properties (see also review by Sutko *et al.*, 1997).

The ryanodine receptor (RyR) has a very high single channel conductance, especially when monovalent cations are the charge carrier (see Table 22). The RyR channel also has a relatively low Ca selectivity (P_{Ca}/P_K ~6 *vs.* 3000 for the sarcolemmal Ca channel, Smith *et al.*, 1988 and see Table 17, pg 109). Indeed, even some relatively large organic monovalent cations can permeate, but the limiting pore diameter appears to be ~3.4 Å (Tinker & Williams, 1993). The length of the RyR pore (i.e. the narrow region where ions must shed their aqueous shell) has been estimated to be ~10 Å, by both streaming potential measurements and use of different length organic divalent cations (Tu *et al.*, 1994; Tinker & Williams, 1995).

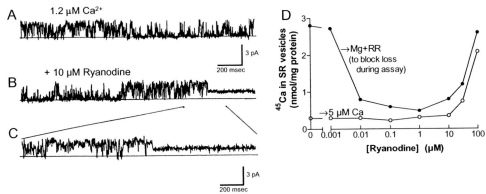

Figure 98. Ryanodine effects on cardiac SR Ca release channel. **A-C.** Recording from a single cardiac Ca release channel incorporated in a lipid bilayer. Currents are shown as upward deflections (from Rousseau *et al.*, 1987, with permission). The *cis* (cytoplasmic) side of the membrane contained 2.5 µM free [Ca] and the *trans* side contained 50 mM Ba as the charge carrier (pH 7.4, 0 mV holding potential). Ryanodine was added 1 min before panel **B** was recorded. **C.** shows the transition from normal gating to a stable subconductance state on an expanded time scale. **D.** Dependence of ^{45}Ca efflux from skeletal muscle SR vesicles on [ryanodine]. Vesicles were passively loaded with ^{45}Ca (100 µM) and incubated for 45 min with ryanodine. They were then diluted into a Mg + ruthenium red (RR) medium, which blocks efflux (unless pretreated with 5 nM - 30 µM ryanodine) or diluted into 5 µM Ca medium which quickly emptied the vesicles (except at high [ryanodine]). Ryanodine causes SR Ca release at 5 nM to ~30 µM, but blocks release at 100 µM (from Meissner, 1986a, with permission).

When Ca is used as the charge carrier, the conductance is lower than for monovalents and ≥50 mM Ca is typically used to obtain clear single channel data. Tinker *et al.* (1993) predicted that under more physiological conditions ([Ca]$_{SR}$=2.4 mM, 120 mM K and 0.5 mM Mg) the single channel Ca current would be 2 pA. This model prediction required extensive extrapolation. Mejia-Alvarez *et al.* (1999) made a concerted effort to approach physiological conditions with their single channel measurements and a unitary current of ~0.30 pA can be inferred (at 2 mM [Ca]$_{SR}$, 150 mM [K], and 1 mM [Mg]). This single channel RyR current is only slightly larger than that of the sarcolemmal Ca channel (~0.2 pA), but this is ~1 million ions/sec or 10^5 times greater than turnover rate of the SR Ca-pump. The typical open time for a RyR is ~3 ms (Tinker *et al.*, 1993).

Molecular Identity and Structure of Ryanodine Receptors

Ryanodine was used as a specific ligand in the purification of the RyR from skeletal muscle (RyR1, Inui *et al.*, 1987a; Campbell *et al.*, 1987; Imagawa *et al.*, 1987b; Lai *et al.*, 1987, 1988a) and cardiac muscle (RyR2, Inui *et al.*, 1987b; Lai *et al.*, 1988b). Mammalian RyR1 has been cloned (MW = 565,223 Da; Takeshima *et al.*, 1989; Marks *et al.*, 1989; Zorzato *et al.*, 1990). The cardiac RyR2 has also been cloned (MW=564,711 Da; Otsu *et al.*, 1990; Nakai *et al.*, 1990) and a third isoform (RyR3) has also been cloned from brain (Hakamata *et al.*, 1992). These RyRs are products of 3 separate genes, but RyR1 & RyR2 are 66% identical and RyR3 is 67-70% identical to RyR1 and RyR2. Amphibian and avian skeletal muscle express α, β and cardiac isoforms and α & β are similar to RyR1 & RyR3 (Sutko & Airey, 1996). Notably, with respect to E-C coupling issues to be discussed in the next chapter α & β isoforms coexist in fast twitch frog skeletal muscle. Moreover, brain expresses both RyR2 and RyR1 in addition to

RyR3 (and the related intracellular Ca release channel, the IP_3 receptor) and there is a very small amount of RyR3 in mammalian skeletal muscle. Knocking out the RyR3 gene in mice does not prevent striated muscle function (Takeshima *et al.*, 1996). However, knocking out RyR1 in mice results in perinatal death (due to skeletal muscle failure, Takeshima *et al.*, 1994). Knockout of RyR2 is embryonically lethal, but this may not be due to defective cardiac E-C coupling at this developmental stage (Takeshima *et al.*, 1998).

Table 22

Cardiac Ryanodine Receptor Permeability and Conductance

	P_x/P_K	Conductance (pS)*	Radius (Å)
K	1.00	723	1.33
Na	1.15	446	0.97
Cs	0.61	460	1.67
Li	0.99	215	0.68
Rb	0.87	621	1.47
Ca	6.5	135	0.99
Ba	5.8	202	1.34
Sr	6.7	166	1.12
Mg	5.9	89	0.66
ammonium	1.42	594	1.7
methylamine	0.67	286	1.9
ethylamine	0.51	105	2.2
dimethylamine	0.09	10	3.1
triethylamine	≤0.04	≤10	3.6

Relative permeability is based on reversal potential shifts in bionic conditions.
*Conductances in 210 mM permeant ion. Data are from Williams (1998).

The tetrameric nature of the ryanodine receptor *in vivo* implies a 2,260,000 Da structure. The protein appears to exist mainly as a homotetramer, based on its quatrefoil appearance (Saito *et al.*, 1988; Lai *et al.*, 1988a; Wagenknecht *et al.*, 1989), gel permeation chromatography (Inui *et al.*, 1987a) and stoichiometry of high affinity ryanodine binding (Lai *et al.*, 1988a, 1989). The large size of this homotetramer has helped to identify it ultrastructurally as the junctional foot process which spans the gap between the SR and sarcolemmal membranes at their junctions. Thus, it traverses the SR membrane providing a channel for SR Ca release and also extends toward the sarcolemmal membrane. This proximity is undoubtedly important in the process of triggering SR Ca release during E-C coupling (see Chapter 8).

Three-dimensional reconstructions of the RyR based on electron microcsopic images have been continuously refined (Wagenknecht *et al.*, 1989; 1994, 1996; 1997; Sasmó *et al.*, 1999; Serysheva *et al.*, 1995, 1999). Figure 99 shows three different views of the RyR. Sites are also indicated where calmodulin and FK-506 binding proteins (FKBP) interact with the RyR (see pg 198). The complex is ~28 nm along each side and ~14 nm high above the SR membrane, which correspond to the width and length of the junctional "feet" observed ultrastructurally in electron micrographs of intact muscle (see Chapter 1). The RyR reconstructions are intriguing because some suggest a channel for Ca flux going through the center of the molecule from the SR lumen and possibly coming out the sides of the RyR into the junctional space (Fig 88 and

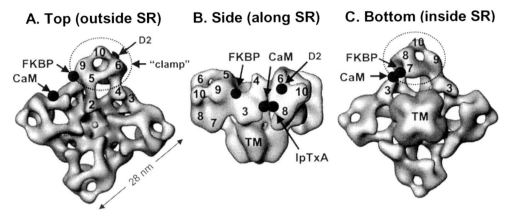

Figure 99 Three-dimensional reconstruction of the skeletal muscle ryanodine receptor. Three views **A.** from top or T-tubule, **B.** from along the plane of the SR membrane and **C.** from within the SR lumen. Selected cytoplasmic domains are numbered. "clamp" (dashed circle) refers to domains 5-10 that form each corners of the cytoplasmic region; TM, transmembrane region; IpTxA, Imperatoxin A ; CaM, calmodulin ; D2, divergency region 2 (amino acids 1303-1406); FKBP, FK506-binding protein. Figure generously provided by T. Wagenknecht.

Serysheva *et al.*, 1999). In Fig 99 the FKBP site is ~9 nm away from the calmodulin site. The FKBP location may be relevant to functional observations which suggest that FKBP is important in coupling monomers within the tetrameric array as well as between tetramers (Brilliantes *et al.*, 1994; Kaftan *et al.*, 1996; Marx *et al.*, 1998a). There is also some initial information about which RyR1 sites might interact with the skeletal L-type Ca channel, α_{1S} or imperatoxin A (Nakai *et al.*, 1998a; Sasmo & Wagenknecht, 1998; Grabner *et al.*, 1999).

The high affinity effects of ryanodine on SR vesicles coupled with observations from more intact preparations (e.g. Sutko *et al.*, 1985) led to the use of ryanodine as a specific ligand in binding studies with SR vesicles (Pessah *et al.*, 1985; Fleischer *et al.*, 1985; Alderson & Feher, 1987; Imagawa *et al.*, 1987b; Inui *et al.*, 1987a; Lattanzio *et al.*, 1987; Meissner & Henderson, 1987). The affinity of the receptor for ryanodine is dependent on [Ca] and the presence of nucleotides (e.g. ATP), but in the conditions typically used K_d values are 4-36 nM.

Figure 100 shows some key RyR domains. The number of suggested transmembrane spanning domains ranges from 4-12 (Takeshima *et al.*, 1989; Otsu *et al.*, 1990) with at least M1-M4 consistent with most data (Balshaw *et al.*, 1999). Results from the related IP$_3$ receptor are more compelling for 6 transmembrane spans (Michikawa *et al.*, 1994; Mignery *et al.*, 1989; Galvan *et al.*, 1999) making 4-6 seem plausible for RyR2 until clearer data are available. A human RyR1 mutation (I4898T) produces central core disease (Lynch *et al.*, 1999; see below) and site directed mutagenesis studies in this M3-M4 region (including GIG, as in Na/Ca exchanger & GYG in K channels) has identified this as the pore loop in RyR2 and RyR1 (Zhao *et al.*, 1999; Balshaw *et al.*, 1999; Gao *et al.*, 2000). This is analogous to the IP$_3$ receptor domain where the channel pore has been shown to reside (the 5th-6th transmembrane spans including an intervening GGVG sequence, Ramos-Franco *et al.*, 1999). Marx *et al.* (2000) demonstrated that the cardiac RyR is really a megacomplex including FKBP12.6, a PKA anchoring protein

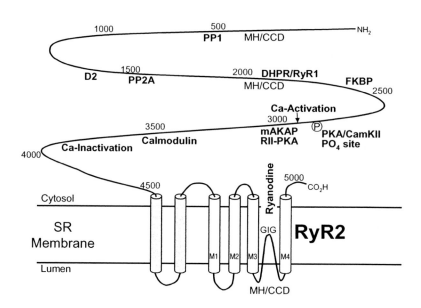

Figure 100 Schematic of domains in cardiac ryanodine receptor sequence. The 4 transmembrane domains M1-M4 are according to Takeshima *et al.*(1989) and there may be 2 more. Approximate locations along the primary structure of several sites of either interaction (e.g. phosphatases 1 & 2A; PP1 & PP2A; mAKAP, kinase anchoring protein), a putative pore region (GIG), PKA/CaMKII phosphorylation site (P) and Ca effector sites. A few sites important in RyR1 are also shown, e.g. mutation sites associated with malignant hyperthermia or central core disease (MH/CCD) and sites where skeletal muscle DHPRs may interact (1635-2636 & 2659-3720, Nakai *et al.*, 1998a). Figure kindly supplied by A.R. Marks.

(mAKAP) and two phosphatases (PP1 & PP2A) in addition to interactions with calmodulin and junctin/triadin described above. These associated proteins will be discussed further below.

Ca sparks: Fundamental Cellular SR Ca Release Events

SR Ca release in the intact myocyte appears to occur via relatively stereotypical local events referred to as Ca sparks (Fig 101, sensed by fluorescent Ca indicators). These Ca sparks (first described by Cheng *et al.*, 1993) occur during rest (at very low frequency) in a stochastic manner, even in the absence of Ca influx. The normal twitch Ca transient in ventricular myocytes is also likely composed of a temporal and spatial summation of thousands of Ca spark events which are synchronized by the AP and I_{Ca} via Ca-induced Ca-release (Cannell *et al.*, 1994,1995; López-López *et al.*, 1994, 1995).

Figure 101A shows two spontaneous Ca sparks in a resting mouse ventricular myocyte during acquisition of a 2-dimensional image. To enhance temporal resolution it is customary to use the line scan mode of the confocal microscope. The whole length of this cell was scanned every 2 ms along a line avoiding nuclei. Figure 101B shows a line scan image with a single prominent Ca spark, where distance along the cell length is shown in the vertical dimension and time along the horizontal dimension. Figure 101C shows the $[Ca]_i$ in the narrow region of the cell where the Ca spark occurs. The surface plot (Fig 101D) shows the time and spatial dependence of local $[Ca]_i$ during this single Ca spark. Ca sparks originate at the T-tubule (Cheng *et al.*,

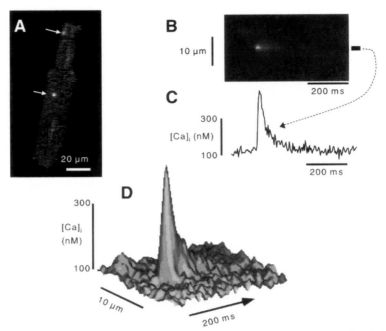

Figure 101 Ca sparks in isolated mouse ventricular myocyte. **A.** Two dimensional laser scanning confocal fluorescence image of myocyte loaded with the Ca-sensitive indicator fluo-3, exhibiting two Ca sparks (arrows). **B.** Line scan image along the long axis of the myocyte (only part is shown). Scans were repeated every 4 ms and stacked from left to right. Distance along the cell is in the vertical direction. **C.** Line graph of [Ca]$_i$ at the spot indicated by the bar in B (~1 μm). **D.** Surface plot of [Ca]$_i$ during a Ca spark, indicating the temporal and spatial spread of Ca (figure kindly supplied by L.A. Blatter).

1996; Parker *et al.*, 1996) and typically reach a peak [Ca]$_i$ of 200-300 nM in ~10 ms, have a spatial spread of ~2 μm (full width half-maximum) and [Ca]$_i$ declines with a time constant of ~25 ms. The decline of local [Ca]$_i$ during the Ca spark is largely due to Ca diffusing away from the site of release. However, we showed that when the SR Ca-ATPase was blocked in rat (by thapsigargin) [Ca]$_i$ decline during a spark was slowed by 26% (and spatial spread also broadened, Gómez *et al.*, 1996). This represents [Ca]$_i$ decline attributable to diffusion away from the source (i.e. both SR Ca-ATPase and Na/Ca exchange were blocked). Conversely, when we stimulated SR Ca-ATPase by PKA activation, local [Ca]$_i$ decline was accelerated by 33% (or 50% compared to diffusion alone). Thus Ca transport rate can effect spatial and temporal spread of Ca sparks and influence their activation of neighboring RyRs via Ca-induced Ca-release.

Quantitative Aspects of SR Ca release Flux

Cheng *et al.* (1993) estimated the Ca flux associated with a single Ca spark as ~2×10^{-19} mol (or 40 fC) and proposed that this might be due to a single RyR channel event (4 pA×10 ms). A more realistic single RyR channel flux is ≤2 fC (0.4 pA × 4 ms, see pg 187). This would be consistent with a cluster of ~20 release channels contributing to a single Ca spark. This is in the range of the clusters of 50-200 feet/RyRs at dyadic junctions in heart (Franzini-Armstrong *et al.*, 1999; see pg 14). Attempts to measure the number of RyRs involved in a Ca spark have been challenging (e.g. measuring smaller events or titrating some of the RyRs with blockers), but have given values in the range of 6-20 (Parker *et al.*, 1996; Lipp & Niggli, 1996; Blatter *et al.*, 1997;

Bridge *et al.*, 1999; Lukyanenko *et al.*, 2000). It is clear now that a Ca spark is due to a cluster of RyRs working as a functional unit (discussed further in Chapter 8).

To explain a resting SR Ca leak rate of 0.3 µmol/L cytosol (Bassani and Bers, 1995) requires about 50 Ca sparks/sec in the cell (or ~2 sparks/pL/sec). This is typical of the resting Ca spark frequency observed in ventricular myocytes (Cheng *et al.*, 1993; Satoh *et al.*, 1997) and is consistent with virtually all of the resting leak of Ca from the SR being attributed to these occasional Ca sparks.

How many RyRs are there in a typical ventricular myocyte? Bers & Stiffel (1993) measured 504, 656, 833 and 1,144 fmol/mg protein RyR in ventricular myocytes from rabbit, guinea-pig, rat and ferret, respectively. This corresponds to 0.08-0.19 µmol/L cytosol RyR or 1.5-3.5 million RyR in a 30 pL myocyte (500 times fewer than SR Ca-pumps). For a resting rate of 50 Ca sparks/sec, only 1,000 RyR need to open each second (or 0.02% of the cell's RyRs). To attain a peak SR Ca release flux of 3 mM/s estimated by Wier *et al.* (1994), would require simultaneous activation of about 40,000 RyR (only ~2% of the cell's complement of RyRs). Furthermore, a total SR Ca release flux of 50 µmol/L cytosol would also require only ~7,500 Ca sparks (based on 40 fC/spark) or ~5% of the cellular RyRs (based on 2 fC/RyR). Thus, normal twitch activation only requires a small fraction of available RyRs to function at any given twitch.

It is of interest to note here that opening of a similarly modest fraction of L-type Ca channels (2-3%) is required to produce the measured whole cell I_{Ca} (pg 114; Lew *et al.*, 1991). For example, there may be ~250,000 dihydropyridine receptors in a 30 pL rat ventricular myocyte, but only ~5,000 Ca channels need to open (with a single channel current of 0.2 pA to produce a peak whole cell current of 1 nA).

Regulation of SR Ca Release

The most direct and compelling data about SR Ca release channel regulation come from measurements of single RyR currents in lipid bilayers. Those studies are challenging and still have the caveats that a) the channels are not in their native physiological environment and b) the behavior of one channel is assumed to be representative of the population of RyRs. For many aspects there is also corroborative evidence from measurements of Ca efflux from heavy SR vesicles, ryanodine binding and cellular experiments. Cellular experiments are necessarily more complex to interpret, but have the advantage of being in a more physiological context. Measurement of ^{3}H-ryanodine binding is simple, but useful because ryanodine binds strongly to the open RyR channel, thus higher ryanodine binding (at sub-B_{max} conditions) can correlate with greater open probability (Xu *et al.*, 1998a), although the inference is indirect. Table 23 shows effects of several factors on RyR gating (see also reviews by Palade, 1987a,b,c; Coronado *et al.*, 1994; Zucchi & Ronca-Testoni, 1997, Shoshan-Barmatz & Ashley; 1998; Xu *et al., 1998a).

Figure 102 shows that Ca activation of the cardiac RyR begins at sub-micromolar [Ca], reaches a broad maximum (at very high P_o) near 100 µM Ca and decreases at very high [Ca] (5-10 mM, Rousseau & Meissner, 1989; Xu *et al.*, 1998a). The skeletal muscle RyR is less strongly activated by Ca alone, requiring more Ca for activation, reaching a lower peak P_o (near 10 µM Ca) and almost completely inactivating by 1 mM Ca. ATP (and other adenine nucleotides) activate cardiac RyR channels, but only if [Ca] is high enough to partially activate the channel

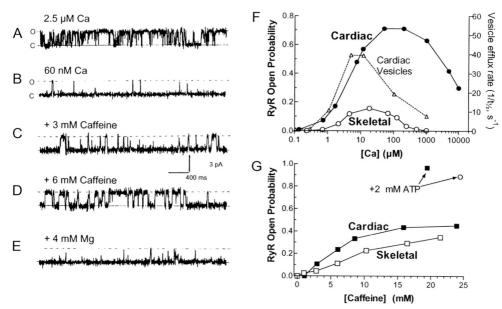

Figure 102. Caffeine, Mg and [Ca]-dependence of RyR gating (channels incorporated into lipid bilayers). **A-E.** Single cardiac Ca release channel records from Rousseau & Meissner (1989) show that lowering *cis*-(cytosolic) [Ca] reduces channel opening (**B**, o=open c=closed), that caffeine activates the channel at low [Ca] (**C & D**) and that Mg blocks the channel (**E**). Current was carried by 50 mM Ca on the *trans* (luminal) side. **F.** Ca dependence of channel open probability (P_o) as in **A-E** (for cardiac and skeletal Ca release channel; data from Xu *et al.*, 1998a) or of the rate of ^{45}Ca efflux from cardiac SR vesicles (Meissner & Henderson, 1987). **G.** Effect of caffeine on cardiac and skeletal RyR in bilayers with ~60 nM *cis* Ca and ~50 mM *trans* Ca as charge carrier. Addition of 2 µM ATP caused the channels activated by caffeine to become almost fully open (P_o ~1; data from Smith *et al.*, 1986; Rousseau *et al.*, 1988).

(Rousseau *et al.*, 1986). In contrast RyR1 can be strongly activated by ATP alone, in the absence of Ca or Mg (Xu *et al.*, 1998a). Mg potently inhibits cardiac RyR opening in the mM range (Fig 102E) and free $[Mg]_i$ is normally 0.5-1 mM in cardiac myocytes. With the cardiac RyR activated by Ca (in the absence of ATP), Mg inhibits P_o half-maximally at 2.3 mM (Xu *et al.*, 1996). However, at physiological [ATP] (5 mM) the inhibitory effect of free [Mg] is modest at 2 mM, and is still only half-inhibited at 5 mM free [Mg]. The precise *in situ* $[Ca]_i$ *vs.* P_o relationship is not known, but ATP shifts activation to the left and Mg shifts it to the right (*vs.* Fig 102F).

While Ca, Mg and ATP are likely to be central physiological modulators of RyR gating, local [ATP] and [Mg] are unlikely to change rapidly during E-C coupling and thus are not likely to be actively involved in the process *per se*. Rather, the local concentrations of ATP and Mg are critical in establishing how the RyR responds to a given physiological Ca signal. For example, while mM Mg inhibits steady state RyR2 open probability (P_o) for any given free [Ca], it also accelerates the decline in P_o induced by a rapid increase in local [Ca] (Valdivia *et al.*, 1995). Free intracellular [Mg] can also increase several-fold during ischemia as [ATP] falls, presumably because ATP is a major buffer of intracellular Mg (Murphy *et al.*, 1989b). Ischemia is also accompanied by intracellular acidosis and RyR2 open probability is reduced by >50% when pH is lowered from 7.3 to 6.5 (Ma *et al.*, 1988; Rousseau & Pinkos, 1990; Xu *et al.*, 1996). Thus, ischemia may greatly depress the responsiveness of the RyR to a given local activating Ca.

Much of the bilayer work is consistent with results from cardiac SR vesicles, where ^{45}Ca efflux rate was stimulated by µM Ca, mM ATP and inhibited by mM Mg ($K_{1/2}$ = 0.3 mM), µM ruthenium red, acidosis and calmodulin (Meissner & Henderson, 1987). Furthermore the Ca flux that they measured is of the order required to activate the myofilaments in the cell.

Caffeine and other methylxanthines (e.g. theophylline, theobromine, pentifylline) activate both the cardiac and skeletal RyR, with cardiac RyR being more sensitive (Fig 102, Rousseau & Meissner, 1989; Rousseau *et al.*, 1988; Liu & Meissner, 1997). Caffeine (1-5 mM) appears to shift the Ca-dependence of RyR gating to ~10 times lower [Ca]. Thus, the RyR in resting cardiac myocytes is strongly activated by caffeine (even at resting [Ca]$_i$). MBED (9-methyl-7-bromoeudistomin D) appears to have caffeine-like effects on RyRs, but is ~1000 times more potent (Seino *et al.*, 1991).

Ryanodine, at 1 nM-10 µM in bilayer studies, causes the RyR to open permanently to a subconductance level (~half of the fully open state, Rousseau *et al.*, 1987). At very high concentration (0.3-2 mM) ryanodine appears to bind to lower affinity sites and completely block the RyR (Rousseau *et al.*, 1987; Lai *et al.*, 1989). Lai *et al.* (1989) demonstrated that there is one high affinity and three low affinity ryanodine binding sites per RyR tetramer. Ryanodine causes similar functional effects on the RyR in isolated SR vesicles (Meissner, 1986a) and in intact cardiac muscle and myocytes (Bers *et al.*, 1987, 1989). The binding of ryanodine to the RyR is very slow and it is practically irreversible. Consequently, the effects of ryanodine are slow to develop. In intact cells and tissues the result is that only a small fraction of RyR are typically activated. This creates a leak which is sufficient to drain the SR of Ca rapidly during rest, but typically the SR can still transiently accumulate Ca (Bers *et al.*, 1987, 1989). In vesicles blocking 99% of the RyRs by ryanodine may reduce Ca loss by ~99% (since there may be ~1 RyR/vesicle). However, in the intact cell, where RyRs are in parallel. blocking 99% of RyRs (with 1% in the open mode) may still result in draining the entire SR. Thus, ryanodine can be trickier to use in intact cells than thapsigargin or caffeine (which is also rapidly reversible).

Higher [Ca]$_{SR}$ intrinsically increases Ca conductance through the RyR2 channel, but higher luminal [Ca] also increases RyR2 open probability (Sitsapesan & Williams, 1994, 1997; Lukyanenko *et al.*, 1996; Tripathy & Meissner, 1996; Xu & Meissner, 1998; Györke & Györke, 1998). Figure 103A shows that increasing [Ca]$_{SR}$ increases the sensitivity of RyR2 to activation by cytosolic Ca. One group suggested that this effect was due to more Ca passing through the channel and acting at the cytoplasmic activating site (Tripathy & Meissner, 1996; Xu & Meissner, 1998). This may well occur, but cannot explain the results of Györke & Györke (1998, Fig 103A), because the [Ca]$_{SR}$ effect was independent of driving voltage direction. This luminal Ca allosteric effect seems genuine. It does require the presence of a cytosolic activator (e.g. ATP or sulmazole) and there may even be more complex Ca allosteric regulation (including a luminal inhibitory site, Ching *et al.*, 2000).

RyR Adaptation or Inactivation

The Ca-sensitivity of RyR2 activation is higher when the [Ca] is raised very rapidly (Fig 103B, Fabiato, 1985b; Györke & Fill, 1993). Abrupt elevation of [Ca] by flash photolysis of caged Ca causes opening of RyR2 in 1-2 ms and after this initial peak the P_o relaxes back to that predicted by the steady state [Ca] dependence (in ~2 sec, Györke & Fill, 1993). This decrease in

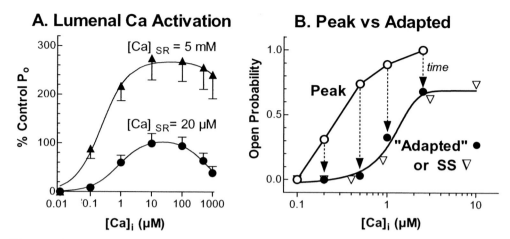

Figure 103. Luminal SR [Ca] and adaptation shift [Ca] dependence of cardiac RyR gating. **A.** Increasing [Ca] on the luminal (*trans*) side of the bilayer (i.e. $[Ca]_{SR}$) shifts the $[Ca]_i$-dependence of RyR P_o. Half activation is shifted by 3.7-fold and maximal P_o is increased 2.7-fold. Data are taken from Györke & Györke, (1998). **B.** Rapid photolytic release of Ca from Ca-DM-nitrophen activates the RyR in 1-2 ms (Peak data). The channel open probability (P_o) gradually decreases (arrows) to a much lower P_o, referred to as the adapted state, which is similar to the steady state (SS) $[Ca]_i$-dependence. Current was carried by 250 mM Cs (from *cis* side). Data from Györke & Fill (1993) was regraphed.

release channel opening is essential for limiting the positive feedback inherent in Ca-induced Ca-release. Györke & Fill referred to this process as adaptation, because after P_o declined the same Ca channel could still be reactivated by a larger Ca pulse. That is, it did not appear to reach an absorbing inactivation state. Very similar results were found by Valdivia *et al.* (1995). However, they found that inclusion of relatively physiological [Mg] accelerated the time course of adaptation so that it occurred in ~100 ms. This brings it closer to the time frame where it could be involved in the turn-off of SR Ca release during a single cardiac contraction.

Several other groups have confirmed a time-dependent decline in RyR2 activation after local [Ca] is raised rapidly (Schiefer *et al.*, 1995; Sitsapesan *et al.*, 1995; Laver & Curtis, 1996). However, some of these studies have been more consistent with an absorbing inactivation state than the adapted state described by Györke and Fill (1993). Whether the term adaptation or inactivation is used to describe this phenomenon, it may serve functionally in the turning off of SR Ca release (which is otherwise inherently regenerative, see pg 227-228). It is also very similar to observations of Fabiato (1985b) in mechanically skinned single ventricular myocytes, where the rate of Ca application was a crucial modulator of SR Ca release produced by a given Δ[Ca] trigger, and where recovery of the E-C coupling process required time (and low $[Ca]_i$).

Zahradníková *et al.* (1999a) showed that rapid jumps of [Ca] produced by flash photolysis mimic the physiological Ca signal produced by abrupt opening of an L-type Ca channel (where local [Ca] rises to 1-20 μM in tens of μs). This rapid rise of [Ca] caused opening of individual RyR2s with a time constant of 0.15 ms and was consistent with activation by ~4 Ca ions. There is still no consensus on the ideal gating scheme for RyR2 (Stern *et al.*, 1999). However, rapid activation appears to favor initially a mode where the open time is longer, and then gating shifts to a mode with shorter openings (possibly accounting for adaptation; Zahradníková *et al.*, 1999b). True RyR2 inactivation might require the very high [Ca] or [Mg] (5-10 mM) at which steady state P_o declines (Fig 102F). This issue will be discussed further in Chapter 8.

Malignant Hyperthermia, cyclic ADP ribose and Toxins

Halothane is used clinically as an inhalation anesthetic and its use can trigger episodes of malignant hyperthermia (MH) in predisposed individuals. MH (and the related central core disease, CCD) is attributed to mutations in RyR1 which, when certain anesthetics are used (e.g. halothane or isoflurane), cause inappropriate RyR activation, SR Ca release, skeletal muscle hypercontracture, massive ATP consumption and consequent potentially fatal elevation in body temperature (Mickelson & Louis, 1996; Loke & MacLennan, 1998). In MH-susceptible human and pig skeletal muscle SR Ca release is more halothane- and Ca-sensitive (Endo *et al.*, 1983; Nelson, 1983; Kim *et al.*, 1984), has higher Ca release rate and greater RyR1 P_o (Mickelson *et al.*, 1988, 1990; Fill *et al.*, 1990, 1991). Dantrolene is a skeletal muscle relaxant which is used clinically to curtail the MH-induced contractures above. Dantrolene blocks SR Ca release, but interestingly has only weak effects on cardiac muscle (Ellis *et al.*, 1976; Van Winkle, 1976; Danko *et al.*, 1985). 4-chloro-*m*-cresol also activates RyRs (Hermann-Frank *et al.*, 1996). It is used diagnostically to distinguish between normal and MH-susceptible muscles.

Cyclic ADP-ribose (cADPR) is a metabolite of β-nicotinamide adenine dinucleotide (NAD), is present in myocytes at 20-200 nM and (along with the related NAADP) releases Ca in sea urchin eggs (Gallione *et al.*, 1991; Walseth *et al.*, 1991; Lee, 1999, 2000). The effect was thought to be mediated by RyR2, but not RyR1 (Mészáros *et al.*, 1993; Galione *et al.*, 1993). Sitsapesan *et al.* (1994) showed that NAD, cADPR and its metabolite ADP-ribose can all activate RyR2. However, at physiological [ATP] no activation was seen at all. They concluded that cADPR, NAD & ADP-ribose compete weakly at the ATP site, but cannot serve as physiological modulators of SR Ca release. Guo *et al.* (1996) also found that flash photolysis of intracellular cADPR caused Ca release in sea urchin eggs, but not in ventricular myocytes.

Toxins isolated from the African scorpion *Pandinus imperator* can selectively activate (IpTx$_A$) or inhibit (IpTx$_I$) SR Ca release channels (Valdivia *et al.*, 1992). Tripathy *et al.* (1998) found that IpTx$_A$ (33 amino acids) alters both RyR1 and RyR2 gating by inducing long-lived subconductance states (28 & 43% of normal conductance), reminiscent of ryanodine-modified or FKBP-depleted channels (see Fig 98C and below). Based on E_m-dependence and enhancement of ryanodine binding, they inferred that IpTx$_A$ binds at a point 23% of the way through the E_m drop into the SR and not at the ryanodine site. Samsó *et al.* (1999) identified the physical location of IpTx$_A$ on the RyR ʹFig 99), 11 nm away from the transmembrane pore and tucked under the crown, away from the sarcolemma. This is relevant because Gurrola *et al.* (1999) found IpTx$_A$ to mimic effects of peptides from the II-III loop of the skeletal muscle DHPR on RyR1 (see Chapter 8). While this would be a long physical reach for this II-III loop (Samsó *et al.*, 1999), it raises intriguing possibilities with respect to protein-protein interactions. Bastidin-10, a macrocyclic compound from the sea sponge *Ianthella basta*, activates RyR1 gating, by stabilizing the channel open state and makes gating almost independent of physiological Ca and

Table 23

Factors Which Alter Ca Release from the SR

	Effective Concentration	Muscle Type	Reference
Enhancers of Ca Release			
Ca	0.3-10 µM	hrt	M & H'87; Rousseau & Meissner,1989
Caffeine	1-10 mM	hrt	Fabiato, 1983; O'Neill et al., 1990a; Rousseau & Meissner, 1989
ATP (or AMP-PCP)	1-5 mM	hrt	Rousseau et al., 1986; M & H'87
Ryanodine	0.01-30 µM	hrt/sk	Rousseau et al., 1987; Meissner, 1986a
Bastadin 10	5 µM	sk	Chen et al., 1999
Bromo-eudistomin D	10 µM	sk	Nakamura et al., 1986
MBED	1-10 µM	hrt/sk	Seino et al., 1991
4-chloro-m-cresol	0.5 mM	hrt/sk	Hermann-Frank et al., 1996; Xu et al., 1998a
cyclic ADP-ribose	2-10 µM	hrt	Mészáros et al., 1993; Sitsapesan et al., 1994
Doxorubicin	7-25 µM	hrt/sk	Zorzato et al., 1985; Nagasaki & Fleischer, 1989; Ondrias et al., 1990
Halothane	~0.5 mM	hrt/sk	Ohnishi, 1979; Su & Kerrick, 1979 Palade, 1987b; Frazer & Lynch, 1992
Imperatoxin A	15 nM	hrt/sk	Valdivia et al., 1992; Tripathy et al., 1998
Polylysine	1-10 µg/ml	sk	Cifuentes et al., 1989
Quercetin	10-300 µM	sk	Kirino & Shimizu, 1982; Palade, 1987b
Sulmazole (AR-L 115BS)	1 mM	hrt	Williams & Holmberg, 1990
Suramin	50 µM	hrt	Sitsapesan & Williams, 1996; Xu et al., 1998a
Sulfhydryl reagents			
$\quad$ AgNO$_3$	0.1-15 µM	sk	Salama & Abramson, 1984
$\quad$ Ag$^+$ or Hg^{2+}	10-25 µM	hrt	Prabhu & Salama, 1990
$\quad$ Cu^{2+}/Cysteine	2-10 µM	sk	Trimm et al., 1986
Nitrosylation (by NO)		hrt	Xu et al., 1998b
Ins(1,4,5)P$_3$	10-30 µM	hrt	Fabiato, 1990
	10-20 µM	sk	Volpe et al., 1985
	0.5 µM	sm	Walker et al., 1987
Inhibitors of Ca Release			
Ca	5-10 mM	hrt	Xu et al., 1998a
Mg	1-3 mM	hrt/sk	M & H'87; Fabiato, 1983
Acidosis	pH 7.5→6.5	hrt	Xu et al., 1996
Ryanodine	>100 µM	hrt/sk	Meissner, 1986a; Jones et al., 1979; Lai et al., 1989
Ruthenium red	10 µM	hrt/sk	M & H'87
Calmodulin	1 µM	hrt	Smith et al., 1989; M & H'87
Dantrolene	2 µM	sk	Danko et al., 1985
Imperatoxin I	1 nM	hrt/sk	Valdivia et al., 1992
Neomycin, gentamycin	60-200 nM	sk	Palade, 1987c
Spermine, spermidine	20-200 µM	sk	Palade, 1987c
Tetracaine, procaine	0.1, 1 mM	hrt/sk	Palade, 1987a; Antoniu et al., 1985; M & H'87, Xu et al., 1998a

M & H'87 is Meissner & Henderson, 1987; hrt=heart, sk=skeletal and sm=smooth muscle, MBED = 9-methyl-7-bromoeudistomin D. This table is based on tables compiled by Fleischer & Inui (1989) and more extensive tables by Palade (1987b, Palade et al., 1989) which were focused on skeletal muscle SR vesicles. This table is intended to focus on cardiac SR Ca release where data are available.

Mg (Chen et al., 1999b). These bastadin-10 effects were abolished if FKBP was displaced from the RyR, suggesting interaction with the RyR-FKBP complex.

Regulation by Protein Kinases, Calmodulin and FKBP

Phosphorylation of RyR2 by cAMP-dependent protein kinase (PKA) produces intriguing effects on channel gating (Valdivia *et al.*, 1995). Basal P_o was decreased by PKA (at 100 nM [Ca]). However, PKA greatly increased peak P_o (to nearly 1.0) during a rapid photolytic increase of local [Ca], while accelerating the subsequent decline in P_o. Thus, phosphorylation by PKA may activate RyR2 gating in the same dynamic way that PKA modifies cardiac contractile force and cellular Ca transients during a twitch (i.e. increasing both amplitude and rate of decline). Marx *et al.* (2000) found that RyR2 phosphorylation by PKA occurs at Ser-2809.

Ca-Calmodulin dependent protein kinase (CaMKII) also phosphorylates the cardiac RyR at Ser-2809 (Witcher *et al.*, 1991). Notably, Witcher *et al.* (1991) found that either endogenous SR CaMKII or exogenous PKA would incorporate 1 PO_4 per RyR2 tetramer, but that exogenous CaMKII could produce higher phosphorylation (4 PO_4 per RyR2 tetramer). Bilayer recordings with skeletal muscle RyR showed that CaMKII either increased or decreased RyR channel openings (Takasago *et al.*, 1991; Wang & Best, 1992). In cardiac RyR CaMKII appears to increase channel P_o (Witcher *et al.*, 1991; Hain *et al.*, 1995), but Lokuta *et al.* (1995) reported that CaMKII decreased RyR2 open probability. This discrepancy may be partly explained by dynamic changes of RyR gating, as discussed above for PKA (but similar data are not available for CaMKII). In voltage clamped myocytes, we found that inhibition of CaMKII prevented a $[Ca]_i$-dependent increase in the fraction of SR Ca released for the same I_{Ca} and SR Ca content (Li *et al.*, 1997b). Introduction of phosphatases (PP1 & PP2A) into myocytes also depresses E-C coupling gain (duBell *et al.*, 1996). Thus, in the intact cardiac cell repeated Ca transients may activate CaMKII, phosphorylate RyR2 and enhance the efficacy of E-C coupling (see pg 268).

A complicating aspect of CaMKII effects on the RyR is that calmodulin (CaM) also has independent effects on the RyR. At [Ca] >100 nM CaM inhibits Ca-induced, caffeine-induced, and AMP-induced Ca release from cardiac and skeletal SR (IC_{50} ~100-200 nM, Meissner, 1986a; Meissner & Henderson, 1987; Plank *et al.*, 1988; Fuentes *et al.*, 1994; Tripathy *et al.*, 1995). These effects were ATP-independent, so CaMKII was not involved. Similarly, Tripathy *et al.* (1995) found that CaM inhibited RyR1 P_o at [Ca] ≥ 1 μM, but stimulated it at [Ca] <100 nM. This dual mode of CaM action was confirmed in skinned skeletal muscle (Ikemoto *et al.*, 1995).

CaM binding to the RyR is also Ca-dependent. Tripathy *et al.* (1995) found that one CaM binds per RyR1 monomer at 100 μM [Ca], but four calmodulins bind per RyR1 monomer at [Ca]<100 nM (K_d ~10 nM). Fruen *et al.* (2000) provided valuable comparative data on effects of calmodulin on RyR1 and RyR2. They found that only 1 CaM binds per RyR1 monomer at both low and high [Ca]. The same is true for RyR2 at 200 μM [Ca], but at 100 nM [Ca] RyR2 binds only 1 CaM per RyR tetramer (and K_d increases from 16 to 84 nM [CaM]). They extended the RyR1 results above, confirming the inhibitory effect of CaM on Ca flux for RyR1 and RyR2 at μM [Ca]. On the other hand, they found no effect of CaM on RyR2 flux or ryanodine binding at 100 nM [Ca] (in the presence or absence of Mg). Thus, it is unclear at this time whether CaM exerts direct functional effects on cardiac RyR (other than activating CaMKII).

FK-506 and rapamycin are immunosuppressant drugs that bind to immunophillin target FK-binding proteins (FKBPs). In T-lymphocytes Ca-CaM normally activates the phosphatase calcineurin which dephosphorylates the nuclear transcription factor NFAT allowing its entry into the nucleus where it stimulates interleukin-2 transcription and T-cell proliferation. The FKBP-FK-506 complex binds to calcineurin preventing its activation and thereby suppressing the immune response (Schreiber & Crabtree, 1992; Marks, 1996). FKBPs are peptide isomerases which also bind to and co-purify with the RyR (Jayaraman *et al.*, 1992; Timerman *et al.*, 1993, 1994, 1996), but the isomerase activity is not essential for RyR effects (Marks, 2000). FKBP-12 (MW 12,000) binds tightly to RyR1 (Fig 99). Heart expresses both FKBP-12 and -12.6 and despite a larger amount of FKBP-12, it is FKBP-12.6 which associates with RyR2 (due to 600× higher affinity, Timerman *et al.*, 1996).

FK-506 and rapamycin cause dissociation of FKBP from the RyR and modify RyR1 and RyR2 gating in bilayer studies (Brilliantes *et al.*, 1994; Ahern *et al.*, 1994; Chen *et al.*, 1994; Kaftan *et al.*, 1996; Barg *et al.*, 1997), although Barg *et al.* (1997) found no effect of FK-506 on RyR2. FKBP removal from RyR1 shows clear appearance of subconductance states (with $\frac{1}{4}$, $\frac{1}{2}$, & $\frac{3}{4}$ of the normal conductance). Kaftan *et al.* (1996) found analogous results with RyR2, where the net effect was an increase in overall P_o (despite the 3 lower conductance states). Indeed, when exogenous recombinant FKBP was added to recombinant RyR in bilayers the normal channel gating properties with FKBP were restored. FK-506 also inhibits RyR2 adaptation (Xiao *et al.*, 1997) and this may relate to altered Ca regulation of RyR2 in the absence of FKBP (below). Complementary measurements in intact cells show that FK-506 increases resting Ca spark frequency and causes resting SR Ca content to decline (McCall *et al.*, 1996a; Xiao *et al.*, 1997). This confirms that the overall enhanced P_o of RyR2 in bilayers after FKBP removal, extends functionally to resting Ca leak in intact ventricular myocytes.

A working hypothesis from this work is that FKBP physically stabilizes the coordinated gating of the 4 RyRs in one homotetramer so that openings go from the fully closed to the fully open state, but with reduced overall P_o for a given [Ca] (e.g. shifting the P_o *vs.* [Ca] relationship to higher [Ca]). The four conductance levels raise an intriguing question about the RyR tetramer, especially in light of the apparent pore(s) down its center (see pg 188): Does each RyR monomer contribute a channel with $\frac{1}{4}$ of the full conductance, or does gating in each subunit contribute to enhancing the conductance of a single central pore by 25%? The former seems more likely. Marx *et al.* (1998a) demonstrated that FKBP may also be involved in physical coupling *between* RyR tetramers. They showed that addition of FKBP induced simultaneous gating of 2 or more full RyR channels, and this effect could be reversed by removal of FKBP with rapamycin. This may be a redundant mechanism which, together with Ca-induced Ca-release, allows individual RyR channels to activate neighboring RyRs and coordinates closure (Bers & Fill, 1998).

FKBP effects may be clinically relevant and FK-506 treatment can be associated with cardiomyopathy (Atkinson *et al.*, 1995). Marx *et al.* (2000) showed that PKA-dependent phosphorylation of RyR2 causes displacement of FKBP from RyR2 and produces the same sort of uncoupled gating as does FK-506 or rapamycin. In heart failure (human & canine) they found that RyR2 is hyperphosphorylated (4 PO_4 per tetramer) with channels showing the FKBP-depleted phenotype (multiple conductances, increased overall flux). The higher phosphorylation could be partly due to less phosphatase (PP1) detected as bound to RyR2 in heart failure (despite higher global PP1 levels). Lower, physiological levels of phosphorylation with PKA (1/tetramer) may increase Ca sensitivity, enhancing E-C coupling (Valdivia *et al.*, 1995). In contrast, hyper-phosphorylation (4/tetramer) could cause persistent diastolic SR Ca leak, limiting SR Ca content and contraction in the failing heart. A puzzling aspect of this work is that CaMKII phosphorylates the same RyR2 site as PKA, but does not produce the same RyR effects as PKA.

Sorcin is a ubiquitous 22 kDa Ca binding protein ($K_{m(Ca)}$=1 µM) reported to associate with both cardiac RyR and DHPR (Meyers *et al.*, 1995, 1998). Lokuta *et al.* (1997) showed that sorcin reduced RyR2 open probability and ryanodine binding (IC_{50} =480-700 nM), but this inhibitory effect could be relieved by PKA-dependent phosphorylation of sorcin. While additional work is required, it is possible that sorcin, like FKBP, serves as a kind of inherent brake on SR Ca release, relievable by PKA-dependent phosphorylation (Valdivia, 1998).

Inositol 1,4,5 trisphosphate (IP₃) Receptor

IP$_3$ is a well documented activator of Ca release from internal stores in non-muscle cells (Berridge, 1987; Berridge & Galione, 1988; Berridge & Irvine, 1989), but the role in cardiac E-C coupling is controversial (see pg 237-243). The IP$_3$ receptor (IP$_3$R) is closely related to the RyR, and these combine to form the superfamily of intracellular Ca release channels. The IP$_3$R was initially isolated from neural tissue (Supattapone *et al.*, 1988) and smooth muscle (Chadwick *et al.*, 1990). The neuronal IP$_3$R was cloned (MW = 313 kDa, Furuichi *et al.*, 1989; Mignery *et al.*, 1989) and there are certain sequence homologies with RyRs. Chadwick *et al.* (1990) showed that the smooth muscle IP$_3$R has the same quatrefoil structure (25×25 nm) as the skeletal muscle ryanodine receptor (despite the smaller molecular weight) and they suggested a similar tetrameric arrangement. There are IP$_3$R subtypes (type-1, type-2 & type-3). Type-1 is the predominant smooth muscle and neuronal IP$_3$R, and it is particularly highly expressed in cerebellar Purkinje neurons. Type-2 and -3 have also been cloned (Südhof *et al.*, 1991; Blondel *et al.*, 1993) and are 69 & 64% identical to type-1. IP$_3$Rs are expressed in a wide variety of tissues, probably constituting the more general SR/ER Ca release channel than RyRs (which are more specific to muscle). In whole heart all three types of IP$_3$Rs are expressed, but in isolated ventricular myocytes only the type-2 IP$_3$R is expressed (Perez *et al.*, 1997). The number of IP$_3$Rs in ventricular myocytes is probably 2-10% of the number of RyRs (Moschella & Marks, 1993; Perez *et al.*, 1997), raising the question (see Chapter 8): what is the function of all of these IP$_3$Rs in ventricular myocytes? The other IP$_3$R types in whole heart are probably in other cell types (e.g. vascular smooth muscle & endothelial). However, cardiac Purkinje fibers seem to express type-1 IP$_3$R and also RyR3 rather than the RyR2 in ventricular myocytes (Gorza *et al.*, 1993).

The IP$_3$Rs have 3 domains going from amino to carboxy ends: 1) ligand binding, 2) coupling and 3) channel (Mignery & Südhof, 1990; Südhof *et al.*, 1991). Despite their sequence and domain similarity, the 3 types of IP$_3$R are differentially regulated by IP$_3$ and Ca. The type-2 IP$_3$R has the highest IP$_3$ affinity (K_d ~25 nM) and this is similar to the $K_{0.5}$ for channel activation (58 nM IP$_3$, Perez *et al.*, 1997; Ramos-Franco *et al.*, 1998). Type-1 has ~4 fold lower affinity and type-3 has ≥10 times lower IP$_3$ affinity than the others (Hagar & Ehrlich, 2000). Figure 104A shows the [IP$_3$]-dependence of channel activation for the three types. IP$_3$R activation is also sensitive to Ca, but the Ca-dependence also differs among the isoforms (Fig 104B). Type-1 IP$_3$R shows a striking bell-shaped Ca-dependence (Bezprozvanny *et al.*, 1991), whereas Type-2 and -3 do not show the prominent decline in P$_o$ at high [Ca] (Ramos-Franco *et al.*, 1998; Hagar *et al.*, 1998). The bell shaped Ca-dependene of type-1 IP$_3$R gating may be functionally important for the generation of Ca waves or oscillations in some cell types (Thomas *et al.*, 1996). That is,

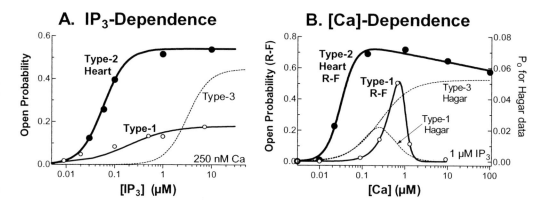

Figure 104. IP_3- and Ca-dependence of IP_3 receptor (IP_3R) activation (**A** and **B** respectively). Single channel data for the type-1, -2 and -3 IP_3R Ca channels was from Ramos-Franco *et al.* (1998, R-F, solid curves) and Hagar (dotted curves, Hagar *et al.*, 1998; Hagar & Ehrlich, 2000). Open probability (P_o) for [IP_3]-dependence of type-3 is scaled up 5.5× so the indicated ratio of maximum P_o for type-3/type-1 is as reported by Ehrlich's group (measured maximum P_o was 0.08, Hagar & Ehrlich, 2000).

the strong inhibition at 1-10 µM Ca may allow local [Ca] to shut off local release. This may also tend to make the IP_3-induced Ca transient more restricted in both time and space with the type-1 IP_3R. Thus, type-1 IP_3R is truly co-regulated by IP_3 and Ca. The type-2 IP_3R in ventricular myocytes is both more sensitive to IP_3 and almost insensitive to [Ca] over the physiological range of $[Ca]_i$ (0.1-10 µM). Thus, the cardiac IP_3R may function more as a pure IP_3 sensor.

The conductance of the IP_3R channel is about half of that seen for the RyR channel, but the selectivity among divalent cations and the P_{Ba}/P_K of 6.3 are similar to that for RyR (see Table 22, Bezprozvanny & Ehrlich, 1994, 1995). The IP_3R, like the RyR, is also modulated by numerous factors, but I will not present as much detail. ATP and non-hydrolyzable ATP analogues potentiate IP_3R channel opening and Ca release (Ferris *et al.*, 1990; Bezprozvanny & Ehrlich, 1993). Heparin is the classical inhibitor of IP_3R channels, but it activates RyR channels, making it a useful diagnostic tool (along with caffeine, which does not activate IP_3R channels). The type-1 IP_3R can also be phosphorylated by protein kinases A, C, G, CaMKII and tyrosine kinase (Ferris *et al.*, 1991a,b, 1992; Komolavilis & Lincoln, 1994; Nakade *et al.*, 1994; Jayaraman *et al.*, 1995). PKA-dependent phosphorylation increases the IP_3-sensitivity of the channel (Burgess *et al.*, 1991), but less is known about regulatory effects of phosphorylation by the other kinases (or for the type-2 IP_3R in general). FKBP binds to IP_3Rs (in a rapamycin- and FK-506-sensitive manner), decreases IP_3-sensitivity and can also form ternary FKBP-IP_3R-calcineurin complexes (Cameron *et al.*, 1995, 1997). Calmodulin also binds to the type-1 IP_3R at a site which also exists in type-2, but not type-3 IP_3R (Yamada *et al.*, 1995). Michikawa *et al.* (1999) also showed that calmodulin may be responsible for mediating the Ca-dependent inhibitory limb of the type-1 IP_3R curve in Fig 104B. This is reminiscent of the role of calmodulin in mediating the Ca-dependent inactivation of L-type Ca channels (see pg 117).

Other SR Channels Related to Ca Release

The permeability of the SR membrane to monovalent ions is very high (Meissner, 1986b). High conductance K- and anion-selective channels exist in the SR membrane (Coronado & Miller, 1979, 1980; Coronado *et al.*, 1980; Hals *et al.*, 1989). Also, there do not appear to be any appreciable concentration gradients of monovalent ions between the inside of the SR and the cytoplasm (Somlyo *et al.*, 1977a,b; Somlyo & Somlyo, 1986). This has three important functional consequences. First, it implies that there is no membrane potential between the cytoplasm and the interior of the SR (which has implications for certain possible models of E-C coupling). Second, it means that flux through the channel will be carried mainly by Ca, despite the poor selectivity of the RyR channel. This is because there is a large driving force for Ca, but not monovalent cations. Third, it allows Ca release to proceed rapidly with monovalent fluxes compensating quickly for the divalent charges (Ca) leaving the SR. Otherwise, the rate of Ca release could be limited, in part by the development of a large negative intra-SR potential (which would oppose further Ca flux from the SR).

In conclusion, it is clear that the SR can accumulate sufficient Ca and release it fast enough to activate cardiac muscle contraction. Indeed, a great deal is now known about how the SR Ca-pump and SR Ca release channel work in isolated systems (such as SR vesicles and in bilayers), and there are often correlates in more intact preparations. The next couple of chapters will focus more directly on the regulation of SR Ca release in the intact cell (E-C coupling mechanisms) and also how the SR Ca transport mechanisms interact with the other Ca transport systems in a dynamic way in the intact cardiac myocyte.

D.M. Bers.
Excitation-Contraction Coupling and Cardiac Contractile Force.
2nd Ed., Kluwer Academic Publishers, Dordrecht, 2001

203

CHAPTER 8

EXCITATION-CONTRACTION COUPLING

Since the classic experiments of Ringer (1883) demonstrated that frog heart would not contract in the absence of extracellular Ca, the crucial nature of Ca in muscle contraction has become increasingly clear. Figure 105A shows a modern version of Ringer's experiment where Ca_o is removed quickly from the medium around a rat ventricular myocyte causing an <u>immediate</u> abolition of contraction (in < 1 sec; Rich *et al.*, 1988). This contrasts strikingly with skeletal muscle (Fig 105B) which can contract for many minutes in the complete absence of extracellular Ca (Armstrong *et al.*, 1972). Figure 106A shows the E_m-dependence of several parameters during voltage-clamp of isolated guinea-pig ventricular myocytes. The E_m-dependence of Ca transients and contractions is bell-shaped, just like I_{Ca} in cardiac preparations (McDonald *et al.*, 1975; London & Krueger, 1986; Cannell *et al.*, 1987; Beuckelmann & Wier, 1988; Callewaert *et al.*, 1988; duBell & Houser, 1989). This is also true for an intrinsic birefringence signal in cardiac muscle which is thought to be associated with SR Ca release (Maylie & Morad, 1984). However, E_m-dependence of intramembrane charge movement (related to Ca channel activation) in heart is sigmoidal (Field *et al.*, 1988; Bean & Ríos, 1989; Hadley & Lederer, 1989, 1991). Thus, in heart, depolarization causes charge movement, resulting in I_{Ca} and Ca transients. At E_m above 10 mV, I_{Ca} is smaller (due to lower driving force) and results in both smaller $\Delta[Ca]_i$ and

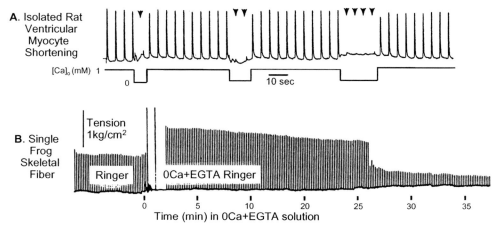

Figure 105. Ca_o-free solution abolishes contractions immediately (< 1 sec) in cardiac myocytes (**A.**), but not for >25 min in single skeletal muscle fibers (**B.**). **A.** $[Ca]_o$ was changed rapidly between stimuli. The cell was stimulated continuously (at 0.2 Hz) and arrowheads indicate stimulations in Ca_o-free solution (from Rich *et al.*, 1988, with permission). **B.** A single frog skeletal fiber stimulated at 0.1 Hz except during the switch to a Ca_o-free solution containing 1 mM EGTA. The eventual decline in force after ~26 min was attributed to gradual membrane depolarization (from Armstrong *et al.*, 1972, with permission).

A. Guinea-Pig Ventricle

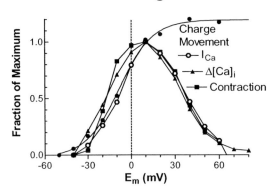

B. Frog Skeletal Muscle

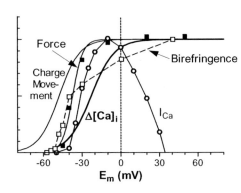

Figure 106*.* Voltage dependence of I_{Ca}, Ca transients, contraction and charge movement in isolated guinea-pig ventricular myocytes (**A**) and frog skeletal muscle (**B**). **A.** Data are from Beuckelmann & Wier, 1988 (I_{Ca} and $\Delta[Ca]_i$ using fura-2), Hadley & Lederer, 1991 (charge movement) and Bers, unpublished (shortening) and are normalized to their maxima (0.9 nA for I_{Ca}, 459 nM for $\Delta[Ca]_i$ and 12 μm for shortening). Charge movement was fit with $Q=Q_{max}/(1+\exp[-(E_m-V^*)/k])$ where Q_{max} was 5 nC/μF, $V^*= 7.5$ mV and $k=11.5$ mV. Holding $E_m \le -40$ mV and test pulses were 20 msec (for Q) and 200-300 msec for other curves. **B.** Skeletal muscle data from Miledi *et al.*, 1977 ($\Delta[Ca]_i$ using arsenazo III), Chandler *et al.*, 1976a (Q), Caputo *et al.*, 1984 (Force), Baylor & Chandler, 1978 (birefringence) and Sanchez & Stefani, 1983 (I_{Ca}). Values were normalized to their maxima (~2 μM for $\Delta[Ca]_i$, 21.5 nC/μF for Q, ~3 kg/cm² for tension and 110 μA/cm² for I_{Ca}). Q_{max} was set to 1, $V^*= 47.7$ mV and $k=8$ mV. The raw $[Ca]_i$ data were fit with the same equation, but with $V^*=23$ mV and $k=9$ mV. Holding E_m was between -100 and -75 mV and pulses were 100 msec for Q, tension and birefringence, 10 msec for $[Ca]_i$ and 1.8 sec for I_{Ca}.

contraction. The parallel nature of I_{Ca} and Ca transient amplitude in heart sometimes makes it difficult to distinguish unequivocally between *direct* effects of Ca entry and the SR Ca release induced by the Ca entry (see Chapter 9). However, three lines of evidence indicate that SR Ca release contributes in a major way to contractile activation in cardiac muscle: 1) the inhibition of cardiac contractions by agents which affect SR Ca (caffeine, ryanodine & thapsigargin), 2) quantitative estimates of Ca entry via I_{Ca} and requirements for myofilament activation, and 3) interpretation of force-frequency relationships. Moreover the bell-shaped E_m-dependence of I_{Ca} and $\Delta[Ca]_i$ is a hallmark of cardiac E-C coupling and the dependence of SR Ca release on Ca influx has led to the moniker, Ca-induced Ca-release (CICR), which will be examined below.

In skeletal muscle charge movement is also sigmoidal as a function of E_m (Fig 106B, Schneider & Chandler, 1973), but $\Delta[Ca]_i$, force and birefringence signal all follow this E_m-dependence, while I_{Ca} remains bell-shaped as in heart. Indeed, since skeletal muscle I_{Ca} activates so slowly (peak I_{Ca} at 22°C is ~200 msec *vs.* ~5 msec for cardiac I_{Ca}), that little I_{Ca} flows during a normal twitch (Sanchez & Stefani, 1978, 1983; Gonzalez-Serratos *et al.*, 1982). This more intrinsically E_m-dependent E-C coupling mechanism in skeletal muscle is referred to as charge-coupled SR Ca release or voltage-dependent Ca release (VDCR) and will be discussed below.

Thus, there are striking fundamental differences in E-C coupling between cardiac and skeletal muscle, despite qualitative similarities discussed in preceding chapters. The following list (and Fig 107) indicates 7 possible mechanisms that have been suggested by various investigators to contribute to SR Ca release in cardiac muscle.

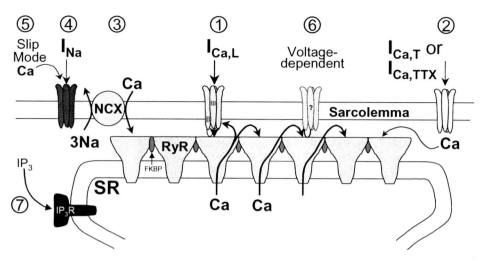

Figure 107. Potential E-C coupling mechanisms in cardiac muscle. Diagram refers to 7 potential mechanisms that have been proposed to contribute to cardiac E-C coupling (see below).

Possible Activators of Cardiac SR Ca release

Ca-induced Ca-release (CICR) variants

1. L-type I_{Ca}.
2. T-type or TTX sensitive I_{Ca} ($I_{Ca,TTX}$).
3. Ca influx via Na/Ca exchange driven directly by E_m-dependence of $I_{Na/Ca}$.
4. Ca influx via Na/Ca exchange driven by local high $[Na]_i$, secondary to I_{Na}.
5. Altered selectivity of Na channels (allowing Ca permeation) with PKA activation.

Ca influx-independent variants

6. Voltage-dependent SR Ca release (VDCR)
7. Inositol (1,4,5)-trisphosphate (IP_3)-iduced SR Ca release (IP_3ICR)

The following sections will discuss three major mechanisms, with focus on the muscle types in which they are most prominent (i.e. VDCR in skeletal muscle, CICR in cardiac muscle and IP_3ICR in smooth muscle). However, I will especially focus on the roles of depolarization-, Ca- and IP_3-induced Ca release in cardiac muscle.

VOLTAGE-DEPENDENT Ca RELEASE (VDCR) & SKELETAL MUSCLE E-C COUPLING

Skeletal muscle activation is strongly E_m-dependent (Hodgkin & Horowicz, 1960) and Schneider & Chandler (1973) described intramembrane charge movement that might drive SR Ca release and hence contraction. This charge movement is recorded as an outward current upon depolarization where all known ionic currents are blocked and linear capacitance current is subtracted (see Fig 108B). It is thought to be membrane delimited because the same amount of charge moves back upon repolarization. This charge movement (charge 1) can be broken down into two components (β, γ) by voltage-clamp protocols, kinetics and pharmacological agents. One component (Q_γ), often apparent as a hump, seems closely related to SR Ca release (Hui, 1983; Ríos $et\ al.$, 1992). Q_γ shows the same threshold (near -60 mV) and steep E_m-dependence as Ca transients (2.5 mV for *e*-fold change, Hui & Chandler, 1990). Ríos & Pizarro (1991) summarized data that has lead to the working model that Q_γ is a result of Ca release rather than causing Ca release. They suggested that locally released Ca (due to RyR1 channels activated by depolarization and Q_β) binds to negative charges on the inside face of the voltage sensor (DHPR) increasing the local E_m, which in turn causes more molecules to undergo the charge movement transition. After several seconds at strongly activating E_m the charge movement goes into an immobilized or inactivated state, where SR Ca release is also prevented. This can cause inequity of on- and off-charge movement (as in Na channel gating) and requires a more negative E_m for charge to return to the resting state (sometimes called charge 2).

Chandler *et al.* (1976a,b) followed up the work of Schneider & Chandler (1973) and proposed a physical "plunger" model by which the charge movement in the T-tubule membrane might activate Ca release from the SR (Fig 108A). In this model, a charged particle $+Z_1$ (valence = +3) would move across the T-tubule membrane, pulling a plunger (spanning the T-tubule-SR gap) out of the SR allowing Ca release to the cytoplasm. The release mechanism could then move more slowly to a refractory state when $-2Z_2$ (total valence more negative than -3) pulls $+Z_1$ back to the position where the channel is plugged. How accurately this conceptual model reflects the physical interaction is unclear, but it was a remarkably prescient idea.

Eisenberg *et al.* (1983) showed that skeletal muscle could be paralyzed by the sarcolemmal Ca channel antagonist, D600, using a specific protocol of cooling and depolarization. Hui *et al.* (1984) showed that charge movement was also inhibited under these conditions. Dihydropyridine Ca channel antagonists (nifedipine and PN200-110) can also inhibit charge movement as well as contraction, particularly in partially depolarized skeletal muscle (Lamb, 1986; Lamb & Walsh, 1987; Ríos & Brum, 1987). Ríos & Brum (1987) suggested that the dihydropyridine receptors (DHPRs) are the voltage sensors for skeletal muscle E-C coupling (and thus are also the locus of the intramembrane charge movement). Since intramembrane charge movement is associated with ion channel gating, the DHPR, which can function as a Ca channel, was a good candidate.

Baylor *et al.* (1983) and Melzer *et al.* (1987) developed a means to estimate the time course of the Ca release flux from the SR of skeletal muscle, based on the measured Ca transient and assumptions about Ca buffering and SR transport. Figure 108B shows a Ca transient, the calculated Ca release flux and the intramembrane charge movement during a voltage-clamp pulse in a frog skeletal muscle fiber (Ríos & Pizarro, 1988). Schneider & Simon (1988) showed that the rapid decline in Ca release (arrows in Fig 108B) depended on [Ca]$_i$. It was unclear whether the transient component of Ca release flux was due to: a) transient CICR activation (and Ca-dependent inactivation) of RyRs due to Ca released from neighboring VDCR release channels or b) Ca-dependent inactivation of some E_m-dependent release channels (Jacquemond *et al.*, 1991; Hollingworth *et al.*, 1992). This issue is not entirely resolved, but at least 3 factors favor an extra CICR component: 1) the transient component can be selectively blocked by low tetracaine concentrations, known to block Ca-dependent RyR channel gating (Pizarro *et al.*, 1992; Shirokova & Ríos, 1997), 2) the physical arrangement of RyRs, where only alternating ones are associated with T-tubule particles (Figs 9, 10 & 109; Block *et al.*, 1988) and 3) the known Ca-dependence of RyRs (Fig 102). These factors make the sum of a steady E_m-dependent plus a

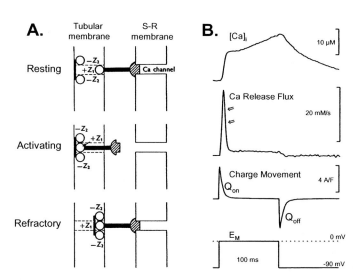

A.
Tubular membrane   S-R membrane

Resting

Activating

Refractory

B.
[Ca]$_i$ 10 µM

Ca Release Flux   20 mM/s

Charge Movement   4 A/F
Q$_{on}$
Q$_{off}$

E$_M$ 0 mV
100 ms   -90 mV

Figure 108. Intramembrane charge movement and SR Ca release in skeletal muscle. **A.** Hypothetical model of how intramembrane charge movement may regulate SR Ca release (from Chandler *et al.*, 1976b, with permission). The "plunger" blocking the SR Ca release channel is pulled out by the voltage-dependent movement of three positive charges ($+Z_1$) across the membrane electrical field (Activating). With maintained depolarization, the slower moving anionic groups (two $-Z_2$, with total charge magnitude > 3) gradually allow the SR release channel to close in a refractory state. **B.** Intracellular Ca transient, calculated Ca release flux and charge movement in response to a depolarizing voltage clamp pulse in frog semitendinosus fiber (from Ríos & Pizarro, 1988, with permission). The charge movement may activate the SR Ca release channel, which in turn partially inactivates during the long pulse (arrows).

transient CICR an attractive working hypothesis (where CICR at unlinked RyRs is triggered by neighboring VDCR at RyRs linked to DHPRs).

It is also interesting to note that the sustained E_m-dependent component of SR Ca release does not show Ca-dependent inactivation. Indeed, Ca release flux in skeletal muscle is also immediately and completely turned off by repolarization. Thus, it may be that the apparent physical linking of RyR1 to overlying DHPRs bestows an E_m-dependence to the RyRs, which also results in lower sensitivity to Ca-dependent inactivation. Interestingly, when skeletal muscle is treated with a low concentration of caffeine, the shut-off of Ca release is not as tightly coupled to repolarization (Simon *et al.*, 1989; Klein *et al.*, 1990). What makes this notable is that low concentrations of caffeine make skeletal SR Ca release more like that in cardiac (in terms of [Ca] sensitivity and RCCs, Endo, 1975b; Rousseau *et al.*, 1988; Sakai, 1965; Konishi *et al.*, 1985). Indeed, CICR can be observed in skinned skeletal muscle (Fabiato, 1984). Thus, while Ca release in skeletal muscle SR appears to be under tight E_m control, VDCR probably coexists with CICR at adjacent RyRs in skeletal muscle.

Shirokova *et al.* (1996) showed that the ratio of peak to steady release flux was higher in frog (4-6) than in mammalian skeletal muscle (~2). They correlated this with the higher ratio of RyR:DHPR measured in frog than mammalian skeletal muscle, suggesting that in frog there may be a larger fraction of RyRs that are not coupled to DHPRs and thus exhibit CICR rather than VDCR. Figure 109 shows the model based on the ultrastructural results of Block *et al.* (1988) in toadfish swimbladder, where alternating RyRs are associated with a tetrad of 4 DHPRs. Since each RyR tetramer has only one high affinity ryanodine binding site, the expected ratio of RyR: DHPR is 2:4 or 0.5. This is just what has been reported for rabbit skeletal muscle (Bers & Stiffel, 1993; Anderson *et al.*, 1994b), while in frog skeletal muscle this value is higher (1-2; Anderson *et al.*, 1994b; Margreth *et al.*, 1993) implying more unlinked RyRs in frog (≥75%) than rabbit (50%). For comparison, this ratio is 4-10 in mammalian ventricle (Bers & Stiffel, 1993), so in heart ≤10-25% of RyR could possibly link to DHPRs (see Fig 10 & below). In frog skeletal muscle there is the additional twist that both α and β RyRs exist (Sutko & Airey, 1996), and the possibility exists that the α-RyR participates in VDCR, while the β-RyR participates in CICR. While most mammalian skeletal muscle contains only RyR1, some tissues contain low levels of RyR3 (e.g. diaphragm and soleus) especially during earlier developmental stages (Conti *et al.*, 1996; Taroni *et al.*, 1997). Several lines of evidence suggest that the RyR3 contributes more to peak SR Ca release and CICR rather than VDCR (Shirokova *et al.*, 1999; Conklin *et al.*, 1999; Ward *et al.*, 2000). Thus, skeletal muscle gating of the RyRs which are physically coupled to DHPRs may be mainly E_m-dependent, whereas the other RyRs may be activated by CICR.

Local SR Ca release events or Ca sparks (pg 191) are also seen in skeletal muscle and initiate from T-tubule/SR junctions (Tsugorka *et al.*, 1995; Klein *et al.*, 1996). In skeletal muscle Ca sparks are more tightly controlled by depolarization (lower stochastic occurrence at resting $[Ca]_i$ and E_m than in heart). Based on prolonged release events induced by ryanodine, $IpTx_A$ and bastadin 10, and their known effects on RyR conductance, González *et al.* (2000) and Shtifman *et al.* (2000) inferred that Ca sparks in skeletal muscle (as in cardiac muscle) are due to more than one RyR, but these groups estimated different values (≥6 or 2-4 RyR per spark).

While E_m directly controls SR Ca release in skeletal muscle, some reports suggested a role for Ca_o (e.g. Frank, 1980), despite the results in Fig 105B. Brum *et al.* (1988a,b) studied the effects of low $[Ca]_o$ on E-C coupling in frog skeletal muscle in detail. They concluded that the effects of low $[Ca]_o$ could be attributed to effects on the T-tubular voltage sensor (or charge movement) rather than on Ca fluxes *per se*. Moreover, in skeletal muscle Ca entry does not have to occur to activate Ca release. Any of group Ia and IIa elements of the periodic table can support charge movement and contraction (Ca > Sr > Mg > Ba >> Li> Na > K > Rb > Cs; Pizarro *et al.*, 1989). This relative affinity sequence is strikingly similar to that reported for the cardiac sarcolemmal L-type Ca channel (see Table 17, page 109), with the notable exception of Mg. Mg does not seem to permeate the cardiac L-type channel (Hess *et al.*, 1986), but can permeate the skeletal muscle L-type Ca channel (McCleskey & Almers, 1985). It is possible that one of these ions must occupy the DHPR/Ca channel structure for the charge movement to occur, but that ionic current flow is not required in skeletal muscle. Indeed, a pore-mutant skeletal Ca channel which does not pass Ca ions can still trigger SR Ca release (Dirkson & Beam, 1999). As we will see below, this is in striking contrast to results in cardiac muscle, where Ca entry appears to be an absolute requirement for SR Ca release.

Murine Muscular Dysgenesis: A Model System

Muscular dysgenesis (*mdg*) is an autosomal recessive genetic mutation in mice that results in failure of E-C coupling in skeletal muscle (e.g. Klaus *et al.*, 1983). It has proven to be a valuable disease model in which to study E-C coupling (Adams & Beam, 1990). Both DHPRs

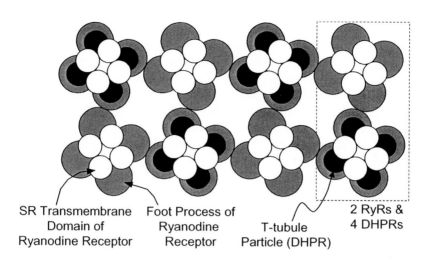

SR Transmembrane   Foot Process of   2 RyRs &
Domain of   Ryanodine   T-tubule   4 DHPRs
Ryanodine Receptor   Receptor   Particle (DHPR)

Figure 109. Spatial relationships between the components at the SR-T-tubule junction in skeletal muscle of toadfish swimbladder. The "foot" processes of the ryanodine receptor (RyR, shaded) span the gap between the SR membrane (in which RyRs are imbedded, white) and the T-tubule membrane in which dihydropyridine receptors (DHPRs) are imbedded (black). Note that DHPR tetrads (made up of 4 α_1 subunits) overlie the RyR tetramers at alternating "feet" (redrawn after Block *et al.*, 1988).

and the α_1 subunit of the Ca channel are lacking in skeletal muscle from *mdg* mice (Pinçon-Raymond *et al.*, 1985; Knudson *et al.*, 1989). The slow Ca current, intramembrane charge movement and ordered arrays of intramembrane particles (tetrads) are also absent in these skeletal muscles (Beam *et al.*, 1986; Beam & Adams, 1990; Shimahara *et al.*, 1990; Takekura *et al.*, 1994). Normal E-C coupling, charge movement, I_{Ca} and tetrads were all restored in *mdg* myotubes by injection of cDNA encoding the normal skeletal DHPR α_{1S} (Tanabe *et al.*, 1988; Adams *et al.*, 1990; Takekura *et al.*, 1994). These results further support the hypothesis that the DHPR is the voltage sensor that produces the charge movement critical to skeletal muscle E-C coupling. It also provides evidence that the intramembrane charge movement, tetrad particles and Ca current are all associated with the same DHPR molecule.

Tanabe *et al.* (1990a,b) also showed that if cDNA encoding the cardiac Ca channel (α_{1C}, rather than the skeletal α_{1S}) was injected into dysgenic myotubes, I_{Ca} and E-C coupling were again restored. However, in this case the I_{Ca} was more like that observed in cardiac muscle (i.e. with faster activation and inactivation kinetics) and E-C coupling was also more like cardiac muscle (e.g. contractions were quickly abolished in the absence of extracellular Ca). Using chimeric cDNA they also found that replacing a single region of the cardiac DHPR with the skeletal counterpart (the cytoplasmic loop between domains II & III, see Figs 51 & 110) was sufficient to cause E-C coupling to be skeletal muscle-type VDCR. Thus, it would seem that the different DHPRs in cardiac and skeletal muscle are sufficient to explain a major difference in E-C coupling in these muscle types. That is, in skeletal muscle the DHPR causes release by virtue of the charge movement (and the mechanical effect which that produces), with the I_{Ca} being incidental. In cardiac muscle the Ca entry via the Ca channel (or DHPR) appears to be the critical event, although charge movement is still important in activation of I_{Ca}.

Skeletal Muscle DHPR-RyR Interaction

The simplest molecular model for skeletal muscle E-C coupling would be that the DHPR is the voltage sensor and translates a signal through direct mechanical interaction to open the RyR (as envisioned by Chandler *et al.*, 1976b). However, there is remarkably little direct biochemical evidence of DHPR-RyR interaction (e.g. crosslinking studies of Murray & Ohendeck, 1997). Caswell *et al.* (1979) showed that SR-T-tubule junctions (triads) disrupted by French Press treatment could reform in cacodylate buffer. Ikemoto *et al.* (1984) showed that such reformed triads also had restored depolarization-induced SR Ca release (presumably due to T-tubule depolarization, see pg 213-214). Triad reformation was also promoted by GAPD (glyceraldehyde 3-phosphate dehydrogenase, Corbett *et al.*, 1985; Caswell & Corbett, 1985). The glycolytic enzymes, GAPD and aldolase, as well as triadin and sorcin have been reported to bind to both DHPRs and RyRs (Thieleczek *et al.*, 1989; Brandt *et al.*, 1990; Kim *et al.*, 1990; Fan *et al.*, 1995; Meyers *et al.*, 1995, 1998) and could bridge between them. However, it is unknown whether any of these proteins play a direct role in E-C coupling.

The chimeric DHPR studies of Tanabe *et al.* (1990a,b) caused particular interest in the DHPR II-III loop and how it might affect RyR properties (see Fig 110). Several groups have shown that peptides from the skeletal II-III loop could alter RyR1 gating in bilayers and also Ca release & ryanodine binding in vesicles (Lu *et al.*, 1994; El-Hayek *et al.*, 1995; Marx *et al.*, 1998b; Dulhunty *et al.*, 1999; Gurrola *et al.*, 1999; Zhu *et al.*, 1999). El-Hayek *et al.* (1995) split the II-III loop into 4 peptides (A-D) and found that only peptide A (Thr^{671}-Leu^{690} or its first 10 residues) altered ryanodine binding to RyR1 and SR Ca release (activating both), and that this effect could be blocked by the C peptide (Glu^{724}-Pro^{760}, see also Saiki *et al.*, 1999). In a more intact system (mechanically skinned skeletal muscle), Lamb *et al.* (2000) showed that peptide A could enhance spontaneous and E_m-dependent SR Ca release and that the triggered release could be partially inhibited by peptide C. Nakai *et al.* (1998b) showed that part of peptide C (residues 711-765) incorporated into an otherwise cardiac DHPR α_{1C} was sufficient to support skeletal type VDCR when expressed in dysgenic myotubes with RyR1, and even just 18 amino acids from skeletal α_{1S} (725-742) produced moderate VDCR.

Nakai *et al.* (1996, 1987, 1998a) also showed that in addition to this orthograde signaling from skeletal DHPR to RyR1, there is a retrograde signal from the RyR1 to DHPR. That is, in dyspedic mouse myotubes (which lack "feet" or RyR1, Takeshima *et al.*, 1994), but which express skeletal DHPRs, there was a normal amount of Ca channel gating charge, but very little I_{Ca} and no E-C coupling. Expression of RyR1 in these dyspedic myotubes restored both E-C coupling (orthograde signal) and also I_{Ca} function (retrograde signal). Expression of cardiac RyR2 was not able to restore either E-C coupling or I_{Ca} via α_{1S}. This suggested that RyR1 feeds directly back on α_{1S} to facilitate the transition from gating charge movement to opening of the Ca channel. Grabner *et al.* (1999) showed that the retrograde signal from RyR1 could be endowed on the cardiac DHPR simply by replacing part of the II-III loop with the skeletal DHPR (720-765). Thus, the DHPR II-III loop appears to be responsible for retrograde as well as orthograde signaling between α_{1S} and RyR1.

So, what about partner regions for the DHPR II-III loop on RyR1? Using RyR chimeras, Nakai *et al.* (1998a) identified 2 large regions of RyR1 which could restore ortho- and retrograde signaling (1635-2636) or retrograde signaling only (2659-3720). Leong & MacLennan (1998a,b)

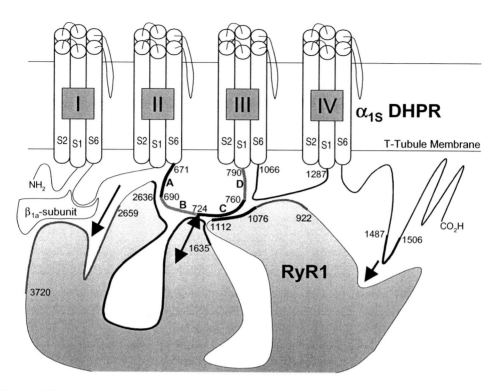

Figure 110. Possible interaction sites between skeletal DHPR and RyR1. Numbers refer to amino acid sequences of α_{1S} and RyR1. Numbered sections have been shown to interact physically or functionally with the other protein, but detailed matching between proteins is fanciful at best. Some long stretches (e.g. 1635-2636 on RyR1) are unlikely to interact throughout, but may include some key sites. Large arrows show orthograde signaling from DHPR to RyR (down) or retrograde from RyR to DHPR (up).

found another potentially important RyR1 region (922-1112) which bound to the II-III loop of α_{1S} (especially 1076-1112 of RyR1) and this region also bound to the III-IV loop of α_{1S}. Notably, this RyR1 region did not bind to II-III or III-IV loops from cardiac α_{1C}. Yamamoto *et al.* (1997) showed that a region of major divergence between RyR1 and RyR2 (known as D2, 1303-1406 in RyR1) was also important in skeletal-type E-C coupling. This elegant ongoing body of work has established that the skeletal muscle DHPR-RyR connection has unique interaction sites and that the highly homologous cardiac α_{1C} or RyR2 cannot functionally substitute with the skeletal counterparts.

While the II-III loop of α_{1S} (especially 681-690) has received a lot of attention as a mediator of skeletal E-C coupling, Proenza *et al.* (2000) found that scrambling this 10 amino acid sequence in α_{1S} expressed in dysgenic myotubes made no difference in restoring E-C coupling (or retrograde I_{Ca} signaling). There is also a 20 amino acid stretch of the DHPR in the proximal carboxy tail (1487-1506 in α_{1S}) that is identical in α_{1C}, and this peptide inhibits ryanodine binding to both RyR1 and RyR2 and reduces RyR1 open probability in bilayers (Slavik *et al.*, 1997). Notably, this region is in the carboxy tail, near sites implicated in Ca- and calmodulin-dependent inactivation and facilitation of cardiac I_{Ca} (see pg 117-120). Mice lacking the normal

Ca channel β subunit gene (β₁ₐ) also lack gating charge movement, I_{Ca} and effective E-C coupling, despite RyR1 expression and replete SR Ca stores (Beurg *et al.*, 1997, 1999a,b). Expression of the cardiac β₂ₐ in these myotubes only partially restored I_{Ca} and Ca transients, but β₁ₐ (especially the carboxy half in chimeras) could completely restore E-C coupling. Thus, there are multiple potential regions of the DHPR complex that might interact functionally with RyR (even if not physically), particularly in skeletal muscle.

Cardiac Muscle DHPR-RyR Interaction?

The situation in cardiac muscle is less clear. While data below support some interaction in heart, the emerging picture is of a much less robust DHPR-RyR interaction than in skeletal muscle. This is entirely consistent in heart with the apparent lack of VDCR (below), the less ordered physical array of DHPR over RyR in junctions (Fig 10) and the 4-10-fold excess of RyR over DHPR (Bers & Stiffel, 1993). This excess of RyR implies that at most 10-25% of RyR could possibly interact with a DHPR. Nevertheless, cardiac DHPRs do appear to be concentrated at sarcolemmal junctions with the SR, albeit not as tetrads (Franzini-Armstrong & Protasi, 1997). El-Hayek & Ikemoto (1998) found that the carboxy half of the II-III loop cardiac peptide A (Ac-10C, KERKKLARTA) could activate RyR1 and Lamb *et al.* (2000) also found that Ac-10C enhanced SR Ca release in skinned skeletal muscle. There is limited data for Ac-10C effects on RyR2, and the effects are in the opposite direction. We found that Ac-10C can inhibit RyR2 open probability in bilayers (IC_{50} ~1 μM, preliminary data only), and when included in the dializing patch pipette this peptide depresses Ca spark frequency by 63% in voltage clamped ventricular myocytes, for the same SR Ca load and diastolic $[Ca]_i$ (Li *et al.*, 1999). As mentioned above the carboxy peptide that is common to α₁C and α₁S inhibits ryanodine binding to RyR2 (Slavik *et al.*, 1997). Thus, it is possible that the analogous cardiac α₁C and RyR2 domains interact, but more work is needed to clarify this.

Bay K 8644, the dihydropyridine L-type Ca-channel agonist, has provided evidence in favor of intermolecular communication between cardiac α₁C and RyR2 in intact ferret ventricular myocytes. Bay K 8644 (100 nM) accelerates resting loss of SR Ca in ventricular myocytes in a manner that is completely independent of Ca influx and which is competitively inhibited by DHP antagonists (Hryshko *et al.*,1989a,b; McCall *et al.*, 1996b; Satoh *et al.*,1998; Katoh *et al.*,2000). This is apparent as a 400% increase in resting Ca spark frequency (e.g. Fig 111A) in the complete absence of extracellular Ca. This effect is maximal within 10 sec of exposure of cells to Bay K 8644, is unaltered by stimulation of APs (in Ca-free solution) and is completely block-ed by nifedipine. Bay K 8644, even at 100 times higher concentration, had no direct effect on cardiac RyR channel gating in bilayer experiments. Another Ca channel agonist which does not bind to the same DHPR site (FPL-64176) had no effect on Ca sparks, but similar effects enhancing I_{Ca}. Bay K 8644 also increased ryanodine binding in intact cells, but not after mecha-nical disruption. Our working hypothesis (Fig 110B) is that Bay K 8644 binds to the DHPR and transmits a Ca-independent signal to the RyR, altering its resting open probability. While this effect appears to be mediated by Bay K 8644 binding to the DHPR, it differs from effects on I_{Ca} which occur both more slowly and in a highly depolarization-dependent manner (Katoh *et al.*, 2000). We concluded that after binding to the DHPR the pathways diverge for the I_{Ca} gating effect and the intramolecular effect on the RyR, manifest as increased resting Ca sparks.

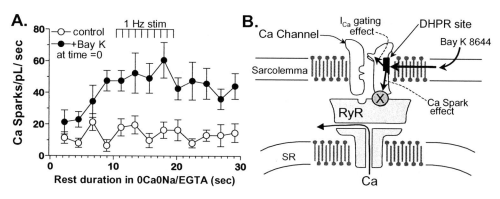

Figure 111. Bay K 8644 alters cardiac RyR2 function in Ca-independent manner. **A.** Ferret ventricular myocytes were stimulated to steady state (1 Hz) in normal Tyrode's and then stimulation was stopped and superfusion switched (in <1 sec) to a Ca-free, Na-free solution with 1 mM EGTA (±Bay K 8644, 500 nM). Ca Spark frequency was monitored for 30 sec. During the middle 10 sec the cells were stimulated at 1 Hz to see if depolarization altered Ca sparks. **B.** Schematic of Bay K 8644 binding to the DHPR and producing divergent effects on I_{Ca} gating and on RyR gating (independent of Ca flux). There may or may not be an intermediate protein $\otimes$ (modified versions of figures in Katoh *et al.*, 2000).

In Fig 111A it is notable that there were Ca sparks in the complete absence of extracellular Ca, emphasizing that Ca sparks are due to SR Ca release which occurs at a very low, but detectable frequency even at diastolic $[Ca]_i$. At this microscopic level it is clear (as in Fig 105A) that action potentials in the absence of $[Ca]_o$ produce no SR Ca release or change in either resting Ca sparks or $[Ca]_i$ (±Bay K 8644). Thus, while these Bay K 8644 studies imply some weak intramolecular link between DHPR-RyR in heart (changing P_o from ~0.0001 to 0.0005), they do not provide any support for VDCR in cardiac muscle. With respect to E-C coupling, it is notable that Bay K 8644 *depresses* E-C coupling (lower Ca release for a given I_{Ca} and SR Ca load; McCall & Bers, 1996; Adachi-Akahani *et al.*, 1999). While one could propose altered RyR Ca sensitivity, this effect is readily explained by the prolonged open times character-istic of Bay K 8644 modified L-type Ca channels (see Fig 61). That is, a comparable whole cell I_{Ca} in the presence of Bay K 8644 will include fewer total channel openings (because some will be open for very long times). Since only the first ms (or so) of opening is needed to trigger SR Ca release, much of the Ca influx will be wasted with respect to triggering SR Ca release (i.e. lower Ca release for a given I_{Ca}). So, there may only be a weak DHPR-RyR link in heart.

Direct Depolarization of the SR?

Peachey & Porter (1959) raised the possibility that skeletal muscle T-tubular depolar-ization could depolarize the SR membrane, causing Ca release. This hypothesis was tested in mechanically skinned skeletal muscle fibers using ionic substitution (Costantin & Podolsky, 1967; Nakajima & Endo, 1973). In this approach, a relatively impermeant anion (e.g. propionate, gluconate or methanesulfonate) is replaced by a permeant one (e.g. Cl), or a permeant cation (e.g. K) is replaced by a relatively impermeant one (e.g. choline, Tris, Li or Na). This could set up a diffusion potential which changes upon the solution switch. Although this can induce Ca release (see Endo, 1985), two major factors make this mechanism seem unlikely physiologically.

First, in these skinned fibers, T-tubules seal off, and with ATP present (required for skinned fiber solutions) they can re-establish the normal transsarcolemmal ion gradients (high [Na] and more positive potential in the sealed off T-tubules). Then ionic substitution can depolarize T-tubules, so that Ca release still depends on charge movement and VDCR as above. A compelling argument for this explanation is that such depolarization-induced Ca release in skinned fibers can be prevented by blocking Na/K-ATPase (preventing T-tubule polarization, Donaldson, 1985; Stephenson, 1985; Volpe & Stephenson, 1986). This argument also holds for heavy SR preparations which may include intact T-tubule-SR junctions. Second, as described at the end of Chapter 7, the permeability of the SR to physiological monovalent ions is very high and there are no appreciable monovalent ion gradients between SR and cytoplasm (Somlyo *et al.*, 1977a,b; Meissner, 1986b; Somlyo & Somlyo, 1986). This makes it likely that $E_m = 0$ across the SR membrane. Fabiato (1985f) also found no evidence for direct SR depolarization-induced SR Ca release in skinned pigeon cardiac myocytes (which lack T-tubules, but exhibit CICR). Thus, a direct SR depolarization-induced Ca release seems untenable.

Mg as a Possible Mediator of VDCR in Skeletal Muscle

Lamb & Stephenson (1990, 1994) and others have extensively used the mechanically skinned skeletal muscle preparations just described above (with sealed off T-tubules) to directly study VDCR in skeletal muscle where the cellular ionic conditions can be readily manipulated. Lamb (2000) made the intriguing proposal that that VDCR works by removing a tonic Mg-dependent inhibition of RyR1 (such that RyR1 gating in Fig 102 looks more like that for cardiac). Note that 1 mM $[Mg]_i$ (or $[Ca]_i$) strongly inactivates skeletal, but not cardiac RyR. Mg also shifts RyR activation curve to higher [Ca]. Thus, depolarization would allow ambient $[Ca]_i$ to activate SR Ca release and repolarization would cause rapid Mg-dependent RyR inhibition.

In conclusion, in skeletal muscle there is clear and compelling evidence for VDCR. The key molecules involved have been identified (DHPR and RyR), these proteins are physically adjoining in the junctional space and active efforts are underway to understand this interaction better in terms of molecular interactions as well as biophysical and theoretical aspects. CICR also occurs in skeletal muscle and may be triggered by the Ca released by VDCR. Thus, while VDCR seems essential to initiate SR Ca release, CICR may boost the initial rate of release.

In cardiac muscle several lines of evidence suggest that VDCR is not functional. 1) The E_m-dependence of $\Delta[Ca]_i$ and contraction follow I_{Ca} and not charge movement (Fig 106). 2) Ca entry seems to be an absolute requirement in cardiac muscle (Figs 105A & see below), 3) Depolarization does not induce SR Ca release by itself and does not appear to modify Ca-induced Ca-release from the SR (Figs 114, 115 & 117), 4) Ca release from cardiac corbular and extended junctional SR is physically too distant for VDCR (if, indeed Ca release from corbular SR occurs physiologically), 5) The exquisite structural DHPR-RyR organization and interaction apparent in skeletal muscle (Fig 109-110) does not seem to exist in heart. Nevertheless, several groups have argued for the presence of VDCR in cardiac muscle, and this possibility will be addressed (pg 235-236) after considering CICR and the evidence for its role in cardiac E-C coupling.

CICR is the more primitive form of E-C coupling from a phylogenetic standpoint. Most invertebrate skeletal muscle (e.g. crayfish) is functionally very similar to mammalian cardiac muscle in this regard (Györke & Palade, 1993, 1994). My perspective is that CICR is very old phylogenetically and has, in general, served well as an adaptive mechanism in heart (where speed of contraction is not of paramount importance). Thus, there may be weak physical interactions (direct or indirect) between cardiac DHPR and RyR, but these function mainly to keep sarco-lemmal Ca channels in the neighborhood of clusters of RyRs. In fast-twitch skeletal muscle, there is considerable adaptive advantage (survival) to high speeds of contraction. The vertebrate skeletal DHPR and RyR1 may have evolved additional points of interaction which are both more robust and also able to transmit the crucial E-C coupling signal very rapidly using the voltage sensor signal, without the need for Ca influx. In this context I_{Ca} in vertebrate skeletal muscle is essentially vestigial (for E-C coupling) and consequently the Ca channel function deteriorated with further evolution. This is consistent with the very slow activation of I_{Ca} (*vs.* charge movement or cardiac I_{Ca}) in vertebrate skeletal muscle. These are just musings, of course.

Ca-INDUCED Ca-RELEASE (CICR)

Ca-Induced Ca-Release in Skeletal Muscle

CICR was first described in skinned skeletal muscle fibers (Endo *et al.,* 1970; Ford & Podolsky, 1970). While CICR exists in both cardiac and skeletal muscle (Chapter 7), the major question is whether it occurs physiologically and how it interacts with other possible mechanisms. Endo (1975a, 1977) argued that CICR was only demonstrable in skeletal muscle fibers at unphysiologically low [Mg], required heavy SR Ca loading and very high trigger [Ca] (e.g. 100 µM Ca with 0.9 mM Mg, or 10 µM Ca with 50 µM Mg). Fabiato (1984, 1985g), however, demonstrated CICR in skeletal muscle with the SR loaded at 100 nM Ca and ~3 mM free [Mg], triggered by a rapid [Ca] increase to 200-600 nM. The preceding section described how CICR and VDCR may coexist and function together in vertebrate skeletal muscle.

Ca-Induced Ca-Release in Mechanically Skinned Cardiac Muscle.

Fabiato & Fabiato extensively characterized CICR in an elegant and formidable series of studies in mechanically skinned single cardiac myocytes (Fabiato & Fabiato, 1973, 1975a,b, 1978a,b, 1979; Fabiato 1981a, 1983, 1985a-c). In a culminating experimental series, Fabiato (1985a-c) used mechanically skinned canine Purkinje fibers because they lack T-tubules (which could reseal and complicate interpretations). The solutions included 5 µM calmodulin (which slightly increased Ca release) and ~3 mM free Mg. The largest CICR was seen in 1-3 mM Mg, although the threshold [Ca] for CICR is higher than at lower [Mg] (Fabiato, 1983). Ca entry via I_{Ca} was simulated by very rapid Ca application, which induced SR Ca release. Solutions of various [Ca] at various rates could be applied as fast as ~1 msec to these skinned cells and SR Ca release was measured using aequorin luminescence and force. Since CICR implies positive feedback, one might expect that Ca release would proceed to completion (as released Ca would cause more and more Ca release). However, a remarkable feature of CICR is that the amount of Ca released is graded with the amount of trigger Ca (Fabiato, 1983, 1985b). Indeed, at higher [Ca] CICR could be inhibited or inactivated (see below).

Figure 112A illustrates Fabiato's approach and shows inactivation of CICR at high [Ca]. In control contractions (C) the 100 nM Ca solution used to load the SR is withdrawn and 250 nM Ca solution applied briefly to activate SR Ca release (note that this [Ca] was insufficient to directly activate contraction; Fig 21A). In the third contraction (test) a higher [Ca] (10 µM) is

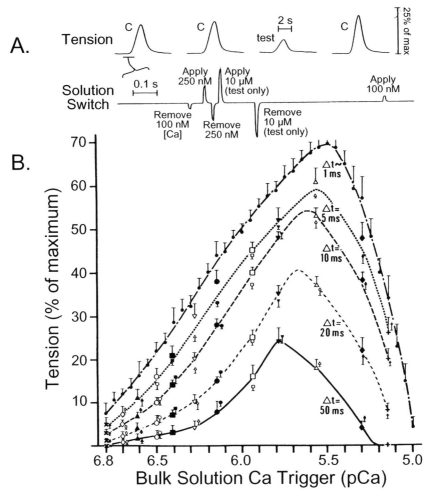

Figure 112. Fabiato's CICR in mechanically skinned canine cardiac Purkinje fiber. **A.** Tension recorded in response to rapid application and removal of experimental solutions of indicated [Ca] (lower trace is expanded time scale, as indicated by bar). In 100 nM [Ca] buffer the SR accumulates Ca. Removal of that solution and application of 250 nM Ca solution for 30 msec induces SR Ca release, peak [Ca] of 1.7 μM and contraction (control traces, C). For the test contraction only, [Ca] was raised to 10 μM for ~150 msec immediately after initiation of Ca release by 250 nM Ca. This extra elevation of [Ca] led to a smaller contraction and peak [Ca] (1.2 μM), indicating Ca-dependent inactivation of SR Ca release. **B.** Relationship between trigger [Ca] for SR Ca release (as pCa= –log [Ca]) and the contraction amplitude resulting from CICR. Experiments were done like the controls in A, except trigger Ca was varied and the time taken to reach the trigger [Ca] was varied from 1 to 50 msec. Ca release depended on both trigger [Ca] and the rate of [Ca] change around the SR (modified from Fabiato, 1985b, with permission).

applied (for ~150 ms) right after the 30 ms pulse of 250 nM Ca. This higher [Ca] results in a <u>smaller</u> contraction and Δ[Ca]$_i$. This indicates that the higher [Ca] inactivates the usual CICR.

Figure 112B shows the trigger [Ca] dependence of the tension transient produced by CICR (Fabiato, 1985b). Data are shown for several different durations taken to reach the indicated trigger [Ca]. It can be appreciated that the Ca released depends on both the trigger [Ca] and the time taken to reach that [Ca]. At high (or supra-optimal) trigger [Ca], the SR Ca release

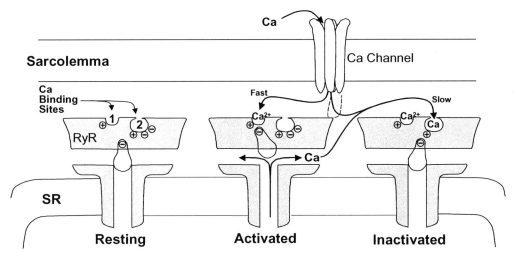

Figure 113. Diagram of CICR based on Fabiato's work. From the resting state (channel closed), Ca may bind rapidly to a relatively low affinity site (1), thereby activating the RyR. Ca may then bind more slowly to a second higher affinity site (2) moving the release channel to an inactivated state. As cytoplasmic [Ca] decreases, Ca would be expected to dissociate from the lower affinity activating site first and then more slowly from the inactivating site to return the channel to the resting state.

was inhibited. CICR also exhibited a refractory period where a second Ca release could not be induced. This was not the case for caffeine-induced Ca-release. Fabiato (1985b) likened this to the inactivation (and recovery from inactivation) described for sarcolemmal Ca channels. He also showed that some steady state inactivation existed at 63 nM Ca, but that this inactivation could be removed by a few seconds at [Ca]= 12 nM (analogous to I_{Ca} inactivation and recovery).

On the basis of these findings Fabiato (1985b) proposed a model (Fig 113) where Ca binds to an activating site with a high *on rate* (but modest affinity) and also binds to a second inactivating site which has a higher affinity, but a slower association constant (~0.7 sec at [Ca]= 63 nM). Thus, when $[Ca]_i$ increases rapidly the activation site is occupied and SR Ca release occurs. The inactivation site binds Ca more slowly to turn off Ca release. Rapid application of very high [Ca] can still produce inactivation more directly since binding to the inactivation site is expected to be proportional to the product of *on rate* and [Ca]. Thus, the very high [Ca] can partially overcome the limitation of the slow *on rate*. This model provides a useful framework for understanding global behavior of E-C coupling at the cellular level in cardiac myocytes.

Ca-Induced Ca-Release: Support from Intact Cardiac Myocytes.

Figure 113 puts the sarcolemmal Ca channel close to the SR Ca release channel (RyR). Thus, Ca entry via I_{Ca} may have ready access to the activation (and inactivation sites) of the SR Ca release channel. The similar E_m-dependence of I_{Ca}, contraction and Ca_i transient in cardiac myocytes (Fig 106A) are classic findings which are consistent with CICR in heart (London & Krueger, 1986; Cannell *et al.*, 1987; Beuckelmann & Wier, 1988; Callewaert *et al.*, 1988; duBell & Houser, 1989). Further support comes from the observation of I_{Ca} "tail transients" (Fig 114, Cannell *et al.*, 1987; Beuckelmann & Wier, 1988). These occur when a cell is first voltage clamped at positive E_m (e.g. +100 mV), where Ca channels are open, but no inward I_{Ca} is seen,

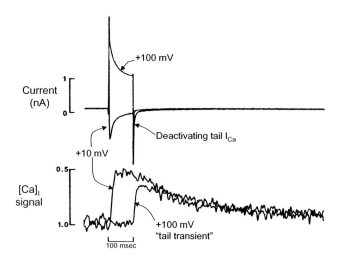

Figure 114. Activation of SR Ca release by tail I_{Ca} during repolarization in a rat ventricular myocyte. Current (top) and $[Ca]_i$ (lower Fura-2 fluorescence traces) in response to depolarization to either +10 mV or +100 mV. Depolarization to +10 mV produces the usual I_{Ca} and $\Delta[Ca]_i$. Depolarization to +100 mV produces no inward I_{Ca} or Ca transient, but upon repolarization to –50 mV, a brief I_{Ca} tail current activates a robust Ca transient due to CICR (modified from Cannell *et al.*, 1987, with permission).

and no Ca transient occurs. Then when E_m is suddenly clamped back to negative E_m (e.g. –50 mV) Ca channels deactivate, but as the Ca channels are closing, a large, short-lived inward I_{Ca} flows through open Ca channels (tail current) and induces a Ca transient and contraction. This is likely to reflect CICR (*vs.* VDCR), although a complex E_m-dependence could be contrived to explain this (Cannell *et al.*, 1987). These "tail Ca_i transients" are not observed in skeletal muscle, where voltage appears to control SR Ca release more directly.

Näbauer *et al.* (1989) provided compelling evidence for CICR (*vs.* VDCR) in rat ventricular myocytes (Fig 115). The first pulse shows a control depolarization with a large I_{Ca} and Ca transient. For the second pulse, 4 mM EGTA was added to decrease $[Ca]_o$ to submicromolar levels. Under these conditions the Ca channel carries a large Na current (see Chapter 5) which inactivates very slowly compared to I_{Ca}. There is no Ca transient associated with this pulse despite the facts that 1) ionic current flowed through the Ca channel, 2) there was presumably charge movement associated with Ca channel activation and 3) there was plenty of SR Ca (as shown by the large caffeine-induced Ca transient). They also showed that Ba current could not induce SR Ca release. Thus, E-C coupling cannot be due to Ca channel charge movement or current *per se*. Ca entry appears to be an absolute requirement for induction of Ca release in cardiac muscle.

Two photolabile Ca chelators Nitr-5 (Adams *et al.*, 1988) and DM-nitrophen (Kaplan & Ellis-Davies, 1988) in which Ca affinity is decreased upon illumination make it possible to produce rapid increases in $[Ca]_i$ in intact cells. Kentish *et al.* (1990) used Nitr-5 to demonstrate CICR in saponin skinned cardiac muscle for comparison with IP_3-induced Ca-release (see pg 241). Valdeolmillos *et al.* (1989) demonstrated that photolysis of Ca-Nitr-5 induced ryanodine-sensitive contractions in rat ventricular myocytes that persisted in the presence of 10 mM Ni

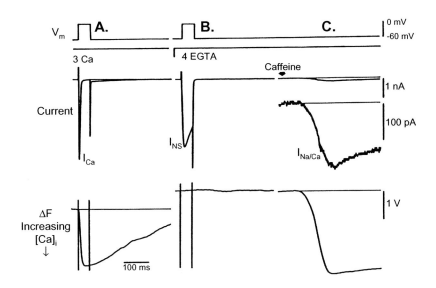

Figure 115. Ca entry is required for induction of SR Ca release in rat ventricular myocytes. **A.** depolarization activates I_{Ca} and a large Ca transient (fura-2 fluorescence). **B.** After replacing extracellular Ca with 4 mM EGTA, depolarization activates Na current through Ca channels (I_{NS}, with characteristically slow inactivation). Na current through the Ca channel does not induce SR Ca release. **C.** Application of 5 mM caffeine induces a large Ca transient (indicating SR Ca available for release) in B, and activates an inward current, likely to be $I_{Na/Ca}$ (from Näbauer *et al.*, 1989, with permission).

(which would block both I_{Ca} and Na/Ca exchange). These contractions probably reflect CICR, but E_m was not measured. Näbauer & Morad (1990) and Niggli & Lederer (1990) performed this type of photolysis experiment in isolated myocytes under voltage clamp. The contractions were largely suppressed by caffeine or ryanodine and were observed at constant E_m (excluding any possibility that the Ca release was depolarization-dependent). Niggli & Lederer (1990) also showed that the CICR was the same whether E_m was -100, 0 or +100 mV, suggesting that CICR in cardiac muscle is not modified by E_m (see also below). Näbauer & Morad (1990) also tried to reproduce Fabiato's experiment (shown in Fig 112A) by increasing $[Ca]_i$ with a flash during the rising phase of the contraction. They did not see any evidence of inactivation of SR Ca release with elevated $[Ca]_i$. They saw only enhancement of contraction. While the $[Ca]_i$ reached by DM-nitrophen photolysis may not have been high enough (or for long enough) to produce inactivation, no intact cellular data have confirmed the result in Fig 112A of CICR inactivation with supra-optimal Ca trigger. CICR inactivation and termination of SR Ca release will be discussed in more detail below (pg 227-230).

Repolarization Induced Turn-off of Ca-Release in Cardiac Muscle?

Cannell *et al.* (1987) showed that the rise in $[Ca]_i$ can be curtailed by repolarization, even after the peak of I_{Ca} has occurred (see Fig 116). They suggested that this might reflect an intrinsic E_m-dependence of the CICR process or that repolarization turned off SR Ca release (as in skeletal muscle). Another possibility is that repolarization hastened Ca extrusion via Na/Ca exchange, thereby limiting the rise of $[Ca]_i$. However, this possibility seems unlikely since Bers

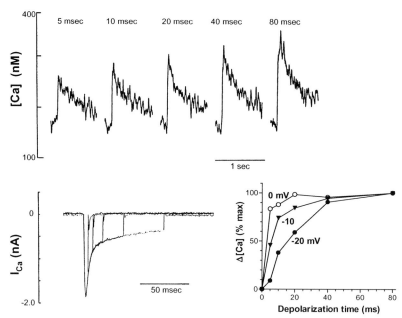

Figure 116. Duration dependence of Ca transients in a rat ventricular myocyte (using indo-1 as Ca indicator). Test pulses to 0 mV (from -50 mV) for the indicated times were given after 5 conditioning pulses to 0 mV to ensure that SR Ca load was the same at each test pulse. Superimposed I_{Ca} traces (leak subtracted) recorded simultaneously are shown. The $\Delta[Ca]_i$ increases despite a constant peak I_{Ca}. Graph shows duration dependence of $\Delta[Ca]_i$ for different test E_m from a different cell in which Na/Ca exchange was prevented by no Na in the pipette or bath solution (from Bers *et al.*, 1990, with permission).

et al. (1990) demonstrated that duration-dependence of $\Delta[Ca]_i$ was still apparent when Na/Ca exchange had been eliminated (in Na-free solutions, Fig 116).

An intrinsic E_m-dependence of CICR is unlikely, based on three types of experiments. First, Niggli & Lederer (1990) found the same contraction at −100, 0 and +100 mV when contraction was initiated by photolysis of Ca-Nitr-5 (see above). Second, in experiments like that in Fig 116, Cleeman & Morad (1991) showed that Ca transients were equally well curtailed when the Ca entry via I_{Ca} was stopped by repolarization to -40 mV (deactivating I_{Ca}) or by further depolarization to +100 mV (preventing Ca influx electrochemically). Third, the E_m-dependence of I_{Ca} is similar to Ca transients and contractions (Fig 106), although substantial Ca transients can be seen with very small I_{Ca} (Cannell *et al.*, 1987). Figure 117 shows another way to look at this type of result. If SR Ca release depended on E_m (in addition to Ca), then one would expect higher $\Delta[Ca]_i$ for a given I_{Ca} at more positive E_m. The opposite is observed in Fig 117 (Beuckelmann & Wier, 1988; Wier *et al.*, 1994; but see pg 233). Less $\Delta[Ca]_i$ is seen at more positive E_m for the same value of I_{Ca}. This is explained by the size of the single channel I_{Ca} (i_{Ca}) at different E_m. That is, at more negative E_m the i_{Ca} amplitude is larger simply because of a greater electrochemical driving force ($E_m - E_{Ca}$, and see Fig 117B). Thus, a Ca channel opening at more negative E_m yields a larger i_{Ca} and is consequently more likely to trigger SR Ca release. This single channel perspective also explains the duration-dependence of E-C coupling shown in Fig 116. The duration-dependence is more prominent at more negative E_m (Fig 116), consistent with longer latencies for single L-type Ca channel opening, especially apparent at E_m just

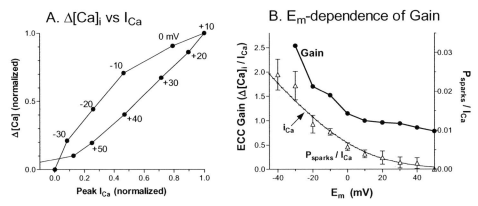

Figure 117. Dependence of Δ[Ca]$_i$ on I$_{Ca}$ and E-C coupling gain in guinea-pig ventricular myocytes. **A.** Data from Beuckelmann & Wier (1988) from Fig 106A. Note that for the same I$_{Ca}$ amplitude the induced Δ[Ca]$_i$ is higher at more negative E$_m$. **B.** The ratio of Δ[Ca]$_i$ to the I$_{Ca}$ needed to induce it is a convenient crude index of E-C coupling gain. The E$_m$-dependence of Ca spark probability (normalized to I$_{Ca}$) is also shown (Data from Santana *et al.*, 1996). The expected E$_m$-dependence of single channel I$_{Ca}$ (i$_{Ca}$), based on the Nernst-Plank equation is similar to both sets of data.

positive to the activation threshold (Rose *et al.*, 1992). Thus, duration-dependence at –20 mV may reflect time-dependent recruitment of SR Ca release units, based on i$_{Ca}$ latency. Together these results strongly suggest that Ca-induced Ca-release is not directly modulated by E$_m$. Higher Δ[Ca]$_i$ for a given I$_{Ca}$ at positive E$_m$ has been reported (e.g. when [Na]$_i$ is elevated, Isenberg *et al.*, 1988), consistent with Ca entry via I$_{Na/Ca}$ or VDCR (see discussion on pg 232-236).

LOCAL CONTROL AND CICR

A more quantitative consideration of CICR requires much more detailed information about the local physical environment in the junction and diffusional limitations in this region. It is useful to consider the [Ca]$_i$ which might be expected in the vicinity of the inner mouth of a sarcolemmal Ca channel. This can be easily done using the solution to the diffusion equation for radial dependence of [Ca] from a point source in a hemisphere (Crank, 1975):

$$[Ca]_{r,t} = [Ca]_{t0} + \frac{q}{2\pi Dr} \times erfc(\frac{r}{2\sqrt{Dr}}) \tag{8.1}$$

where [Ca]$_{t0}$ and [Ca]$_{rt}$ are the initial [Ca]$_i$ and the [Ca]$_i$ at a radial distance r, from the channel mouth at time t after a current q is activated, and D is the diffusion coefficient.

Figure 118A shows [Ca]$_i$ as a function of radial distance from the inner mouth of a sarcolemmal Ca channel (for two different D values). Inclusion of Ca binding to the inner sarcolemmal surface delays the steady state, but does not change the final value (Bers & Peskoff, 1991). The [Ca] rises to very high values near the channel (r ~0.2 nm) and is 10-100 μM at the SR side of the junctional cleft (r ~15 nm) where RyR Ca binding sites may be. For r <20 nm local [Ca]$_i$ is at its steady state value in <1 msec (the last factor in eq. 8.1 is ~1). This means that Ca diffusion away from this region is "keeping up" with Ca entry via the channel. It is thus implicit that [Ca]$_i$ in this region will decrease rapidly when I$_{Ca}$ stops. This may partly explain rapid deactivation of SR Ca release when I$_{Ca}$ is stopped by early repolarization.

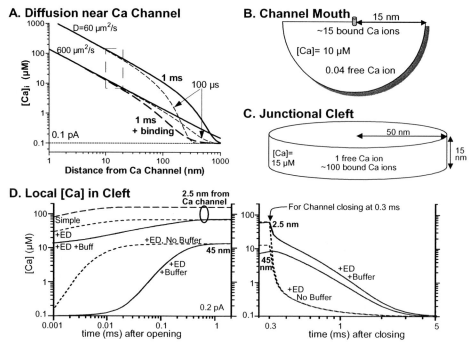

Figure 118. Predicted [Ca]$_i$ near the inner mouth of a Ca channel and junctional cleft. **A.** Solid curves are from Eq. 8.1 (q =0.1 pA, [Ca]$_{to}$ =100 nM, t= 1 ms). Thin broken curves are at 100 µs and the thick broken curve includes linear Ca binding to the inner sarcolemmal surface (as in Bers & Peskoff, 1991). **B.** Within a 15 nm radius of a Ca channel mouth for free [Ca]=10 µM there is less than one free Ca ion and only ~ 15 bound to the membrane. **C.** For the whole junctional cleft (at 15 µM free [Ca]) there is only 1 Ca ion free and ~100 bound. **D.** [Ca] predicted in the junctional cleft by Soeller & Cannell (1997) for a Ca channel opening at the cleft center (0.2 pA), including local membrane Ca buffering and electrodiffusion (ED). Right panel assumes that the channel closes at 0.3 ms (data for D kindly supplied by M.B. Cannell).

It is worth considering the actual numbers of Ca ions in the hemisphere around a Ca channel or in the dyadic cleft space. Figure 118B shows that at 10 µM [Ca] there is less than one free Ca ion (0.04) within this small hemisphere and ~15 Ca ions bound to the membrane. For the whole dyadic cleft (Fig 118C) at 15 µM [Ca] there is still only 1 Ca ion total (and ~100 Ca ions surface bound). Thus, one should think about [Ca] in this environment as a stochastic probability, rather than as an extensive quantity.

Langer & Peskoff (1996) and Soeller & Cannell (1997) extended our work on diffusion near Ca channels, by including important geometric constraints, local buffering and electro-diffusion. Figure 118D shows that inclusion of electrodiffusion (+ED) limits steady state [Ca] (due to charge repulsion by higher local [Ca]). Without buffers, local [Ca] rises throughout the cleft to the steady state value in <10 µs. Even with buffers [Ca] throughout the cleft is >10 µM in < 1 ms (Soeller & Cannell, 1997). When the Ca channel closes (typically after 0.3 ms, Rose *et al.*, 1992) the local [Ca] falls more slowly with Ca buffers, but still within ~5 ms. Cannell & Soeller (1997) extended this simulation to activation of RyRs and illustrated how the junctional geometry contributes to the optimal tuning of the E-C coupling process.

The notion of local control of RyR by Ca in cardiac E-C coupling was a logical extension from Fabiato's 1985 work, where the rate of [Ca] change in the RyR environment could activate or inactivate SR Ca release.   This, combined with the apparent junctional colocalization of DHPR with RyRs and simple diffusional modeling, made local control appealing.   Leblanc & Hume (1990) brought the issue into sharp focus by results suggesting that Na entry via I_{Na} could raise local submembrane $[Na]_i$ to cause local elevation of $[Ca]_i$ (via Na/Ca exchange) and consequent triggering of SR Ca release.   Lederer *et al.* (1990) coined the term "fuzzy space" for the junctional cleft, emphasizing the importance of local spatial concentration gradients in this restricted junctional space and their consequences.   This captured the spirit which was apparent in many papers and labs at about that time; clearly the field had collectively embraced the importance of local concentration gradients in E-C coupling.   Stern (1992) crystallized some key aspects in a series of mathematical models which indicated that common pool models (where trigger [Ca]=global [Ca]) could not explain the graded nature of CICR.   To obtain a reasonable amplification factor required the common pool system to teeter on the brink of spontaneous release. He also considered two models of local control: 1) a "Ca-synapse" where 1 DHPR triggers only 1 RyR, and 2) a "cluster bomb" where 1 DHPR triggers a cluster of RyRs.   Either model could explain both graded release and high gain, but the synapse model required an unrealistically large single RyR Ca flux.

The initial observation of localized SR Ca release events (Ca sparks) by Cheng *et al.* (1993) was timely and gave immediate physical evidence for elementary Ca release events that were restricted in space (see pg 190-192).   Ca sparks initiate along z-lines, raise local [Ca] by ~200 nM (rise in 10 ms, fall with τ~ 25 ms) and have a spatial spread of ~2 μm (Cheng *et al.*, 1993, 1995, 1996; López-López *et al.*, 1994, 1995; Cannell *et al.*, 1994, 1995; Shacklock *et al.*, 1995; Gómez *et al.*, 1996; Satoh *et al.*, 1997).   It should be noted that the scale of these optical signals (~1 μm) is 100 times larger than the depth of the junctional cleft (and 10,000 times larger volume).   So even Ca spark measurements, while quite valuable, still don't directly reflect local $[Ca]_i$ in the cleft.   Ca sparks occur randomly at very low frequency in the resting cell (~100/s, independent of Ca entry), but several thousand Ca sparks can be synchronized by I_{Ca} (and CICR) during depolarization, and the released [Ca] summates in time and space to produce the whole cell Ca transient.   To visualize discrete Ca sparks during a twitch requires the almost complete blockade of I_{Ca} (by nifedipine, D600 or Cd) so that there are fewer local signals to overlap in time and space (which normally obscures their resolution).   Cheng *et al.* (1993) initially proposed that Ca sparks might represent single RyR events, but it now seems likely that a cluster of RyRs (6-20) function in concert to produce a Ca spark (see pg 191-2).   However, the precise number of RyR is not known and how they are synchronized is still not completely clear.   Of course local CICR within a cluster of RyRs almost surely occurs, but RyRs within a cluster may also be physically linked and undergo simultaneous coupled gating, providing redundancy of control (Marx *et al.*, 1998a; Bers & Fill, 1998).   Thus, the data seem to suggest that the cluster bomb model is most appropriate.

In the local control theory of Stern (1992) it is acceptable that within a cluster of RyRs (perhaps a junctional region or couplon) Ca release can be effectively all-or-none. That is, the release within a cluster can be regenerative.   However, the physical separation between clusters and the high local [Ca] required to ignite a cluster prevents one cluster from activating another.

This is really the heart of local control theory. Indeed, Ca sparks normally do not trigger Ca sparks in neighboring region (except during Ca waves). Parker *et al.* (1996) showed that occasionally a Ca spark can activate a lateral neighbor along a z-line (~0.76 μm away), but never longitudinally from one z-line to the next (~1.8 μm), despite the observed slower Ca diffusion in the lateral *vs.* longitudinal direction. Thus, CICR gradation comes largely from the recruitment of different numbers of RyR clusters, rather than varying the flux at each release cluster.

SR Ca release can also be induced by Ca entry via Na/Ca exchange and by flash photolysis of caged Ca (López-López *et al.*, 1995; Lipp & Niggli, 1996, 1998). These Ca triggers are not necessarily as localized to the junctional region, nor are they likely to produce as large a rise in local $[Ca]_i$. Interestingly these approaches can produce SR Ca release which also appears more spatially uniform (*vs.* Ca sparks), leading Lipp & Niggli (1996) to propose unresolvable events or "Ca quarks," several times smaller than Ca sparks. It is not clear why RyRs activated this way do not produce a locally regenerative Ca spark (cluster bomb). Niggli (1999) speculated that there may be 2 classes of RyRs in the cleft: 1) those immediately apposed to DHPRs which may have low Ca-sensitivity, but large release flux and 2) the others with higher Ca-sensitivity, but lower Ca release flux (e.g. very brief openings). When I_{Ca} is activated the first class of RyR is readily activated and the large release flux recruits the neighbors in the cluster (a Ca spark). With a weaker global elevation of $[Ca]_i$ a few of the second class of RyRs might fire, but not produce a strong enough trigger to activate the first class or a Ca spark (hence producing only a Ca quark). Its not clear if this conceptual model would work, but it is an interesting notion that is yet to be tested.

Gain and Fractional SR Ca release

So what is the real amplification factor of CICR? This is often referred to as gain, where a measure of SR Ca release is divided by the Ca trigger signal that produces it. In the most literal sense it should be the amount of total SR Ca released (or rate of release) divided by the integrated triggering I_{Ca} (or influx rate). Moreover, one should correct for the contribution of I_{Ca} to the Ca transient, so gain = $(\Delta[Ca]_{tot} - \int I_{Ca}dt)/ \int I_{Ca}dt$. Wier *et al.* (1994) reported a gain of ~16 at E_m =0 mV in rat ventricle (using peak flux rates), which varies with E_m as in Fig 117B (higher at more negative E_m, due to higher unitary i_{Ca}). We find a gain of 3-8 in rabbit using total Ca fluxes at E_m= 0 mV, which varies with SR Ca load (Shannon *et al.*, 2000b). These values are generally consistent with the overall Ca fluxes in these species (Chapters 3 & 9). Many investigators use variations on this gain factor which are also quite useful, but require less detailed quantitative analysis of Ca fluxes (e.g. $\Delta[Ca]_i$/peak I_{Ca} or $d[Ca]_i/dt$/peak I_{Ca}). This is a reasonable simplification to allow comparison of gains under different conditions (especially when varying Ca trigger at constant SR Ca load).

Since the amount of SR Ca release also depends on the amount of available SR Ca, gain would be expected to vary as a function of SR Ca load, even if the intrinsic E-C coupling process is not changed. Thus, we also use fractional release as an index of the efficacy of E-C coupling, especially when SR Ca load is being varied (Bassani *et al.*, 1993b, 1995b; Shannon *et al.*, 2000b). Notably, knowledge of SR Ca load is required for fractional release measurements. Figure 119 shows both gain and fractional release determined from the same data. We showed that during a normal twitch the SR releases 43, 35 & 55% of its Ca in intact rabbit, ferret and rat

A. Gain of E-C Coupling

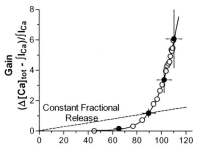

B. Fractional SR Ca Release

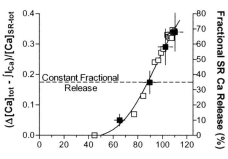

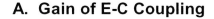

SR Ca load (μmol/l cytosol)

Figure 119. Gain of E-C coupling and fractional SR Ca release in rabbit ventricular myocytes. Data from voltage clamp studies measuring I_{Ca}, $[Ca]_i$ (indo-1) and SR Ca load (as in Fig 93). Na-free solutions were used to prevent Na/Ca exchange from complicating I_{Ca} measurements. **A.** Gain was measured in individual cells as total amount of SR Ca released / total $\int I_{Ca}$ (typical maximal gain was 6-10). To illustrate the SR Ca load-dependence of gain for all pulses in all cells the definition was relaxed as shown. **B.** Fractional SR release (total Ca release flux/ SR Ca load) was sometimes >100% at very highest loads (i.e. some released Ca was taken up and re-released during a pulse). The maximal % SR Ca depletion during a twitch was rarely >50% at any time. Left axis chosen (as for A) to define the shape of the curve, right axis is approximate for true fractional release. Dotted lines indicate expectations if fractional release was unchanged by SR Ca load (data are taken from Shannon *et al.*, 2000b).

ventricular myocytes, for SR Ca contents of ~100 μmol/L cytosol (Bassani *et al.,* 1993b, 1995b; Delbridge *et al.,* 1997). The fractional release changes in parallel to the I_{Ca} amplitude (for a given SR Ca load), as expected for the graded nature of CICR (Bassani *et al.,* 1995b). When SR Ca load is varied a striking finding is that fractional release (& gain) become almost zero at an SR Ca content which is still ~50% of normal (see Fig 119). That is, I_{Ca} cannot release this Ca, but caffeine can. We suspect that this is an effect of low luminal $[Ca]_{SR}$ to reduce the sensitivity of the RyR to trigger I_{Ca}. This would serve to prevent further SR Ca depletion and also encourage refilling, but it is remarkable that CICR seems to shut off at moderate $[Ca]_{SR}$. This modulation of Ca release flux by $[Ca]_{SR}$ may even be involved in the termination of normal SR Ca release (see below). At high SR Ca load both gain and fractional release increase steeply, and this may be due to high $[Ca]_{SR}$ causing sensitization of RyR gating to cytosolic [Ca] (see Fig 103A). Thus, there may be a continuous modulation of SR Ca release by luminal Ca. This would also explain the apparent "spontaneous" release of Ca associated with SR Ca overload. At very high $[Ca]_{SR}$, the RyR may be sufficiently sensitized so that even diastolic $[Ca]_i$ is sufficient to activate SR Ca release, which may propagate as a wave (because neighboring RyR clusters are also sensitized). In this sense spontaneous SR Ca release may really be triggered by high $[Ca]_{SR}$. Under these conditions diastolic $[Ca]_i$ is often elevated as well and could conspire with $[Ca]_{SR}$ to cause SR Ca release (Edgell *et al.,* 2000). This increased fractional release with SR Ca load (Bassani *et al.,* 1995b; Shannon *et al.,* 2000b) is consistent with the effects of $[Ca]_{SR}$ on single RyR gating (pg 194) and work in intact myocytes (Han *et al.,* 1994b; Spencer & Berlin, 1995).

The frequency of Ca sparks certainly increases with increasing SR Ca load and at a certain point macrosparks (more than one locus firing together) and Ca waves are seen (Cheng *et al.,* 1996; Satoh *et al.,* 1997). It also seems that the Ca spark frequency declines at lower SR Ca load at unaltered $[Ca]_i$ (Satoh *et al.*, 1997) and this is consistent with a continuous modulation of RyR gating by $[Ca]_{SR}$. However, at low $[Ca]_{SR}$ this point is complicated because Ca spark amplitude decreases, making them more difficult to detect (Song *et al.*, 1997). Thus, high $[Ca]_{SR}$ may increase a) individual RyR open probability in bilayer recording, b) Ca spark frequency during rest in intact cells and c) fractional SR Ca release due to CICR during E-C coupling.

Activation of SR Ca Release and Time Course of Ca Release Flux

The E_m-dependence and latency of Ca spark activation match that of I_{Ca} activation near the threshold for activation (López-López *et al.*, 1995; Cannell *et al.*, 1995; Santana *et al.*, 1996; Collier *et al.*, 1999). These studies uniformly demonstrated that the opening of a single L-type Ca channel is sufficient to activate a Ca spark. It is more controversial how many Ca ions must bind to activate SR Ca release. López-López *et al.* (1995) showed that the probability of Ca sparks (P_{sparks}) as a function of E_m was roughly that expected for single channel Ca current (i_{Ca}). Since local [Ca] in the cleft is expected to be proportional to i_{Ca} (Soeller & Cannell, 1997), this would be consistent with a direct dependence of P_{sparks} on local [Ca] and thus activation of a spark by one Ca ion. Whole cell $[Ca]_i$ data of Fan & Palade (1999) also seemed to support this. Santana *et al.* (1996) followed up this issue with additional Ca spark data and divided P_{sparks} by I_{Ca}, which can intrinsically correct for the E_m-dependence of I_{Ca} gating. Then the E_m-dependence of P_{sparks}/I_{Ca} should be linear if one Ca ion is required, but their data showed E_m-dependence like i_{Ca}, indicating that two Ca ions are needed for activation (see i_{Ca} in Fig 117B). The single RyR2 in bilayers seems to require ~4 Ca ions to be activated (Zahradníková, 1999a). Thus, the opening one Ca channel can trigger a Ca spark and 1 - 4 Ca ions are probably required to bind to an RyR to start a Ca spark, in which a cluster of RyRs are recruited by CICR (or coupled gating).

During a strong activation of I_{Ca}, as during the AP, there is rapid activation of SR Ca release (as Ca sparks) and there appears to be very little delay (perhaps < 1 ms) between peak I_{Ca} and the peak of SR Ca release flux (pg 122). Figure 120 shows the time course of SR Ca release measured by several different approaches. The slowest SR Ca release flux signal is based on deconvolution of the whole cell Ca transient (Sipido & Wier, 1991; Wier *et al.*, 1994; Shannon *et al.*, 2000b). This is not surprising because it uses a global $[Ca]_i$ signal (even though we correct the signal for dye kinetics). This global signal may be what the myofilaments sense and is thus functionally important, but it represents a damped and distorted version of the release flux produced by the RyRs. Measuring the timing of Ca spark occurrence during a Ca transient provides a closer optical signal and one can differentiate that to get a rather rapid release flux time course (López-López *et al.*,1995; Cannell *et al.*, 1995; Blatter *et al.*, 1997; Collier *et al.*, 1999; Bridge *et al.*, 1999). However, the Ca spark is still distributed over a relatively large area of the sarcomere, so this signal is still too slow. Song *et al.* (1998) devised a "Ca spike" approach to measure SR Ca release flux, using a combination of a low affinity fast Ca indicator (Oregon Green 488 BAPTA-5N or OG-5N; at 1 mM) plus 4 mM EGTA (a slow high affinity Ca buffer) in the patch pipette. As Ca is released it binds rapidly to OG-5N increasing fluorescence, but as it diffuses away from the source Ca binds to EGTA, limiting spatial spread of the fluorescence signal (see also Cleeman *et al.*, 1998). Song *et al.* (1998) showed that the time course of these Ca spikes was similar to $d[Ca]_i/dt$ during a Ca spark.

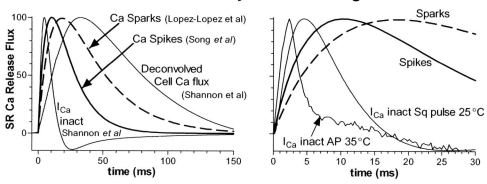

Figure 120. SR Ca release flux measured by different approaches in ventricular myocytes. The slowest curve is based on quantitative deconvolution of total Ca fluxes and global [Ca]$_i$ measures in rabbit with kinetic corrections for Ca binding to indicators and buffers (Shannon *et al.*, 2000b). Ca sparks curve is based on the occurrence of Ca sparks in guinea-pig ventricular myocytes reported by López-López *et al.* (1995). The time course of Ca spikes in rat is taken from the work of Song *et al.* (1998). Time course of SR Ca release-dependent inactivation of I$_{Ca}$ is also shown for rabbit ventricular myocytes during square voltage clamp pulses at 25°C (Shannon *et al.*, 2000b) and AP-clamp pulses at 35°C (Puglisi *et al.*, 1999; see Fig 60 for methods). Right panel is on an expanded time base.

In addition to these optical signals, SR Ca release causes I$_{Ca}$ inactivation and this can be used as an indicator of Ca release rate (see Figs 60 & 120, Puglisi *et al.*, 1999; Shannon *et al.*, 2000b). This electrophysiological signal is not subject to indicator kinetics and uses a sensor (the L-type Ca channel) which is perfectly positioned to detect local [Ca] changes in the cleft. With an AP at 35°C the peak SR Ca release flux may occur as early as 2.5 ms and coincide with the peak I$_{Ca}$ (i.e. with no detectable delay). The disadvantage of this I$_{Ca}$ signal is that it may be nonlinear and cannot be calibrated. With the simplifying assumption that all of the integrated Ca release flux from the global Ca measurements is compressed into the more rapid kinetics of the local I$_{Ca}$ signals, the peak release flux would be 3-10 times higher than the value of ~3 mmol/L cytosol/s for the deconvolved global Ca (Wier *et al.*, 1994; Shannon *et al.*, 2000b). Thus, the apparent Ca release flux sensed by global Ca indicators (and the myofilaments) is slower and lower than that sensed locally near the RyRs. This would also increase the required fraction of the cell's RyRs needed to explain the measured Ca release flux, from ~2% (pg 192) to ~6-20%.

Termination of SR Ca Release

Since CICR has intrinsic positive feedback, what turns off SR Ca release? In principle there are 3 possibilities: 1) local depletion of SR Ca, 2) inactivation (or adaptation) and 3) stochastic attrition (e.g. Stern, 1992; Sham *et al.*, 1998 Lukyanenko *et al.*, 1998). Stochastic attrition means that if the L-type Ca channel and all relevant RyRs in a junction happen to be closed at the same moment (as channels gate stochastically), the local [Ca]$_i$ would fall very rapidly (Fig 118D) which could interrupt the otherwise regenerative release. This could work well if only one DHPR and one RyR are involved, but the larger the number of RyRs responsible for a Ca spark, the less likely it will be that they all close at once. SR Ca depletion is not the key factor because when cells are treated with ryanodine or caffeine, very long lasting local [Ca]$_i$

elevations (>200 ms) are seen and these do not decline with time (Cheng *et al.*, 1993; Satoh *et al.*, 1997). If local SR Ca could be depleted on the time scale of a Ca spark one would expect $[Ca]_i$ to sag during long events. Thus, diffusion from other regions of the SR may prevent local SR Ca depletion. However, during a global Ca transient the entire $[Ca]_{SR}$ declines. Given the evidence supporting a modulatory role of $[Ca]_{SR}$ on RyR gating, $[Ca]_{SR}$ depletion might play some role in shutting off global SR Ca release during a twitch. This may be why we do not find SR depletion to much greater than ~50% during large Ca releases (Shannon *et al.*, 2000b), which coincides with the SR Ca load where gain and fractional release are zero (Fig 119, and see Bassani *et al.*, 1995b). However, as stated above, this can't explain why Ca sparks turn off, so depletion is not the main factor controlling termination of SR Ca release.

Sham *et al.* (1998) addressed termination of SR Ca release in an elegant Ca spike study. They confirmed that SR Ca depletion was not the cause. Early L-type channel openings produced Ca spikes, but reopenings (or prolonged opening) of L-type Ca channels did not reactivate SR Ca release. Even large tail I_{Ca} (due to the Ca channel agonist FPL-64176) did not seem to induce local Ca release, unless the region hadn't already fired. These results argue strongly against stochastic attrition and suggest that some sort of inactivation process must occur. The inability to re-activate with large tail I_{Ca} would also favor a more absorbing inactivation, rather than adaptation as seen in isolated RyRs (Györke & Fill, 1993; pg 194-5). Functionally, it may not matter in the intact cell whether inactivation is absorbing or not, especially if the local $[Ca]_i$ cannot be physiologically driven high enough to reactivate the RyR (as in bilayers).

Ca spikes are a clever strategy to monitor Ca release flux more directly. However, trapping the Ca which leaves the SR has several major consequences which may alter the time course of SR Ca release. First, it prevents released Ca from potentially activating neighboring RyRs, tending to reduce release time and spatial spread. Second, it lowers local $[Ca]_i$ around the RyR, which may either reduce local activation (reducing release) or limit inactivation (enhancing Ca release). Third, it greatly delays reuptake of Ca by the SR which, may make local $[Ca]_{SR}$ depletion more severe (reducing total Ca release). This could be due to the electrochemical effect of lower $[Ca]_{SR}$ on release flux, but also the possible regulatory effect of $[Ca]_{SR}$.

While it is clear that RyR Ca flux inactivates, the mechanism is unresolved. While there is evidence for Ca-dependent inactivation (and adaptation; Chapter 7), models which include a fateful inactivation linked to activation (independent of Ca) can also explain cellular experiments (Stern *et al.*, 1999). There may even be two Ca-dependent steps 1) Ca-dependent adaptation, causing reduced mean open time (Zahradníková *et al.*, 1999b), and 2) a separate absorbing Ca-dependent inactivation caused only by very high [Ca] (1-10 mM, see Figs 102-3) on the downward side of the RyR2 P_o dependence on [Ca]. However, since local [Ca] would rarely reach this very high level, this absorbing state might not be readily achieved.

Recovery from Inactivation/Adaptation

Whether RyRs turn off by inactivation or adaptation, there must be some time required for these channels to return to their initial Ca sensitivity. This is analogous to recovery from inactivation for I_{Ca} or I_{Na}. Figure 121 shows an AP and Ca transient along with the recovery of I_{Ca}, SR Ca content, RyR availability and tension. Full recovery of contractile force in mammalian ventricle generally requires ~1-2 sec depending on temperature, species and other

A. AP and Ca transient

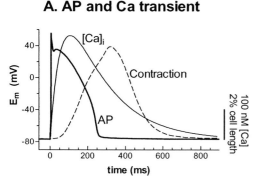

B. Recovery of E-C Coupling

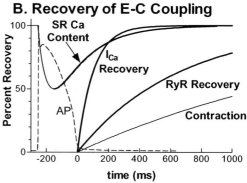

Figure 121. Recovery of E-C coupling in heart. **A.** AP, Ca transient and contraction recorded in rabbit ventricular myocyte at 37°C (by K. Schlotthauer). **B.** The AP is shown with time=0 reset to the end of repolarization. The SR Ca content is plotted as the reciprocal of the Ca transient assuming ~50% SR Ca release (recovery τ ~200 ms). An adjacent dashed curve (barely discernible) shows a 5 ms lag between SR Ca uptake and availability for release. I_{Ca}, RyR and tension recovery are described by τ=100 ms (Fig 57) τ=650 ms and τ=1.7 s, respectively, starting after AP repolarization.

conditions (Gibbons & Fozzard, 1975; Edman & Jóhannsson, 1976; Wolfhart, 1979; Lipsius *et al.*, 1982; Yue *et al.*, 1985; Wier & Yue, 1986).

I_{Ca} recovers from inactivation with a time constant (τ) of ~100 msec at –80 mV, but recovery is slower at more positive E_m (Fig 57, e.g. Kass & Sanguinetti, 1984; Josephson *et al.*, 1984; Lee *et al.*, 1985; Fischmeister & Hartzell, 1986; Hadley & Hume, 1987; Fedida *et al.*, 1987a; Tseng, 1988; Argibay *et al.*, 1988). I_{Ca} recovery can also overshoot and this may be related to Ca-dependent I_{Ca} facilitation (see pg 119). Early AP restitution may also influence I_{Ca} due to its E_m-dependence (e.g. see Boyett & Jewell, 1978, 1980).

The SR Ca content also recovers rapidly. Figure 121B shows that SR Ca content falls and recovers during the Ca transient (and SR Ca uptake is largely reflected in $[Ca]_i$ decline). In some early models of the force-frequency relationship it was supposed that time was required for Ca to move from an uptake to a release compartment (e.g. from longitudinal to junctional SR, Morad & Goldman, 1973; Edman & Jóhannsson, 1976; Wolfhart, 1979; Yue *et al.*, 1985). This hypothetical construct was useful in explaining the observed 1-2 sec delay between $[Ca]_i$ decline and ability to release Ca during an AP. However, Ca diffusion from longitudinal SR to junctional SR (< 1 μm) without membrane barriers should take << 5 msec (shown in Fig 121B as a broken curve, lagging the SR Ca content curve by 5 ms). Indeed, we now know that the Ca in the SR can be released in < 200 ms by application of caffeine or cold solution, despite a much longer recovery time for responsiveness to I_{Ca} or rapid Ca application (Fabiato, 1985b; Bers *et al.*, 1987; Sham *et al.*, 1998). Thus, the SR Ca release channel is refractory to activation via CICR, but not to activation by caffeine or cooling.

Fabiato (1985b) showed that recovery time of RyRs was accelerated by low $[Ca]_i$ in much the way I_{Ca} recovery is hastened by more negative E_m (Fig 57). Cheng *et al.* (1996) showed this recovery process (Fig 122) by triggering a depolarization-induced SR Ca release in the wake of a Ca wave passing through the cell. Figure 122 shows that for cell regions where the Ca wave passed before the image started (top) the local Ca transient has fully recovered and is uniform along the cell length. However, at the bottom of the cell, where the Ca wave has recently passed, the local RyRs are refractory to activation. The τ of recovery of local E-C coupling (Fig 122C) was ~650 ms. DelPrincipe *et al.* (1999) found that cellular CICR triggered by flash photolysis of caged Ca recovered with a τ of 320 ms, but after a localized SR Ca release they could not detect local refractoriness after 250 ms. They concluded that global SR depletion and rebinding of Ca to key intra-SR sites might be involved in the restitution process. The local Ca transient ends in <100 ms compared to >1 s for the global Ca transient. I suspect that Ca-dependent recovery (as proposed by Fabiato) is still important in restitution of E-C coupling, but intra-SR Ca may also be an important modulator. There may also be a slower phase of recovery of some RyRs from inactivation both macroscopically and microscopically, which takes several seconds (Satoh *et al.*, 1997). That will be discussed with respect to rest potentiation in Chapter 9 (Fig 138).

Thus, it appears that locally the gating of the RyR in the intact ventricular myocyte is governed by three key intrinsic factors: 1) local $[Ca]_i$ via CICR, inactivation and recovery, 2) $[Ca]_{SR}$, perhaps by modulating the $[Ca]_i$-dependence of channel gating and 3) recent history, reflecting inactivation and recovery from inactivation (which are both time- and Ca-dependent).

Spontaneous SR Ca Release, Cyclic Contractions and Ca Waves

In general, the inactivation of SR Ca release and time required for recovery from inactivation limit positive feedback of CICR, allowing cardiac relaxation and stabilizing resting $[Ca]_i$. Indeed, immediately after a twitch there is a reduction in Ca spark frequency which slowly recovers during rest without changes in $[Ca]_i$ or SR Ca load (Satoh *et al.*, 1997). However, when SR Ca load is increased above a certain level (e.g. by raising $[Ca]_o$) Ca spark frequency is greatly increased and many Ca sparks appear immediately after the twitch. These can trigger Ca waves which propagate through the cell via CICR (Cheng *et al.*, 1996; Satoh *et al.*, 1997). Clearly elevation of SR Ca content can partially defeat the intrinsic E-C coupling safeguards against the positive feedback inherent in CICR. High $[Ca]_{SR}$ may alter RyR gating in two ways: 1) it may increase the sensitivity to activation by $[Ca]_i$ (Fig 103A), and 2) it may greatly hasten the recovery of RyRs from inactivation (allowing Ca waves). These effects could be interdependent and should be incorporated into future refinements of RyR gating schemes.

Cheng *et al.* (1996) detected discrete Ca sparks which initiate Ca waves, and for slowly propagating waves, Ca sparks could be detected along the wavefront. Thus, Ca waves, like normal global Ca transients, are still caused by the temporal and spatial summation of Ca sparks (although they are not temporally synchronized during waves). The combination of reduced refractoriness and increased Ca-sensitivity of the RyRs allow longitudinal Ca wave propagation by CICR, which normally does not occur (Parker *et al.*, 1996). The shortening of refractory period cannot be complete, because when two Ca waves approach each other from opposite directions they almost invariably annihilate each other on contact (i.e. they don't pass through each other; Lipp & Niggli, 1993). While these Ca waves can be arrhythmogenic and contribute to mechanical dysfunction (see Chapter 10), they are also beneficial in limiting Ca overload. This is because spontaneous SR Ca release at resting E_m gives the Na/Ca exchanger a thermodynamic advantage in extruding Ca from the cell (Chapter 6), and 15-20% of the SR Ca content is extruded during a wave (Díaz *et al.*, 1997a,b). This means that if the cell can extrude

A. Cell

B. Line Scan

C. Recovery

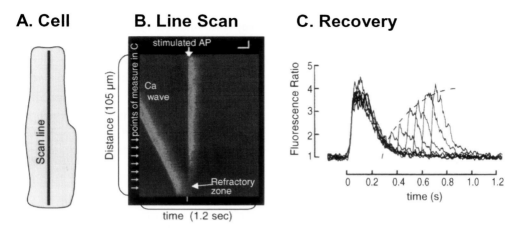

Figure 122. Microscopic recovery of E-C coupling in a rat ventricular myocyte. **A.** schematic cell showing a longitudinal scan line. **B.** Ca wave (measured with fluo-3) is propagating from the top of the cell toward the bottom at constant velocity (angle implies ~120 μm/s). At the point indicated an AP is stimulated causing a spatially uniform Δ[Ca]$_i$ in the top half of cell, but the region near the bottom is partially refractory due to the recent passage of the wave there. **C.** [Ca]$_i$ measured at the points indicated in B, time aligned to the wave front. Note the uniform and large local [Ca] during the wave at each point and the progressive increase in Δ[Ca]$_i$ as the local RyRs recovery from prior activation/inactivation during the wave. Data from Cheng *et al.* (1996); image kindly supplied by W.J. Lederer.

Ca, these waves will tend to progressively decline. However, when Na/Ca exchange is inhibited (e.g. by Na-pump blockade or [Na]$_o$ removal) waves can continue repeatedly as oscillations.

Fabiato & Fabiato (1972) showed that elevated [Ca] in skinned cardiac myocytes induced cyclic contractions. These are also observed in intact myocytes and muscles, where they are also manifest as contractile or Ca waves (propagating at 100->2000 μm/s) or as a series of aftercontractions (Kass *et al.*, 1978; Orchard *et al.*, 1983; Stern *et al.*, 1983; Wier *et al.*, 1983; Allen *et al.*, 1984b; Kort & Lakatta, 1984; Capogrossi *et al.*, 1986a,b; Mulder *et al.*, 1989; Backx *et al.*, 1989; Takamatsu & Wier, 1990). In general these phenomena are observed where Ca overload is expected (e.g. high [Ca]$_o$, low [Na]$_o$, high stimulation frequency, Na-pump inhibition, long depolarizations and reduced sarcolemmal permeability barrier). Fabiato (1985b) argued that cyclical Ca release is mechanistically different from CICR, partly because it is seen at [Ca] where CICR can be inactivated (e.g. 30 μM Ca). He also argued that they represent a purely pathological state of Ca overload. Indeed, the lack of spontaneous contractions is often used as a criterion for healthy isolated cardiac myocytes. O'Neill *et al.* (1990b) showed that the normal systolic Δ[Ca]$_i$ cannot propagate in rat ventricular myocytes without Ca overload. While Ca waves may be pathophysiological, I prefer to think of the behavior of CICR in a continuum, where very high [Ca]$_{SR}$ modulates intrinsic RyR properties (increasing [Ca]$_i$-sensitivity and decreasing refractoriness), allowing local release to propagate.

Ca waves could propagate by saltatory conduction of CICR via Ca sparks, as above. An alternative would be that a heavily Ca loaded SR region reaches its limit first (dumping its Ca to the cytoplasm), then extra Ca uptake in neighboring SR could contribute to activation of release in the next region by raising [Ca]$_{SR}$ (Takamatsu & Wier, 1990). By blocking the SR Ca-ATPase Lukyanenko *et al.* (1999) showed that this sort of Ca uptake by the SR ahead of the wave front is not important in wave propagation. Moreover, they showed that sensitizing the RyR to $[Ca]_i$ by low [caffeine], allowed propagating Ca waves to be observed at much lower SR Ca loads. Thus, sensitization of CICR to $[Ca]_i$, abbreviated refractoriness and the inherent larger rate of Ca release at higher $[Ca]_{SR}$ must be the predominant factors in allowing propagating Ca waves in cardiac myocytes.

In conclusion, CICR triggered by $I_{Ca,L}$ is probably the central means by which SR Ca release is controlled in cardiac muscle. However, some other sources of trigger Ca, VDCR and IP$_3$ICR have also been proposed to play roles. These are considered below.

OTHER E-C COUPLING MECHANISMS IN HEART

Alternative Ca Triggers in Cardiac CICR

There can be little doubt that $I_{Ca,L}$ is a robust and sufficient Ca trigger in cardiac E-C coupling via CICR. There are several other ways that Ca can enter the cell during depolarization that might also contribute: 1) $I_{Ca,T}$, 2) Na/Ca exchange (either driven by E_m or by local $[Na]_i$ secondary to I_{Na}) and 3) $I_{Ca,TTX}$ or Ca entry via Na channels.

T-type I_{Ca} ($I_{Ca,T}$) is undetectable in most ventricular myocyte types, but can be significant in Purkinje and some atrial cells (see pg 102). It is also unknown whether T-type Ca channels are located at the sarcolemmal-SR junctions. Thus, $I_{Ca,T}$ cannot be a major player in CICR in most ventricular myocytes. Even in guinea-pig ventricular myocytes $I_{Ca,T}$ is small compared to $I_{Ca,L}$. In principle, $I_{Ca,T}$ could work like $I_{Ca,L}$ if the T-type Ca channels were preferentially localized at junctions, and the effectiveness of a given $I_{Ca,T}$ trigger would be expected to be comparable to that of $I_{Ca,L}$. This was directly tested by Sipido *et al.* (1998a) in guinea-pig ventricular myocytes and Zhou & January (1998) in canine Purkinje fibers. They measured SR Ca release induced by comparable (and measured) $I_{Ca,T}$ and $I_{Ca,L}$. SR Ca release triggered by $I_{Ca,T}$ was greatly delayed in onset and also slower than that triggered by a comparable $I_{Ca,L}$ trigger. Indeed, the $\Delta[Ca]_i$ induced by a larger $I_{Ca,T}$ (at -40 mV) was ~6 times smaller than for a smaller $I_{Ca,L}$ (at -30 mV, Sipido *et al.*, 1998a). These results suggest that T-type Ca channels are <u>not</u> preferentially located in junctional regions in these cells. Thus, $I_{Ca,T}$ can trigger SR Ca release, but obviously not in ventricular myocytes which lack $I_{Ca,T}$. Even in cells which exhibit $I_{Ca,T}$, it is probably only a very minor contributor to cardiac E-C coupling, overshadowed by $I_{Ca,L}$.

˙Ca influx via Na/Ca exchange might also trigger SR Ca release, as suggested by our earlier work with elevated $[Na]_i$ (Bers *et al.*, 1988). Leblanc & Hume (1990) showed a tetrodotoxin-sensitive component of contraction. Their data gave credence to the hypothesis that Na influx via Na channels raised local $[Na]_i$ and that this caused Ca entry via Na/Ca exchange to trigger SR Ca release (see Fig 74). Subsequent studies have supported these results (Levesque *et al.*, 1994; Lipp & Niggli, 1994; Vites & Wasserstrom, 1996). However, other results suggest that this mechanism does not contribute appreciably to the physiological activation of SR Ca release (Sham *et al.*, 1992; Bouchard *et al.*, 1993; Sipido *et al.*, 1995b). They suggested that the above observations were due to either E_m-escape during voltage clamp or gradual changes in SR Ca load. Before dismissal of this hypothesis, it would be valuable to know how large and how long-lasting local elevation of $[Na]_i$ produced by I_{Na} might be, and whether it occurs in the junctional cleft (see Fig 74).

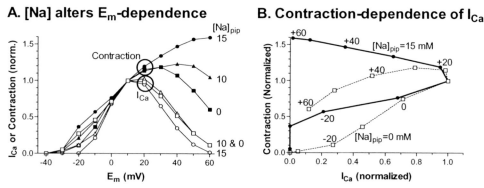

Figure 123. [Na]$_i$ and E$_m$-dependence of contraction. **A.** E$_m$-dependence of contraction and I$_{Ca}$ in voltage clamped rabbit ventricular myocyte (E$_m$ steps from −50 mV to the indicated E$_m$) with different [Na] in the patch pipette ([Na]$_{pip}$), normalized to the value at +10 mV. **B.** I$_{Ca}$-dependence of contraction for data in A. Note that for the same I$_{Ca}$ amplitude the contraction is higher at more positive E$_m$ (mean data from Litwin *et al., 1998* are replotted).

Ca entry via Na/Ca exchange can also be activated directly by depolarization (Chapter 6). The reversal potential for this Na/Ca exchange current at rest is typically −30 to −80 mV. Thus, during the rapid upstroke of the action potential to +50 mV Ca influx via outward I$_{Na/Ca}$ is favored thermodynamically. Several labs have provided evidence that this Ca entry via Na/Ca exchange can trigger SR Ca release and contraction, especially at large positive E$_m$ and in the absence of I$_{Ca,L}$ (Levi *et al.,* 1994; Baartscheer *et al.,*1996; Wasserstrom & Vites, 1996; Litwin *et al.,* 1998). Figure 123 shows that with higher [Na] in the dialyzing patch pipette the E$_m$-dependence of contraction becomes less bell-shaped (*vs.* Fig 106A and 117). Thus, there is greater contraction and presumed SR Ca release for a given I$_{Ca}$ at more positive E$_m$ (Fig 123B), especially with high pipette [Na]. This is what would be expected for Ca entry via I$_{Na/Ca}$ (Chapter 6). Surprisingly this was even true with zero Na in the pipette.

Sipido *et al.* (1997) found the usual (pg 203, Fig 106) bell-shaped E$_m$-dependence of both peak I$_{Ca}$ and Δ[Ca]$_i$ during the first 20 ms, even with 20 mM [Na] in the patch pipette. I$_{Ca}$ triggered a rapid [Ca]$_i$ rise (Fig 124B) and an additional very slow [Ca]$_i$ rise at positive E$_m$ (likely due to Ca entry via I$_{Na/Ca}$). The eventual peak [Ca]$_i$ (at ~250 ms with 20 mM [Na]$_i$) showed an E$_m$-dependence like that in Fig 123A for 10-15 mM [Na]$_{pip}$. These two kinetic components of [Ca]$_i$ rise are difficult to resolve in contraction records. With I$_{Ca}$ blocked, Sipido *et al.* (1997) showed that outward I$_{Na/Ca}$ could trigger SR Ca release at positive E$_m$. At E$_m$ = +70 mV, I$_{Na/Ca}$-induced Ca release rate was almost as high as that induced by I$_{Ca}$ at +10 mV (Fig 124A-B). However, the I$_{Na/Ca}$-induced Ca release was delayed, requiring 60-120 ms (*vs.* 10 ms for I$_{Ca}$), and the efficacy of a given Ca influx in triggering SR Ca release was ~4-fold lower for I$_{Na/Ca}$ *vs.* I$_{Ca}$ (Fig 124C-D). The apparent delay is important, because it means that even at +60 mV, I$_{Ca}$ activates CICR long before the I$_{Na/Ca}$-mediated Ca influx is sufficient to activate release. Thus, when both I$_{Ca}$ and I$_{Na/Ca}$ triggers are functional CICR is controlled almost entirely by I$_{Ca}$. It may be noted that this is even the case for this unphysiologically high [Na]$_i$, using 20 mM [Na] in the dialyzing pipette. Normal [Na]$_i$ is less than half of that in rabbit ventricular myocytes.

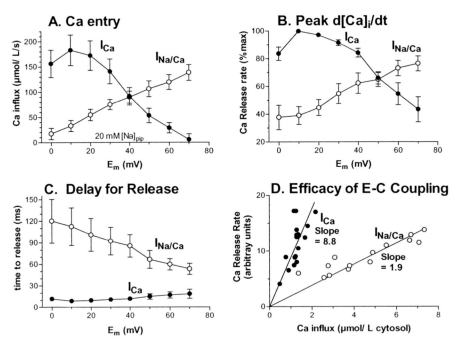

Figure 124. Comparison of I_{Ca} and $I_{Na/Ca}$ in triggering SR Ca release. Data are from voltage clamped guinea-pig ventricular myocytes (225 ms depolarizations from $E_m = -45$ mV) with K-aspartate and 20 mM Na in the pipette. **A.** E_m-dependence of Ca entry via I_{Ca} or $I_{Na/Ca}$. **B.** Maximal rate of rise of $[Ca]_i$ (from fluo-3 signal), normalized to the maximum in the same cell. **C.** Time from depolarization to maximum rate of $[Ca]_i$ rise. **D.** E-C coupling efficacy of Ca influx via I_{Ca} *vs.* $I_{Na/Ca}$. Fluxes were converted assuming 6.44 pF/pL (data from Sipido *et al.*, 1997, kindly supplied by K.R. Sipido).

Indeed, when an L-type Ca channel opens (early in the AP) high local $[Ca]_i$ can prevent further Ca influx via Na/Ca exchange (see Fig 74). Thus, Ca entry via $I_{Na/Ca}$ may provide a back-up or redundant system for activation of SR Ca release, or one that allows gradual rise of local $[Ca]_i$ that works synergistically with the L-type Ca channel opening. López-López *et al.*, (1995) found that Ca entry via Na/Ca exchange produced slow uniform rise in $[Ca]_i$ throughout the cell (rather than Ca sparks). Thus, Na/Ca exchange may help set local junctional $[Ca]_i$ for local I_{Ca} activation, or may bring some Ca in during the latent time before a particular Ca channel opens.

Initial studies reported that Na/Ca exchangers reside mainly in T-tubules (Frank *et al.*, 1992) or uniformly in the sarcolemma (Kieval *et al.*, 1992). Scriven *et al.*, (2000) found that the Na/Ca exchanger was not co-localized with either Na channels or RyRs, whereas DHPRs were highly colocalized with RyRs (Table 4). This suggests that the Na/Ca exchanger is not in the ideal place for either responding to I_{Na} or directly triggering SR Ca release. In addition, the unitary flux though the Na/Ca exchanger is perhaps 1000 times lower than $I_{Ca,L}$. Thus, a Ca influx trigger comparable to a single L-type Ca channel would require ~1000 Na/Ca exchanger molecules. This would place physical constraints on the ability of Na/Ca exchange to produce a comparable localized Ca trigger signal for E-C coupling (requiring $>10^4$ exchangers/μm^2 in the junction; see pg 146). Thus, Ca influx via Na/Ca exchange can trigger SR Ca release, but the physiological role is unclear. On the other hand, Na/Ca exchange may become more important in

E-C coupling when I_{Ca} is reduced, $[Na]_i$ is increased or Na/Ca exchange expression is upregulated as in heart failure (Chapter 10).

Ca entry via tetrodotoxin-sensitive Ca current ($I_{Ca,TTX}$) was reported in the absence of $[Na]_o$ and attributed to a distinct subpopulation of Na channels (LeMaire *et al.*,1995; Aggarwal *et al.*, 1997). While this $I_{Ca,TTX}$ could mediate CICR, it is unclear that any appreciable Ca entry occurs in the presence of physiological $[Na]_o$. Santana *et al.* (1998; Cruz *et al.*, 1999) showed provocative data to suggest that cardiac Na channel selectivity could be altered dramatically by either β-adrenergic agonists, ouabain or digoxin. Based on shifts of the I_{Na} reversal potential they inferred that Na channel P_{Ca}/P_{Na} increased from essentially zero to >1, making the Na channel prefer Ca over Na (termed "slip-mode conductance"). This TTX-sensitive Ca entry appeared able to trigger SR Ca release. The authors proposed this as a novel mechanism explaining the inotropic effects of β-adrenergic agonists and cardiac glycosides (effects generally attributed to increased I_{Ca} & SR Ca-pump activity for β-adrenergic agonists, or to Na/K-ATPase inhibition and Na/Ca exchange for glycosides). Nuss & Marbán (1999) found no evidence at all for altered P_{Ca}/P_{Na} in cells with heterologous expression of cardiac α and $β_1$ Na channel subunits, although Cruz *et al.* (1999) in similar heterologous expression experiments found effects which were quite like their results in cardiac myocytes (Santana *et al.*, 1998). The provocative finding of a huge change in Na channel selectivity induced by cAMP or ouabain has eluded detection by other groups and is not widely accepted. For example, DelPrincipe *et al.* (2000) could not detect any Ca influx via I_{Na} with β-adrenergic agonists (using optical measurement of Ca influx), indicating a maximal P_{Ca}/P_{Na} of 0.04 for I_{Na}. Chandra *et al.* (1999) found $P_{Ca}/P_{Na} = 0.017$ for cardiac I_{Na}, which was unchanged by adrenergic stimulation. We also find no effects at all of ouabain or digoxin in myocytes which have been depleted of intra- and extracellular Na, to prevent Na/Ca exchange (Altamirano *et al.*, 1999). It is also unclear whether $I_{Ca,TTX}$ and slip-mode conductance are related (Wier & Balke, 2000). Further clarification would be useful.

In conclusion, the central physiological Ca trigger in CICR appears to be $I_{Ca,L}$. T-type channels are either not present at all or not localized at the junction, making them weak substitutes. Ca entry via Na/Ca exchange can induce SR Ca release, but in normal physiological conditions it brings in too little Ca, too late, and again, not as well focused at the RyR, when compared to $I_{Ca,L}$. However, Na/Ca exchange may modulate E-C coupling and under certain conditions its role in CICR may be enhanced. TTX-sensitive Ca entry will require further study. For now I consider its role in E-C coupling as speculative.

Voltage-Dependent Ca Release (VDCR) in Heart

Previous sections provide compelling evidence for VDCR in skeletal muscle and overwhelming experimental evidence against VDCR in cardiac muscle (even though some RyRs might interact with DHPRs, see pg 212-213). Despite this evidence a series of studies have suggested a VDCR mechanism in cardiac myocytes, similar to that in skeletal muscle, with an E_m-dependence negative to the normal $I_{Ca,L}$ activation and this VDCR is apparently not blocked by nifedipine (Ferrier & Howlett, 1995; Hobai *et al.*, 1997b; Howlett *et al.*, 1998; Ferrier *et al.*, 1998, 2000; Mason & Ferrier, 1999). Depolarization appears to require intracellular cAMP, but not Ca influx to trigger SR Ca release. On the other hand, this VDCR (unlike that in skeletal muscle) requires extracellular Ca and this Ca-dependence makes it somewhat less compelling as a Ca-influx independent E-C coupling mechanism. Most of these studies have focused on a two-step E_m protocol to separately activate VDCR and CICR. The first step to –40 mV activates VDCR and the second step from –40 to 0 mV activates CICR. They reported that the VDCR component was more sensitive to 30 nM ryanodine and 200 µM tetracaine (opposite to skeletal muscle) and that CICR was more sensitive to block by Cd and nifedipine. There are several issues that have limited the widespread acceptance of VDCR in heart, despite these intriguing observations.

First, extracellular Ca is required and other divalent or trivalent cations do not substitute. This certainly differs from VDCR in skeletal muscle where many mono- and divalent cations readily support VDCR (pg 208). Being able to demonstrate VDCR without Ca would allow clearer distinction from CICR. Moreover, since CICR is very selective for Ca over all other ions, the similar high Ca-selectivity of putative VDCR is a concern. Second, cardiac VDCR requires strong stimulation of cAMP or PKA. The powerful stimulation of I_{Ca} by cAMP makes it very difficult to completely block I_{Ca} and the shift of I_{Ca} activation to more negative E_m (Fig 64) means that I_{Ca} will indeed be activated during the VDCR step to –40 mV. It might also explain why they find apparent VDCR activation and availability at E_m negative to that for basal I_{Ca} activation. These studies use K-containing solutions, making it particularly difficult to verify complete block of I_{Ca} (an essential point to rule out CICR). Indeed, cAMP broadens the normal bell-shaped $\Delta[Ca]_i$-dependence (Hussain & Orchard, 1997; Piacentino et al., 2000) such that a very small fraction of maximal I_{Ca} can trigger a large SR Ca release (at more positive and negative E_m). This relates to the next point. Third, the SR Ca load in the myocytes is very high where VDCR is reported (due to PKA phosphorylation of phospholamban and enhanced SR Ca uptake). The high SR Ca content strongly sensitizes SR Ca release to trigger Ca (seen in Fig 119, even without PKA). Thus, even a tiny fraction of unblocked I_{Ca} can lead to substantial SR Ca release and the efficacy of a single channel opening at –40 mV to trigger Ca release is very high (Fig 117B). Since cAMP is such a powerful promoter of CICR, this makes it harder to isolate any VDCR. Fourth, if VDCR is important in cardiac E-C coupling it should be very robust, and not require special conditions to be observed (e.g. high cAMP). Many investigators over the years have used very similar (if not identical) conditions and found only evidence supporting CICR and refuting VDCR in heart (see CICR section). We have never seen results consistent with VDCR in heart in my lab. Piacentino et al. (2000) made a concerted effort to mimic the conditions used in Ferrier & Howlett's work and saw no evidence for VDCR. All of their data were fully explained by CICR. In conclusion, some of the data suggesting VDCR in heart are interesting, but I am not convinced that VDCR is functional in cardiac myocytes.

Other E-C Coupling Proposals

Alkalosis was proposed as an SR Ca release activator (Nakamura & Schwartz, 1972) and can increase RyR open probability (Ma et al., 1988), but also increases SR Ca accumulation (Fabiato, 1985e). It seems unlikely that alkalosis is a physiological activator of SR Ca release, although the pH sensitivity of SR Ca uptake and release may modify SR Ca content, Ca release and contraction (Orchard & Kentish, 1990). Early observations of Na effects on Ca uptake in SR vesicles raised the possibility that local elevation of $[Na]_i$ during the cardiac action potential might directly induce Ca release from the SR (Palmer & Posey, 1967; Vassort, 1973; Caillé et *al.*, 1979). However, cardiac SR vesicle and skinned fiber studies showed this to be unlikely (Jones *et al.*, 1977; Fabiato, 1986c). These phenomena may be related to displacement of Ca bound at the inner sarcolemmal surface by mM Na (see pg 51), or local $[Na]_i$ elevation near the sarcolemma due to I_{Na} (Akera *et al.*, 1976). However, these are still variants of CICR (see pg 232-235) and contractions are abolished in the absence of Ca_o, despite maintained Na entry (Figs 105A & 115). Heavy metals (Ag^+, Hg^{2+}, Cu^{2+}, Zn^{2+}, Cd^{2+}) and sulfhydryl oxidation can induce rapid Ca release in isolated SR vesicles (Abramson *et al.*, 1983, 1987; Salama & Abramson, 1984; Trimm *et al.*, 1986; Prabhu & Salama, 1990). These may certainly modulate RyR gating (see pg 197), but surely are not the normal driving factors in cardiac E-C coupling.

IP_3-INDUCED Ca RELEASE (IP_3ICR)

Inositol(1,4,5)-trisphosphate Induced Ca Release in Smooth Muscle

IP_3 induces endoplasmic reticulum (ER) Ca release in many cell types (Berridge, 1987, 1993, 1995; Berridge & Galione, 1988; Berridge & Irvine, 1989). In smooth muscle IP_3 induces SR Ca release in both skinned fibers and SR vesicles (Suematsu *et al.*, 1984; Carsten & Miller, 1985; Smith *et al.*, 1985b; Somlyo *et al.*, 1985; Yamamato & van Breemen, 1985; Watras & Benevolensky, 1987). IP_3-activated Ca channels have also been described in SR vesicles from brain, smooth muscle and cardiac muscle (see pg 200-201; Ehrlich & Watras, 1988). The IP_3 activated Ca release in smooth muscle appears to be large enough and fast enough to explain adrenergic agonist induced E-C coupling (Somlyo *et al.*, 1985, 1988; Walker *et al.*, 1987).

A challenge in studying IP_3ICR in isolated muscles is overcoming diffusional limitations such that IP_3 concentration rises very quickly at the SR surface (and is not degraded on its way to the SR). The experiments in Fig 125 overcome these limitations in permeabilized smooth muscle by laser photolysis of caged IP_3 and caged phenylephrine (an α_1-adrenergic agonist; Somlyo *et al.*, 1988). The release of ~1 µM IP_3 activated contraction with a 0.4 sec lag. This latency is less

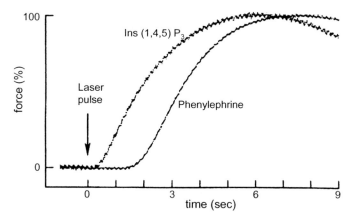

Figure 125. Activation of contraction in guinea-pig smooth muscle strips by photolysis of caged IP_3 or caged phenylephrine (from Somlyo *et al.*, 1988, with permission). Portal vein strips were depolarized (143 mM KCl) for the phenylephrine experiment or permeabilized (50 mg/ml saponin) for the IP_3 experiment (~10% of the 50 µM phenylephrine & 10 µM IP_3 were released by a 50 nsec laser pulse).

than when the muscle was activated by release of ~5 μM phenylephrine (1.8 sec). These results are consistent with the relatively slow contractile activation of smooth muscle and the additional steps involved with phenylephrine activation (e.g. receptor activation of phospholipase C which forms IP_3 and diacylglycerol). Smooth muscle also has a well developed metabolic pathway for production of IP_3 (coupled to adrenergic receptors and G-proteins) and also for degradation of IP_3 (Sasaguri *et al.*, 1985; Saida & Van Breeman, 1987; Walker *et al.*, 1987; Somlyo *et al.*, 1988). Heparin, which blocks the IP_3 receptor (Worley *et al.*, 1987), can also inhibit phenylephrine and IP_3-induced contractions in smooth muscle (Kobayashi *et al.*, 1988, 1989). Thus, IP_3ICR is clearly physiologically important in smooth muscle (especially in the case of pharmaco-mechanical coupling).

CICR is also apparent in smooth muscle (Saida, 1982) and there are ryanodine-sensitive Ca pools in vascular smooth muscle (Ito *et al.*, 1986; Hwang & van Breemen, 1987; Ashida *et al.*, 1988; Kanmura *et al.*, 1988). Iino *et al.* (1988) showed that guinea-pig smooth muscle has two intracellular Ca pools: one which is both IP_3 and caffeine/ryanodine sensitive and a second which is only IP_3 sensitive. Thus, IP_3ICR and CICR mechanisms coexist in SR regions in smooth muscle. The importance of both IP_3ICR and CICR in smooth muscle E-C coupling is compelling (Somlyo *et al.*, 1988; van Breemen & Saida, 1989; Somlyo & Himpens, 1989; Somlyo & Somlyo, 1990, 1994; Himpens *et al.*, 1995; Van Breeman *et al.*, 1995; Bolton *et al.*, 1999; Austin & Wray, 2000; Jaggar *et al.*, 2000). However, it is not as clear exactly how these two mechanisms interact. Indeed, the relative predominance of IP_3ICR and CICR varies in different smooth muscle cell types. IP_3R and RyR are each located in both superficial and deep SR in smooth muscle myocytes (Nixon *et al.*, 1994; Lesh *et al.*, 1998) and in intestinal smooth muscle there are ~10 times as many IP_3Rs as RyRs (Wibo & Godfraind, 1994).

Smooth muscle is activated by receptor agonists (pharmacomechanical coupling, independent of E_m) as well as by action potentials and tonic depolarizations. This additional heterogeneity makes it particularly difficult to generalize, and I will not go into detail here with respect to smooth muscle (for more detail see the reviews cited above). Some smooth muscles, like urinary bladder, exhibit phasic contractions triggered by APs (Heppner *et al.*, 1997). In these muscles, there appears to be prominent CICR via RyR as in cardiac muscle (contributing ~70% of the activating Ca). In tonic smooth muscle (e.g. arteries) the majority of activating Ca appears to come from Ca influx via L-type Ca channels, probably as a window current at depolarized E_m (Knot & Nelson, 1998; Knot *et al.*, 1998). There are also receptor-operated channels (typically non-selective cation channels) which can initiate depolarization (pharmaco-electrical coupling). This can result in either an AP in phasic smooth muscle (with I_{Ca} causing the AP upstroke), or bring E_m into the range where a significant Ca window current occurs (−40 to −20 mV, Fig 57) allowing some steady Ca entry.

Ca activated K currents carried by big conductance K channels (BK_{Ca}) are involved in negative feedback by causing hyper- or repolarization, thereby turning off further Ca entry. BK_{Ca} channels are known to be responsible for spontaneous transient outward current spikes (STOCs) observed in smooth muscle cells (Benham & Bolton, 1986). These STOCs and the high [Ca] required to activate BK_{Ca} channels (2-10 μM), led to the suggestion that local submembrane $[Ca]_i$ may transiently be much higher than bulk $[Ca]_i$ (see review by Jaggar *et al.*, 2000). This would

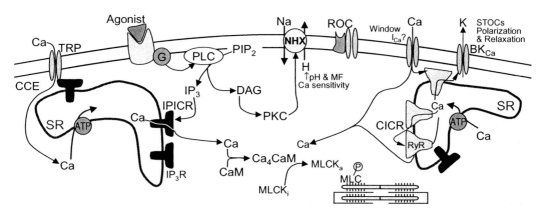

Figure 126. E-C coupling in smooth muscle (IP$_3$ICR & CICR). Receptor agonist (e.g. α_1-adrenergic)
activate the receptor and a GTP-binding protein coupled to that receptor activates phospholipase C (PLC),
which produces IP$_3$ and diacylglycerol (DAG). IP$_3$ stimulates SR Ca release and DAG activates protein
kinase C (PKC) which can modify contractile proteins, ion channels and Na/H exchange. Depolarization
can be initiated by receptor activated channels (ROC) which can promote L-type Ca channel opening.
CICR also occurs via RyRs in smooth muscle and can contribute to propagating Ca waves. SR Ca release
via RyRs as Ca sparks also opens Ca-activated K channels (BK$_{Ca}$), which produce spontaneous transient
outward currents (STOCs), which can hyperpolarize E$_m$ and thereby deactivate I$_{Ca}$. Depletion of SR Ca
stores can also activate capacitative Ca entry (CCE) via a mechanical signal from the IP$_3$R to the TRP
(transient receptor potential) channel. Ca activates smooth muscle contraction by binding to calmodulin
(CaM), which activates myosin light chain kinase (MLCK) to phosphorylate myosin light chain (MLC) such
that actin and myosin to interact. This contrasts with striated muscle where Ca activates myofilaments by
direct binding to troponin C (TnC).

also be consistent with a diffusion restricted space between the SR and sarcolemma, similar to
that proposed in the superficial buffer barrier hypothesis (van Breeman *et al.*, 1995).

Figure 126 shows E-C coupling in smooth muscle (Kamm & Stull, 1989; Somlyo &
Himpens, 1989; Somlyo & Somlyo, 1990, 1994; van Breemen *et al.*, 1995; Bolton *et al.*, 1999;
Jaggar *et al.*, 2000). Pharmacomechanical coupling is started by a receptor agonist, rather than
an action potential as in striated muscle. Agonist occupied receptor activates a GTP binding
protein which stimulates phospholipase C to cleave phosphatidylinositol-(4,5)-bisphosphate
(PIP$_2$) into IP$_3$ and 1,2-diacylglycerol (DAG). DAG activates PKC which stimulates Na/H
exchange causing alkalosis and increased myofilament Ca sensitivity. PKC also phosphorylates
myofilament proteins and membrane channels directly to modulate their function. Depolarization can be induced by receptor activated channels (or depolarization in a neighboring
electrically coupled cell). This can activate L-type Ca channels, and in these cells with large
surface: volume ratio a given Ca flux (pA/pF) can have a strong impact on [Ca]$_i$. Ca entry can
trigger CICR involving RyRs, and RyRs and IP$_3$Rs can interact in producing both Ca waves and
Ca oscillations in smooth muscle. Smooth muscle myofilaments are activated by Ca differently
than striated muscle. Ca binds to calmodulin to activate a myosin light chain kinase (MLCK).
Phosphorylation of the regulatory myosin light chains then allows actin-activation of myosin
ATPase activity. Crossbridge cycling is also much slower in smooth muscle, which allows tonic
force (attached crossbridges) at relatively low energy cost. Several chemical reactions must

occur along the E-C coupling pathway, accounting for the slow onset of force development in smooth muscle compared to striated muscle.

Ca sparks in Smooth Muscle: SR Ca Release can Contribute to Relaxation

Nelson *et al.* (1995) demonstrated Ca sparks in vascular smooth muscle cells. These Ca sparks are longer in duration than those in cardiac myocytes (20 ms rise time and 50-60 ms half-decay time). It is now clear that Ca sparks are seen in most smooth muscle and are undoubtedly the direct cause of the STOCs which are mediated by BK_{Ca} channels (Jaggar *et al.*, 2000). A particularly intriguing aspect of this work is that local SR Ca release as Ca sparks can serve to relax smooth muscle by local activation of BK_{Ca} channels and STOCs which hyperpolarize the whole cell (thereby shutting off Ca entry via I_{Ca}). Thus, a local $[Ca]_i$ rise which does not appreciably alter global $[Ca]_i$ or contractile activation, can induce global $[Ca]_i$ decline and relaxation. That is, local CICR can lead to global relaxation (rather than contraction as in cardiac muscle). BK_{Ca} channels have a very large unitary conductance (120 pS) and one channel may contribute a ~10 pA current in the cell. Thus a cluster of 10-100 BK_{Ca} channels can produce 100-1000 pA of outward current. With the high input impedance of smooth muscle cells, this can strongly hyperpolarize the cell.

There are also small conductance Ca activated K channels (SK_{Ca}) which may participate in this negative feedback loop and Ca-activated Cl channels which can contribute to depolarization (but of course can only raise E_m as far as E_{Cl}), and activation of these Cl channels can lead to spontaneous transient inward currents (STICs). Although STOCs and STICs can even coexist in the same cells (ZhuGe *et al.*, 1998), STOCs decays much faster than STICs. This is presumably due to the lower $[Ca]_i$ required to activate $I_{Cl(Ca)}$ in smooth muscle (365 nM, Pacaud *et al.*, 1992; note that this differs markedly from cardiac $I_{Cl(Ca)}$, pg 85). BK_{Ca} channels would only be briefly activated while local $[Ca]_i$ is > 1 μM. Blocking RyR (or BK_{Ca} channels) can lead to ~10 mV depolarization and an increase in tonic force in cerebral arteries (Knot *et al.*, 1998), consistent with a tonic basal contribution of Ca spark- and BK_{Ca}-dependent hyperpolarization in this tissue. Thus, there is a complex interplay of factors in smooth muscle, but clearly CICR from RyRs can contribute either in a positive way to E-C coupling (especially in phasic muscles) or in negative feedback producing relaxation. There do not appear to be Ca-activated K channels in cardiac myocytes.

Capacitative Ca entry in Smooth Muscle

Depletion of intracellular Ca stores in a wide variety of cell types results in the activation of Ca influx, known as capacitive Ca entry (CCE, Putney, 1986, 1997; Putney & Ribeiro, 2000; Berridge, 1995). Hoth & Penner (1992, 1993) showed that the Ca entry pathway was a Ca-selective current, which they called I_{crac} (Ca-release activated current). CCE does not occur in cardiac muscle, but has been seen in several vascular smooth muscle preparations (Missiaen *et al.*, 1990; Baró & Eisner, 1992; Blatter, 1995). There was substantial controversy about whether the signal from the SR/ER was mediated by a diffusible messenger molecule or by direct conformational coupling between an ER/SR Ca store sensor and the I_{crac} channel (see Putney & Ribeiro, 2000, for review). Hardie & Minke (1993) suggested that the *Drosophila* transient receptor potential (TRP) channel protein might be invlved in CCE. Kiselyov *et al.* (1998, 1999) showed that IP$_3$R and TRP3 directly interact, that the IP$_3$R (even added exogenously) could activate 66 pS TRP3 channels and that the N-terminal IP$_3$ binding domain was sufficient to activate TRP3. Additionally, an endogenous Ca channel was similarly modified by IP$_3$ and IP$_3$R (Zubov *et al.*, 1999). The N-terminal of the IP$_3$R may activate TRP channels, but when the ER/SR is Ca-loaded the activation is repressed. Thus, the IP$_3$R might serve as a sensor of the ER/SR [Ca] and transmit this signal to the cytoplasmic side of the IP$_3$R where it transmits regulatory information to the TRP channel Fig 126). This may relate to the apparent luminal [Ca]$_{SR}$-dependence of RyR2 gating (Pg 194-195, 225) and to the retrograde molecular feedback from RyR1 to the skeletal muscle DHPR (pg 211). Indeed, like cardiac cells and isolated RyR2, the SR Ca release via RyR in smooth muscle and via IP$_3$R seems to be sensitive to luminal [Ca] (ZhuGe *et al.*, 1999; Missiaen *et al.*, 1994; Berridge, 1997). The precise role of CCE in smooth muscle and its interaction with CICR, IP$_3$ICR and other Ca channels will require further study.

IP$_3$ Induced Ca Release in Skeletal Muscle

The possibility that IP$_3$ is involved in skeletal muscle E-C coupling was raised by observations that application of IP$_3$ could induce SR Ca release in skinned skeletal muscle fibers and SR vesicles (Vergara *et al.*, 1985; Volpe *et al.*, 1985; Donaldson *et al.*, 1987). IP$_3$ production was increased during tetanic contractions (Vergara *et al.*, 1985) and the enzymes required for IP$_3$ synthesis and degradation are present (Vergara *et al.*, 1985, 1987; Hidalgo *et al.*, 1986; Hidalgo & Jaimovich, 1989; Varsanyi *et al.*, 1989; Lagos & Vergara, 1990). It has also been suggested that the effect of IP$_3$ on skeletal muscle is [Ca] and E$_m$-dependent (Volpe *et al.*, 1986; Donaldson *et al.*, 1988).

On the other hand, numerous reports show that IP$_3$ does not induce SR Ca release in skeletal muscle (Scherer & Ferguson, 1985; Lea *et al.*, 1986; Mikos & Snow, 1987; Palade, 1987c). Using photolysis of caged IP$_3$ (as in Fig 125), Walker *et al.* (1987) showed that IP$_3$-induced contractions were too small and much too slow to be physiologically relevant. Indeed, the rapid turn-off of SR Ca release with repolarization (Simon *et al.*, 1989) is several orders of magnitude faster than degradation of the IP$_3$ (Somlyo *et al.*, 1988). The enzymes and substrates involved in rapid IP$_3$ turnover are present, but not at levels which would make this feasible (Walker *et al.*, 1987; Somlyo *et al.*, 1988; Hidalgo & Jaimovich, 1989; Varsanyi *et al.*, 1989). Blinks *et al.* (1987) found apparent IP$_3$ICR in detubulated skeletal muscle, proposing that IP$_3$ could induce depolarization of sealed off T-tubules, but not in intact fibers. Finally, blocking the IP$_3$ receptor with intracellular heparin produced no effect on skeletal muscle E-C coupling (Pape *et al.*, 1988), in contrast to the profound depression seen in smooth muscle (Kobayashi *et al.*, 1988). In conclusion, IP$_3$ICR is unlikely to play any substantial role in skeletal muscle E-C coupling. However, there are IP$_3$R in skeletal muscle, and more recent work seems to point to a perinuclear localization and a possible role in nuclear Ca signaling (Jaimovich *et al.*, 2000).

IP$_3$ Induced Ca Release in Cardiac Muscle

Hirata *et al.* (1984) first showed IP$_3$ICR from cardiac SR vesicles. However, Movsesian *et al.* (1985) found no effect of IP$_3$ in isolated cardiac SR or in myocytes permeabilized by saponin. Nosek *et al.* (1986) found that IP$_3$ potentiated spontaneous and caffeine-induced Ca-release in cardiac muscle. Vites & Pappano (1990) showed IP$_3$ induced contractions in small

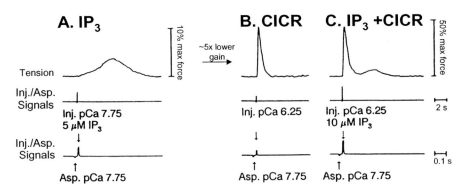

Figure 127. IP$_3$ and Ca-induced Ca-release in a mechanically skinned rat ventricular myocyte (from Fabiato, 1986b, with permission). Rapid injection (Inj.) of 5 µM IP$_3$ induced a small and slow contraction (**A**), compared to that induced by a rapid increase in [Ca] from 20 nM to 560 nM (i.e. via CICR in **B**). Note different tension scales. Simultaneous application of these two stimuli produced a contraction in which the major part was not much different than with CICR (**C**). Aspiration (Asp.) of 20 nM precedes injections.

skinned multicellular preparations from chick atria which were caffeine- and ryanodine-sensitive. Fabiato (1986a,b, 1990) showed that rapid application of IP$_3$ to skinned rat myocytes could induce SR Ca release, but that it was much smaller and slower than that induced by CICR (Fig 127). Kentish *et al.* (1990) confirmed this in skinned rat ventricular muscle, using flash photo-lysis of caged Ca and caged IP$_3$. Very high [IP$_3$] could induce SR Ca release, but the rate and extent of Ca release was much lower than for CICR.

These studies made it clear that IP$_3$ICR is not centrally important in cardiac E-C coupling. However, IP$_3$ could still serve as a modulator of CICR (Nosek *et al.*, 1986; Suarez-Isla *et al.*, 1988). Activation of cardiac α_1-adrenergic and muscarinic receptors increases IP$_3$ production as well as contractile force (Gilmour & Zipes, 1985; Brown & Jones, 1986; Poggioli *et al.*, 1986; Jones *et al.*, 1988; Otani *et al.*, 1988; Scholz *et al.*, 1988). On the other hand, the increase in Ca transients and contractions in response to α-adrenergic activation in mammalian ventricle appear to be mediated mainly by PKC, rather than IP$_3$ (Endoh, 1996; Mattiazzi, 1997; Gambassi *et al.*, 1998). Thus, while it is clear that several cardiac membrane receptors stimulate phospholipase C to produce both IP$_3$ and diacylglycerols (DAG), the DAG stimulation of PKC appears to predominate in alteration of acute contractile function.

Kijima *et al.* (1993) found IP$_3$ binding sites in ventricular homogenates. In membrane fractionation studies, RyR was enriched in SR/sarcolemmal fractions, while IP$_3$R was especially enriched in a different fraction that included intercalated disks. This agreed with their immuno-localization, suggesting IP$_3$R preferentially at intercalated disks rather than in SR. Perez *et al.* (1997) found that the IP$_3$R expressed in ventricular myocyte is the type-2 isoform (while other cells in ventricular homogenate express type-1 IP$_3$R). The number of IP$_3$R is as much as 10% of the number of RyR. Lipp *et al.* (2000) confirmed that cardiac myocytes express type-2 IP$_3$R and found six times higher IP$_3$R expression in atrial than ventricular myocytes. They found atrial myocyte IP$_3$Rs to be sub-sarcolemmal and apparently co-localized with surface RyRs. They found that IP$_3$ could produce SR Ca release in skinned atrial cells and that a membrane permeant

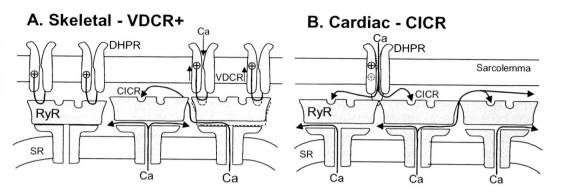

A. Skeletal - VDCR+

B. Cardiac - CICR

Figure 128. E-C coupling in skeletal and cardiac muscle (VDCR & CICR). **A.** In skeletal muscle the physical link between the sarcolemmal Ca channel (or DHPR) is critical for VDCR. Ca released by VDCR can then activate uncoupled RyRs via CICR. Ca influx is not required in skeletal muscle E-C coupling and Ca cycles mainly between the SR and the cytoplasm. **B.** In cardiac muscle Ca entry via I_{Ca} activates RyR via CICR. Ca from I_{Ca} or one RyR can activate a neighboring RyR via CICR. Physical links between the sarcolemmal and SR Ca channels in cardiac muscle probably do not transmit a signal for VDCR.

IP$_3$ analogue enhanced Ca spark frequency and twitch $\Delta[Ca]_i$ in intact atrial myocytes. They suggested that IP$_3$ might interact with RyR-mediated CICR in atrial myocytes. However, a specific role for IP$_3$ICR in ventricular myocytes is still not clear.

Preliminary immunolocalization studies with type-2-specific IP$_3$R antibodies show a perinuclear localization in ventricular myocytes (with G.A. Mignery, unpublished). We speculate that such perinuclear IP$_3$R may be activated by neurohumoral agents known to cause increased [IP$_3$] (e.g. α-adrenergic agents or endothelin). The IP$_3$ might activate local Ca-dependent processes at or in the nucleus (e.g. CaMKII) due to high local [Ca] near the IP$_3$R. This could contribute to transcriptional regulation that is also seen with these agents. This possibility seems attractive, because it would allow cardiac myocytes to distinguish between the regular global dynamic [Ca]$_i$ signals and those neurohumoral signals that might regulate cardiac transcription in a Ca-dependent manner (Ramirez *et al.*, 1997). There is evidence for ion channels in nuclei of cardiac myocytes (Rousseau *et al.*, 1996) and other cell types (Stehno-Bitel *et al.*, 1995; Humbert *et al.*, 1996) and there is considerable evidence for Ca-dependent transcriptional regulation (Karin & Hunter, 1995; Cahill *et al.*, 1996; Malviya & Rogue, 1998). While an appealing possibility, I should emphasize that this is mainly speculation at present. On balance, IP$_3$ICR might play a minor modulatory role in cardiac E-C coupling (especially in atrial cells), but CICR is clearly the primary mechanism of cardiac E-C coupling.

SUMMARY

In a simplified manner the 3 muscle types can serve as models of the 3 main mechanisms of SR Ca release (i.e. VDCR in skeletal, CICR in heart and IP$_3$ICR in smooth muscle, Figs 128 & 126). It should be emphasized that this is an oversimplification since there is some evidence in support of every permutation of mechanism and muscle type. For example, VDCR appears to be the crucial initiating process in skeletal muscle. However, there are at least twice as many RyRs as T-tubule/DHPR tetrads in skeletal muscle and CICR may be crucial in recruiting the RyRs which are not physically coupled to T-tubule tetrads. IP_3 can also induce Ca release in skeletal muscle under some circumstances, although the physiological relevance of this pathway is not yet clear. In cardiac muscle CICR is the main E-C coupling mechanism. However, IP_3 may modulate cardiac Ca release, and there is some evidence for a functional direct link between the sarcolemma and the SR (and possibly VDCR). Whether this DHPR-RyR link is important, aside from just bringing the RyR and DHPR close together, is not known. In smooth muscle there is compelling evidence for both IP_3ICR and CICR. There is even evidence that the IP_3R interacts with a different plasma membrane Ca channel (TRP) involved in CCE where the signal is retrograde from IP_3R to TRP.

D.M. Bers.
Excitation-Contraction Coupling and Cardiac Contractile Force.
2nd Ed., Kluwer Academic Publishers, Dordrecht, 2001

CHAPTER 9

CONTROL OF CARDIAC CONTRACTION BY SR AND SARCOLEMMAL Ca FLUXES

Both Ca influx and SR Ca release are important elements in E-C coupling and Ca from both sources can contribute to the activation of contraction. In this chapter I will try to clarify the dynamic interplay of transsarcolemmal and trans-SR Ca fluxes in different cardiac muscle preparations and under different experimental situations.

While Ca entry via I_{Ca} triggers SR Ca release in cardiac E-C coupling, Ca entry may also contribute to $[Ca]_i$ elevation during contraction. Since SR Ca release depends on I_{Ca}, it can be difficult to distinguish unequivocally between the direct effects of Ca entry $vs.$ effects of Ca entry on SR Ca release. For example, interventions which increases I_{Ca} typically increase $\Delta[Ca]_i$ and contraction. How can we distinguish whether this is due to: a) the direct effect of Ca entry, b) an increased fractional SR Ca release (due to higher I_{Ca}) or c) an increase in SR Ca load? One cannot simply block Ca entry to study the contribution of SR Ca to contraction, because CICR will also be blocked. On the other hand, one can inhibit the SR Ca function (with caffeine, ryanodine or thapsigargin) to study the activation of contraction by I_{Ca} in the absence of a functional SR contribution. This approach is especially valuable because while SR Ca release is clearly capable of activating the myofilaments (pg 186), this is less clear for I_{Ca} (pg 120).

SPECIES, REGIONAL AND DEVELOPMENTAL DIFFERENCES

Figure 129 shows the effects of caffeine and ryanodine on steady state twitch contractions in several cardiac preparations. Variation is apparent among different species (frog $vs.$ rabbit $vs.$ rat), at different stages of development, (neonatal $vs.$ adult) and regionally in the heart (rabbit ventricle $vs.$ atrium). While caffeine can prevent net SR Ca uptake by making the SR extremely leaky to Ca (Weber & Herz, 1968), it has side effects at the mM concentrations that are required for SR effects. For example, caffeine increases myofilament Ca sensitivity (Wendt & Stephenson, 1983, see Chapter 2), can increase Ca influx (Bers, 1983; Tseng, 1988) and inhibits phosphodiesterases (Butcher & Sutherland, 1962), thereby elevating cyclic AMP. These other caffeine effects tend to increase force and may be partly why the values for caffeine are typically higher than for ryanodine. Ryanodine is much more specific in its interaction with the SR (the K_d is nM), but its action is more complex (Sutko $et\ al.$, 1985; Bers $et\ al.$, 1987; see pg 183-185). The concentration dependence of these agents does not vary in different tissues, despite the difference in maximal effect (Sutko & Willerson, 1980; Shattock & Bers, 1987). Thus, the variation in tension depression among cardiac tissues in Fig 129 by caffeine and ryanodine indicates the relative requirement for SR Ca release for myofilament activation.

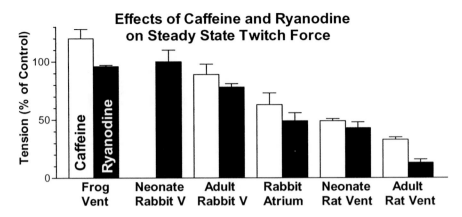

Figure 129. The effect of caffeine (10 mM) or ryanodine (100 nM) pretreatment on steady state twitch contractions (0.5 Hz at 30°C or 23°C for frog) in various cardiac muscle preparations (Data are from Bers, 1989; Haddock *et al.*, 1999, and unpublished observations).

However, the 20-30% reduction of twitch contractions by ryanodine in rabbit ventricular muscle cannot be taken to mean that under normal conditions the SR contributes only 20-30% of the Ca required for myofilament activation. It simply means that in the absence of a functional SR, Ca influx <u>can</u> supply sufficient Ca to activate a nearly normal amplitude contraction. Under normal conditions, SR Ca release raises $[Ca]_i$, which decreases slightly the gradient for Ca influx (a minor effect), but more importantly inactivates I_{Ca} and shortens the action potential. Figure 60 (pg 122) showed that preventing SR Ca release doubles the amount of Ca influx via I_{Ca} during the same AP (e.g. from 6 to 12 µmol/L cytosol). Preventing SR Ca release also prolongs AP duration (e.g. in rabbit ventricle from 222 to 305 ms at 37°C, Shattock & Bers, 1987), which could also increase Ca influx by another 10% or so (based on Fig 59). In addition, the lower Ca transient in the absence of SR Ca release will allow more Ca influx to occur via Na/Ca exchange (Fig 74).   Thus, preventing SR Ca release indirectly increases Ca influx, and so would underestimate the normal contribution of SR Ca release to the twitch.

On the other hand, ryanodine can diminish the ability of a given Ca influx to activate contraction. This is because some of the Ca entering the cell may also be transiently accumulated by the SR (see pg 183-185). Indeed, in the presence of ryanodine the SR can accumulate a similar amount of Ca as under control conditions, albeit only very transiently (Bers *et al.*, 1987; MacLeod & Bers, 1987). This transient Ca uptake by ryanodine-treated SR is especially notable at post-rest contractions. In this case the SR is Ca-depleted, such that the net SR Ca accumulation may more closely keep pace with Ca influx via I_{Ca} (which is also reduced during post-rest depolarizations, Fig 58, pg 119). Indeed, ryanodine, even at very low concentrations, preferentially depresses post-rest contractions (Fig 130; Hajdu & Leonard, 1961; Bers, 1985; Malécot & Katzung, 1987). So, ryanodine can allow the SR to still function as a transient Ca buffer.

Caffeine can prevent SR Ca accumulation altogether (since RCCs are abolished even at very short rest intervals, Bers *et al.*, 1987). Thus, with caffeine the SR may be more effectively short-circuited such that Ca entry has more direct access to the myofilaments. At high ryanodine

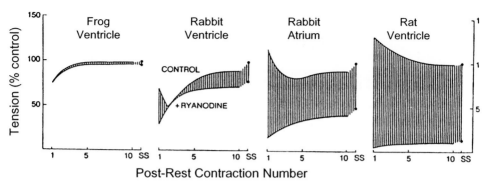

Figure 130. Recovery of twitch force after 30 sec rest in frog, rabbit and rat ventricle and rabbit atrium in the absence (top) and presence (bottom) of 100 nM ryanodine. Steady state twitch tension is shown by the end points of each curve (SS). Shading indicates ryanodine-sensitive force (redrawn from Bers, 1985).

concentrations (>10 μM) or after long exposure times, there is often some recovery of twitch contraction despite a Ca-depleted SR (Sutko & Willerson, 1980; Bers, 1985; Lewartowski *et al.*, 1990). This probably reflects a higher percentage of ryanodine-modified (leaky) SR release channels, such that the effect is more like caffeine (i.e. the transient buffering ability is lost).

Thapsigargin, which blocks the SR Ca-ATPase, also progressively depresses twitch contractions as SR Ca is gradually depleted. However, acutely blocking the SR Ca-ATPase can <u>increase</u> twitch contraction and Ca transients. This is true both when the SR Ca content is low (so SR Ca release does not occur, Bassani *et al.*, 1993b; Janczewski & Lakatta, 1993) or when SR Ca content and release are normal (Fig 133C; i.e. if SR Ca loss is prevented during pump-blockade, Bassani *et al.*, 1994a). The explanation is that the SR Ca-ATPase actively transports Ca as soon as [Ca]$_i$ rises, and is rapid enough to limit the peak [Ca]$_i$ attained during the twitch. In conclusion, complete SR Ca-ATPase blockade by thapsigargin can prevent both SR Ca uptake and release, and may most directly indicate the ability of Ca influx to activate contraction (but only after the SR is Ca-depleted). However, Ca influx will still be higher than during a normal twitch with SR Ca release (as above), and it can be difficult to block the pump completely with thapsigargin in multicellular preparations (Baudet *et al.*, 1993; see pg 169).

There are ultrastructural correlates to these pharmacological dissections. For example, the SR network is most highly-developed in adult rat ventricle, somewhat less in rabbit atrium and ventricle, and is the most sparse and poorly developed in frog ventricle (Chapter 1). Furthermore, the small diameter of frog ventricular myocytes (and hence high surface:volume ratio) makes Ca entry a more plausible mechanism for activation in frog. Therefore, the virtual insensitivity of frog ventricle to ryanodine is not especially surprising and in frog ventricular muscle it is possible that the myofilaments can be activated entirely by Ca entering from outside the cell at each contraction (Morad & Cleeman, 1987; Chapman, 1983).

Fabiato & Fabiato (1978a; Fabiato, 1982) also found variation in CICR among different preparations, consistent with the above interpretation. For example, CICR could not be observed in frog or prenatal rat ventricle, but was most prominent in adult rat ventricular myocytes. This developmental transition to relative SR dependence is also apparent in other mammalian cardiac preparations (Penefsky, 1974; Maylie, 1982; Seguchi *et al.*, 1986; Haddock *et al.*, 1999). This

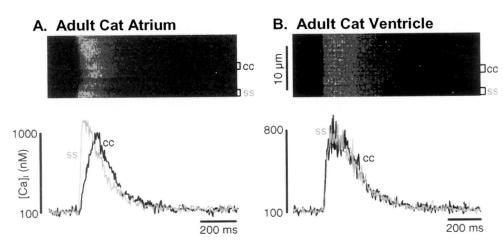

Figure 131. Spatial [Ca]$_i$ gradients in atrial myocytes. **A.** Transverse line scan in a cat atrial myocyte, showing that [Ca]$_i$ rises earlier in the subsarcolemmal (ss) region than the cell center (cc). **B.** Similar transverse line scan and Ca transients in a cat ventricular myocyte, showing simultaneous [Ca]$_i$ rise across the cell. Lower traces show superimposed ss and cc traces (figure kindly supplied by L.A. Blatter).

agrees with ultrastructural results which indicate that the T-tubule/SR system is gradually developing from the prenatal period through the first few weeks of life, albeit at different rates in different species (Scheibler & Wolff, 1962; Legato, 1979; Olivetti *et al.*, 1980; Hoerter *et al.*, 1981; Page & Beucker, 1981; Penefsky, 1983; Goldstein & Traeger, 1985; Artman, 1994). Furthermore, SR Ca uptake in vesicles increases over this developmental period in rat, rabbit and sheep ventricle (Nayler & Fassold, 1977; Nakanishi & Jarmakani, 1984; Mahony & Jones, 1986; Pegg & Michalak, 1987). An interesting twist on this variation is that in chipmunks that hibernate, the ventricle appears to function like rat ventricle during hibernation, but more like rabbit ventricle when not hibernating (Kondo & Shibata, 1984; Kondo, 1986, 1988).

Spatial [Ca]$_i$ gradients are generally not observed during twitches in adult ventricular myocytes (Figs 131, 132). This is because T-tubules conduct depolarization axially to the center of the cell and local CICR throughout the cell is synchronized by I$_{Ca}$ activation. This synchrony also occurs along the myocyte length (Fig 122). Both adult atrial and neonatal ventricular myocytes lack appreciable T-tubules, and the [Ca]$_i$ rises first at the cell periphery and then spreads to the center of the cell (Figs 131, 132; Berlin, 1995; Hüser *et al.*, 1996; Haddock *et al.*, 1999). In both atrial and neonatal ventricular myocytes there are RyRs transversely arranged at the level of the Z-line, despite a lack of T-tubules (Sedarat *et al.*, 2000). In atrial muscle, SR Ca release appears to propagate transversely via CICR, because the peak [Ca]$_i$ at the center can be as high as the subsarcolemmal [Ca]$_i$, and ryanodine depresses both central and subsarcolemmal Ca transients. Furthermore, local [Ca]$_i$ at the center can exceed subsarcolemmal [Ca]$_i$, which is not expected for simple Ca diffusion from the subsarcolemmal region. The ability of CICR to propagate axially also depends on local SR Ca content, and propagation fails when central SR Ca load is low (Hüser *et al.*, 1996). This reflects the SR Ca-load-dependence of SR Ca release (pg 225).

In neonatal rabbit ventricular myocytes the Ca transient (subsarcolemmal or central) does not seem to involve appreciable SR Ca release, but appears to reflect mainly diffusion from the

A. Adult Rabbit Ventricle   B. Neonatal Rabbit Ventricle

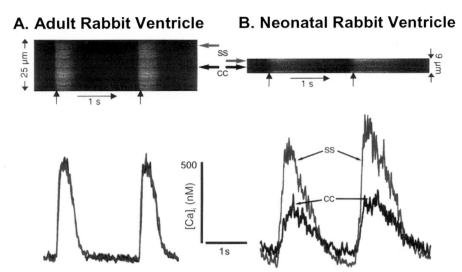

Figure 132. Spatial $[Ca]_i$ gradients in neonatal rabbit ventricular myocytes. **A** (top). Transverse line scan in a rabbit ventricular myocyte (25 μm wide) showing uniform Ca transients in the subsarcolemmal (ss) region and the cell center (cc). At bottom are superimposed ss (grey) and cc (black) Ca transients from A. **B**. Similar transverse line scan and Ca transients in a 9 μm wide neonatal rabbit ventricular myocyte, with. superimposed ss and cc traces. Data are from study of Haddock *et al.* (1999).

subsarcolemmal region to the center (Fig 132; Haddock *et al.*, 1999).   In adult myocytes thapsigargin decreases the rate of rise of $[Ca]_i$ for both subsarcolemmal and central location by 80%. In neonatal myocytes the rate of subsarcolemmal and central $[Ca]_i$ rise is 44% and 12%, respectively of that in adult myocytes, but thapsigargin has no effect at all on the neonatal myocyte Ca transient (peak, rate of rise or spatial gradient). There is, however, Ca stored in the neonatal myocyte SR, because caffeine-induced Ca transients and contractures are robust, and are spatially homogeneous (Balaguru *et al.*, 1997; Miller *et al.*, 1997; Haddock *et al.*, 1999). However, this SR Ca does not seem to participate in E-C coupling. Ca sparks are seen in the neonatal myocytes, but preferentially in the subsarcolemmal region. We speculated that RyRs in neonates may not be clustered or as sensitive to Ca (especially non-junctional RyRs), such that they are not normally activated during E-C coupling (Haddock *et al.*, 1999).

If neonatal rabbit ventricular myocytes don't have SR Ca release to boost the Ca influx signal, how is there enough Ca to activate the myofilaments? The density of I_{Ca} (in A/F) is actually lower by ~50% in neonatal ventricular myocytes (*vs.* adult; Osaka & Joyner, 1991; Wetzel *et al.*, 1991; Akita *et al.*, 1994). The higher surface:volume ratio in neonatal cells (which have smaller diameters and lack T-tubules), would increase the impact that a given I_{Ca} (in pA/pF) has on $[Ca]_i$ by a factor of ~2-3 (Haddock *et al.*, 1997). Neonatal myocytes also have a longer AP than adult (especially in rat). Thus, I_{Ca} may still bring in 5-10 μmol/L cytosol in neonatal myocytes. Na/Ca exchanger expression and current are ~5-fold higher (in pA/pF) in neonatal than adult rabbit ventricular myocytes (Boerth *et al.*, 1994; Artman *et al.*, 1995; Haddock *et al.*, 1997). Haddock *et al.* (1997) showed that 9-14 μmol/L cytosol enters the neonatal myocyte via $I_{Na/Ca}$ during a 300 ms pulse at +60 mV (*vs.* 1-2 μmol/L cytosol for adult) and this produced 10% cell shortening (*vs.* <<1% in adult). The lack of SR Ca release allows greater Ca entry via $I_{Na/Ca}$

in the neonate.   Thus, Ca influx might be 15-20 µmol/L cytosol, with 67-75% due to $I_{Na/Ca}$ (consistent with modest twitch inhibition by blockade of I_{Ca}, Wetzel *et al.*, 1995).   Intracellular Ca buffering power is also 2-3 times lower in neonatal ventricular myocytes (Bassani *et al.*, 1998), consistent with the lower amount of myofilament and SR Ca-ATPase at this stage of development.   This means that neonatal myocytes need only 33-50% as much activator Ca to reach the same state of activation as adult cells.   Thus, Ca influx of 17-25 µmol/L cytosol in neonatal cells may activate as effectively as a combined Ca influx & SR Ca release of 50 µmol/L cytosol in adult cells.   In conclusion, neonatal rabbit ventricular myocytes appear to depend on Ca influx by $I_{Na/Ca}$ + I_{Ca}. This Ca influx by itself may be sufficient to support contraction because of high Na/Ca exchange expression, high surface:volume ratio and lower cytosolic Ca buffering.

Based on results from several sources a rough sequencing of cardiac muscle preparations from most to least SR reliant is (V, ventricle; A, atrium): calf Purkinje fiber > adult mouse V ≥ adult rat V > dog V ~ ferret V > cat V > neonate rat V ~ rabbit A > human V > rabbit V ≥ failing human & rabbit V > guinea-pig V > neonate rabbit V > fetal V (human, cat & rabbit) > trout V > frog V ~toad V (Penefsky, 1974; Sutko & Willerson, 1980; Sutko & Kenyon, 1983; Bers, 1985; Malécot *et al.*, 1986; Seguchi *et al.*, 1986; El-Sayed & Gesser, 1989; Schlotthauer *et al.*, 1998; Pieske *et al.*, 1999a; Haddock *et al.*, 1999).   In a given species, atrial muscle is typically more SR Ca-dependent (with more active CICR, Fabiato, 1982), and has faster [Ca]$_i$ decline, due in part to lower phospholamban content.   Shorter atrial AP duration may also limit Ca entry via I_{Ca} or Na/Ca exchange.   Of course this sequence is only approximate, and the relative importance of the SR Ca release also varies under different conditions (e.g. changes in frequency, drugs, etc.).

Ca Removal Fluxes

The amount of Ca which enters the myocyte at each steady state twitch must also be extruded from the cell; otherwise the cell would be gaining or losing Ca (i.e. not in steady state, see also pg 52-55 & 152-156).   Although there are 4 Ca removal systems (SR Ca-ATPase, Na/Ca exchange, sarcolemmal Ca-ATPase and mitochondrial uniporter), the analysis of Ca removal fluxes can be more direct than that for activator Ca.   Bassani *et al.* (1994a) developed a quantitative method which determines the specific contributions of these Ca transport systems to relaxation and [Ca]$_i$ decline in rabbit and rat ventricular myocytes (below & Figs 133-5).

First, Ca transients are recorded with selective inhibition of Ca removal systems (Fig 133).   In Fig 133A only the slow systems (mitochondrial Ca uptake and sarcolemmal Ca-ATPase) can remove [Ca]$_i$, because Na was not present anywhere and SR Ca uptake was blocked by either caffeine or thapsigargin.   Both caffeine-induced Ca transients and those evoked by an action potential (with SR Ca-pump completely blocked by thapsigargin) declined with a τ ~12 s. This was true in both rat and rabbit ventricular myocytes indicating that the combined action of the mitochondrial Ca uptake and sarcolemmal Ca-pump were comparable in these species. Moreover, the AP-induced twitch (with thapsigargin) only released about half of the SR Ca load (which could all be released by caffeine).   This is consistent with the findings that ~50% of the SR Ca content is released during a normal twitch.   These results also emphasize that the mitochondria and sarcolemmal Ca-ATPase require >20 s to bring [Ca]$_i$ down to diastolic levels.

Figure 133B shows that the [Ca]$_i$ decline during the normal rabbit ventricular twitch is slowed by 30% when Na/Ca exchange is blocked.   In this case [Ca]$_i$ decline depends on the

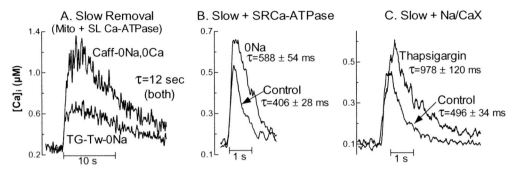

Figure 133. Ca transients in rabbit ventricular myocytes with selective Ca transporter block. **A.** Twitch and caffeine-induced Ca transient (Caff) where both SR Ca uptake and Na/Ca exchange were prevented. Caff was applied in 0Na,0Ca solution. Twitch in thapsigargin (TG-Tw) was evoked after pre-depletion of Na$_i$ (and in Na-free solution). The SR Ca-ATPase was completely inhibited by thapsigargin, but SR Ca content normal (i.e. prior to gradual SR Ca depletion). **B.** Twitches evoked in either control or Na-free solution (in both cases Na$_i$ was predepleted to prevent Ca entry via Na/Ca exchange). **C.** Twitches evoked in either control or with the SR Ca-ATPase completely blocked by thapsigargin (in both cases cells were incubated in 0Na, 0Ca solution ±TG to maintain SR Ca while SR Ca-pump blockade was instituted. Data are regraphed from Bassani *et al.* (1994a) and time constants τ are shown for mean data.

combined action of the slow systems plus the SR Ca-ATPase. When the SR Ca-ATPase is selectively blocked by thapsigargin (Fig 133C), [Ca]$_i$ decline is slowed by 50%, indicating that the combined slow systems plus Na/Ca exchange can restore diastolic [Ca]$_i$ in ~2 s. Notably peak twitch [Ca]$_i$ is higher than control when either the SR Ca-ATPase or the Na/Ca exchanger is blocked. This indicates that in rabbit ventricle Ca removal by the SR Ca-ATPase and Na/Ca exchange can actually curtail the peak of the Ca transient, because removal begins as soon as [Ca]$_i$ rises. This was also true in rat ventricular myocytes with respect to SR Ca-pump blockade, but not Na/Ca exchange inhibition.

To analyze Ca fluxes, the free [Ca]$_i$ during [Ca]$_i$ decline must be converted to total cytosolic [Ca] ([Ca]$_{Tot}$), as in Fig 29 or 87. Then the rate of total Ca removal from the cytosol (d[Ca]$_{Tot}$/dt) can be graphed as a function of [Ca]$_i$ for each point in time (see Fig 87 or 134A). This transport rate must be the sum of the individual transport rates given by

$$d[Ca]_t/dt = J_{SR} + J_{Na/CaX} + J_{Slow} - Leak \qquad (9.1)$$

where the three J terms refer to flux through the SR Ca-ATPase, Na/Ca exchange and the combined slow Ca transport by mitochondria and sarcolemmal Ca-ATPase. Leak is considered to be small compared to other fluxes during [Ca]$_i$ decline. For simplicity J$_{SR}$, J$_{Na/CaX}$ and J$_{Slow}$ can be empirically described as simple [Ca] dependent fluxes via a Hill equation:

$$J_x = \frac{V_{max}}{1 + (K_m/[Ca]_i)^n} \qquad (9.2)$$

J$_{Slow}$ is first fit by using the decline of [Ca]$_i$ when other systems are blocked (Fig 133A), where J$_{SR}$ and J$_{NaCaX}$ are zero in Eq 9.1. We then assume that this [Ca]$_i$-dependence of J$_{slow}$ (with a V$_{max}$, K$_m$ and *n*) is valid for other Ca transients in that species. Similarly, parameters for J$_{NaCaX}$ can be measured during a twitch in thapsigargin (or a caffeine-induced Ca transient) where d[Ca]$_t$/dt = J$_{Na/CaX}$ + J$_{Slow}$ (Fig 133C-thapsigargin). Likewise parameters for J$_{SR}$ are measured using the

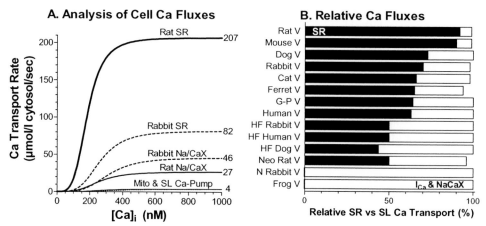

Figure 134. $[Ca]_i$-dependence of Ca transport in ventricular myocytes. **A.** Ca transport functions derived from Ca transients in intact rabbit and rat ventricular myocytes. Ca transport rates as functions of $[Ca]_i$ for the SR Ca-ATPase, Na/Ca exchange (NaCaX) and combined slow systems (Mito & SL Ca-pump) were determined as described in the text and with respect to equations 9.1 & 9.2. Independent values obtained for J_{SR}, $J_{Na/CaX}$ and J_{Slow} respectively were: V_{max} (given at the end of each curve in μmol/L cytosol/sec); K_m (in nM) = 264, 316, and 362 in rabbit and 184, 257 and 268 in rat; n = 3.7, 3.7, 3.2 in rabbit and 3.9, 3.4 an 3.5 in rat. (based on data from Bassani *et al.*, 1994a). **B.** Relative Ca fluxes in different ventricular (V) preparations based on analyses like Fig 134A and 135 (see also Table 20, pg 153). Black bars are % activation and extrusion by SR, white bars are % supply by I_{Ca} and removal by NaCaX.

twitch where Na/Ca exchange is blocked (Fig 133B-0Na). This analysis can be checked to see if total Ca removal during the normal twitch Ca transient is well described by the sum in Eq 9.1 (and this is the case). Figure 134A shows the resulting Ca flux functions estimated in this way for rabbit and rat. V_{max} for the SR Ca-ATPase in rat is larger than in rabbit, but the situation is reversed for Na/Ca exchange. J_{Slow} is quite small compared even to the J_{NaCaX}. It should also be noted that the Hill function (Eq 9.2) used to describe J_x does not necessarily have to be a good mechanistic descriptor of the flux (e.g. it is not for Na/Ca exchange). What is important is that it provides a reasonably good empirical fit to the dependence of $d[Ca]_i/dt$ on $[Ca]_i$ over the $[Ca]_i$ range of interest.

The final piece of this analysis (Fig 135) is to calculate how these systems compete dynamically and simultaneously during a normal twitch. Here we use the free $[Ca]_i$ during that twitch to calculate the instantaneous individual fluxes through each system (Eqs 9.1 & 9.2). Ideally, this analysis would include the backfluxes for each of these transporters as described for the SR Ca-pump and Na/Ca exchange (pg 174 and 149), but that was not done by Bassani *et al.* (1994a). This would allow net flux via these systems to more closely approach zero as free $[Ca]_i$ returns to the resting level. Accounting for local spatial distributions of both Ca transporters and buffering sites could also make this sort of analysis more comprehensive (e.g. Fig 74).

Figure 135 shows that during a normal twitch the fractions of Ca transported by the SR, Na/Ca exchange and slow systems are 70, 28 and 2% respectively in rabbit and 92, 7 and 1% in rat myocytes. This 28% estimate of Ca flux by Na/Ca exchange in rabbit agrees with the 25-33% estimated based only on the ratio of time constants of relaxation or $[Ca]_i$ decline (pg 52-54). The 7% value for rat also agrees with very similar experimental results in rat by Negretti *et al.*

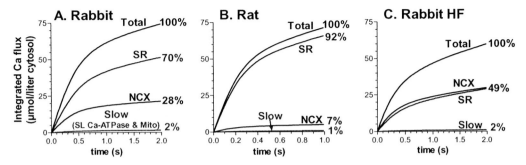

Figure 135. Integrated Ca fluxes during twitch relaxation in rabbit and rat ventricular myocytes. Free [Ca]$_i$ during twitch relaxation was used as a driving function to calculate Ca flux via each system, using the functions in Fig 134A. Percents indicate the fraction of the total cytosolic Ca removal attributable to each system when they dynamically interact in the cell. Data in **A** and **B** are from Bassani *et al.* (1994a). For **C** rabbit heart failure (HF) the V$_{max}$ for NCX was increased 116% and SR Ca-ATPase was reduced by 24% as indicated by Pogwizd *et al.* (1999).

(1993). Thus, there are clear species differences in this competition between the SR Ca-ATPase and the Na/Ca exchange. In heart failure the expression of SR Ca-ATPase can be down-regulated and the Na/Ca exchange up-regulated (see Chapter 10). This shifts the balance of fluxes during [Ca]$_i$ decline. In a rabbit heart failure model, we found that Na/Ca exchange was increased ~2-fold at the mRNA, protein and functional level, while SR Ca-ATPase function was reduced by up to 24% (Pogwizd *et al.*, 1999). This resulted in an almost unchanged rate of [Ca]$_i$ decline and twitch relaxation. We interpreted this as a large increase in Na/Ca exchange offsetting a small decrease in SR Ca-ATPase function. However, as in Fig 135C, this creates a situation where SR Ca-ATPase and Na/Ca exchange contribute almost equally to [Ca]$_i$ decline in heart failure. We also showed that this shift may occur in human heart failure (Schlotthauer *et al.*, 1998; Pieske *et al.*, 1999a). Table 20 (pg 153) and Fig 134B shows data for several species.

Ca influx must match Ca efflux

If 28% of Ca removal during twitch relaxation is due to Na/Ca exchange in rabbit (Fig 135A) we would expect Ca influx and SR Ca release in rabbit to supply roughly 28 & 70% of the activating Ca respectively (and 7 and 92% in rat). This would be required to maintain cellular and SR Ca balance and prevent net gain or loss of Ca. Delbridge *et al.* (1996, 1997) assessed Ca influx and SR Ca release quantitatively in rabbit and rat (see Fig 31, pg 55). We measured Ca influx via I$_{Ca}$, the SR Ca content by caffeine-induced I$_{Na/Ca}$ integral and used measurements of fractional SR Ca release (Bassani *et al.*, 1993b, Delbridge *et al.*, 1997). Table 24 summarizes quantitative analysis of data from rabbit and rat ventricular myocytes. After making corrections for surface:volume ratios, the integrated I$_{Ca}$ in rabbit myocytes is sufficient to increase [Ca]$_{Tot}$ by 9.7 µM and the SR Ca content is 87 µmol/L cytosol. Using 43% of SR Ca released during a twitch we have 9.7 plus 43% of the SR Ca content (43 × 87) giving 47 µmol/L cytosol activating the twitch, with 23% coming from I$_{Ca}$ and 77% from SR Ca release. These numbers are in good agreement with the experiments in Fig 135, where 28% of Ca extrusion was due to Na/Ca exchange and 70% due to SR Ca uptake. Similar analysis for the rat twitch in Table 24 also agrees with ~7-8% of activating Ca coming across the sarcolemma with 92% from the SR.

Table 24

Fraction of Activator Ca from I_{Ca} and SR Ca release

	Rabbit		Rat	
	I_{Ca}	SR ($I_{Na/Ca}$)	I_{Ca}	$I_{Na/CaX}$ (SR)
$\int I\,dt$ (fC/pF)	221 ± 14	860 ± 118	185 ± 12	851 ± 70
$\Delta[Ca]_{Tot}$ (μM)	9.7 ± 0.5	77 ± 11	6.5 ± 0.3	120 ± 8
SR Ca (μmol/L cytosol)		87 ± 13[†]		138 ± 9[†]
Twitch $\Delta[Ca]_i$ (μmol/L cytosol)	9.7	87×0.43	6.5	138×0.55
Total (μmol/L cytosol)	= 47		= 82	
Activator Ca (%)	23 ± 2%	77 ± 2%	7.9%	92%

Data are from Delbridge *et al.* (1996) for rabbit and Delbridge *et al.* (1997) and Yuan *et al.* (1996) for rat ventricular myocytes. Columns labeled SR ($I_{Na/Ca}$) show integrated $I_{Na/Ca}$ to derive SR Ca content (first 3 lines) and the amount of SR Ca release contributing to the twitch (*vs.* Ca influx via I_{Ca} (last 3 lines; see Table 2 & 9). [†]Increase from 77 to 87 (& 120 to 138) reflects correction for non Na/Ca exchanger-mediated Ca removal during caffeine-induced contracture (Table 20).

Terracciano & MacLeod (1997) used a slightly different approach to measure Ca entry during AP-clamp. In rat ventricular myocytes they found that Ca entry via I_{Ca} was 3.5% of the SR Ca content. This is equivalent to the above 7% results in rat (assuming a 50% fractional SR Ca release). They also studied guinea-pig ventricular myocytes at both 0.5 and 0.2 Hz and found that the Ca influx via I_{Ca} was a much larger fraction of the SR Ca content at lower frequency (~30 and 50% respectively). This is consistent with the higher transsarcolemmal Ca flux dependence in guinea-pig in Fig 134B. At the lower frequency, the SR Ca content was lower while I_{Ca} was slightly higher (secondary to less Ca-dependent inactivation of I_{Ca}). Consequently the ratio of I_{Ca} to SR Ca load was higher at lower frequency. Given the different methodologies and limitations ([Ca]$_i$ decline *vs.* current integration), this agreement seems remarkably good.

What about Ca entry via Na/Ca exchange during the cardiac action potential? I have focused here on I_{Ca}, but early in the AP some Ca entry via Na/Ca exchange may occur (see Fig 74, pg 151). However, the amount of Ca entry during a normal Ca transient is likely to be <1 μmol/L cytosol (pg 149-151), much less than 10% of that entering via I_{Ca}. Thus, under normal conditions it is expected that most of Ca influx is via I_{Ca} and only a very small fraction (<10%) is via Na/Ca exchange (see also Grantham & Cannell, 1996). On the other hand, when [Na]$_i$ is high, as with digitalis-induced inhibition of the Na/K-ATPase, this situation can change and substantial Ca can enter during the AP and activate contraction (see Fig 72 and Chapter 10).

BIPHASIC CONTRACTIONS

Under certain conditions two phases of contraction can be seen, where the first component is often attributed to SR Ca release and latter to Ca influx. Indeed, biphasic contractions have been reported under a variety of conditions, especially when cAMP is increased or when the SR is relatively Ca-depleted (Braveny & Sumbera, 1970; Coraboeuf, 1974; Allen *et al.*, 1976; Beresewicz & Reuter, 1977; Seibel *et al.*, 1978; Bogdanov *et al.*, 1979; Endoh *et al.*, 1982; King & Bose, 1983; Reiter *et al.*, 1984; Honoré *et al.*, 1986, 1987; Malécot *et al.*, 1986).

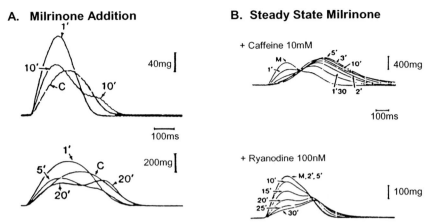

A. Milrinone Addition   **B. Steady State Milrinone**

Figure 136. Biphasic contractions in ferret ventricular muscle induced by 240 μM milrinone (at 28°C and 0.5 Hz). **A.** Addition of milrinone to two different muscles, C is control and numbers refer to time after milrinone addition (in min). **B.** Steady state biphasic contractions in milrinone (M) and changes in contractions after addition of 10 mM caffeine (top) or 100 nM ryanodine (bottom) for the times indicated. Both of these agents depress the first phase of contraction and caffeine also increases the second component. (from Malécot *et al.*, 1986, with permission of the American Heart Association).

Figure 136 shows biphasic contractions induced by the cardiotonic drug milrinone. Milrinone increases I_{Ca} (due to phosphodiesterase inhibition) and exerts a mild caffeine-like action on the SR (Malécot *et al.*, 1986; Rapundalo *et al.*, 1986) Initially, contractions are increased in amplitude and shortened in duration, probably due to cAMP-induced enhancement of I_{Ca}. Over the next few minutes the fast peak decreases and a second component becomes increasingly apparent. We attributed this to a milrinone-induced SR Ca leak (like low [caffeine]), such that the larger Ca entry via I_{Ca} can activate contraction directly (but more slowly). Figure 136B shows that the early component is suppressed by either caffeine or ryanodine. The second component is relatively unaffected by ryanodine, but is enhanced by caffeine. Since caffeine increases myofilament Ca sensitivity, these results are consistent with the first component of biphasic contractions being due to SR Ca release and the second component being due to Ca influx.

Slow or tonic contractions can be readily seen when depolarization is prolonged by voltage clamp pulses in frog and mammalian heart, even when SR Ca transport is blocked (see Figs 71, 75 & 78, Morad & Trautwein, 1968; Braveny & Sumbera, 1970; Goto *et al.*, 1971; Léoty & Raymond, 1972; Coraboeuf, 1974; Horackova & Vassort, 1976, 1979; Chapman & Tunstall, 1981; Chapman, 1983; Eisner *et al.*, 1983; Isenberg & Wendt-Gallitelli, 1989). These tonic contractions can be due to either sustained Ca entry via Na/Ca exchange or a Ca window current. Those due to Ca entry via Na/Ca exchange are sensitive to the [Na] gradient and are more prominent at positive potentials (Fig 71). Those due to window I_{Ca} are more commonly observed at $E_m = -30$ to 0 mV and still occur in the absence of Na (Fig78).

REST DECAY AND REST POTENTIATION

Here I will discuss dynamic changes in SR Ca content Ca influx and SR Ca release in non-steady state conditions (e.g. during rest and upon resumption of stimulation after rest).

Early Electrical and Mechanical Restitution

Immediately after a contraction, some time is required before another contraction of the same amplitude can be activated. This early phase of recovery of contraction (~1 s) is often termed mechanical restitution and is essentially a relative refractory period. Several systems contribute to this finite restitution period, but the predominant factor after the first 200 ms is recovery of the RyR from an inactivated or adapted state (see Chapter 8, pg 228-230).

This explanation for early mechanical restitution also explains the well known functional response in cardiac muscle known as post-extrasystolic potentiation (PESP, Hoffman *et al.*, 1956). This is where activation occurs prior to full mechanical restitution, such that only a weak contraction occurs (extrasystole), but the subsequent contraction is potentiated (PESP). If I_{Ca} recovers (even partially) before the extrasystole, some Ca will enter the cell at the extrasystole. If SR Ca release is refractory, normal Ca release will not occur, resulting in a weak contraction, and the lower $[Ca]_i$ will allow more Ca influx via I_{Ca} (due to less Ca-induced inactivation) and less Ca efflux via Na/Ca exchange. The net gain in Ca during the extrasystole will enhance SR Ca content. Then, at the next beat, when the SR Ca release channel has recovered, there is a greater SR Ca release and contraction (PESP). In the intact heart a premature ventricular contraction (PVC) would cause this same chain of events. However, the reduced ventricular filling time will further reduce the contraction at the extrasystole (and may not raise ventricular pressure sufficiently to open the aortic valve). In contrast, at the post-extrasystolic beat the ventricular preload is higher than normal (especially after a compensatory pause for a missed sinus beat). The increased preload enhances myofilament Ca sensitivity and contractile force (Chapter 2) and works synergistically with the enhanced Ca transient to produce a very strong PESP. This creates the sensation of the heart "skipping a beat."

Mechanical alternans, where even at a constant frequency, contraction amplitude alternates from one beat to the next (Wolfhart, 1982) may also be explained this way. If the normal refractory period for the SR Ca release channel is prolonged (e.g. due to elevated $[Ca]_i$ or low temperature) then Ca release and $\Delta[Ca]_i$ would be small (but Ca influx would still occur). By the next pulse the SR may no longer be refractory (and at higher Ca load), so a larger than normal Ca release may occur. The larger Ca transient inactivates I_{Ca} faster (limiting Ca influx), and enhances Ca extrusion via Na/Ca exchange. This results in a lower Ca content for the next contraction. Thus, the smaller contraction might be smaller for two reasons: 1) because the SR has less Ca and 2) due to refractoriness of the SR release mechanism (see Fig 143).

Slow Ryanodine Receptor Recovery and Rest Potentiation

In addition to the rapid restitution above (and pg 228-230), which occurs in the first second after a twitch, there is a slower phase which occurs over many seconds. This phase may be largely responsible for rest potentiation, which refers to the increase in contraction amplitude observed after a rest period of 10-120 sec (e.g. in rat ventricle, see top trace in Fig 137B). Figure 137B shows that rest potentiation develops in rat to a maximum of ~130% of control with a τ of ~8 sec and stays elevated for 5 min (Twitch NT). The enhanced contraction (and Ca transient) occurs despite no change in SR Ca content (assessed by caffeine application, Caff NT).

Rabbit (and guinea-pig) ventricle typically exhibit rest decay rather than rest potentiation (see Fig 137A, Twitch NT), but as discussed below this is primarily due to a decrease in SR Ca

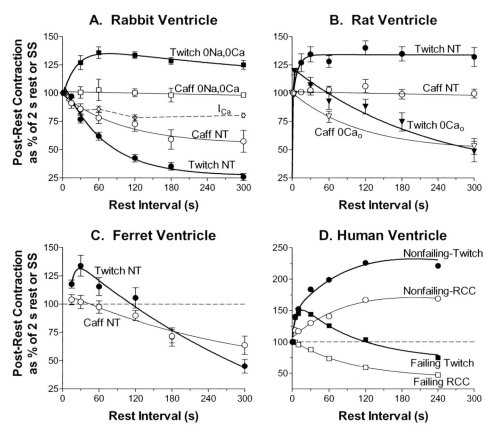

Figure 137. Rest decay of twitch contraction, SR Ca content and peak I_{Ca}. Post-rest twitches, caffeine-induced contractures (Caff) or RCCs were measured in normal Tyrode's solution (NT) or when Na/Ca exchange was blocked by 0Na,0Ca during only the rest (in **A**), or after pre-depleting $[Na]_i$ and rest in Ca-free NT (to stimulate Ca efflux via Na/Ca exchange, $0Ca_o$ in **B**). SR Ca load data (Caff & RCC) were fit to $[Ca]_{SRC} = a \cdot \exp(-t/\tau_{RD})(1-\exp(-t/\tau_{RF})) + b$, where t is time, τ_{RD} & τ_{RF} are time constants of rest decay of SR Ca content & rest-dependent filling (used to explain SR Ca increase or delays in SR Ca decline), and a and b are constants for scaling and baseline respectively. Twitch data were fit with the expression $c[Ca]_{SRC}(1-\exp(-t/\tau_{ECC})) + d$, where τ_{ECC} is the time constant for recovery of E-C coupling (20, 8, 7, & 7 s for rabbit, rat, ferret and human) and c and d are scaling and baseline constants. A small second τ was included to describe the slow decline in twitch in rabbit ventricle after long rests in 0Na,0Ca. Data are at 23°C except for human (37°C) and pre-rest steady state (SS) stimulation was 0.5 Hz except for human (1 Hz). Data are from Hryshko & Bers (1990), Bers *et al.* (1993), Bassani & Bers (1994) and Pieske *et al.* (1999a).

content (Caff NT). If the loss of SR Ca is prevented by exposure to 0Na,0Ca solution during the rest (Caff 0Na,0Ca), rabbit ventricular myocytes exhibit the same rest potentiation as observed in rat ventricular myocytes (Twitch-0Na,0Ca, Bassani & Bers, 1994). The amplitude of the I_{Ca} trigger at the post-rest twitch is typically smaller by 5-20% due to the loss of Ca-dependent I_{Ca} facilitation (I_{Ca} trace; see also pg 119). Thus, this slow phase of rest potentiation develops with a τ of 5-10 sec, can occur without any increase in SR Ca load or I_{Ca} and indicates a time-dependent increase in fractional SR Ca release.

This slow recovery of SR Ca release can also be seen at the microscopic level using Ca sparks (Satoh *et al.*, 1997). Immediately after a twitch in rat ventricular myocytes, there is a

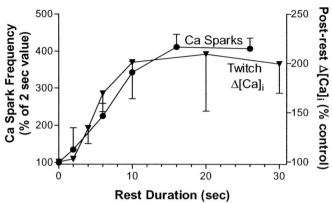

Figure 138. Recovery of Ca spark frequency and rest potentiation in rat. After stimulation at 0.5 Hz, rat ventricular myocytes were rested for various periods and Ca spark frequency was observed using confocal microscopy and post-rest potentiation of Ca transients was also recorded by field stimulation. There was no change in SR Ca content during this period (assessed by caffeine-induced Ca transients) Time constants fit to the data were 5 & 7 sec for twitch and Ca spark frequency. Data are from Satoh *et al.* (1997).

period where spontaneous resting Ca sparks are nearly abolished, but then Ca spark frequency gradually recovers back to a steady state level. Figure 138 shows that recovery of Ca sparks parallels that of rest potentiation (Satoh *et al.*, 1997). Therefore, this slow recovery of SR Ca release appears to be an intrinsic property of individual RyRs (or at least of RyR clusters).

At high SR Ca content this quiet period with respect to Ca spark frequency can be overcome (Satoh *et al.*, 1997). This may be due to the effects of luminal SR [Ca] on the gating properties of the cardiac RyR (pg 194-195, 225). This may encroach on a restitution-dependent, intrinsic safety factor against spontaneous SR Ca release between beats and may contribute to delayed afterdepolarizations and triggered arrhythmias at high SR Ca loads.

Since this slow recovery phase takes several seconds to develop, it may seem irrelevant to the normal physiological situation with heart rates of ≥ 1 Hz. Nevertheless, the experimental study of post-rest contractions has increased our overall understanding of how E-C coupling functions in the intact cell and this will be more apparent in subsequent sections in this Chapter. It should also be appreciated that if some fraction of RyRs are unavailable for SR Ca release for several seconds after activation, then at steady state heart rates of ≥ 1 Hz, there will be a certain fraction of RyRs which are in a refractory state and unable to participate in E-C coupling. Moreover, this fraction will be expected to change with heart rate or stimulation frequency (see Force-Frequency Relationship below, pg 267).

Rest Decay and SR Ca Depletion

Rest decay refers to the rest-dependent decline in the amplitude of the first post-rest twitch with increasing rest duration, and is apparent in many mammalian cardiac preparations (Fig 137A, Twitch NT; Allen *et al.*, 1976). During rest, there is a finite leak of Ca from the SR (~0.3 μmol/L cytosol/sec in both rabbit and rat ventricular myocytes; Bassani & Bers, 1995) and this may occur primarily as Ca sparks, due to occasional stochastic RyR openings (see pg 192). Once Ca leaks into the cytosol, it is subject to the same competition among Ca transport systems as discussed above for twitch relaxation and [Ca]$_i$ decline (i.e. mainly the SR Ca-ATPase and

Na/Ca exchange). If Ca extrusion is prevented by 0Na,0Ca solution, there is no serious competitor with the SR Ca-pump, and consequently the Ca which leaked from the SR is mainly taken back up by the SR, preventing net loss of SR Ca (see Fig 137A, Caff 0Na,0Ca). However, in rabbit ventricular myocytes, there is normally a substantial thermodynamic gradient favoring Ca extrusion via Na/Ca exchange (see Fig 72). Thus, some Ca leaked from the SR during rest is extruded from the cell, while the remainder is taken back up by the SR. The Ca which leaves the cell during rest typically exceeds the transsarcolemmal Ca leak and results in a net loss of cellular and SR Ca. Quantitatively, if 33-50% of the leaked SR Ca (0.3 µmol/L cytosol/sec) is extruded by Na/Ca exchange the cell would lose 6-10 µmol/L cytosol/min, such that an SR Ca load of 100 µmol/L cytosol could be half-depleted in ~5 min (as in Fig 137A). This decline in SR Ca load is the main explanation for rest decay as seen prominently in rabbit and guinea-pig ventricular muscle and myocytes (Fig 137A, NT traces). The amplitude of RCCs also declines as a function of rest duration in a manner parallel to that of stimulated twitches (Bridge, 1986; Bers, 1989). Guinea-pig (Fig 79) behaves similar to rabbit ventricle (with somewhat faster rest decay) and mouse behaves very similarly to rat ventricle.

In addition to the progressive loss of SR Ca available for release during rest decay, a smaller I_{Ca} may also make a minor contribution during the first 10 sec of rest. The ability of a given I_{Ca} trigger to cause SR Ca release may also affect rest decay in two opposing ways. On one hand, we expect fractional SR Ca release to increase during rest as described above for rest potentiation. On the other hand, as SR Ca content declines, the lower $[Ca]_{SR}$ decreases fractional SR Ca release, and this can be profoundly inhibitory at low SR Ca content (see Fig 119). Several factors may be involved at early times, but the decreased SR Ca content and fractional SR Ca release are increasingly dominant factors at later times. At some point as SR Ca falls (even before the SR becomes fully depleted), the SR may stop participating in E-C coupling. This may occur at an SR Ca load of 30-40 µmol/L cytosol (as in Fig 119). The so called "rested-state contraction" (where further rest makes no difference) reflects a state in rabbit and guinea-pig where the contraction is largely due to Ca influx, rather than SR Ca release (not the case for rat).

It is important to appreciate that the decline in SR Ca content need not be complete after long rest intervals. $[Ca]_{SR}$ may simply establish a new steady state, where at low SR Ca content, there is both a reduction in SR Ca leak and enhanced ability of the SR Ca-pump to compete with Na/Ca exchange. The reduced leak may be due to low $[Ca]_{SR}$, which decreases Ca spark frequency and also lowers Ca flux through open Ca release channels. The enhanced SR Ca-pump competition with Na/Ca exchange may be due to higher net SR Ca-pump rate at low $[Ca]_{SR}$ (less backflux, pg 173-177) and also to de-activation of the Na/Ca exchanger at low $[Ca]_i$ (pg 139-140). Indeed, Terracciano & MacLeod (1996) found that after caffeine-induced SR Ca depletion in guinea-pig ventricular myocytes (which behave much like rabbit myocytes) there was spontaneous SR refilling during rest, to ~50% of the steady state seen at 0.2 Hz stimulation.

An implication from this framework is that anything which inhibits SR Ca-pumping (e.g. thapsigargin) or increases SR Ca leak (e.g. ryanodine), would shift the competition toward extrusion by Na/Ca exchange and be expected to accelerate rest decay. This is seen with both thapsigargin and ryanodine (Figs 79 & 96; Bassani & Bers, 1995; Sutko *et al.*, 1986; Bers *et al.*, 1987,1989). Furthermore, anything which inhibits Ca extrusion via Na/Ca exchange would bias the competition toward the SR Ca-pump and slow rest decay. This effect is clearly seen for elevated $[Na]_i$ (with Na/K-ATPase inhibition), reduced $[Na]_o$ (Sutko *et al.*, 1986) and the extreme case where Na/Ca exchange is completely blocked by 0Na, 0Ca (Figs 137A, 79-80 & 95).

These implications may also explain why rat (& mouse) ventricle typically do not exhibit rest decay of twitches or SR Ca content (Fig 137B, NT traces). That is, in rat *vs.* rabbit the SR Ca-Pump activity is higher and Na/Ca exchange is less able to extrude Ca (see Fig 134A). Indeed, for the rat, this inability of the Na/Ca exchanger to extrude Ca may be a consequence of a relatively high resting $[Na]_i$ in rat and mouse myocytes (Shattock & Bers, 1989; Yao *et al.*, 1998), which means that there is little or no driving force for Ca extrusion at diastolic E_m and $[Ca]_i$ (see Fig 140). However, we can deplete rat cells of $[Na]_i$ by incubation in 0Na,0Ca solution, and then returning to Ca-free normal Tyrode's for the rest interval (0Ca$_o$ in Fig 137B). This shifts the driving force on the Na/Ca exchange, such that it can compete better with the SR Ca-pump. Fig 137B shows that in rat ventricular myocytes this results in clear rest decay of both SR Ca (Caff 0Ca$_o$) and twitches evoked immediately after restoring Ca$_o$ (Twitch 0Ca$_o$). Thus, there is a critical and dynamic balance between SR and sarcolemmal Ca transporters which is crucial in determining SR Ca available for release.

In the simplest quantitative terms, the amplitude of the post-rest contraction depends mainly on two factors: 1) the amount of SR Ca available for release ($[Ca]_{SRC}$ in Fig 137 legend), multiplied by 2) fractional SR Ca release (which depends on time and $[Ca]_{SRC}$). In many cardiac preparations $[Ca]_{SRC}$ declines during rest, due to the balance of SR Ca transport and Na/Ca exchange as described above. While $[Ca]_{SRC}$ is declining, the slow phase of post-rest recovery of E-C coupling is increasing (τ_{ECC} ~7 sec in Fig 137 legend). This can lead to transient rest potentiation which is commonly seen in ferret ventricle (Fig 137C), and many other cardiac preparations (including failing human ventricle, Fig 137D). At longer times the rest potentiation (τ_{ECC}) factor may be maximal, but as $[Ca]_{SRC}$ continues to decline with time, the product of $[Ca]_{SRC} \times$ fractional release will progressively decline. The fractional release factor (assuming the Ca trigger is unchanged) will increase at short times, but if SR Ca stays high (as in rat), then fractional release may not change further. If $[Ca]_{SRC}$ declines, it will also reduce fractional release and can exacerbate the rest decay of twitch contraction (i.e. both factors decline).

So in ferret ventricle (Fig 137C) there is typically rest potentiation which lasts for up to 2 min, but then rest decay becomes more dominant as $[Ca]_{SRC}$ declines monotonically. In non-failing human ventricle, $[Ca]_{SRC}$ appears to increase during rest (Fig 137D, Pieske *et al.*, 1999a). In this case post-rest twitches are greatly enhanced, because both $[Ca]_{SRC}$ and fractional release factors are increasing. This has also been reported in some cases for rat ventricle (Bers, 1989; Bers & Shattock 1989; Lewartowski & Zdanowski, 1990; Banijamali *et al.*, 1991; Maier *et al.*, 2000). We interpret this in the following manner for the rat (and possibly human). If $[Na]_i$ increases during pacing (from 's already high value in rat), the reversal potential for $I_{Na/Ca}$ may fall below the diastolic E_m, such that net Ca entry occurs during diastole. This implies that net Ca extrusion occurs during systole in rat. As we will see, this actually occurs (Fig 139). Thus, rat $[Ca]_{SRC}$ may increase, remain unchanged or even decrease during rest. Indeed, when $[Na]_i$ is low in individual rat myocytes rest decay can occur (Fig 137B; Frampton *et al.*, 1991). This emphasizes the importance of specific ionic conditions in driving the delicate balance of Ca fluxes across the sarcolemmal and SR membrane. In ferret ventricle, an unusually strong sarcolemmal Ca-ATPase can partially substitute for Na/Ca exchange in mediating cellular Ca extrusion during rest decay (Bassani *et al.,* 1994b, 1995a). In this specific case 0Na, 0Ca solution during rest does not abolish rest decay of SR Ca content (as in Fig 137A), but only slows this rest decay partially (see Fig 80).

In human heart failure, there is decreased SR Ca-ATPase expression and increased Na/Ca exchanger expression (e.g. Hasenfuss, 1998a). This shifts the competition between the SR Ca-ATPase and Na/Ca exchange more in favor of the Na/Ca exchanger during rest. Consequently, failing human ventricle exhibits rest decay of $[Ca]_{SRC}$, and only a transient rest potentiation is seen. As in ferret, this occurs during the time when the positive effect of RyR recovery is sufficient to more than offset the initial small loss in $[Ca]_{SRC}$.

Clearly this is a simplified consideration of diastolic Ca fluxes since it neglects other possible Ca fluxes (e.g. mitochondrial Ca fluxes and sarcolemmal Ca leak and Ca-pump). However, the mechanisms considered above appear to be the most important ones and suffice to explain the main features of diastolic changes in SR Ca content. Thus, the process of rest decay in cardiac muscle appears to depend upon Ca extrusion via Na/Ca exchange and the balance of SR Ca-pump and leak.

Ca Influx and Efflux in Rabbit and Rat Ventricle

The above results suggest major fundamental differences in transsarcolemmal Ca fluxes in rat *vs.* rabbit ventricle during both rest and contraction. Shattock & Bers (1989) compared Ca fluxes in rat *vs.* rabbit ventricle during the cardiac cycle using extracellular Ca microelectrodes. We demonstrated that during the twitch in rabbit ventricle net Ca influx occurs, but that during the twitch in rat ventricle net Ca efflux occurs (see Fig 139). Since Na/Ca exchange is the main mechanism by which Ca is extruded from cardiac cells, we suggested that the large Ca efflux seen in rat was due to Ca released by the SR and extruded by Na/Ca exchange. Indeed, Ca efflux recorded in rat ventricle was caffeine sensitive and larger at the first large post-rest contraction. We also compared resting intracellular Na activity (aNa_i) and found that aNa_i was significantly higher in rat (12.7 mM or $[Na]_i$ =16 mM) than rabbit ventricle (7.2 mM or $[Na]_i$ =9 mM).

In rabbit ventricle Ca extrusion via Na/Ca exchange is thermodynamically favored at rest because the predicted reversal potential for Na/Ca exchange ($E_{Na/Ca}$) is positive to E_m (see Fig 140). During the action potential E_m exceeds $E_{Na/Ca}$ (even though $[Ca]_i$ is elevated) such that there may be a modest driving force favoring Ca entry during the AP (see also Figs 72 & 74). This, together with I_{Ca}, explains the transient Ca_o depletions seen during contractions in rabbit ventricle (Fig 139A) and Ca loss during diastole (as in rest decay). The rate of diastolic Ca extrusion is small, despite the large thermodynamic driving force. This is because inward $I_{Na/Ca}$ is limited by the low resting $[Ca]_i$, both kinetically and due to deavtivation (Weber *et al.*, 2001).

The resting $[Na]_i$ in rat ventricle is high enough that the $E_{Na/Ca}$ is near the resting E_m (Fig 140). In particular, after a train of stimuli aNa_i would be higher still, such that $E_{Na/Ca}$ *would* be negative to E_m and net Ca uptake would be favored. This can explain the above described rest-dependent increase in SR Ca sometimes seen in rat ventricle and could contribute to rest potentiation. While Bassani *et al.* (1994a) found no difference in diastolic $[Ca]_i$ in rat *vs.* rabbit, DuBell & Houser (1987) reported higher resting $[Ca]_i$ in rat than in cat ventricular myocytes. In rat ventricle the AP duration is also very short (compared to rabbit ventricle), and normally lacks

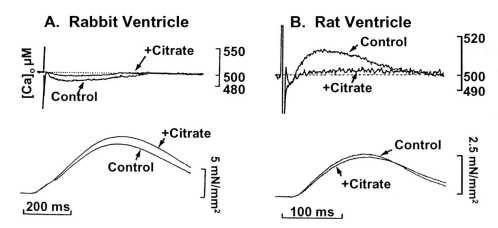

Figure 139. Changes in [Ca]$_o$ measured with double barreled Ca-selective microelectrodes during individual contractions in rabbit (**A**) and rat (**B**) ventricular muscle (0.5 Hz, 30°C). The traces show [Ca]$_o$ (top) and tension (bottom) in the absence and presence of 10 mM citrate (which limits Ca$_o$ depletion by buffering [Ca]$_o$ (but it can also inhibit I$_{Ca}$, Bers *et al.*, 1991). The bath [Ca]$_o$ = 0.5 mM and is indicated by the dotted line. (A is redrawn from Shattock & Bers, 1989, with permission.).

an appreciable plateau phase (see Fig 140). Thus, during the contraction, when [Ca]$_i$ is high, E$_{Na/Ca}$ is positive to E$_m$, so that there is a large driving force favoring Ca extrusion via Na/Ca exchange. In this way the competition between the SR Ca-pump and the Na/Ca exchanger is biased toward the latter, and net Ca efflux occurs during the contraction (compare Fig 139B and 140B). During a potentiated post-rest contraction a larger Ca efflux will occur and the SR Ca content will be lower at the next contraction until a new steady state is achieved (where Ca influx and efflux must again be equal over a complete cardiac cycle). This may contribute to the decrease in contraction amplitude during post-rest recovery and also to the well known negative "staircase" or force-frequency relationship in rat ventricle (see below).

If the depolarization in a rat ventricular myocyte is prolonged near 0 mV by a voltage clamp pulse (to resemble that in rabbit ventricle), the negative "staircase" can be converted to a positive "staircase" (Spurgeon *et al.*, 1988), as would be expected from Fig 140. Figure 141 shows a similar result in guinea-pig ventricle which behaves much like rabbit ventricle. Increasing pulse duration leads to a positive staircase, while reduction of pulse duration to 100 msec leads to a negative staircase (Isenberg & Wendt-Gallitelli, 1989). Thus, prolonging the duration of depolarization can increase intracellular (and SR) Ca loading by two means: 1) limiting the extrusion of Ca via Na/Ca exchange and 2) allowing continued Ca entry via sarcolemmal Ca channels (and possibly via Na/Ca exchange, depending on conditions).

Ryanodine greatly accelerates rest decay of RCCs in rabbit ventricle (t$_{1/2}$ ~1 sec, Fig 96), but does not completely abolish RCCs in rat ventricle (Bers & Christensen, 1990). This is consistent with the foregoing discussion, since the low transsarcolemmal [Na] gradient may limit Ca extrusion via Na/Ca exchange (so that even a "leaky" SR may be able to retain some Ca). Furthermore, by manipulating [Na] and [Ca] gradients, rabbit ventricle can be made to behave more like rat ventricle, and *vice versa* (Bers & Christensen, 1990; Bassani & Bers,1 994). For example, in Fig 137A-B, limiting Ca extrusion by 0Na,0Ca in rabbit ventricle causes rest

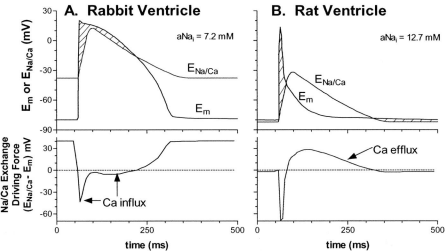

Figure 140. Schematic diagram of the estimated changes in the reversal potential of the Na/Ca exchange ($E_{Na/Ca}$) that accompany the action potential and Ca_i transient in rabbit and rat ventricle (top) . The estimated changes in the net electrochemical driving force for Na/Ca exchange ($E_{Na/Ca}-E_m$) are shown in the bottom panels. We assumed a stoichiometry of 3Na:1Ca for the Na/Ca exchanger, aNa_i values as actually measured in these preparations (Shattock & Bers, 1989) and, for simplicity, the Ca transient accompanying the contraction has been assumed to be the same for both species. Resting $[Ca]_i$ was assumed to be 150 nM, rising to a peak of 1 μM, 40 msec after the AP upstroke. The shape of the Ca transient was calculated as described by Bers (1987b). Note the similarity between the lower panels and the $[Ca]_o$ traces in Fig 139. (Top panels were redrawn after Shattock & Bers, 1989, with permission).

potentiation as seen in rat ventricle. Conversely, boosting Ca extrusion via Na/Ca exchange in rat causes rest decay which resembles that in rabbit.

While depolarization alters transsarcolemmal Ca fluxes, Ca extrusion via Na/Ca exchange can also modify the AP. Schouten & ter Keurs (1985) demonstrated that removal of $[Na]_o$ suppressed a slow component of the rat ventricular AP which was most prominent at large contractions where $[Ca]_i$ is high (see Fig 142). They attributed the late low plateau AP phase to inward $I_{Na/Ca}$ (i.e. 3 Na influx for 1 Ca extruded). Hilgemann & Noble (1987) simulated this

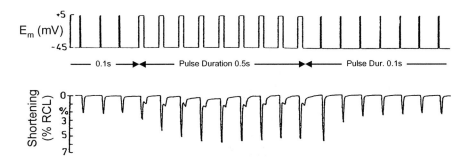

Figure 141. Duration of depolarization determines the direction of the contraction staircase in guinea-pig ventricular myocyte. E_m and shortening as a percent of resting cell length (RCL) under voltage-clamp (37°C, $[Ca]_o=1.8$ mM). (From Isenberg & Wendt-Gallitelli, 1989, with permission).

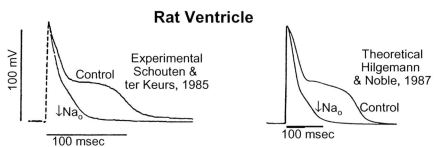

Figure 142. Action potentials recorded from rat ventricular muscle (left) stimulated at low frequency where contractions are large in control superfusate and after reduction of [Na]$_o$ from 150 to 30 mM. This behavior could be simulated in an AP model simply by reducing the effective [Na] for Na/Ca exchange (right). (from Schouten & ter Keurs, 1985 and Hilgemann & Noble, 1987, with permission).

effect in their model of the rat ventricular action potential (Fig 142).

APs are also influenced by Ca fluxes during paired-pulse stimulation and mechanical alternans (Wolfhart, 1982; Hilgemann, 1986a,b). Figure 143 shows extracellular Ca depletion, E_m and force in rabbit atrium during paired-pulse stimulation (Hilgemann, 1986b). As the large contraction develops, [Ca]$_o$ reaches a nadir (maximal influx), but net Ca efflux is evident by the end of the contraction. This is analogous to the result with rat ventricle in Fig 139B where high [Ca]$_i$ drives Ca efflux via Na/Ca exchange. The small paired-pulse beat produces progressive net Ca$_o$ depletion, a more prominent AP plateau and only a tiny contraction. As for the extrasystole above, SR Ca release may be refractory at the small beat, such that no SR Ca is released. Thus [Ca]$_i$ remains low during the AP, which allows more Ca influx (explaining the larger Ca$_o$ depletion and the higher AP plateau). The low [Ca]$_i$ limits I_{Ca} inactivation and Ca extrusion via Na/Ca exchange during the small beat. The net result is that the SR is more Ca loaded (and non-refractory) at the time of the next pulse. In this case inward $I_{Na/Ca}$ may limit rapid repolarization at the large beat. However, the persistent inward I_{Ca} at the small beat may more than offset the

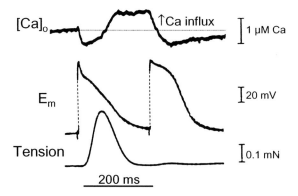

Figure 143. Paired-pulse stimulation of rabbit atrium in the presence of 2 mM 4-aminopyridine (to suppress transient outward K currents). The [Ca]$_o$ is assessed by the absorbance of the extracellular Ca indicator, tetramethylmurexide. Free [Ca]$_o$ is 150 µM, the basic frequency is 0.5 Hz and the smaller paired-pulse beat is evoked 200 msec after the main pulse (from Hilgemann, 1986b, with permission).

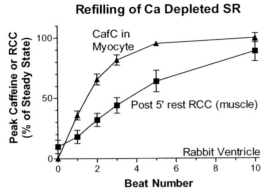

Figure 144. Refilling of the SR with Ca after depletion in rabbit ventricle.. The SR Ca content was depleted by either a 5 min rest period in ventricular muscle (at 30°C) or by a 10 s exposure to 10 mM caffeine in myocytes (at 23°C). Recovery of SR Ca content upon resumption of stimulation at 0.5 Hz was assessed by a second caffeine-induced contracture in myocytes or by an RCC in muscle (data are taken from Bers, 1989 and Bassani *et al.*, 1993b).

lower inward $I_{Na/Ca}$ at the small beat (with respect to E_m). Since there is little Ca efflux during the small paired-pulse (where SR Ca release is refractory) one could consider the integrated I_{Ca} to be "injected" into the SR. Once the Ca which enters has been pumped into the SR, the SR then has an extra aliquot of Ca available for the next contraction (as for the PESP on pg 256).

SR Ca Refilling and Post-Rest Recovery

After long rests in rabbit ventricular muscle or after sustained caffeine application, the SR is depleted of Ca. Thus, when contractions are resumed the SR gradually refills to the steady state level. Figure 144 shows the time course of SR Ca refilling in rabbit ventricle (using caffeine or RCCs to assess SR Ca). In general, the recovery of twitches and SR Ca are similar. However, SR Ca can recover back to steady state faster than stimulated twitches (especially after long rest intervals). Thus, most, but not all of the twitch recovery is due to refilling of the SR. Indeed, if 10-15 μmol Ca/L cytosol enters via I_{Ca}, it would take 5-10 beats to restore SR Ca content to 60-100 μmol/L cytosol (see Fig 145).

The half-time for refilling the SR is 2-4 beats and it reaches steady state in 10-15 beats. This agrees with results from extracellular Ca_o depletion studies in rabbit ventricle (Bers & MacLeod, 1986; MacLeod & Bers, 1987; Bers, 1987b). These Ca_o depletions, which reflect net Ca uptake by the cells, reach a maximum in 6-12 contractions upon resumption of stimulation after a rest with the half-maximum typically occurring at beat 4-5 (see Figs 97 & 165). I_{Ca} amplitude also increases toward steady state during the first 5-10 post-rest pulses (see Fig 58). However, this I_{Ca} staircase is small and its contribution to the post-rest recovery is not clear.

Figure 145 shows an elegant quantitative procedure to assess Ca fluxes during refilling of the SR, after Ca depletion induced by caffeine application in a voltage clamped ferret ventricular myocyte (Trafford *et al.*, 1997). They use the reasonable simplification that during a pulse from – 40 to 0 mV, inward current indicates Ca influx via I_{Ca}, and that upon repolarization

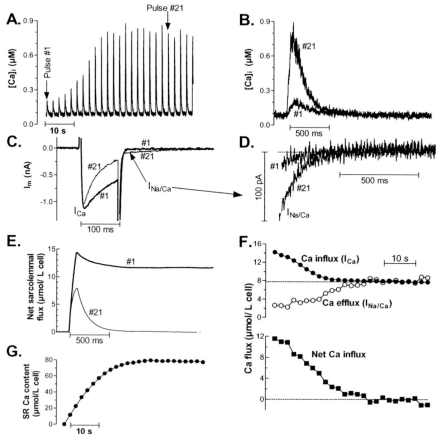

Figure 145. Ca fluxes and SR Ca content during refilling after depletion. Induced by caffeine. **A.** Ca transients during the first 25 voltage clamp pulses from –40 to 0 mV for 100 ms (27°C). **B.** Expanded time scale of selected Ca transients. **C.** Currents for the 1st and 21st pulse. **D.** Enlarged $I_{Na/Ca}$ traces from C. **E.** Evolution of net integrated transsarcolemmal Ca flux for pulse 1 & 21 (corrected for surface:volume ratio). **F.** Unidirectional Ca fluxes and net Ca influx (influx – efflux), based on integrals of data in panels C-E. **G.** Cumulative cellular Ca gain, which is assumed to be nearly all taken up by the SR. Data from Trafford *et al.* (1997, kindly supplied by the authors) were regraphed.

the slow inward tail current indicates Ca extrusion via $I_{Na/Ca}$ (Fig 145C). Panel A shows the recovery of Ca transients during 100 ms pulses at 0.5 Hz. Panels B & C show details of [Ca]$_i$ and current for the 1st and 21st pulses. As the SR reloads the Ca transient is larger and I_{Ca} inactivates more rapidly, gradually decreasing the integrated I_{Ca} influx to a steady state value (Panels C & F; see also Fig 60). As the Ca transients increase, the Ca extrusion by $I_{Na/Ca}$ also increases (enlarged in panel D) to a steady state where Ca efflux via $I_{Na/Ca}$ is equal to Ca influx via I_{Ca} (8 μmol/L cell! = 12 μmol/L cytosol, panel F). Thus, at pulse #21 Ca influx = Ca efflux, and no net gain or loss of cell Ca occurs (panels E & F). In contrast, at pulse #1 Ca influx far exceeds Ca efflux and the cellular Ca content rises by ~12 μmol/L cell (panel E and F). Since diastolic [Ca]$_i$ doesn't change, it is reasonable to assume that the cellular Ca gain reflects a gain in SR Ca (panel G). Thus, over these 21 beats the SR Ca content rises from 0 to 80 μmol/L cell (120 μmol/L cytosol).

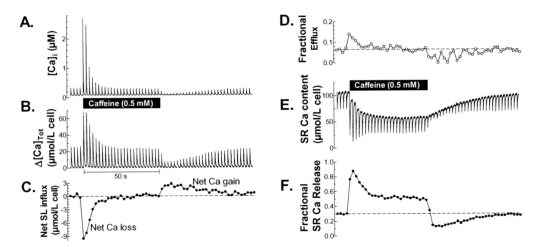

Figure 146. Increased SR Ca release enhances Ca transients only transiently. Adding 0.5 mM caffeine enhances CICR and abruptly increases twitch $\Delta[Ca]_i$ & $\Delta[Ca]_{Tot}$ (**A,B**), but this increases Ca extrusion via $I_{Na/Ca}$ (**C,-D**) and reduces SR Ca content (**E**). Despite a maintained elevation of fractional SR Ca release (**F**) twitch $\Delta[Ca]_i$ returns to control (where Ca influx and efflux are again equal, **C**). At this point I_{Ca} is unchanged, and since $\Delta[Ca]_i$ is the same, so is $I_{Na/Ca}$ ($[Ca]_o$=0.5 mM, pulses are from –40 to 0 mV for 100 ms at 0.5 Hz). Data from Eisner *et al.* (2000) & Trafford *et al.* (2000) was kindly supplied by the authors.

SR Ca refilling occurs with a time course similar to that in Fig 144, but the data in Fig 145 provide valuable detailed information about the underlying transsarcolemmal Ca fluxes.

Eisner *et al.* (1998, 2000) also argue that enhancing (or partially inhibiting) RyR release can only produce transient changes in contractility, but not steady state changes. This is based on results as in Fig 146 with low caffeine concentrations (~0.5 mM, which enhances CICR, O'Neill *et al.*, 1990a; Trafford *et al.*, 2000), with tetracaine (which depresses CICR, Overend *et al.*, 1997, 1998), and the following rationale. If SR Ca release (or CICR) is abruptly enhanced, the SR will release more Ca at the first twitch or two, but the larger $\Delta[Ca]_i$ increases Ca extrusion via $I_{Na/Ca}$ (and will limit Ca entry via I_{Ca}), resulting in a reduction of SR Ca content at the next twitch. The lower SR Ca content causes $\Delta[Ca]_i$ and fractional SR Ca release to decline at subsequent twitches. These twitches could still have a higher Ca transient than control, but this would cause SR Ca load to decline further. In the steady state in Fig 146, twitch $\Delta[Ca]_i$ comes back essentially to the control level, but this occurs with a lower SR Ca content and a higher fractional SR Ca release. This is because sarcolemmal Ca efflux and influx must come back into balance at steady state. Thus, if Ca influx is not changed, Ca efflux must be unchanged and the same $\Delta[Ca]_i$ would be required to drive the same Ca extrusion via $I_{Na/Ca}$. Exactly the converse was found with inhibition of CICR by tetracaine (or caffeine withdrawal, later in the Fig 146 traces). This sort of autoregulation of Ca transients emphasizes the integral role of SR Ca content in the regulation of SR Ca release. It also indicates that alteration of RyR gating, by itself is not a robust way to modulate contractility for more than a few beats. However, if combined with stimulation of the SR Ca-pump (as occurs with β-adrenergic activation), this can create a much faster and stable inotropic change than can be accomplished by SR Ca-pump activation alone (which would otherwise require 5-20 twitches to reach a new higher SR Ca content and inotropic state, Eisner *et al.*, 1998).

This paradigm is conceptually instructive and appropriate over a limited linear range, but must not be extrapolated too broadly. Clearly, if CICR is completely blocked, no SR Ca release occurs and smaller steady state contractions would result. Likewise, if CICR were hypersensitized (as for caffeine concentrations, >5 mM), the SR is becomes completely Ca-depleted, and again there is no SR Ca release, and depressed steady state twitches (e.g. see Figs 129-130). Of course, the lack of SR Ca release will allow Ca influx to rise, but this may not compensate for the lack of Ca from the SR. Changes in the time course of the AP or Ca transient, and continued alteration of SR Ca release during diastole can also complicate this analysis.

FORCE-FREQUENCY RELATIONSHIPS

The relationship between stimulation pattern and contractile force has attracted study since the early work of Bowditch (1871) and Woodworth (1902). This force-frequency relationship has been reviewed (e.g. Kruta, 1937; Braveny & Kruta, 1958; Blinks & Koch-Weser, 1961; Koch-Weser & Blinks, 1963; Wood *et al.*, 1969; Allen *et al.*, 1976; Edman & Jóhannsson, 1976; Johnson, 1979; Wolfhart & Noble, 1982; Lewartowski & Pytkowski, 1987; Schouten *et al.*, 1987). However, we can now better address the cellular mechanisms involved than was possible in some of these classic reviews. Most of the key fundamental mechanisms have been addressed above with respect to mechanical restitution, rest decay (and potentiation), post-rest recovery, paired-pulses, alternans and post-extrasystolic potentiation. We can draw on those mechanisms to explain most features of the force-frequency relationship.

Figure 147 shows a classical response to a transient increase in stimulation frequency in rabbit ventricular muscle. The first pulse at 1.5 Hz is smaller, probably reflecting insufficient time for the SR Ca release channel recovery from inactivation. Continued pacing at 1.5 Hz leads to a progressive positive staircase (which overcomes the continued infringement on restitution). At least three factors could contribute to this increase: 1) increased I_{Ca}, 2) higher diastolic $[Ca]_i$ (due to greater Ca influx/sec and also less time between contractions for Ca extrusion), and 3) increased SR Ca load available for release (as a consequence of the above, and the higher average $[Ca]_i$). The higher average $[Ca]_i$ may also stimulate CaMKII, which can increase fractional SR Ca release (Li *et al.*, 1997b). Additionally, higher frequency raises $[Na]_i$ (Cohen *et al.*, 1982; January & Fozzard, 1984; Ellis, 1985; Boyett *et al.*, 1987). This shifts the Na/Ca exchange balance further toward less Ca extrusion and more Ca influx. The result is that there is more Ca in the cell and in the SR. This is confirmed by extracellular Ca depletions and larger RCCs when stimulation frequency is increased in rabbit ventricle (Bers & MacLeod, 1986; Bers, 1989; Maier *et al.*, 2000). Figure 148A shows that SR Ca rises with increasing frequency in rabbit and guinea-pig ventricle (based on RCCs), in parallel with changes in twitch force.

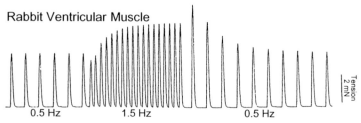

Rabbit Ventricular Muscle

0.5 Hz   1.5 Hz   0.5 Hz

Tension 2 mN

Figure 147. Frequency-dependent changes in twitch force in rabbit ventricular muscle (30°C).

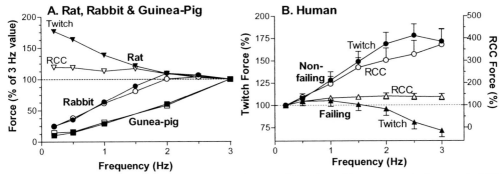

Figure 148. Force-frequency relationship in rabbit, rat, guinea-pig and human ventricular muscle (37°C). Effect of frequency on twitch force (filled symbols) and SR Ca content (open symbols, assessed by RCCs initiated within 5 sec of the last steady state stimulated contraction). Data for rabbit and rat are from Maier *et al.* (2000), guinea-pig from Kurihara & Sakai (1985) and human from Pieske *et al.* (1999a).

In Figure 147, switching back to 0.5 Hz results in a large first contraction. This probably reflects a combination of the relatively high SR Ca content (described above) and also a greater fraction of SR Ca released (due to the greater time available for recovery from inactivation of the SR release channel). This large SR Ca release and longer diastolic interval stimulates substantial Ca extrusion via Na/Ca exchange, and limits Ca entry via I_{Ca}. Consequently there is a progressive decline in the amount of Ca in the SR until the initial steady state is re-attained (e.g. where Ca efflux via Na/Ca exchange over one cycle matches Ca influx via I_{Ca}). Stepwise declines from potentiated contractions have also been used as an index of the fraction of released Ca that is resequestered (or recirculated) into the SR (Wolfhart & Noble, 1982; Schouten *et al.*, 1987). That is, if the second contraction is 70% of the potentiated one, then one might say that ~70% of the Ca released was recycled to the SR. Using "recirculation fraction" this way tacitly assumes that Ca influx is negligible, trigger Ca is unchanged and that the relation between SR Ca released and peak force is linear. This limits the true quantitative value of these recirculation fraction values, but they may be helpful empirically.

Figure 148 shows force-frequency relationships in several types of ventricular muscle, along with measures of SR Ca content (measured on-line in the same muscles using RCCs). Rabbit, guinea-pig and nonfailing human ventricle all show classic positive force-frequency relationships, accompanied by parallel increases in SR Ca content. Thus, despite encroachment on restitution time in these preparations as frequency increases, the increase in SR Ca appears to more than compensate, such that the product $[Ca]_{SRC} \times$ fractional release is increased.

In rat and mouse ventricle, SR Ca content is often relatively high, even at very low stimulation frequencies (as in post-rest contractions, Fig 137B). This may be due in part to relatively high $[Na]_i$ which limits Ca extrusion via Na/Ca exchange (Shattock & Bers, 1989; Yao *et al.*, 1998). Thus, increasing frequency in rat (Fig 148A or mouse) usually causes little or no further increase in, or even a slight decrease in SR Ca content (Bers, 1989; Shattock & Bers, 1989; Bouchard & Bose, 1989; Banijamali *et al.*, 1991; Maier *et al.*, 2000). This makes the dominant frequency-dependent effect in rat (& mouse) the encroachment into full recovery time of E-C coupling. This is why rat and mouse myocytes often show negative force-frequency relationships. On the other hand, rat ventricle can also exhibit a positive force-frequency relationship (Schouten & ter Keurs, 1986; Layland & Kentish, 1999; Kassiri *et al.*, 2000), presumably when cells start with low SR Ca content at low frequency (such that [Na]$_i$ and SR Ca can increase with frequency, Frampton *et al.*, 1991; Layland & Kentish, 1999).

In the failing human heart (Fig 148B), SR Ca content increases only slightly with increasing frequency (mostly between 0.2 and 1 Hz), and this is associated with some increase in twitch force. However, SR Ca load does not increase further at higher frequency, and so the relationship from 1 to 3 Hz is dominated by the intrinsic depressant effect of higher frequency on fractional SR Ca release. This results in a flat or negative force-frequency relationship. This would, of course, limit the functional reserve of the failing human heart and could be a direct consequence of reduced levels of SR Ca-ATPase and increased levels of Na/Ca exchange expression in the failing heart (see Chapter 10; Pieske *et al.*, 1999a). Another limiting factor in the intact heart (normal or failing) is reduced diastolic filling time at higher heart rates.

Thus, a largely positive force-frequency relationship is expected for normal mammalian cardiac muscle, except for those tissues which have either high SR Ca load at low frequency or possibly those with short AP duration (such as rat & mouse ventricle and some atrial preparations). In this case large Ca efflux may occur during the twitch as in rat ventricle (Figs 139-140). Even for these exceptions one can find conditions where a positive staircase is demonstrable (e.g. rat ventricle at low [Ca]$_o$, low [Na]$_i$ or high frequency, Forester & Mainwood, 1974; Henry, 1975; Frampton *et al.*, 1991; Schouten & ter Keurs, 1986; Layland & Kentish, 1999; Kassiri *et al.*, 2000). The potential physiological importance of a positive force-frequency relationship in maximizing cardiac output at high heart rates, makes the rat and mouse ventricle results of some concern. Indeed, some investigators (who typically record positive force-frequency relationships in rat) have suggested that this is the true physiological condition, and that the negative force-frequency relationship often observed in rat and mouse ventricle result from effects of tissue or cell isolation (which cause increased SR Ca load at low frequency).

The competition between the SR Ca-ATPase and Na/Ca exchange may also change as a function of frequency. We used paired RCCs (as described in Fig 76) to determine the ratio of RCC2/RCC1 at 37°C (Pieske *et al.*, 1999a; Maier *et al.*, 2000). If all Ca released at RCC1 is re-sequestered by the SR during relaxation of RCC1 this ratio is 100%. In rabbit and nonfailing human heart RCC2/RCC1 increases monotonically as twitch frequency increases from 0.25 Hz to 2 Hz (28 to 65% in rabbit and 37 to 74% in human). A simple explanation for this effect could be that as frequency increases, the gradual increase in [Na]$_i$ (Cohen *et al.*, 1982; Maier *et al.*, 1997a) limits the ability of the Na/Ca exchange to compete with the SR Ca-ATPase. In addition, increasing frequency also accelerates [Ca]$_i$ decline due to an increased rate of SR Ca transport, possibly due to CaMKII (see next section). Thus, the SR Ca-ATPase becomes increasingly dominant over the Na/Ca exchanger in transporting Ca from the cytosol at higher frequencies. In both rat and failing human ventricle the RCC2/RCC1 ratio was high even at low frequency, and did not change appreciably with frequency. We interpreted this as a reflection of the strong dominance of the SR Ca-ATPase in rat at all frequencies, and to a limitation in SR Ca-ATPase in the failing human heart.

Frequency-dependent acceleration of relaxation (FDAR)

Mammalian ventricular muscle shows a marked frequency-dependent acceleration of relaxation (FDAR, Fig 149; Schouten, 1990; Pieske *et al.*, 1995; Hussain *et al.*, 1997). This

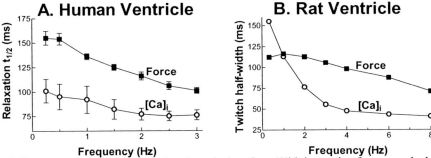

Figure 149. Frequency-dependent acceleration of relaxation. With increasing frequency the half-time (or half-width) of relaxation and [Ca]$_i$ decline get shorter. Data at 37°C are taken from Pieske *et al.* (1995) for human (**A**) and from Layland & Kentish (1999) for rat (**B**).

FDAR is also readily apparent when comparing twitch relaxation at a steady state (SS) frequency (e.g. 1 Hz) *vs.* a post-rest twitch, and is independent of β-adrenergic activation (Fig 150; Bassani *et al.*, 1995c). From a physiological standpoint this effect may be very important in speeding relaxation at high heart rates, allowing the heart to refill more rapidly between beats. Schouten (1990) hypothesized that faster relaxation of the SS *vs.* post-rest beat was due to CaMKII-dependent phosphorylation of phospholamban (PLB). That is, with stimulation at SS (or higher frequency), the average [Ca]$_i$ is higher and that could activate CaMKII to phosphorylate phospholamban and thus accelerate SR Ca-ATPase, [Ca]$_i$ decline and relaxation. With a long rest or lower frequency, PLB may be dephosphorylated, causing slower [Ca]$_i$ decline. We tested this in rat, ferret and mouse myocytes and found that the CaMKII inhibitors (KN-62 & KN-93), could abolish the acceleration of relaxation and [Ca]$_i$ decline during SS *vs.* post-rest twitches (Bassani *et al.*, 1995c; Li *et al.*, 1997b, 1998). It takes several beats at 1 Hz for the acceleration in [Ca]$_i$ decline to develop (Fig 150A; τ ~5 s) and FDAR was lost during rest with a biexponential time course (τ = 3.4 and 69 s), consistent with known kinetics of CaMKII activation, deactivation and slow deactivation of autophosphorylated CaMKII (Braun & Schulman, 1995; De Konnick & Schulman, 1998). Furthermore, phosphatase inhibitors prevented (or delayed) the post-rest slowing of twitch [Ca]$_i$ decline (Fig 150C). The accelerated twitch [Ca]$_i$ decline was SR-dependent, because the effect was abolished or reversed if SR Ca uptake was prevented with thapsigargin or caffeine (such that relaxation was via Na/Ca exchange, Fig 150B). However, PLB phosphorylation is not essential for FDAR, because it still occurs in the PLB knockout mouse, and is still abolished by KN-93 (Li *et al.*, 1998; DeSantiago & Bers, 2000). Thus, it appears that accelerated relaxation at high heart rates is due to CaMKII-dependent stimulation of SR Ca transport, but does not require phospholamban.

This issue is not yet mechanistically resolved. Some groups found that KN-62 or KN-93 do not abolish FDAR (Hussain *et al.*, 1997; Layland & Kentish, 1999; Kassiri *et al.*, 2000). Bluhm *et al.* (2000) found that FDAR of isometric force was lower in PLB-KO mice. Hagemann *et al.* (2000) also showed frequency-dependent phospholamban phosphorylation (at [16]Thr) which correlated with FDAR. It is possible that direct CaMKII-dependent phosphorylation of the cardiac SR Ca-ATPase (Xu *et al.*, 1993) occurs, but this has been challenged (Odermatt *et al.*, 1996; Reddy *et al.*, 1996). So, even the appropriate CaMKII target involved in accelerating SR Ca transport during FDAR in ventricular myocytes is not yet identified unequivocally.

A. Twitch-Dependent Acceleration of Relaxation

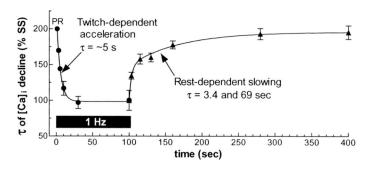

B. FDAR depends on SR   C. FDAR depends on CaMK

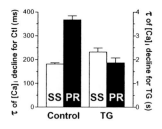   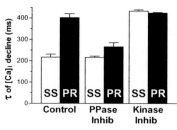

Figure 150. Frequency-dependent acceleration of relaxation (FDAR) at steady state (SS) *vs.* post-rest (PR) contractions. **A.** Build up of FDAR at 1 Hz, and dissipation during rest. Time constant (τ) of $[Ca]_i$ decline is shown for the PR contraction and ensuing 100 twitches at 1 Hz. Stimulation was then stopped at 100 sec and a single twitch was evoked after different periods of rest (2-300 s). After resumption of SS, another rest period was tested. **B.** FDAR was observed for SS *vs.* PR in control twitches, but not when the SR Ca-ATPase was blocked by thapsigargin (TG). In this case, relaxation depends on Na/Ca exchange (note 10-fold slower τ values in TG) **C.** Inhibition of phosphatase activity by okadaic acid (10 μm) prevented slowing of $[Ca]_i$ decline at the PR twitch. Inhibition of CaMKII alone (by KN-62) or together with PKA inhibition (by H-89, as shown) prevented the acceleration of $[Ca]_i$ decline from PR to the SS. Data are in rat ventricular myocytes and are from Bassani *et al.* (1995c).

In conclusion, there is great variation in details of $[Ca]_i$ regulation in different cardiac muscle preparations and conditions. However, this apparent complexity can be largely understood by considering a small number of common systems which interact and a few key functional properties that differ among cardiac preparations. Ca influx can activate substantial contractions in some mammalian as well as amphibian hearts, but under normal conditions the SR is the major source of Ca for activation of adult mammalian cardiac muscle. Ca influx can serve to trigger SR Ca release and also contribute to the loading of the SR for the next contraction. Ca released from the SR can either be re-accumulated by the SR or extruded from the cell via Na/Ca exchange. In the steady state, however, the Ca extruded by Na/Ca exchange during one cardiac cycle is balanced with the Ca influx via I_{Ca} (and possibly Na/Ca exchange). The Ca content of the SR can be gradually depleted by the sarcolemmal Na/Ca exchange during rest, and can also be quickly refilled during post-rest recovery by the Ca entering via I_{Ca} in 5-10 contractions. Depending on the transsarcolemmal [Na] gradient, rest can either deplete the SR or fill the SR with Ca. Clearly a dynamic yet delicate balance exists in the control of intracellular Ca in the heart and changes in these -systems can lead to inotropic and lusitropic changes.

D.M. Bers.
Excitation-Contraction Coupling and Cardiac Contractile Force.
2nd Ed., Kluwer Academic Publishers, Dordrecht, 2001

CHAPTER 10

CARDIAC INOTROPY AND Ca MISMANAGEMENT

In this chapter I will discuss some general mechanisms involved in cardiac inotropy and their relationship to cellular Ca overload and mismanagement. It is not intended as a comprehensive review of either inotropic agents or cardiac pathophysiology. I will start by considering five different means of cardiac inotropy: 1) hypothermia, 2) β-adrenergic activation, 3) α-adrenergic activation, 4) CaMKII activation and 5) cardioactive steroids (digitalis glycosides). Then I will discuss the ways in which cellular Ca regulation can go awry, with particular emphasis on Ca overload and heart failure. Finally, I will address strategic sites for induction of cardiac inotropy. This discussion may help to bring some of the characteristics of specific cellular systems discussed in preceding chapters into a more integrative picture of cellular Ca regulation.

CARDIAC INOTROPY

Hypothermic Inotropy

Reduction of temperature from 37°C in mammalian cardiac muscle results in an increase in developed force (Kruta, 1938; Sumbera *et al.*, 1966; Blinks & Koch-Weser, 1963; Langer & Brady, 1968). This hypothermic inotropy results in a remarkable 400-500% increase in force at 25°C (see Fig 151). Much of this large inotropic effect occurs immediately, when temperature is abruptly changed between twitch contractions (see Fig 152). This rapid change suggests that alteration in SR Ca content or relatively slow biochemical changes are unlikely to be critical for most of this inotropic effect. Additionally, hypothermic inotropy of similar amplitude is still observed when normal SR function is depressed by ryanodine or caffeine (Fig 151B, Shattock & Bers, 1987). Myofilament Ca sensitivity and maximal force are both decreased by cooling, albeit only moderately at 29 *vs.* 36°C (see Fig 20, pg 29; Harrison & Bers, 1989a). This suggests that $[Ca]_i$ must either increase dramatically or come to more complete equilibration with the myofilaments at cooler temperature. Figure 60 (pg 122) shows that cooling from 35 to 25°C reduces peak I_{Ca} (Q_{10} ~3, Cavalié *et al.*, 1985) and increases action potential duration (e.g. from ~220 to ~370 msec in rabbit ventricle; Shattock & Bers, 1987; Puglisi *et al.*, 1999). Interestingly, the lower peak I_{Ca} is compensated by slower Ca channel inactivation at 35°C, such that total Ca entry via I_{Ca} is essentially the same at 25 *vs.* 35°C (Fig 60; Puglisi *et al.*, 1999).

If peak I_{Ca} is reduced, we would also expect less Ca-induced SR Ca-release (particularly as SR Ca load is unlikely to change between two consecutive twitches in Fig 152). On the other hand, since cooling increases the open probability of the cardiac SR Ca release channel (by increasing the duration of openings, Sitsapesan *et al.*, 1991), a greater fraction of the SR Ca content might be released for a given I_{Ca} trigger. Whether this effect would be sufficient to compensate for the lower peak I_{Ca} is not completely clear. However, peak $[Ca]_i$ is much larger

Hypothermic Inotropy in Rabbit Ventricle

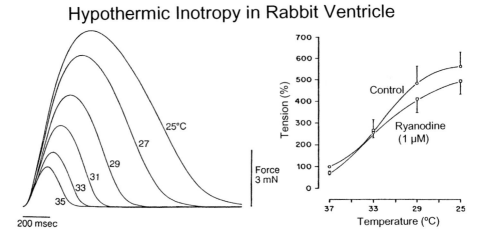

Figure 151. Hypothermic inotropy in rabbit ventricular muscle (0.5 Hz). Steady state contractions are shown at the indicated temperatures (left). Pre-equilibration with 1 µM ryanodine does not prevent this hypothermic inotropy in rabbit or rat (right panel is from Shattock & Bers, 1987, with permission).

during steady state twitches at 25 *vs.* 35°C (Puglisi *et al.*, 1996). The maximum rate of rise of force (+dF/dt) is also not decreased at the first contraction at 25°C in Fig 152C, indicating that SR Ca release is at least as large as at 35°C. Otherwise the slower development of contractile force expected from the myofilaments at l+ow temperature (for any given [Ca]) should lead to a smaller +dF/dt. So peak [Ca]$_i$ *is* increased at lower temperature. While this might reflect higher fractional SR Ca release, an alternative explanation should be considered.

Relaxation is greatly delayed at 25 *vs.* 35°C (Fig 152) and the Ca transport systems which drive relaxation are slowed by cooling. Indeed, the halftimes for twitch relaxation and [Ca]$_i$ decline in rabbit ventricular myocytes are more than doubled (from 50 to 130 ms and 117 to 252 ms respectively) upon cooling from 35 to 25°C (Puglisi *et al.*, 1996). This creates a greatly prolonged time to peak tension and this allows the myofilaments to more closely approach a steady state level of activation by [Ca]$_i$. It also allows peak [Ca]$_i$ to reach a higher level, simply because Ca transport out of the cytosol is slowed, analogous to the increased peak twitch [Ca]$_i$ when either the SR Ca-pump or Na/Ca exchange are blocked (Fig 133). Thus there is a prolonged "active state" where the myofilaments are being activated. Moreover, at 25°C there is a more distinct separation between the activation and relaxation phase. Note that the delay between maximum +dF/dt and –dF/dt in Fig 152C is ~200 ms at 35°C and ~950 ms at 25°C.

We also analyzed Ca fluxes via SR Ca-ATPase and Na/Ca exchange during relaxation and [Ca]$_i$ decline at 25 *vs.* 35°C, as described in Figs 133-135 (Puglisi *et al.*, 1996). The SR Ca-ATPase, Na/Ca exchange and slow systems (sarcolemmal Ca-ATPase plus mitochondrial Ca uniporter) are all slowed by 2-3-fold upon cooling from 35 to 25°C, so each system has a functional Q$_{10}$ of 2-3. This is consistent with the 2-3 times slower relaxation half-time at 25°C. However, the relative competition between these Ca transport systems is not appreciably changed, such that in rabbit the SR Ca-ATPase is still responsible for 70-75% of [Ca]$_i$ decline, and the Na/Ca exchanger 20-25%. This parallel slowing of all Ca transporters was also seen in

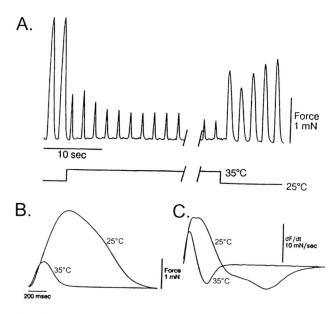

Figure 152. Hypothermic inotropy in rabbit ventricular muscle is rapidly induced. A quick change in temperature shows that most of the hypothermic inotropy take place rapidly. The muscle was stimulated at 0.5 Hz with temperature switch >90% complete in ~300 ms (using the same set-up as for RCCs). In **A**, the break in the force record is ~2 min. Force (**B**) and dF/dt (**C**) are shown for the first contraction after cooling to 25°C and the last contraction at 35°C from panel A.

ferret and cat ventricular myocytes. With the prolonged AP duration at 25°C, this could especially delay the functional contribution of Na/Ca exchange to [Ca]$_i$ decline, creating a slight additional bias toward the SR *vs.* extrusion from the cell.

In the steady state at lower temperature the Na-pump is inhibited (Q$_{10}$ ~3, Eisner & Lederer, 1980) and [Na]$_i$ rises (Shattock, 1984; Chapman, 1986). The rise of [Na]$_i$ will also shift Ca fluxes via Na/Ca exchange and tend to increase cellular and SR Ca content and Ca influx. Indeed, in the steady state SR Ca content is increased by cooling to 23-25°C, measured by caffeine-induced Ca transients and RCCs (Shattock & Bers, 1987; Puglisi *et al.*, 1996). The Ca loading effect may be responsible for much of the slower phase of hypothermic inotropy which develops over a minute or two (in contrast to the more immediate changes discussed above).

β-Adrenergic Agents and Cardiac Inotropy

β-adrenergic receptor (β-AR) activation is particularly important to consider, because it is the physiological means by which the inotropic, lusitropic and chronotropic states of the heart are controlled via sympathetic stimulation. Indeed, sympathetic nerve endings and β-ARs are broadly distributed throughout the heart. Isoproterenol, a β-adrenergic agonist, can produce large increases in cardiac contraction, Ca transient amplitude and the rates of relaxation and [Ca]$_i$ decline (see Fig 153). Four effects of β-adrenergic agents have already been discussed: 1) decreased myofilament Ca sensitivity due to troponin I phosphorylation (Chapter 2), 2) increased I$_{Ca}$ (Chapter 5), 3) enhanced SR Ca-ATPase rate (Chapter 7) and 4) altered RyR gating (Chapter 7). Activation of β$_1$-ARs can cause all of the major cardiac adrenergic effects (inotropy,

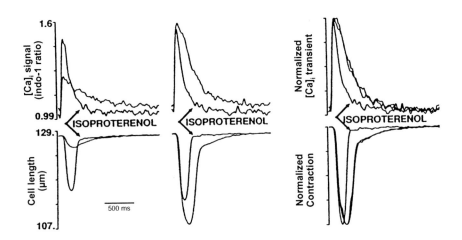

Figure 153. Effect of the β-adrenergic agonist, isoproterenol (0.5 mM) on Ca$_i$ transients (top) and shortening of rat ventricular myocytes at 23°C. At left [Ca]$_o$=1 mM in the presence and absence of isoproterenol. Center panel traces are a different cell with [Ca]$_o$ = 3 mM Ca$_o$ or 1 mM Ca$_o$ plus 0.5 µM isoproterenol, so that similar peak [Ca]$_i$ was reached in both cases (note smaller contraction with isoproterenol). Right panel shows traces normalized traces from control and isoproterenol (from middle panel). Note the faster time course with isoproterenol (from Spurgeon *et al.*, 1990 with permission).

lusitropy and chronotropy) and I will focus on that pathway. β$_2$- and β$_3$-ARs will be discussed on pg 280. β-adrenergic agonists stimulate adenylyl cyclase (see Fig 65, pg 129), elevating cyclic AMP, which activates cyclic AMP-dependent protein kinase (PKA) and which phosphorylates several key proteins, including: 1) troponin I (reducing Ca affinity of TnC), 2) sarcolemmal Ca channels (increasing I$_{Ca}$), 3) phospholamban (increasing SR Ca pump rate) and 4) SR Ca release channels (modifying RyR gating). The stimulation of I$_{Ca}$ and SR Ca uptake causes Ca transients to be larger and faster after β-adrenergic agonists (Figs 153 & 154).

In the presence of a β-adrenergic agonist, more Ca enters the cell at each excitation (due to increased I$_{Ca}$) and the SR accumulates a larger fraction of the cytosolic Ca pool during relaxation (due to SR Ca-pump stimulation). Thus, a larger SR Ca load is expected. The increased I$_{Ca}$ (and SR Ca) may also increase the fraction of SR Ca which is released. The result is a much larger peak [Ca]$_i$ during contraction with isoproterenol (see Figs 153 & 156). Of course, the SR Ca-pump stimulation also accelerates relaxation and leads to a shorter time to peak tension an [Ca]$_i$, and more rapid relaxation and [Ca]$_i$ decline. If Na/Ca exchange is unaltered, the SR Ca-pump stimulation will also bias the competition between these two mechanisms in favor of the SR Ca-pump (even though the higher peak [Ca]$_i$ will also stimulate Ca extrusion via Na/Ca exchange, see Fig 145). This bias toward the SR Ca-pump (*vs.* Na/Ca exchange) can also explain why isoproterenol can abolish the negative post-rest staircase in rat ventricular myocytes (Fig 154A, Raffaeli *et al.*, 1987). That is, if less Ca is not extruded via Na/Ca exchange at the large contractions (because the SR Ca-pump competes more effectively), the SR Ca load will not decrease progressively from beat to beat as discussed on page 267. It is also possible that isoproterenol shortens the time for the SR Ca release process to recover from inactivation. This could also contribute to the loss of the negative staircase.

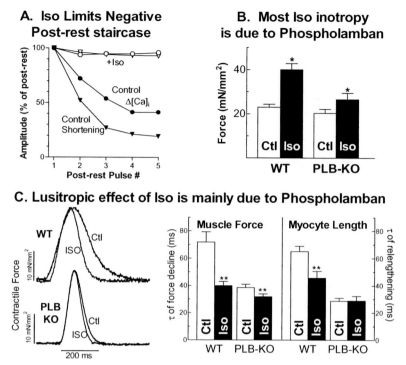

Figure 154. Isoproterenol (Iso) effects on inotropy and lusitropy at 23°C. **A**. Iso abolishes the negative staircase observed upon resumption of 0.2 Hz stimulation after rest in rat ventricular myocytes at 23° (Data taken from Raffaeli *et al.*, 1987). **B**. Iso nearly doubles contractile force in wild type (WT) mouse ventricle, but only increases force by 30% in the phospholamban knockout (PLB-KO) mouse. **C**. In WT mouse, Iso reduces relaxation time constant (τ) by nearly 50%, whereas in PLB-KO myocyte relaxation was unaffected by Iso. In PLB-KO muscles developing force, there was a small lusitropic effect of Iso. [Ca]$_o$ or sarcomere length was adjusted to match twitch amplitude (±Iso) in C. Data in B & C are from Li *et al.*, 2000).

β-adrenergic activation also decreases myofilament Ca sensitivity (due to phosphorylation of TnI, see Chapter 2), but the dramatic increase in Ca transients more than compensates for this, so contractions are increased substantially (but less so than Ca transients, Fig 156). It had been thought that the lower myofilament Ca sensitivity (and Ca-affinity) might contribute to the more rapid relaxation (or lusitropic effect) observed with β-adrenergic agonists (due to faster Ca dissociation from troponin C). However, data of McIvor *et al.* (1988) and Endoh & Blinks (1988) suggested that the lusitropic effect of isoproterenol was attributable mainly to SR Ca-pump stimulation, rather than decreased myofilament Ca sensitivity. Mechanical factors, such as the rate of cross-bridge detachment and geometric considerations might also be involved in the β-adrenergic induced acceleration of relaxation (Hoh *et al.*, 1988). We quantitatively compared the contributions of TnI and phospholamban phosphorylation in the lusitropic effect of isoproterenol (Fig 154C, Li *et al.*, 2000). In mice lacking phospholamban (PLB-KO), isoproterenol had no effect at all on myocyte or muscle twitch relaxation, despite a substantial increase in TnI phosphorylation. However, this was only the case when relengthening was measured in the absence of an external mechanical load (at right). When muscles from these PLB-KO mice developed isometric force, the amount of lusitropic effect observed with isoproterenol was directly related to the amount of force development (left). This emphasizes the dynamic interplay between force, myofilament properties and Ca transients. Nevertheless, the lusitropic effect of isoproterenol in the PLB-KO mice was still very small, compared to wild type mice. We estimated that at maximal force, ~85% of the lusitropic effect is due to phospholamban phosphorylation and acceleration of SR Ca-pumping, while only 15% could be due to TnI phosphorylation.

PKA-dependent phosphorylation of the cardiac RyR can also increase RyR sensitivity to activation by a Ca trigger in lipid bilayers (Valdivia *et al.*, 1995; Marx *et al.*, 2000). Thus isoproterenol might be expected to directly increase SR Ca release during the twitch by an effect on the RyR. On the other hand, preliminary data in intact myocytes indicate that when we control for changes in SR Ca load and I_{Ca}, isoproterenol does not increase SR Ca release (Ginsburg & Bers, 2001). Thus it is not yet entirely clear how important the PKA-dependent phosphorylation of the cardiac RyR is in the inotropic response to catecholamines.

Interestingly, there is still a significant inotropic effect of isoproterenol in the PLB-KO mouse (though much less than in wild type mice or other ventricular myocytes (Wolska *et al.*, 1996b; Li *et al.*, 2000). This may be mainly due to the large increase of I_{Ca}, which progressively increases SR Ca content in the absence of phospholamban (by simple mass action). That is, there is more Ca influx, higher average $[Ca]_i$ and consequently higher SR Ca-pump rate. The higher I_{Ca} may also increase contractility by increasing fractional SR Ca release (in WT & PLB-KO).

The enhanced I_{Ca} with β-adrenergic agonists tends to elevate the plateau phase of the cardiac action potential, but β-adrenergic agonists also increase cardiac K conductance (e.g. I_{Ks}, Gadsby, 1983; Walsh & Kass, 1988, 1991) which shortens the AP and tends to hyperpolarize the diastolic E_m. I_{Ca} also inactivates faster because of the high $\Delta[Ca]_i$. β-adrenergic agonists also activate the CFTR Cl current in cardiac myocytes (pg 84; Harvey & Hume, 1989). The net result of effects on Ca, K and Cl currents is that AP duration can be increased, decreased or unchanged depending on species and experimental conditions (Tsien, 1977; Tsien *et al.*, 1986). However, under physiological conditions AP shortening is typical, and is consistent with the positive chronotropic effect of β-adrenergic agonists. That is, shorter AP duration allows channels to recover from refractoriness, thereby allowing higher heart rates. Earlier repolarization will also indirectly stimulate Ca extrusion via Na/Ca exchange (Fig 140).

β-adrenergic agonists also influence the inward pacemaker current I_f (pg 86-87), which is activated by hyperpolarization. β-adrenergic agonists shift the E_m-dependence of I_f activation to more depolarized potentials (see Fig 42), resulting in a more rapid diastolic depolarization (DiFrancesco, 1986; DiFrancesco *et al.*, 1986). β-adrenergic agonists also accelerate the decline in potassium conductance (g_K, Bennett *et al.*, 1986; Connors & Terrar, 1990) which may contribute to pacemaker activity (especially in cells with more positive diastolic potentials, such as sino-atrial nodal cells (Noble, 1985; Noma, 1996). Stimulation of SR Ca uptake may also increase spontaneous SR Ca release in pacemaker cells, activating inward (depolarizing) current (pg 95). Thus, several effects contribute to the positive chronotropic effect of β-AR stimulation.

This increase in heart rate can increase cardiac output independent of β-adrenergic agonists. That is, increased frequency by itself would increase contractility (and speed relaxation), based purely on the force-frequency relationship and frequency-dependent acceleration of relaxation discussed in Chapter 9 (i.e. independent of the β-adrenergic activation). Thus, the increase in contractility *in vivo* with β-adrenergic agonists is a combination of the intrinsic inotropic & lusitropic effect of increased frequency and the PKA-mediated effects, which are directly attributable to β-adrenergic activation (e.g. increased I_{Ca} and SR Ca pumping). Thus, cardiac output can be greatly enhanced by β-adrenergic agonists.

Sarcolemmal Na/K-ATPase is also affected by β-adrenergic agonists (see pg 90). While some results indicated that β-adrenergic agonists can stimulate Na/K-ATPase and reduce $[Na]_i$ (Wasserstrom *et al.*, 1982; Lee & Vassalle, 1983; Désilets & Baumgarten, 1986; Kockskämper *et al.*, 2000), Gao *et al.* (1996, 1997c, 1998a) provided compelling evidence for Na/K-ATPase inhibition by β-adrenergic agonists and PKA. Na/K-ATPase inhibition would cause $[Na]_i$ to rise, further limiting the ability of Na/Ca exchange to compete with the SR Ca-ATPase. This could also contribute to greater cellular and SR Ca load. It could also exacerbate the rise in $[Na]_i$ caused by the accompanying physiological increase in heart rate. Thus, PKA-dependent regulation of the Na/K-ATPase may contribute indirectly to the enhanced Ca transients and inotropy induced by activation of PKA, but the net effect is somewhat controversial.

Activation of β-ARs also increases metabolism and glycogenolysis (via PKA, that activates phosphorylase b kinase, which in turn activates phosphorylase b, resulting in glycogen breakdown, Hayes & Mayer, 1981). The increased metabolic energy demand, in combination with the large demands due to the increased inotropic state and frequency, can increase O_2 consumption dramatically (Rolett, 1974). This is a shortcoming of β-adrenergic agonists as inotropic agents. That is, in energetic terms (and in terms of O_2 requirement) increasing contractility and heart rate via β-adrenergic agonists is expensive. β-ARs are also down-regulated or removed from the membrane during chronic activation and in the failing human heart (Watanabe *et al.*, 1982; Stiles *et al.*, 1984; Bristow *et al.*, 1982, 1986). This makes β-adrenergic agonists more useful for acute rather than chronic inotropic therapy.

β-ARs are members of the 7-transmembrane domain receptor family that couple to heterotrimeric GTP-binding proteins (with α & βγ subunits); in the case of $β_1$-AR it is G_s (Figs 65, 155). The third intracellular loop of the receptor interacts with the carboxy-terminal of the $G_α$-subunit. When the β-AR is activated by a ligand, bound GDP is exchanged for GTP, and the $G_{sα}$ subunit is activated (until GTP is hydrolyzed to GDP). Activated $G_{sα}$ dissociates from the ternary complex (agonist-receptor-G-protein) and can activate adenylyl cyclase to produce cAMP. The amount of adenylyl cyclase may be a rate-limiting step in the cascade (Gao *et al.*, 1998b), and the main isoforms in heart are types V & VI (Ishikawa *et al.*, 1994). β-ARs can become desensitized (or uncoupled) in seconds to minutes, and this process involves phosphorylation of a serine on its carboxy-terminal tail, by a G-protein coupled receptor kinase (GRK) or PKA (Post *et al.*, 1999). Two GRKs appear to be involved in heart, GRK2 (also called β-AR kinase-1, or βARK-1) and GRK5. After β-AR phosphorylation, another protein (β-arrestin) can bind to the β-AR, and prevents further interaction with G_s (Lefkowitz, 1993). β-arrestin can also interact with clathrin and this results in the internalization of β-ARs (Goodman *et al.*, 1996; Ferguson *et al.*, 1996). Once internalized the receptors can either be recycled to the membrane in a re-sensitized form (after dephosphorylation, Krueger *et al.*, 1997) or degraded as a final step in receptor down-regulation. Interestingly, this down-regulation and loss of cell surface β-ARs, which occurs importantly in heart failure (Bristow *et al.*, 1982), is accompanied by reduction in β-AR mRNAs due to decreased message stability (Hadcock *et al.*, 1989).

The stimulatory effect of β-adrenergic agonists on adenylyl cyclase and cAMP production can be inhibited by another G-protein (G_i) which is activated by muscarinic M_2 receptors (and some other receptors). Thus, parasympathetic release of acetylcholine can diminish the effect of sympathetic stimulation of β-ARs. While this clearly occurs in the sino-atrial node, and is important in the control of heart rate, there are fewer parasympathetic nerve endings in ventricular muscle (Löffelholz & Pappano, 1985). Thus, parasympathetic activation may have less anti-adrenergic effect on contractility than on heart rate. Nevertheless, there are muscarinic (and other) receptors in ventricular myocytes which can mediate G_i-dependent limitation of adenylyl cyclase activation. Histamine and serotonin receptors can also couple to G_s and enhance contractility via stimulation of adenylyl cyclase (Brodde *et al.*, 1998)

$β_2$- and $β_3$-ARs are also present in mammalian ventricle (see Table 25). $β_1$-AR are more numerous than $β_2$-AR in ventricle (~75% of total β-ARs) and $β_1$-AR also are more sensitive to the physiological agonist norepinephrine than are $β_2$- or $β_3$-ARs (Brodde, 1993; Lafontan, 1994; Post *et al.*, 1999). Thus, the majority of β-AR response is likely to be mediated by $β_1$-AR. Consistent with this idea, knockout of the $β_1$-AR gene in mice, results in prevention of both inotropic and chronotropic response to isoproterenol (although most of these knockout mice die *in utero*; Rohrer *et al.*, 1996). On the other hand, there is compelling data that $β_2$- and $β_3$-AR can alter ventricular myocyte function. There is even evidence that $β_2$-AR are more effectively coupled to adenylyl cyclase than $β_1$-ARs (Bristow *et al.*, 1989; Kaumann *et al.*, 1989).

$β_2$-AR activation can produce the same effects as discussed above for $β_1$-ARs. However, there is evidence to suggest that $β_2$-ARs can couple to both G_s and G_i in rat and dog ventricular myocytes (Xiao *et al.*, 1995, 1999; Kuschel *et al.*, 1999b; Chen-Izu *et al.*, 2000). They found that $β_2$-AR stimulation induced a PKA-dependent inotropy and increase of I_{Ca}, but did not raise global cAMP levels or phosphorylate phospholamban, TnI or protein C (all of which were seen with $β_1$-AR activation). Moreover, Ca channels in a cell attached patch could be activated by $β_1$-AR agonist outside the patch (diffusive signaling), but the $β_2$-AR agonist zinterol only activated I_{Ca} if it was included in the patch pipette (local signaling only). However, pertussis toxin treatment (disrupting G_i regulation) allowed $β_2$-AR agonist to also activate I_{Ca} via diffusive signaling (zinterol outside the pipette). Thus the apparent G_s/G_i coupling of $β_2$-ARs may create very localized PKA activation which can phosphorylate nearby Ca channels, but not distant targets like phospholamban and TnI. Perhaps co-activation of G_i limits the amount of cAMP produced, creating a very local stochastic PKA activation. This intriguing pathway is still controversial. For example, La Flamme & Becker (1998) found no evidence that $β_2$-AR activation modulates Ca handling in rat ventricular myocytes, even with pertussis toxin.

$β_2$-AR overexpression in transgenic mice (by >100-fold) appears to fully activate the PKA-mediated inotropic state, even in the absence of β-adrenergic agonists (Milano *et al.*, 1994; Bond *et al.*, 1995). This has been taken as evidence that the $β_2$-AR can shift back and forth between a resting state and a stochastically rare active state (stimulating G_s). Thus even though a very small fraction of unoccupied $β_2$-ARs are in this active state, the massive overexpression allows strong basal activation and cAMP production. This work also illustrated nicely the

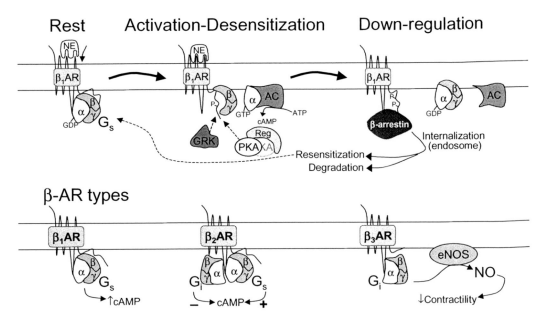

Figure 155. β-adrenergic receptor signaling in ventricular myocytes. Top shows the process of activation by norepinephrine (NE), $G_{s\alpha}$-activation of adenylyl cyclase (AC) and production of cAMP (which activates PKA). PKA phosphorylates key functional targets (see Fig 65), and along with GRK2 & GRK5 phosphorylates (P) the β-AR to cause desensitization. Then β-arrestin binds to the phosphorylated β-AR, causing internalization. Bottom shows differences in coupling of β_1-, β_2- & β_3AR to G-proteins (G_s and/or G_i) and different consequences. Note that the β_3AR lacks the GRK phosphorylation sites that lead to desensitization and down-regulation (see also Fig 65, pg 129).

principle of *inverse agonism*. That is, drugs that can shift this equilibrium toward the resting state (e.g. the β_2-AR inverse agonists ICI 118,551) can prevent this basal agonist-independent activation in the β_2-AR transgenic mouse. This differs from classical receptor antagonists, which block binding and activation by an agonist.

β_3-AR activation in ventricular myocytes appears to produce negative inotropic effects (Gauthier *et al.*, 1996, 1998, 1999, 2000; Varghese *et al.*, 2000). These negative inotropic effects are sensitive to pertussis toxin (implicating G_i/G_o rather than G_s) and appear to be mediated by nitric oxide (NO) produced by endothelial NO synthase (NOS3, which is constitutively expressed in ventricular myocytes). NO production in ventricular myocytes stimulates guanylyl cyclase, cGMP production, and protein kinase G activation. This cascade produces negative inotropic effects in heart, but the molecular mechanisms are not as clearly identified. Nitric oxide can decrease myofilament Ca sensitivity via PKG-dependent phosphorylation of TnI, just as seen for PKA (Pfitzer *et al.*, 1982; Lincoln & Corbin, 1978; Shah *et al.*, 1994, Kaye *et al.*, 1999). Nitric oxide can also decrease I_{Ca} (Méry *et al.*, 1993; Sumii & Sperelakis, 1995; Wahler & Dollinger, 1995). β_3-ARs lack the carboxy-tail serines that are the target for phosphorylation by βARK-1 (or GRK5 or PKA) and thus do not appear to exhibit desensitization and down-regulation as seen for β_1- and β_2-AR. This may be particularly important in heart failure, where the normally dominant β-AR (β_1-AR) is down-regulated. In this case, the negative inotropic effect of β_3-AR may become unmasked (i.e. it is normally masked by the positive effect of β_1- &

β_2-AR, which are more numerous and have higher affinity for noreipnephrine). Nevertheless, most (if not all) of the β-AR response of ventricular muscle to the physiological agonist norepinephrine, appears to be mediated by β_1-AR.

α-Adrenergic Agents and Cardiac Inotropy

Inotropy can also be mediated by α-adrenergic receptors (α-ARs) in the heart, and in some hearts α-AR are comparable in number to β-ARs (Bode & Brunton, 1989; Benfey, 1990; Brodde & Michel, 1999). These α-ARs are 7 transmembrane domain G-protein-coupled receptors, and cardiac myocytes appear to express only the α_1-AR subtype (α_2-ARs are primarily involved in presynaptic inhibition of norepinephrine release, Brodde & Michel, 1999). Table 25 (pg 287) shows densities of receptors and ion transporters in whole tissue (fmol/mg homogenate protein) and also the estimated surface density ($/\mu m^2$) on the sarcolemma (or on the SR). Schümann *et al.* (1974, 1975) demonstrated inotropic effects attributable to α-AR activation, and this inotropic pathway has gradually become better appreciated (reviewed by Endoh, 1996). In addition to the inotropic effects, α_1-AR activation is involved in ventricular hypertrophic signaling (Simpson, 1985; see pg 312). The inotropic and hypertrophic effects are largely mediated via the G-protein G_q. There are strong parallels between the downstream effects of α_1-AR activation and some other G_q-coupled receptors, such as endothelin (ET-1) and angiotensin II receptors (ET$_A$ & AT$_1$, Endoh, 1996), but I will restrict the discussion here mainly to α_1-AR.

Three subtypes of α_1-ARs are expressed in heart (α_{1A}, α_{1B} & α_{1D}). The pharmacologically defined α_{1A}-AR subtype turned out to be the clone originally known as α_{1c}AR, but to avoid confusion these are now both referred to as α_{1A}-AR (Zhong & Minneman, 1999). The α_{1A}-AR is selectively activated by the agonist A61603, and blocked by the selective antagonists WB-4101, (+)-niguldipine, 5-methylurapidil and KMD-3123 (Brodde & Michel, 1999), although WB-4101 can also block α_{1D}-AR with high affinity. The α_{1B}-AR is preferentially alkylated by chloroethylclonidine (CEC), which creates an irreversible block. The α_{1D}-AR can be selectively blocked by BMY-7378, but this agent is also a partial agonist at serotonin (5-HT$_{1A}$) receptors (Goetz *et al.*, 1995). The α_{1D}-AR is also intermediate between α_{1A}- and α_{1B}-AR in sensitivity to CEC and 5-methyurapidil. Phenylephrine, methoxamine and cirazoline are non-selective α_1-AR agonists, and phenylephrine is the most widely used. The hypertrophic response appears to be mediated via the α_{1A} receptor subtype, while the inotropic (action is mediated mainly by the α_{1B}-AR subtype, with some contribution by α_{1A}-AR (Minneman *et al.*, 1988; Minneman, 1988; Simpson *et al.*, 1990; Michel *et al.*, 1990; Knowlton *et al.*, 1993; Endoh, 1996; Gambassi *et al.*, 1998; Brodde & Michel, 1999; Rohde *et al.*, 2000). In rabbit ventricle the $\alpha_{1A/B}$-AR pool is 40% α_{1A}-ARs and 60% α_{1B}-AR, while in rat it is 20:80% (Gross *et al.*, 1988; Takanashi *et al.*, 1991; Sallés *et al.*, 1994). The α_{1D}-AR numbers and functional impact are small in comparison to α_{1A}- and α_{1B}-AR (Deng *et al.*, 1996; Yang & Endoh, 1997; Wolff *et al.*, 1998).

The magnitude of the inotropic effect of α-AR activation varies in different ventricular preparations, with rabbit >rat >ferret > guinea-pig > human >> dog (Hartmann *et al.*, 1988; Hescheler *et al.*, 1988; Hiramoto *et al.*, 1988; Jakob *et al.*, 1988; Endoh, 1996) and a similar sequence is seen for ET-1 and angiotensin-II (Endoh, 1996). Figure 156 shows Ca transients and force during α- and β-AR activation in rabbit ventricle where the maximal α-AR-induced inotropy is ~50-60% of the maximal β-adrenergic response (the same is true for ET-1 &

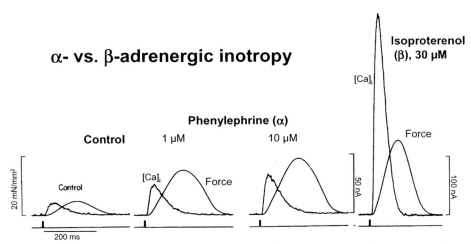

Figure 156. The influence of α-adrenergic activation and β-adrenergic activation on contractions and Ca$_i$ transients (the earlier peaks, measured with aequorin) in rabbit ventricular muscle at 37.5°C, stimulated at 1 Hz and equilibrated continuously with 1 μM bupranolol (a β-adrenergic blocker). Several [phenylephrine] were applied and then washed out. Then isoproterenol was added at a high enough concentration to overcome most of the β-adrenergic blockade by bupranolol. Note that the Ca$_i$ transient in the presence of isoproterenol was recorded at reduced gain (modified from Endoh & Blinks, 1988, with permission).

angiotensin-II in rabbit ventricle, Endoh & Blinks, 1988; Endoh, 1996). With α-AR activation the Ca transient amplitude is increased (but less than for β-AR), and there is no acceleration of [Ca]$_i$ decline (as for β-AR). Despite the smaller increase in Δ[Ca]$_i$ with phenylephrine *vs.* isoproterenol, the contraction amplitude is comparable. This is consistent with the reduced myofilament Ca sensitivity classically observed with β-AR/PKA activation (see Fig 157A). However, α$_1$-AR does just the opposite (i.e. they increase myofilament Ca sensitivity; see Fig 157B; Endoh & Blinks, 1988). This causes a modest negative lusitropy (slowed relaxation), again contrasting to the prominent positive lusitropy with β-AR activation.

Enhanced myofilament Ca sensitivity explains part of the α$_1$-AR inotropic effect, but higher myofilament Ca affinity would tend to decrease the Ca transient amplitude (since more Ca would bind). Thus, the increase in Δ[Ca]$_i$ implies that some other changes must also occur (e.g. more Ca entry or SR release). Despite early suggestive results (Brückner & Scholz, 1984) α-AR activation does not appear to increase I$_{Ca}$ (Hescheler *et al.*, 1988; Hartmann *et al.*, 1988; see pg 130). In contrast, α-AR agonists can even stimulate cAMP phosphodiesterase activity, reducing cAMP (Buxton & Brunton, 1985). Thus, increased I$_{Ca}$ cannot explain the enhanced Δ[Ca]$_i$.

AP duration is typically increased by α$_1$-AR activation in parallel to the positive inotropic effect (Endoh *et al.*, 1991). This may be due primarily to decreased K-currents. For example, I$_{to}$ is decreased by α$_1$-AR activation in rat and rabbit (Fedida *et al.*, 1990; Apkon & Nerbonne, 1988; Ravens *et al.*, 1989; Williamson *et al.*, 1997; Homma *et al.*, 2000). This can prolong the AP, especially in rat myocytes where I$_{to}$ is a critical determinant of AP duration. α$_1$-AR stimulation also decreases I$_{K1}$ in rabbit ventricle (Fedida *et al.*, 1991). This would both prolong AP duration and destabilize diastolic E$_m$, which could increase the likelihood of triggered arrhythmias. In guinea-pig ventricle which lacks I$_{to}$, α$_1$-AR shortens AP duration and produces a PKC-dependent increase in delayed rectifier K current (Dirksen & Sheu, 1990)

A. β-AR Reduces MF Ca sensitivity   B. α₁-AR Increases MF Ca sensitivity

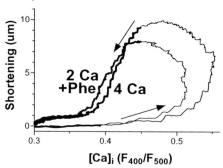

Figure 157. β-ARs decrease, while α₁-ARs increase myofilament Ca sensitivity. **A.** Rabbit ventricular myocyte contraction was plotted as a function of $[Ca]_i$ for each time point during a twitch (23°C, 0.5 Hz). Arrows show the direction of time. $[Ca]_i$ rises ahead of shortening, but during the relaxation phase (bold) the relationship between shortening and $[Ca]_i$ provides a crude dynamic index of myofilament Ca sensitivity (Spurgeon *et al.*, 1992). Note the right shift induced by isoproterenol (Iso), indicating decrease d myofilament Ca sensitivity. In control $[Ca]_o$ was increased to 8 mM to match peak shortening seen with Iso (2 mM $[Ca]_o$). **B.** Phenylephrine (Phe) produces the opposite shift in myofilament Ca sensitivity, and this effect was blocked by the PKC inhibitor calphostin C ($[Ca]_o$ was 4 mM in control, to match contraction with that in Phe). Data were provided by J. DeSantiago (DeSantiago *et al.*, 1998).

consistent with PKC-mediated stimulation of I_{Ks} (pg 81; Walsh & Kass, 1991). Thus, α₁-AR effects may be species-dependent, but the AP prolongation seen in most myocytes would tend to increase Ca influx (by I_{Ca} and possibly $I_{Na/Ca}$) and also decrease Ca efflux via Na/Ca exchange (allowing greater SR Ca uptake). This could contribute to the enhanced Ca transients seen with α₁-AR, but let's look at the signaling cascade initiated by α₁-AR activation (Fig 158).

α-AR activation causes G_q to activate phospholipase C (PLC), which splits phospha-tidylinositol 4,5-bisphosphate (PIP₂) into IP₃ and diacylglycerol (DAG) (Fig 158, Brown & Jones, 1986; Poggioli *et al.*, 1986; Jones *et al.*, 1988; Otani *et al.*, 1988; Scholz *et al.*, 1988). DAG activates protein kinase C (PKC), while IP₃ can activate or modulate Ca release. There is little evidence for IP₃ causing enhanced Ca transients in ventricular myocyte (see Chapters 7 & 8). Indeed, most groups find that the α₁-AR-induced increase in $\Delta[Ca]_i$ and inotropy are abolished by inhibition of PKC, even though IP₃ production remains (Endoh, 1996; Gambassi *et al.*, 1998; DeSantiago *et al.*, 1998). My current speculation (pg 243 & Fig 158) is that IP₃ activates SR/ER Ca release near (or in) the nucleus (without impact on global $[Ca]_i$) and that this may activate nearby CaMKII selectively. This may explain the apparent link between CaMKII activation and transcriptional regulation in the hypertrophic phenotype pathway (Ramirez *et al.*, 1997). Thus, IP₃ may not be involved in the inotropic effects of α₁-AR activation.

PKC activation in response to α₁-AR activation stimulates Na/H exchange to extrude protons (Wallert & Frölich, 1992). This Na/H exchange causes both intracellular pH and $[Na]_i$ to rise (Gambassi *et al.*, 1990, 1998). The alkalinization is mainly responsible for the increased myofilament Ca sensitivity (see Chapter 2, Fig 157), and the rise in $[Na]_i$ contributes to the increase in Ca transients via Na/Ca exchange (see next section). Thus, α₁-AR activation

α-Adrenergic Regulation

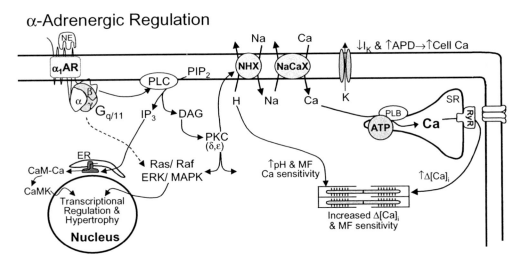

Figure 158. α_1-AR transduction pathway in ventricular myocytes. The α_1-AR activates the G-protein G_q, which activates phospholipase C (PLC) and D. PLC produces IP_3 and diacylglycerol (DAG) and these products have divergent effects leading to positive inotropy and hypertrophy (see text).

increases both $\Delta[Ca]_i$ (less than β-AR) and myofilament Ca sensitivity, without accelerating Ca transport. The result is a positive inotropy, with modest negative lusitropy.

α_1-AR agonists, endothelin and angiotensin-II can also exert negative inotropic effects, resulting in sometimes bi- or triphasic changes in force upon application. These effects may be mediated by stimulation of Na/K-ATPase   (pg 90), I_{Ks} (shortening AP duration, above), $I_{K(ACh)}$ (Kurachi *et al.*, 1989). In rat ventricular myocytes phenylephrine caused acidification when α_{1A}-ARs were blocked (rather than alkalinization seen with phenylephrine alone or when α_{1B}-AR are blocked, Gambassi *et al.,* 1998). Thus α_{1B}-AR may cause a decrease in pH_i (still PKC-dependent) that limits the increase in pH_i induced by activation of the α_{1A}-AR. PKC can also phosphorylate the PKA sites on TnI (Ser^{23} & Ser^{24}, which reduce myofilament Ca sensitivity) and also Ser^{42} & Ser^{44}, which reduce myofilament ATPase rate and unloaded shortening in response to α_1-AR activation (Noland *et al.*, 1995, 1996; Strang & Moss, 1995). PKC has multiple isoforms and other targets in heart (including other myofilament proteins, channels and transporters). These effects help explain multiphasic responses sometimes seen with α_1-AR, ET-1 and angiotensin-II. These agents also stimulate a hypertrophic signaling cascade (see pg 314).

Physiological norepinephrine (and epinephrine) release activates both α- and β-ARs, but the inotropic effect is mediated mainly by β-adrenergic activation. However, in species with a prominent α-adrenergic response (e.g. rabbit), up to one-third of the inotropic response to norepinephrine can be attributed to α_1-AR activation (Aass *et al.*, 1983; Nawrath, 1989; Endoh, 1996; Brodde & Michel, 1999).

Ca-Calmodulin dependent protein kinase (CaMKII)

The previous sections have described how PKA and PKC modulate contractility. CaMKII is modulated by changes in $[Ca]_i$ (associated with altered frequency or inotropic states). Little is known quantitatively about dynamic changes in activation state of CaMKII during the cardiac cycle. Indeed, one may expect Ca-CaM to change during the Ca transient (Fig 29), which may activate CaMKII in a cyclical manner. However, activated CaMKII also becomes auto-phosphorylated, and thus stays active in an autonomous manner, independent of $[Ca]_i$ (Braun & Schulman, 1995; De Koninck & Schulman, 1998). This gives the CaMKII system memory and the ability to integrate $[Ca]_i$ signals (e.g. increasing activation state with increasing frequency, see pg 271).

Local $[Ca]_i$ near the mouth of the L-type Ca channel causes inactivation by binding to calmodulin (pg 117), and the frequency-dependent facilitation of I_{Ca} appears to require CaMKII (pg 119). Thus, CaMKII activation can increase I_{Ca}. Phospholamban is also phosphorylated by CaMKII and this can stimulate the SR Ca-ATPase (pg 167) and CaMKII can thus increase SR Ca content. The ryanodine receptor (RyR) is also phosphorylated by CaMKII, and both calmodulin and CaMKII alter RyR gating in a complex manner, even in isolation in bilayer studies (Pg 198). To assess whether CaMKII has any intrinsic effect on E-C coupling, we used voltage clamped ventricular myocytes and controlled SR Ca load (keeping it constant) and measured SR Ca release as a function of I_{Ca} (Li *et al.*, 1997b). We found that the CaMKII inhibitor KN-93 prevented a Ca-dependent increase in SR Ca release for the same SR Ca load and I_{Ca} trigger. That is, if the conditioning pulses did not elevate $[Ca]_i$ very much, there was no effect of KN-93. Thus, endogenous CaMKII may have stimulatory effects on I_{Ca}, SR Ca uptake and E-C coupling, and could contribute to dynamic regulation during changes in heart rate and inotropic state.

Cardioactive Steroids: Glycoside Inotropy

Digitalis is the oldest cardiac inotropic agent. Withering (1785) described its use in heart failure, known then as dropsy, and the related cardioactive steroids are still among the most efficacious inotropic agents. Since ouabain and digitalis glycosides were recognized as specific

---

Table 25 compiled with help of M.T. Ziolo, includes the following abbreviations: V=ventricle; A=atrium; L=left; R=right; HF= heart failure, DCM=dilated cardiomyopathy, ICM= ischemic cardiomyopathy, G-Pig= guinea-pig CGP=CGP-12177; ICYP=iodocyanopindolol, isradipine=PN200-110, QNB, quinuclidinyl benzilate; SL, sarcolemma; E-PO4, Phosphoenzyme.

* SL B_{max} values for saxitoxin (678 fmol/mg) and ouabain (365 pmol/mg) were divided by the purification factor ($35\times$ & $\sim60\times$ respectively). Colvin *et al.*, (1985) & Doyle *et al.* (1985) estimated SL ouabain and saxitoxin site density at 330 and 3.6-7.6/μm^2 respectively, using different assumptions.

‡Assuming 120 mg homogenate protein/g wet weight.

†B_{max} are from microsomes. Extrapolation to SL surface density uses 2-fold enrichment, 120 mg pn/ g wet wt, 2.43 g wet wt/L cytosol, 7 pF/pL and 1 $cm^2/\mu F$ (or fmol/mg $\times$ 0.125, see pg 6, & 42). For DHPR and RyR 109 mg cell pn/ ml cell volume was used. For the SR Ca-pump 1.96 μm^2 SR/μm^3 was used, and for the RyR 0.18 μm^2 junctional SR/μm^3 cell was used (Table 1). Maximal possible density for 27 nm square RyRs would be 1400/μm^2 and for a 12 nm wide SR Ca-ATPase $\sim$6000/μm^2.

a Endoh *et al.*, 1991
b Anthonio *et al.*, 2000
c Maurice *et al.*, 1999
d Tse *et al.*, 2000
e Böhm *et al.*, 1990
f Brodde, 1996
g Rohrer *et al.*, 1996
h Musser *et al.*, 1993
i Kompa *et al.*, 1995

j Brodde & Michel, 1999
k Steinfath *et al.*, 1992
l Sallés *et al.*, 1994;
   Gross *et al.*, 1988
m Takanashi *et al.*, 1991
n Kobayashi *et al.*, 1999
o Pieske *et al.*, 1999b
p Vatner *et al.*, 1988
q Ishihata & Endo, 1995

r Nozawa *et al.*, 1994
s Regitz-Zagrosek *et al.*, 1995
t Doyle *et al.*, 1985
u Colvin *et al.*, 1985
v Cheon & Reeves, 1988
w Bers& Stiffel, 1993
x Levitsky *et al.*, 1981

Table 25
Hormone receptors and Ion Transporters in Cardiac Muscle

	Ligand	K_d (nM)	B_{max} (fmol/mg)	Density ($/\mu m^2$)		
β-adrenergic receptors					$\beta_1/(\beta_1 + \beta_2)$	
Rat LV	CGP	0.83	60 [a]	8	60% [b]	
Rabbit LV	"	1.1	133 [a]	17	77% [c]	
Dog LV	"	2.5	125 [a]	16	72% [d]	
Human V	"	0.52	100 [e]	13	73% [f]	
Human V (DCM)	"	0.57	31 [e]	3.2	57% [f]	
Human V (ICM)	"	0.58	41 [e]	3.8	75% [f]	
Mouse V	ICYP	0.08	50 [g]	6.5	72% [g]	
G-Pig V	"	0.01	59 [h]	8	93% [i]	
α-adrenergic receptors					$\alpha_{1B}/(\alpha_{1A}+\alpha_{1B})$	α-AR/β-AR
Rat LV	prazosin	0.14	112 [a]	14	80% [l]	1.86 [a]
Rabbit LV	"	0.25	19 [a]	2.4	60% [m]	0.15 [a]
Dog LV	"	0.26	26 [a]	3.2		0.21 [a]
Human V	"		10 [j]	1.3		0.1
Human V (HF)	"	0.063	11 [k]	1.4		0.29
Mouse V	"	0.05	15 [k]	1.9		0.3
G-Pig Heart	"	0.05	16 [k]	2		0.27
Endothelin-1					$ET_A/(ET_A+ET_B)$	
Rat V	ET-1	0.030	155 [n]	19	91% [n]	
Rat V (HF)	"	0.029	243 [n]	30	86% [n]	
Human	"	0.013	63 [o]	8	63% [o]	
Human (HF)	"	0.028	122 [o]	15	73% [o]	
Muscarinic (M₂)						
Dog	QNB	0.12	157 [p]	20		
Dog (HF)	"	0.13	121 [p]	15		
Human	"	0.58	275 [e]	34		
Human (DCM)	"	0.5	201 [e]	25		
Human (ICM)	"	0.47	249 [e]	31		
Angiotensin II	"				$AT_2/(AT_1+ AT_2)$	
Rat, ferret	AngII	1.5	21, 37 [q]	3-5		
Rabbit, dog	"	1-2	37, 76 [q]	5-9		
Human V	"	1.1	6 [r]	0.7	67% [r]	
Human RA	"	0.5	11 [s]	1.4	69% [s]	
Human RA (HF)	"	0.7	4 [s]	0.5	64% [s]	
Adenosine (A₁)					A/V	
Rat V	DPCPX	1.5	12 [h]	1.4	1.5 [h]	
Rabbit V	"	1.9	9 [h]	1.1	1.7 [h]	
G-Pig	"	3	34 [h]	4.3	2.2 [h]	
Na Channel						
Sheep V	Saxitoxin*	0.22	20 [t]	3		
Na/K-ATPase (SL)						
Bovine V	Ouabain*	33	6000 [u]	1032		
Na/Ca exchanger						
Dog V	Rate	-	1087 [v]	187		
DHPR (SL Ca Channel)						
Rabbit V my	isradipine	1	137 [w]	16		
Rat V my	"	1	114 [w]	14		
G-P V my	"	1	151 [w]	18		
Ferret V my	"	2	112 [w]	13		
RyR (SR Ca release channel)					RyR/DHPR	
Rabbit V my	Ryanodine	3	504 [w]	184	4	
Rat V my	"	4	833 [w]	304	7	
G-P V my	"	2	656 [w]	240	5	
Ferret V my	"	4	1144 [w]	418	10	
SR Ca-ATPase						
G-P V	E-PO₄‡	-	49,000 [x]	2600		

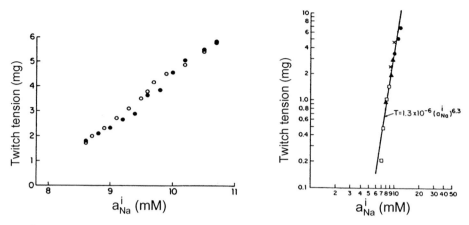

Figure 159. Twitch tension in dog Purkinje fiber depends on aNa$_i$ (measured with Na-selective micro-electrodes, 36°C, 1 Hz). At left, measurements were made during the onset (•) and washout (o) of inotropy induced by 1 μM strophanthidin in one fiber. The right panel shows data from the same fiber (×) and from 3 other fibers on a log-log plot (from Lee & Dagostino, 1982 and Lee, 1985, with permission).

inhibitors of the Na/K-ATPase (Glynn, 1964; Skou, 1965), it has become increasingly clear that this action is primarily responsible for the positive inotropic effects (as well as negative inotropic and arrhythmogenic effects which limit glycoside utility, see pg 294-300).   There were indications that very low glycoside concentrations could stimulate Na/K-ATPase, and reduce [Na]$_i$, while still producing inotropy (Blood, 1975; Cohen *et al.*, 1976; Godfraind & Ghysel-Burton, 1977; Noble, 1980).   However, this may be secondary to autonomic catecholamine secretion and stimulation of β-ARs (Hougen *et al.*, 1981). The powerful cardiovascular effect of Na-pump inhibitors and other results fueled the search for, and discovery of endogenous ouabain (a natriuretic factor, which may contribute to hypertension; Hamlyn *et al.*, 1991, 1996).   Here, I will focus here on the mechanisms by which glycosides lead to cardiac inotropy and Ca overload.

Inhibition of the Na-pump by strophanthidin or acetylstrophanthidin (ACS, rapid acting & reversible) increases aNa$_i$ and contractility (Figs 159 & 161).   Indeed, the aNa$_i$-dependence of twitch force can be very steep, particularly in cardiac Purkinje fibers where force can double with ~1 mM rise of aNa$_i$ (with Hill coefficients of 3-6, Lee & Dagostino, 1982; Wasserstrom *et al.*, 1983; Im & Lee, 1984; Eisner *et al.*, 1984).   In ventricular muscle the relationship is less steep, probably because of a ceiling effect.   That is, in rabbit ventricle at ~29°C and 0.5 Hz, control twitches are ~40% of the maximum myofilament force (Harrison & Bers, 1989a).

Glynn (1964), Repke (1964) and Langer (1965) first suggested that reciprocal Na and Ca movements might be involved in this inotropic effect.   This was before Na/Ca exchange was demonstrated, after which this hypothesis was more clearly stated (Reuter & Seitz, 1968; Baker *et al.*, 1969; Langer & Serena, 1970).   Now it is quite clear that relatively small increases in [Na]$_i$ can have a large impact on the balance of Ca fluxes mediated by Na/Ca exchange.   For example, an increase of [Na]$_i$ from 9 mM to 12 mM would shift the reversal potential for Na/Ca exchange ($E_{Na/Ca}$, by −30 mV; see Fig 72).   This will tend to increase Ca influx via Na/Ca exchange during the AP and also limit Ca extrusion via Na/Ca exchange during relaxation and diastole.   The result

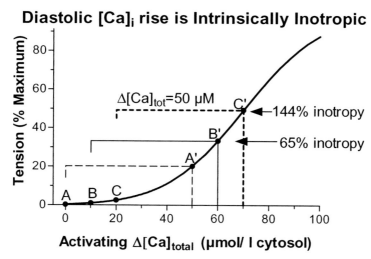

Figure 160. Increased diastolic $[Ca]_i$ increases developed tension, for the same amount of activating Ca. Tension-dependence on total cytosolic Ca ($[Ca]_{Tot}$), where Force=$100/(1+(600/[Ca]_i)^4)$ and $[Ca]_{Tot}$= $(244/(1+673/[Ca]_i))-44.5$. A, B and C ($[Ca]_{Tot}$=0, 10 & 20 μmol/L cytosol) correspond to diastolic $[Ca]_i$ levels (150, 193 & 241 nM) and A', B' and C' correspond to tension and $[Ca]_{Tot}$ reached when 50 μmol/L cytosol is added to A, B and C respectively ($[Ca]_i$ = 425, 504 & 595 nM).

is that resting $[Ca]_i$ can increase (Lee *et al.*, 1980; Marbán *et al.*, 1980; Bers & Ellis, 1982; Sheu & Fozzard, 1982; Allen *et al.*, 1984a; Weingart & Hess, 1984; Wier & Hess, 1984). Let's consider the impact of elevated diastolic $[Ca]_i$ on contraction, if all other things are equal.

Figure 160 shows how force depends on total cytoplasmic Ca (see also Fig 28). In this case, three diastolic $[Ca]_i$ values are indicated: control (A=150 nM) and values expected during inotropic effects of Na-pump inhibition (B=193 nM & C=241 nM), which are at or below the threshold for myofilament activation. If we assume that activation adds a "bolus" of 50 μmol Ca/L cytosol, then A goes to A', B to B' and C to C' (peak $[Ca]_i$ ~600 nM). Thus, increasing resting $[Ca]_i$ from A to either B or C would increase developed force (by 65 or 144%), despite an exactly constant $\Delta[Ca]_{tot}$ and a $\Delta[Ca]_i$ increase of only 13 and 28%. Therefore increased diastolic $[Ca]_i$ can contribute significantly to the inotropic effect of cardiac glycosides.

The rise in $[Na]_i$ and shift in $E_{Na/Ca}$ will limit the ability of the Na/Ca exchange to compete with the SR Ca-pump during relaxation, thereby increasing SR Ca uptake. Along with the higher diastolic and mean $[Ca]_i$ under these conditions, higher SR Ca load is expected. Indeed, SR Ca content assessed by RCCs is increased with Na-pump inhibition (Fig 161B). Of interest, the RCC amplitude remains high at high ACS concentration, despite a progressive decline in the amplitude of twitch contractions. This negative inotropic effect of high concentrations of cardioactive steroids will be addressed below (pg 294-300). The increase in SR Ca content with glycosides results in greater SR Ca release (Wier & Hess, 1984; Allen *et al.*, 1985b), and contributes to the glycoside inotropy. Indeed, some investigators attribute the entire glycoside inotropy to an increased SR Ca release (Morgan, 1985; Akera, 1990). While SR Ca loading is likely to be a dominant contributor to the inotropic effect, it may not be that simple.

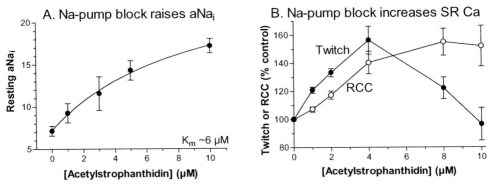

Figure 161. Effect of Na-pump inhibition by acetylstrophanthidin (ACS) on aNa$_i$, twitch tension and SR Ca content in rabbit ventricular muscle (30°C, 0.5 Hz). **A**. Resting aNa$_i$ measured with Na-selective microelectrodes (data from Shattock & Bers, 1989). **B**. Steady state twitch tension and RCCs induced immediately after a twitch (to assess SR Ca content; data from Bers & Bridge, 1988).

For example, if the SR is inhibited by caffeine or ryanodine, the inotropic effect of ACS can be just as large as under control conditions (Fig 162). While increased SR Ca load is surely important in glycoside inotropy, this result demonstrates that the inotropy can still occur without a normally functioning SR. Thus, changes in diastolic [Ca]$_i$ and transsarcolemmal Ca fluxes may also contribute to the glycoside inotropy.

Na-pump inhibition and elevation of [Na]$_i$ are expected to favor Ca influx via Na/Ca exchange and make Ca extrusion less favorable. Under normal conditions the amount of Ca influx via Na/Ca exchange is insufficient to activate appreciable contraction (pg 150, Fig 74). This can also be appreciated in Fig 163, where the Ca channel antagonist nifedipine virtually abolished twitch force under control conditions (and in the presence of caffeine or ryanodine). However, when [Na]$_i$ is increased by ACS (with the SR suppressed by caffeine or ryanodine) contraction is much less sensitive to nifedipine, despite a large decrease in AP duration (Fig 163). Increasing AP duration back to control under these conditions also returned twitches to

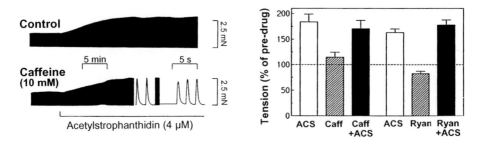

Figure 162. Acetylstrophanthidin (ACS) increases twitch force, even with caffeine or ryanodine. Rabbit ventricular muscle (at 30°C, 0.5 Hz, 4 μM ACS). After washout, and equilibration with 10 mM caffeine, ACS was applied again. The ACS-induced increase in force was similar in control and after treatment with 10 mM caffeine or 500 nM ryanodine (right, adapted from Bers, 1987b, with permission).

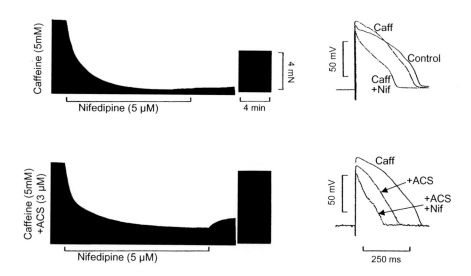

Figure 163. The Ca channel blocker nifedipine nearly abolishes control twitch tension, either by itself (not shown) or in the presence of 5 mM caffeine (top). However, after Na-pump inhibition (by ACS), nifedipine does not abolish tension, despite reduction in AP duration (right). Experiments were with rabbit ventricular muscle at 30°C, stimulated at 0.5 Hz (adapted from Bers *et al.*, 1988, with permission).

control levels (Bers *et al.*, 1988). This indicates that when [Na]$_i$ is elevated, enough Ca can enter the cell via Na/Ca exchange to activate contraction directly. It was also suggested that Ca influx via Na/Ca exchange can trigger SR Ca release (Bers *et al.*, 1988; Leblanc & Hume, 1990). While this triggering action is still controversial (see Fig 71, 74 & pg 232-4), it is clear that with high [Na]$_i$ large amounts of Ca can enter the cell via Na/Ca exchange. But *does* Ca influx via Na/Ca exchange increase measurably with Na-pump inhibition?

I studied the influence of ACS on sarcolemmal Ca fluxes in rabbit ventricle using extra-cellular Ca microelectrodes (Bers, 1987b). ACS sometimes increased Ca$_o$ depletion (or net Ca uptake) in a simple manner (Fig 164A). At other times ACS increased the initial Ca$_o$ depletion rate, but then gave way to net Ca efflux during the contraction (Fig 164B, trace 2). This may have the same cellular basis as the Ca efflux observed during twitches in rat ventricle (Fig 139), or upon abrupt application of low [caffeine] (Fig 146). That is, the large SR Ca release (contraction was 225% of control in Fig 164B) and the shorter AP duration in ACS may stimulate Ca extrusion via Na/Ca exchange, analogous to rat ventricle in Fig 140 (see Fig 164C).

The fact that Ca efflux occurs during contraction and probably overlaps temporally with Ca influx, makes it hard to assess changes in unidirectional Ca influx. To limit this problem, I studied the effect of ACS on Ca influx under conditions where Ca efflux is initially minimized (Fig 165). This occurs at the first few post-rest contractions in the presence of ryanodine (as discussed on pg 183-5) or after SR Ca depletion (Fig 145). Ryanodine causes rapid SR Ca depletion at rest, which is reflected by the rapid rise in [Ca]$_o$ when stimulation is stopped in Fig 165C *vs.* A. Thus, during the first post-rest contraction, the SR begins empty and may accumulate much of the Ca which enters the cell. This post-rest contraction is small and the low [Ca]$_i$ will not stimulate much Ca efflux via Na/Ca exchange. Therefore only Ca influx is

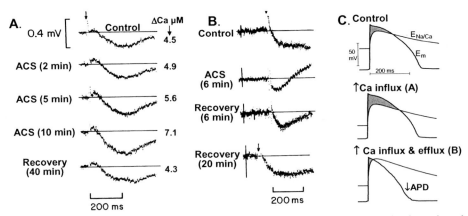

Figure 164. Extracellular Ca depletions in rabbit ventricle measured with Ca-selective microelectrodes (30°C, 0.5Hz, $[Ca]_o$=0.3 mM). **A.** Na-pump inhibition (by ACS) increased the ΔCa_o (see numbers at right), reflecting more Ca influx. **B.** ACS increased the initial rate of Ca_o depletion, but then Ca started to come out of the cells, indicated by the increase in $[Ca]_o$ (from Bers, 1987b, with permission). **C.** Conceptualized explanation of differences in A and B, based on driving forces as in Figs 72 & 140.

appreciable during the first two post-rest contractions and Ca_o depletion occurs without recovery between beats (Fig 165C or E). During the first few pulses, the amount of Ca_o depletion increases at each beat, consistent with the I_{Ca} staircase (Fig 58) and possibly more Ca entry via Na/Ca exchange.

Addition of ACS in control (Fig 165B) prevents SR Ca loss during rest (i.e. slows rest decay) and no slow rise in $[Ca]_o$ is seen. Since the SR and cell did not lose Ca during rest, the post-rest contraction is large, and no cumulative Ca_o depletion occurs (i.e. the SR is already Ca loaded). With ACS in the presence of ryanodine (Fig 165D), the SR is emptied rapidly during rest, although more slowly than with ryanodine alone (Fig 165C). ACS slows the ryanodine-induced SR Ca loss in rabbit ventricle (assessed by RCCs; Bers & Christensen, 1990).

With the background above we can now compare the effect of ACS on Ca influx in Fig

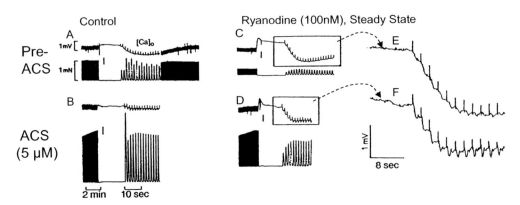

Figure 165. Acetylstrophanthidin (ACS) increases twitch force, even with caffeine or ryanodine. Rabbit ventricular muscle (at 30°C, 0.5 Hz, 4 μM ACS). After washout and equilibration with 10 mM caffeine, ACS was applied again. The ACS-induced increase in force was similar in control (**A** *vs.* **B**) and after treatment with 500 nM ryanodine (**C-F**; adapted from Bers, 1987b, with permission).

165E *vs.* F, where Ca efflux has been minimized. At the first post-rest contraction, ACS greatly increases the initial rate and extent of Ca_o depletion (~6- and 2-fold, respectively). As steady state is approached (where Ca influx = Ca efflux over each cycle), both Ca influx and Ca efflux appear to be increased by ACS. The greater Ca influx is via Na/Ca exchange favored by the elevated $[Na]_i$. The greater efflux results from the increased peak $[Ca]_i$ during the twitch which drives Ca efflux via Na/Ca exchange (and overcomes the shift in $E_{Na/Ca}$ favoring Ca influx). Ryanodine helps to temporally separate Ca influx and efflux phases since peak $[Ca]_i$ occurs later. This allows us to conclude that Na-pump inhibition can lead to increased Ca influx and efflux during the AP (although Pizarro *et al.,* 1985 did not detect strophanthidin effects on Ca depletion in frog ventricle). Le Grand *et al.* (1990) showed that ouabain increases both L- and T-type Ca currents. It is possible that the higher average $[Ca]_i$ in the presence of Na-pump inhibition contributes to this increase of I_{Ca} as suggested by Marbán & Tsien (1982). This I_{Ca} facilitation may be related to the I_{Ca} staircase phenomenon shown in Fig 58.

Two additional Na/Ca exchange-independent modes of glycoside inotropy have been proposed. First, ouabain has been shown to increase the open probability of single RyR channels in lipid bilayers (McGarry & Williams, 1993; Rardon & Wasserstrom, 1990). However, this might be expected to only produce a transient elevation of SR Ca release as seen for low caffeine concentrations (Fig 146). Second, it has been suggested that ouabain or digoxin changes the selectivity of cardiac Na channels, such that they become equally permeant to Ca ions (the so-called slip-mode conductance, Santana *et al.,* 1998; see pg 235). This would increase the Ca influx signal in CICR and enhance SR Ca release. Although these two results are intriguing, I am skeptical that either of these pathways contribute significantly to glycoside inotropy, for the following simple reason. If cells are depleted of $[Na]_i$ and studied in completely Na-free solutions, we find that glycosides have no effect at all (transient or otherwise) on contractions (under conditions where inotropy is seen in normal Na-containing solutions, Altamirano *et al.,* 1999). Thus, glycoside inotropy appears to depend on the presence of Na, and is presumably due to Na/K-ATPase inhibition and consequent alterations of $[Na]_i$ and $[Ca]_i$.

There are intriguing data indicating that Na/K-ATPase isoforms are differentially distributed on the sarcolemma of cardiac and smooth muscle cells (McDonough *et al.,* 1996; Juhaszova & Blaustein, 1997). In rat ventricular myocytes, the α_1-isoform is preferentially localized to T-tubules, while the α_2-isoform is ubiquitous. In smooth muscle the low ouabain-affinity α_1-isoform is ubiquitously distributed, while the higher ouabain-affinity α_2- and α_3-isoforms are preferentially localized in regions overlying the SR. Ouabain augmented Ca transients without raising global $[Na]_i$ in smooth muscle (Arnon *et al.,* 2000). This work indicates that local junctional microdomain $[Na]_i$ and $[Ca]_i$ may be controlled more by local Na/K-ATPase and Na/Ca exchange molecules. Su *et al.* (2001) also showed that abrupt Na/K-ATPase inhibition in guinea-pig ventricular myocytes increases the efficacy of a given I_{Ca} to trigger SR Ca release. Thus, a normally functioning Na/K-ATPase may maintain $[Na]_i$ and $[Ca]_i$ in the junctional cleft at lower values than bulk cytosolic, and this may limit CICR. Goldhaber *et al.* (1999) found that abrupt $[Na]_o$ removal increased resting Ca spark frequency, attributing this block of tonic Ca removal from the junctional cleft by Na/Ca exchange (although Ca entry via Na/Ca exchange may have contributed to this effect).

Glycosides limit Ca efflux via Na/Ca exchange and also favor Ca influx via Na/Ca exchange. It is hard to distinguish which mode of transport is causing inotropy. Satoh *et al.* (2000) used KB-R7943 to selectively block outward $I_{Na/Ca}$ (Ca entry). KB-R7943 did not prevent the inotropic effect of strophanthadin, but prevented the spontaneous activity characteristic of glycoside toxicity and cellular Ca overload. We suggested that slowing Ca extrusion via Na/Ca exchange is sufficient for the inotropic effect, but that Ca overload and toxicity occur when $[Na]_i$ rises to the level where net Ca influx occurs via outward $I_{Na/Ca}$ (blocked by KB-R7943).

In conclusion, glycoside inotropy can be attributed primarily to Na-pump inhibition and consequent shifts in Na/Ca exchange, making Ca influx more favorable and Ca efflux less favorable. During individual contractions this can occur by increasing diastolic $[Ca]_i$, increasing SR Ca content (and release) and increasing Ca influx early in the contraction. These are, of course, all interrelated and it is difficult to determine unequivocally the fractional contribution of each effect. When the cell gains too much Ca due to the shift in Na/Ca exchange, negative inotropic and arrhythmogenic effects occur. These will be discussed in the next section.

Ca MISMANAGEMENT AND NEGATIVE INOTROPY

Ca Overload and Spontaneous SR Ca Release

At high glycoside concentrations the positive inotropic action gives way to a negative inotropic effect (Figs 161B and 166). Other toxic effects of glycosides also become apparent: 1) elevated resting force, 2) oscillatory after-contractions and 3) oscillatory or delayed afterdepolarizations (DADs, Fig 166). It now seems clear that all of these effects are secondary to cellular Ca overload and spontaneous Ca release from the SR during diastole.

Fabiato & Fabiato (1972) observed spontaneous cyclical contractions due to SR Ca release in skinned rat ventricular myocytes when bathing [Ca] was >100 nM. In intact rat ventricle Lakatta & Lappé (1981; Lappé & Lakatta, 1980) reported scattered light intensity fluctuations (SLIF) attributed to spontaneous SR Ca release-induced local contractions, and these were enhanced by high $[Ca]_o$ or ouabain. Resting rat ventricle often shows spontaneous SR Ca release, SLIF and a high Ca spark frequency at rest, whereas rabbit ventricle only shows them at high $[Ca]_o$ or with Na-pump inhibition (Kort & Lakatta, 1984, 1988a,b; Capogrossi & Lakatta, 1985; Capogrossi *et al.*, 1986a; Díaz *et al.*, 1996, 1997a; Satoh *et al.*, 1997). This is consistent with rat ventricle having high resting SR Ca load, because resting $[Na]_i$ is high (Chapter 9). Furthermore, Ca sparks, spontaneous oscillations and SLIF in rat ventricle are suppressed for several seconds after a stimulated synchronous contraction.

In intact single cells spontaneous SR Ca release events can propagate as Ca waves, especially when SR Ca load and $[Ca]_i$ are very high (see pg 230-2). Local $[Ca]_i$ during a wave is comparable in amplitude and kinetics to that during a twitch (Fig 122). However, when whole cell $[Ca]_i$ is measured, the $\Delta[Ca]_i$ amplitude appears to be smaller and slower, because of the lack of spatial uniformity. While the negative consequences of these Ca waves will be discussed below, there is also a beneficial effect. The high $[Ca]_i$ and negative E_m drives Ca extrusion from the cell via Na/Ca exchange, and this unloads the cell and SR of Ca. Díaz *et al.* (1997a) found that Ca waves occur at a threshold SR Ca load of ~100 μmol/L cytosol, and that a typical Ca wave in rat ventricular myocytes causes extrusion of ~15 μmol/L cytosol (and we find similar

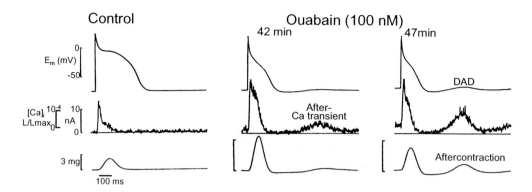

Figure 166. Ouabain-induced delayed afterdepolarizations (DADs) and aftercontractions in a canine cardiac Purkinje fiber at 35°C, 1 Hz. Addition of the Na-pump inhibitor decreased AP duration, increased the Ca transients (assessed by aequorin luminescence) and increased contractile force. Diastolic force eventually rises and developed force declines as DADs and aftercontractions become more apparent (modified from Wier & Hess, 1984, with permission).

values in rabbit). This allows SR Ca load to fall below threshold. Indeed, if Ca extrusion via Na/Ca exchange is prevented the cell will continue to oscillate (as observed in skinned cells where the Ca has nowhere to go). Once the cell has extruded this ~15 μmol/L cytosol, it may then take several seconds for cellular Ca to increase back to the point where spontaneous Ca release occurs again. With higher Ca overload this delay can be abolished and SLIF, Ca waves and Ca sparks can be elevated immediately after the twitch (Kort & Lakatta, 1988a; Díaz *et al.*, 1996; Satoh *et al.*, 1997). Caffeine and ryanodine abolish both the $[Ca]_i$ and tension fluctuations in all of these cases, confirming that the SR is the source.

The functional consequence of spontaneous SR Ca releases are serious at both the cellular and tissue level (and both mechanically and electrophysiologically). When a stimulated twitch occurs soon after a spontaneous release, the stimulated Ca transient and contraction are depressed (Allen *et al.*, 1985b; Capogrossi *et al.*, 1986b; Capogrossi & Lakatta, 1985). The weaker Ca release can result from a combination of incomplete mechanical restitution (e.g. refractoriness of the SR Ca release channel, Fig 122, Ishide *et al.*, 1990) and a net loss of Ca from the cell (as discussed above). In multicellular preparations such spontaneous Ca release can occur in random cells, but as the number of Ca overloaded cells increases a progressive decline in contractile force is expected. The negative inotropic effect in multicellular preparations is much more severe than this simple additive expectation. This is because the cells are not independent, but linked mechanically in series. A weakly activated cell will have high compliance and be stretched by more fully activated cells. Such a fully activated cell will also produce less force and shortening velocity as a consequence of its shorter sarcomere length. Additionally, the shortening that was required to stretch the more compliant cell will not contribute to external work. Thus, the negative consequences of these inhomogeneous spontaneous Ca releases are greatly amplified. These spontaneous contractions can limit the inotropic effect of increasing Ca load (e.g. by cardioactive steroids, reduced $[Na]_o$, elevated $[Ca]_o$ etc.). This also emphasizes the importance of the normal syncytial behavior of cardiac muscle.

While twitch force falls in Fig 161B at high [ACS], RCC amplitude is not reduced. This may be due to synchronous SR Ca release at an RCC and the fact that RCCs reflect the sum of SR Ca released plus cytosolic Ca. The plateau RCC amplitude at high [ACS] in Fig 161B may be because mean cellular Ca (SR + cytosolic) does not decrease. Progressive Ca loading may be expected, but could be limited by Ca extrusion during local Ca releases when [Ca]$_i$ is high.

As discussed in Chapter 8 (pg 230-2), the mechanism for these spontaneous SR Ca releases and waves in cardiac myocytes is probably via propagated Ca-induced Ca-release (Mulder et al., 1989; Backx et al., 1989; Takamatsu & Wier, 1990; Lukyanenko et al., 1999). Both elevated [Ca]$_i$ and high [Ca]$_{SR}$ contribute to the propagation of waves. Ca waves in single cells can readily propagate through the whole cell (at ~100 µm/s), but in multicellular preparations they generally do not propagate through gap junctions from one cell to the next (Wier et al., 1997; Lamont et al., 1998; Kaneko et al., 2000). In intact beating rat heart, Kaneko et al. (2000) found no diastolic Ca waves, unless the heart rate was slowed. Then sporadic Ca waves at low frequency were seen (4 /cell/min), with only 6% propagating to a neighboring cell. Raising [Ca]$_o$ from 2 to 4 or 6 mM increased wave frequency, even during the diastolic interval during 1 Hz pacing. Some regions with higher average [Ca]$_i$ produced "Ca-overload" waves with much higher wave frequency (28 /cell/min) and 23% propagated to neighboring cells. This may especially enhance arrhythmogenesis (see below). A third variety (agonal waves) occurred in severe Ca overload regions (133 waves/cell/sec). These appeared to immediately precede cell death, and the wave propagation to other cells was again lower (9%), perhaps due to reduced gap junction conductance at high local [Ca]$_i$ and low pH$_i$. Thus, three types of Ca waves were observed (sporadic, Ca-overload and agonal), and they may contribute differently to arrhythmogenesis and contractile dysfunction. All of these waves propagated at 80-120 µm/s. Higher rates of wave propagation (200-8000 µm/s) have been seen in trabeculae, but these rates may well require a concomitant mechanical or electrophysiological component of propagation (in addition to CICR).

Spontaneous SR Ca releases can be relatively synchronized among cells right after electrical stimulation and can produce the aftercontractions and delayed afterdepolarizations (DADs) which are commonly associated with Ca overload and digitalis toxicity (see Fig 166). Synchronization is probably because the Ca release events are initiated by SR Ca uptake during twitch relaxation, when a point is reached where the combination of SR Ca load, [Ca]$_i$ and recovery from refractoriness initiate SR Ca release (which can be similarly timed in many cells). Thus, the initial Ca release and wave occurrence can be relatively synchronous in many cells. However, at subsequent spontaneous releases the cells vary as to the timing, amount of SR Ca release, wave duration and the amount of Ca that was extruded by Na/Ca exchange. Then whether a second wave occurs (and at what time) will be much more variable from cell to cell. The result is that a second aftercontraction is usually smaller and broader in time course.

This progressive decline in amplitude of oscillatory aftercontractions (see Fig 166) may be partly due to desynchronization. It may also be due to the progressive decrease in SR Ca load. That is, fewer cells continue to oscillate and those that do will produce smaller Ca transients. If Na/Ca exchange is prevented from extruding Ca, oscillatory aftercontractions can continue with minimal decrement, and this same situation can be seen in skinned cells where Ca efflux cannot

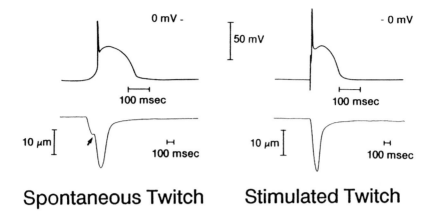

Spontaneous Twitch   Stimulated Twitch

Figure 167. Membrane potential and cell length during a twitch resulting from a multifocal spontaneous Ca release (left) and an electrically driven twitch (right) in a rat ventricular myocyte (at 37°C). These contractions are considered to be multifocal whenever two waves are moving in one cell, even if they both originated from a single site near the middle of the cell. Multifocal contractions more often depolarize the cell sufficiently to trigger an action potential (from Capogrossi *et al.*, 1987, with permission).

occur (Fabiato & Fabiato, 1978b). In addition to mechanical problems, there are also important electrophysiological consequences associated with these aftercontractions.

Afterdepolarizations and Triggered Arrhythmias

Aftercontractions are associated with delayed afterdepolarizations (DADs), and it is clear that SR Ca release is responsible for both. That is, SR Ca release activates the myofilaments (aftercontraction), but also activates a transient inward current (I_{ti}) which is responsible for DADs (Lederer & Tsien, 1976; Kass *et al.*, 1978). These I_{ti} and DADs are responsible for the oscillatory afterdepolarizations observed with Ca overload and these can, in turn, lead to triggered arrhythmias in the heart (Ferrier & Moe, 1973; Rosen *et al.*, 1973a,b; Ferrier, 1977; Wit & Rosen, 1992). The process of Ca overload can lead to triggered arrhythmias via a fairly well defined sequence of events.

Three different Ca-activated currents have been proposed to contribute to I_{ti}: 1) Na/Ca exchange current ($I_{Na/Ca}$), 2) Ca-activated chloride current ($I_{Cl(Ca)}$) and 3) a nonselective cationic current ($I_{NS(Ca)}$, Colquhoun *et al.*, 1981, Cannell & Lederer, 1986; Wit & Rosen, 1992; Zygmunt *et al.*, 1998; Schlotthauer & Bers, 2000). Most recent work has not supported a significant role for $I_{NS(Ca)}$ in I_{ti} or DADs of ventricular myocytes, favoring instead key roles for $I_{Cl(Ca)}$ and $I_{Na/Ca}$ (Fedida *et al.*, 1987b; Papp *et al.*, 1995; Laflamme & Becker, 1996; Szigeti *et al.*, 1998; Zygmunt *et al.*, 1998; Egdell & MacLeod, 2000; Schlotthauer & Bers, 2000). In dog ventricular myocytes Zygmunt *et al.* (1998) attributed 60% of I_{ti} to $I_{Na/Ca}$ and 40% to $I_{Cl(Ca)}$. There is clearly $I_{Cl(Ca)}$ in rabbit ventricular myocytes at 37°C (Zygmunt & Gibbons, 1991; Laflamme & Becker, 1996; Puglisi *et al.*, 1999), but we find that >90% of the Ca-activated current in rabbit ventricular myocytes at 23 or 37°C is $I_{Na/Ca}$ and not $I_{Cl(Ca)}$ (Delbridge *et al.*, 1996; Schlotthauer & Bers, 2000; Pogwizd *et al.*, 2001, but see also Szigeti *et al.*, 1998). $I_{Na/Ca}$ also seems to dominate in guinea-pig ventricular myocytes (Fedida *et al.*, 1987b; Kimura, 1988). In human ventricular myocytes the [Ca]$_i$-dependent inward current is almost entirely $I_{Na/Ca}$, although atrial myocytes exhibit some

$I_{NS(Ca)}$ (Koster *et al.*, 1999; Schlotthauer *et al.*, 2000). Thus, I_{ti} is mainly $I_{Na/Ca}$, but $I_{Cl(Ca)}$ (and even $I_{NS(Ca)}$) may play a small variable role in certain tissues or conditions.

The contributions of aforementioned currents to DAD generation may differ from those during an I_{ti} (where E_m is clamped constant), because E_m changes dynamically during DADs and alters the electrochemical driving force (most notably for $I_{Cl(Ca)}$). Consider that if $E_{Cl} = -60$ mV, a DAD from -80 to -70 mV reduces the Cl driving force by 50%. For $I_{Na/Ca}$ the $E_{Na/Ca}$ may be -40 mV at rest, but as $[Ca]_i$ rises $E_{Na/Ca}$ rises to about $+10$ mV (see Fig 140), thereby more than offsetting the effect of a 10 mV depolarization. Thus, voltage clamp studies will overestimate the role of $I_{Cl(Ca)}$ in DADs. Figure 168 shows caffeine-induced DADs (or cDADs), used to measure the quantitative relationship between SR Ca release and depolarization (Schlotthauer & Bers, 2000; Pogwizd *et al.*, 2001). This sort of quantification would not be practical with spatially inhomogeneous spontaneous Ca waves. APs were activated at different frequencies (to vary SR Ca load), and then caffeine was rapidly applied to release SR Ca and trigger a cDAD. With increasing SR Ca load (and $\Delta[Ca]_i$) larger cDADs were observed until the point where SR Ca release triggered an AP. Figure 168B shows how ΔE_m increases with $\Delta[Ca]_i$ and in rabbit cells APs are triggered at $\Delta[Ca]_i \sim 500$ nM (requiring $\Delta[Ca]_{Tot} \sim 80$ μmol/L cytosol).

This amount of Ca might be released during a spontaneous Ca release, but its ability to trigger an AP may be limited by several factors. First, spontaneous SR Ca release normally occurs in waves, which are not spatially homogeneous, such that the Ca-activated I_{ti} would have a lower peak, but be of longer duration. Even if the integrated I_{ti} is the same, spreading it out over a longer time reduces the cDAD amplitude and increases the amount of I_{ti} required to trigger an AP (Schlotthauer & Bers, 2000). This effect may nearly double the amount of Ca release needed to trigger an AP (requiring $\sim 100\%$ of SR Ca content). Second, during a spontaneous SR Ca release, Ca reuptake by the SR is not prevented by caffeine. Thus the inward $I_{Na/Ca}$ in rabbit or human will only remove 30% of the released Ca at negative E_m (Table 20, and less than this in rat & mouse). This would affect the integrated I_{ti} more than its peak, but could provide an additional safety margin in a normal ventricular myocyte. Thus it may be difficult for spontaneous SR Ca release to trigger an AP, but it can occur, especially when more than one Ca wave occurs simultaneously in a cell (Fig 167; Capogrossi *et al.*, 1987).

In the whole heart there is an additional stabilizing effect because neighboring cells will act as current sinks, limiting the ΔE_m produced by a given local $I_{Na/Ca}$. However, the cellular changes which cause either more SR Ca release (Ca overload) or greater local depolarization for a given $\Delta[Ca]_i$ (below) would tend to increase the propensity for triggered arrhythmias. That is, there would be a greater chance for a cell cluster that is local enough, synchronous enough and large enough to overcome the 3-dimensional current sink limitation and trigger a propagating arrhythmia.

In heart failure (HF) there is ~ 2-fold increase in the expression and function of Na/Ca exchange (Hasenfuss *et al.*, 1999; Pogwizd *et al.*, 1999), which means that any given $[Ca]_i$ will produce about twice as much inward $I_{Na/Ca}$. In addition, if there is also reduced SR Ca-ATPase function in HF, the Na/Ca exchanger will extrude a larger fraction of the released Ca (further increasing I_{ti}). There is also a 50% reduction in the inward rectifier K current (I_{K1}) which is responsible for stabilizing diastolic E_m (Beuckelman *et al.*, 1993; Kääb *et al.*, 1996; Puglisi *et al.*,

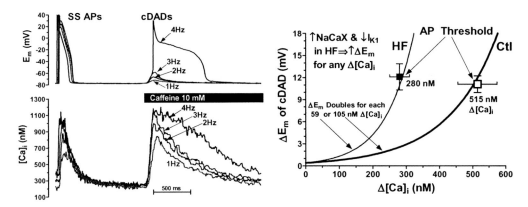

Figure 168. Caffeine-induced Ca transients and delayed afterdepolarizations (cDADs). Rabbit ventricular myocytes were studied at 37°C under current clamp. Steady state (SS) APs were induced at different frequencies, resulting in altered twitch and caffeine-induced Δ[Ca]$_i$. Larger Δ[Ca]$_i$ caused larger cDADs and at some point trigger APs. Mean subthreshold data are fit by 0.4exp(kΔ[Ca]$_i$), such that ΔE$_m$ doubles for each Δ[Ca]$_i$ of ln(2)/k (as indicated). Large squares indicate threshold for triggering APs. Data at left are redrawn from Schlotthauer & Bers (2000) and at right from Schlotthauer *et al.* (2000).

2000; Pogwizd *et al.*, 2001). Reduced I$_{K1}$ would also mean that any given I$_{ti}$ would produce a greater depolarization, and be more likely to trigger an AP. These factors greatly increase the propensity for arrhythmias to be triggered by Ca overload and DADs in HF.

Indeed, in a non-ischemic rabbit model of HF with I$_{Na/Ca}$ and I$_{K1}$ changes as above, we find that the threshold Δ[Ca]$_i$ during a cDAD required to trigger an AP is reduced by ~50% from control (Fig 168B; Pogwizd *et al.*, 1999, 2001). Moreover, these HF rabbits develop runs of non-sustained ventricular tachycardia (not seen in control) which initiate by a non-reentrant mechanism (e.g. DADs) based on 3-dimensional mapping studies (Pogwizd, 1995). Mapping studies in nonischemic human HF have shown that almost all arrhythmias initiate by non-reentrant mechanisms, whereas ~50% of those in ischemic HF initiate by non-reentrant mechanisms (Pogwizd *et al.*, 1992, 1998). These arrhythmias in the failing rabbit model above are inducible by infusion of β-AR agonists, and aftercontractions (like those in Fig 166) were readily induced by isoproterenol in isolated HF myocytes as well (Pogwizd *et al.*, 1999, 2001). Our working hypothesis for arrhythmogenesis in HF is the following (see Fig 175). In HF SR Ca content is typically reduced (due to increased Na/Ca exchange and/or reduced SR Ca-ATPase function), and this by itself would make spontaneous SR Ca release less likely. However, when SR Ca load is increased by β-AR activation (via phospholamban phosphorylation) spontaneous SR Ca release can occur and produce more I$_{ti}$ (due to greater I$_{Na/Ca}$) and that I$_{ti}$, in turn causes much greater depolarization (due to reduced I$_{K1}$). On a related note, sudden cardiac death due to arrhythmias occurs commonly in moderately severe HF, but much less commonly in the latest stages of HF when β-AR responsiveness is lost, but ventricular function continues to decline (Bristow *et al.*, 1982; Kjelshus, 1990). Thus, without the β-AR-induced boost in SR Ca loading, spontaneous SR Ca release and DADs may not occur, but contractile function may be severely depressed by the low SR Ca content.

While Ca overload and aftercontractions or DADs secondary to Na-pump inhibition are perhaps the most extensively studied, the same sequelae occur with other causes of cellular Ca overload. These may include reduced $[Na]_o$, increased Na permeability (e.g. monensin), elevated $[Ca]_o$, Ca channel agonists, large/long depolarizations, high frequency stimulation, decreased membrane Ca or Na permeability barrier or decrease in energy supply required to maintain normal ionic gradients. In summary, Ca overload causes spontaneous SR Ca release which can contribute to:

1) High mean resting $[Ca]_i$ (basal and also average from spontaneous SR Ca releases),
2) Increased diastolic force,
3) Greater inactivation of Ca-induced Ca-release at a normal pulse,
4) Asynchrony of Ca release (due to refractoriness in areas of recent Ca release),
5) Reduced twitch force
6) Partial synchronization of spontaneous release after systole
     (due to the bolus of Ca influx and maybe synchrony of RyR inactivation & recovery),
7) Added series compliance (refractory cells) that contracting cells must stretch,
8) Ca_i-dependent increase of inward I_{ti} (mainly $I_{Na/Ca}$),
9) Depolarization (afterdepolarization),
10) Triggered arrhythmias

Acidosis

For more than 100 years acidosis has been known to depress myocardial contractility (Gaskell, 1880), and it is important to consider because acidosis is a major consequence of myocardial ischemia and contributes to the ischemic decline in force. The situation is potentially complicated by the fact that changing pH can modify virtually every cellular system involved in Ca regulation and force development. Nevertheless, some important conclusions can be drawn from experimental work aimed at evaluating this complex problem with respect to $[Ca]_i$ and force (see Orchard & Kentish, 1990; Hulme & Orchard, 1998; Choi *et al.*, 2000).

Respiratory acidosis (increasing extracellular CO_2) produces more rapid decline in pH_i and contraction than does metabolic acidosis which is induced by decreasing $[HCO_3]_o$ or applying weak acids such as acetic or butyric acids (Fry & Poole-Wilson, 1981). This has been taken as evidence that the major negative inotropic effect is due to intracellular (rather than extracellular) acidosis. Thus, even though low pH_o can inhibit I_{Ca} (Irisawa & Sato, 1986; Krafte & Kass, 1988), which would decrease contraction, that effect must be minor. Reduced pH_i can also decrease I_{Ca} (Sato *et al.*, 1985; Irisawa & Sato, 1986; Kaibara & Kameyama, 1988), although Hulme & Orchard (1998) found unchanged I_{Ca} with acidosis.

Ca transport by several systems is depressed at low pH_i, including SR Ca-ATPase (Fabiato & Fabiato, 1978a; Mandel *et al.*, 1982), RyR gating (Xu *et al.*, 1996; Kentish & Xiang, 1997) and Na/Ca exchange (Philipson *et al.*, 1982; Doering & Lederer, 1993). It is therefore somewhat surprising that acidosis increases (or fails to depress) Ca transient amplitude, but decreases contractile force (see Fig 169, Allen & Orchard, 1983; Orchard, 1987; Allen *et al.*, 1989; Hulme & Orchard, 1998). This indicates that the negative inotropic effect of acidosis is mainly at the level of myofilament responsiveness to $[Ca]_i$ (*vs.* reduction of Ca transients).

Acidosis does indeed decrease both myofilament Ca sensitivity and maximum force production (Fig 170, Donaldson & Hermansen, 1978; Fabiato & Fabiato, 1978a; Kentish &

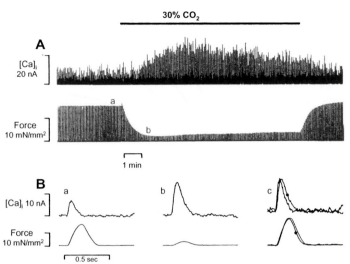

Figure 169. Respiratory acidosis depresses force, but not Ca transients. **A.** In a ferret papillary muscle pH_o was reduced from 7.4 to 6.7 by increasing $[CO_2]$ at 30°C and 0.33 Hz). Tension falls rapidly, but partially recovers. $[Ca]_i$ was measured using aequorin, which may exagerate changes in peak $[Ca]_i$ and is not highly sensitive to diastolic $[Ca]_i$ (due to exponential dependence of light on $[Ca]_i$). **B.** Averaged aequorin and force traces before (a) and after 1.5 min of acidosis (b), and with those traces scaled and superimposed (c where • denotes the trace during acidosis, from Orchard and Kentish, 1990, with permission).

Nayler, 1979; Blanchard & Solaro, 1984). Blanchard & Solaro (1984) concluded that much of the shift in myofilament Ca sensitivity could be attributed to a decrease in the affinity of ^{45}Ca binding to cardiac TnC. The effect of pH on Ca binding to troponin C is also amplified by a pH-sensitive change in the affinity of TnI for TnC (El-Saleh & Solaro, 1988; Solaro *et al.*, 1989). The reduction in maximum force appears to be a separate effect and also amplifies the depressant effect of acidosis on force development (Orchard & Kentish, 1990). Acidosis decreases maximum force much more than it does myofibrillar ATPase activity (Kentish & Nayler, 1979; Blanchard & Solaro, 1984). This may mean that acidosis decreases the maximum force (and efficiency) of each crossbridge as well as the turnover rate of the ATPase. These myofilament effects are the major cause of the negative inotropic effect of acidosis.

Neonatal ventricular (and skeletal) muscle is less sensitive to the depressant effects of acidosis than is adult ventricular muscle, and this is due primarily to a much smaller shift in myofilament Ca sensitivity (Solaro *et al.*, 1988). Reducing pH from 7 to 6.5 produced a 4-fold decrease in Ca affinity in adult rat (K_{Ca} increased from 1.5 to 4 µM), but only a 1.8-fold decrease in neonate rat myofilaments (K_{Ca} increased from 0.7 to 1.2 µM). Neonatal myofilament Ca sensitivity is also higher than adult, even at pH 7.0 (see Fig 21D). The smaller pH dependence in neonatal hearts appears to result, in part, from the different TnI isoform expressed in the fetal and newborn heart (slow skeletal TnI; see pg 32-33). This may help to protect the perinatal heart from ischemic stresses during development and at birth.

Ca transient amplitude during abrupt acidosis can be initially increased, unchanged or decreased (e.g. Orchard & Kentish, 1990; Hulme & Orchard, 1998; Choi *et al.*, 2000). However, in almost all reports there is then a progressive increase in twitch $\Delta[Ca]_i$, and this causes a partial recovery of contractions. Acidosis also leads to a gradual increase of diastolic $[Ca]_i$ (Bers &

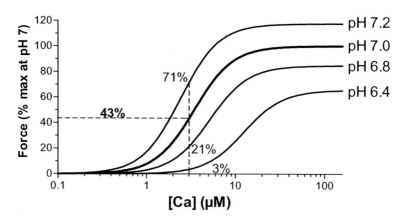

Figure 170. The effect of pH on the myofilament Ca sensitivity in triton-skinned guinea-pig ventricular muscle at 30°C. Note that a [Ca]$_i$ that produces 43% activation at pH 7.0 produces much less force at pH 6.8 and 6.4 (vertical broken line and numbers). Curves are redrawn, based on Orchard & Kentish (1990).

Ellis, 1982; Kohmoto *et al.*, 1990, Nakanishi *et al.*, 1990). As presented in Fig 160, this could contribute to the progressive force recovery and increase in peak Ca transient during acidosis. The increased diastolic [Ca]$_i$ may be partly due to proton competition at intracellular Ca buffering sites, such as TnC (Bers & Ellis, 1982; Vaughan-Jones *et al.*, 1983; Blanchard & Solaro, 1984) . This reduced Ca buffering could result in a greater Δ[Ca]$_i$ for a given addition of total Ca. To simulate a pH change from 7.0 to 6.5, I reduced TnC affinity in Table 10 and Fig 26 by 4-fold (based on Fig 170). Then the same increment in total Ca (75 μmol/L cytosol) would increase peak [Ca]$_i$ from 500 to 640 nM. Looked at another way, this reduces the amount of total Ca required to raise [Ca]$_i$ to 1 μM (from 117 to 101 μmol/L cytosol). This is a modest decrease in overall Ca buffering, but is consistent with the non-significant decrease (from 121 to 109) in buffering power measured by Choi *et al.* (2000). More importantly, for the same Δ[Ca]$_i$ (500 nM) developed force would decrease almost 10-fold (from 50% of maximum at pH 7 to 6%).

    Low intracellular pH also stimulates proton extrusion via Na/H exchange, especially when pH$_o$ is relatively normal. Indeed, for acid loads, cardiac cells appear to rely mainly on Na/H exchange for pH$_i$ regulation, while for alkali loads the Cl/HCO$_3$ exchange appears to be more important (Vaughan-Jones, 1982; Piwnica-Worms *et al.*, 1985; Ellis & MacLeod, 1985). Thus, extrusion of protons via Na/H exchange increases [Na]$_i$, particularly at normal pH$_o$ (Deitmer & Ellis, 1980; Bountra & Vaughan-Jones, 1989). While the Na/K-ATPase might be expected to reduce [Na]$_i$ back toward the control level, decreasing pH below 7.5 also inhibits the Na-pump (e.g. Sperelakis & Lee, 1971). The result is that [Na]$_i$ increases during respiratory acidosis with a time course similar to the slow recovery phase of contraction (Fig 171, Harrison *et al.*, 1992b). Thus, the increase in [Na]$_i$ may contribute to the slow recovery of contractile force via a shift in Na/Ca exchange and increase in [Ca]$_i$. Under conditions where extracellular pH was held constant, Bountra & Vaughan-Jones (1989) showed that reduced pH$_i$ could lead to an increase in [Na]$_i$ and twitch tension in guinea-pig papillary muscle. They attribute this positive inotropic effect to shifts of Na/Ca exchange which were sufficient to overcome the

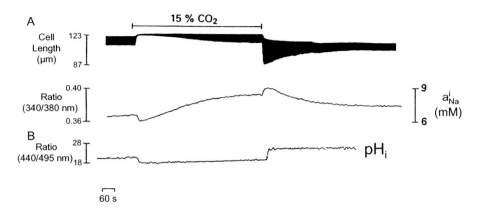

Figure 171.   Respiratory acidosis decreases contraction (**A**), and pH$_i$ (**B**, assessed by BCECF fluorescence) in a rat ventricular myocyte at 26°C, stimulated at 1 Hz. Intracellular Na activity (assessed by SBFI fluorescence) gradually increases during acidosis. This increase aNa$_i$ may contribute to the contractile recovery (via a shift in Na/Ca exchange). The initial decrease in the SBFI fluorescence trace was attributed to a pH effect on SBFI (from McCall *et al.*, 1990, with permission).

largely depressant effects of intracellular acidosis. Thus, it seems likely that the gain in cellular Na (and consequently Ca) contributes to the increased Ca transient observed with acidosis.

Na/Ca exchange is also inhibited by low pH (Philipson *et al.*, 1982). Together with the increased [Na]$_i$ discussed above, the ability of the cell to extrude Ca via Na/Ca exchange may be severely compromised. As with cardiac glycosides, this may also contribute to increased SR Ca loading (see below) and larger Ca transients seen during acidosis, but could also lead to Ca overload and consequent arrhythmias (Coraboeuf *et al.*, 1976; Kurachi, 1982). If spontaneous SR Ca release occurs during acidosis, negative inotropic effects would be exacerbated (as discussed on pages 295-300).

Acidosis also decreases cardiac SR Ca uptake in both isolated SR vesicles and skinned myocytes (see Chapter 7, Shigekawa, 1976; Mandel *et al.*, 1982; Fabiato & Fabiato, 1978a; Fabiato, 1985e). Indeed, the rate of the twitch [Ca]$_i$ decline in intact cells and muscle is slowed by acidosis (Fig 169, Hulme & Orchard, 1998). However, the increased diastolic [Ca]$_i$ and cellular Ca loading described above more than compensate for the slower SR Ca uptake at low pH$_i$. This explains the increased SR Ca content, which has been clearly documented during acidosis (Harrison *et al.*, 1992b; Hulme & Orchard, 1998; Choi *et al.*, 2000). Ca sparks in myocytes and RyR channel gating in bilayers are inhibited by acidosis (Ma *et al.*, 1988; Rousseau & Pinkos, 1990; Xu *et al.*, 1996; Balnave & Vaughan-Jones, 2000). Fabiato (1985e) showed that the optimal free [Ca] trigger for CICR was higher at low pH, and Hulme & Orchard (1998) showed that acidosis reduced fractional SR Ca release. Indeed, variability in the initial Δ[Ca]$_i$ response to abrupt acidosis might depend on how extensively E-C coupling is depressed (this effect may be more dramatic in cases where there is an initial decrease in Ca transients (Choi *et al.*, 2000). Moreover, if SR Ca release in inhibited, this will cause further gain in cellular and SR Ca (as in the case of partial block of the RyR by tetracaine, pg 267). As SR Ca load rises, there is a progressive increase of SR Ca release during the twitch. Thus the increase in SR Ca load (due to the combination of RyR block and elevated [Na]$_i$ & [Ca]$_i$) would gradually increase twitch $\Delta[Ca]_i$ and contraction during acidosis. The result is that there is less fractional release of Ca from the SR at low pH, but this can be more than offset by a larger SR Ca content.

As mentioned above, during acidosis the time constant of twitch $[Ca]_i$ decline is slowed. However, as diastolic $[Ca]_i$ and $\Delta[Ca]_i$ increase during sustained acidosis, Nomura *et al.* (2000) showed that the time constant of $[Ca]_i$ decline recovers significantly. Moreover, they found that this recovery could be prevented by the CaMKII inhibitor KN-93. This is consistent with work by Vittone *et al.* (1998). They showed that in the absence of PKA activation, CaMKII-dependent phospholamban phosphorylation at Thr[17] occurred with elevated Ca transients, but only at acidic pH (possibly due to phosphatase inhibition, pg 167). Thus, accelerated SR Ca-pumping could explain the faster $[Ca]_i$ decline and partially overcome the direct inhibitory effect of acidosis. This CaMKII-dependent acceleration of $[Ca]_i$ decline is reminiscent of the frequency-dependent acceleration of relaxation (FDAR) discussed on pg 270-272. While PLB is not required for FDAR, it is unknown whether PLB is required for this secondary regulation during acidosis.

The increase in $[Na]_i$ via Na/H exchange at low pH_i can be limited if extracellular pH is low, as in ischemia (Bountra & Vaughan-Jones, 1989). If pH_o is suddenly returned to normal while pH_i is still low (as during reperfusion after ischemia), there is a large outwardly directed $[H^+]$ gradient. This is precisely the condition where Na/H exchange can extrude protons rapidly, but with the consequence that $[Na]_i$ rises rapidly (Bountra & Vaughan-Jones, 1989). The high $[Na]_i$ increases cell and SR Ca content via Na/Ca exchange and can be arrhythmogenic. Lazdunski *et al.* (1985) hypothesized that this mechanism is responsible for the large cellular Ca accumulation associated with reperfusion after ischemia, and there is much evidence supporting this view (see *Ischemia* below, and Karmazyn *et al.*, 1999).

In conclusion, the effects of acidosis on cellular Ca and force production are complex, but some important aspects seem clear. Reduced myofilament Ca sensitivity and maximum force are the main factors responsible for the negative inotropic effect of acidosis. Acidosis also depresses RyR sensitivity to Ca, but this is offset (progressively) by an increase in cellular and SR Ca content. This gain in cell Ca is attributable mainly to proton extrusion via Na/H exchange & Na/K-ATPase inhibition, which together elevate $[Na]_i$, and this consequently raises Ca due to shifts in Na/Ca exchange (or simply depressed Ca extrusion via Na/Ca exchange). Decreased myofilament Ca binding may also reduce Ca buffering slightly. The increased cellular and SR Ca load can contribute to the progressively larger Ca transients (but still with reduced force), and can also lead to cellular Ca overload.

Before leaving this subject it is worth briefly reviewing pH buffering and the transporters which are responsible for regulating pH_i (e.g. Leem & Vaughan-Jones, 1998; Leem *et al.*, 1999: Pucéat, 1999). As mentioned on pg 46, cardiac intracellular pH buffering is very high (β=20-90 mM/pH unit). In the absence of CO_2/HCO_3 Leem *et al.* (1999) described intrinsic pH_i buffering with two classes of buffers: B_{max1}=84 mM, pK_{a1} = 6.03 and B_{max2} =29 mM, pK_{a2} = 7.57. Thus intrinsic pH_i buffering power falls biphasically from ~50 at pH 6 to ~20 at pH 7.6. In contrast, buffering by CO_2/HCO_3 increases with increasing pH (from ~11 at pH 6.9 to 48 at pH 7.3), and the overall buffering power is about doubled in the presence of CO_2/HCO_3. So at a normal pH_i of 7.04 in CO_2/HCO_3 buffer (*vs.* 7.07 in Hepes buffer), total cellular buffering power is ~45.

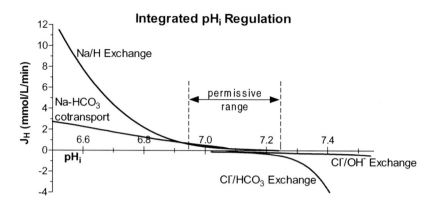

Figure 172. Acid transporters involved in pH_i regulation. Acid efflux (positive) or influx (negative) on each of the four transport systems is indicated for different pH. The range for normal pH_i is indicated as the permissive range. Curves were drawn from equations in Leem *et al.* (1999).

There are also four ion transport mechanisms involved in regulating pH_i. Two are acid extruders, Na/H exchange (which removes H) and Na-HCO$_3$ cotransport (which brings in HCO$_3$). These are activated at low pH_i (Fig 172). The other two bring acid into the cell, Cl$^-$/HCO$_3^-$ exchange (or anion exchanger, which extrudes HCO$_3^-$) and Cl$^-$/OH$^-$ exchange (which extrudes OH$^-$). Figure 172 shows the relative acid flux mediated by each of these systems in a guinea-pig ventricular myocyte (Leem *et al.*, 1999). In the presence of an acid load, the Na/H exchange is more strongly activated than is Na-HCO$_3$ cotransport, and during alkalosis Cl$^-$/HCO$_3^-$ exchange is more strongly activated than Cl$^-$/HCO$_3^-$ exchange. At normal resting pH_i all four systems may produce similar non-zero flux (~0.15 mM/min).

Hypoxia and Ischemia

The effects of hypoxia and ischemia on Ca and force development will only be discussed briefly here (see Downey, 1990; Reimer & Jennings, 1992; Jennings *et al.*, 1995; Goldhaber, 1997; Opie, 1998). In a simplistic sense acidosis can be considered a stepping stone toward understanding pathological changes associated with the more clinically relevant situations of hypoxia and ischemia. Indeed, acidosis is an early consequence of hypoxia (due to shifting of metabolism to glycolysis and lactic acid production) and ischemia (where lactic acid and other metabolites are also not washed away). In this context much of the acidosis discussion above may be extended to hypoxia and ischemia. To simplify, we can consider 4 main attributes of ischemia: 1) acidosis (as above), 2) hypoxia, 3) altered high energy phosphates ([ATP]/[ADP][P$_i$]) and 4) elevated [K]$_o$. While ischemia creates dire conditions by itself, reperfusion after ischemia can suddenly make things even worse. I will briefly discuss a few key issues which are most related to the theme of this book, but cannot review in any comprehensive way here the extensive field of ischemia and reperfusion.

As discussed above, acidosis decreases myofilament Ca sensitivity and maximum force. During ischemia (or hypoxia with inhibition of glycolysis) high energy phosphates are gradually depleted and inorganic phosphate (P$_i$) can increase from ~1 mM to 20 mM (Allen & Orchard,

1987). This high [P_i] by itself depresses the Ca sensitivity of the myofilaments (Herzig & Rüegg, 1977; Kentish, 1986). In combination with intracellular acidosis, myofilament Ca sensitivity can be profoundly depressed. The combination may work synergistically if, as in skeletal muscle, the inhibitory form of P_i is diprotonated (H_2PO_4, Nosek *et al.*, 1987). This form would make up a higher fraction of the total P_i pool at lower pH and could exert a more powerful depressant effect. Thus, the decline in force generation in ischemia, as in acidosis, is probably largely attributable to decreased myofilament activation. Again, as with acidosis, force can be severely depressed while Ca transients remain large (Lee *et al.*, 1988; Allen *et al.*, 1989).

While we typically think of [ATP] when considering energetic limitations, ΔG_{ATP} also depends on [ADP] and [P_i], as $\Delta G_{ATP} = \Delta G^\circ + RT \cdot \ln\{[ADP][P_i]/[ATP]\}$, where $\Delta G^\circ = -30$ kJ/mol. So, even though ATP is well buffered and a decline of [ATP] from 11 to 10 mM would seem inconsequential, this may result in an increase of [ADP] from 50 μM to 350 μM, and a 10-fold change in [ADP][P_i]/[ATP] (for [P_i]=4-5 mM). This reduces the energy available from ATP hydrolysis by 10%. While this may contribute to dysfunction at the myofilament level, it will also affect ion transport. As pointed out on pg 62, the Na/K-ATPase and SR- and sarcolemmal Ca-ATPases all function at relatively high energetic efficiency. However, when the ΔG_{ATP} declines, the maximal [Na] and [Ca] gradients that can be established by these ATPases will be lower. This can be appreciated by inspection of Fig 89 (pg 174). For the above 10% reduction of ΔG_{ATP}, the maximal [Ca]$_{SR}$/[Ca]$_i$ gradient would be reduced by 50%. This would lower both the maximal SR Ca content achievable and also slow the terminal phase of [Ca]$_i$ decline mediated by the SR Ca-pump (which would elevate diastolic [Ca]$_i$, for both thermodynamic and kinetic reasons). This energetic issue can limit cardiac contractile reserve (Tian & Ingwall, 1996; Tian *et al.*, 1997, 1998). The lower [Ca]$_{SR}$ decreases both the Ca available for release and the fraction released during E-C coupling (Fig 119). This ΔG_{ATP} effect on Na/K-ATPase could also contribute to the increase in [Na]$_i$, with its array of consequences discussed above.

As ischemia progresses and creatine phosphate becomes depleted, [ATP] declines more rapidly, [P_i] continues to rise and [ADP] rises more steeply (Fig 173). This can dramatically reduce the energy available from ATP (ΔG_{ATP}) and that can affect all ATP dependent processes, including myofilament ATPase as well as ion transport ATPases. This can depress intrinsic myofilament contractile parameters and reduce the maximal [Ca] gradient across the SR and [Ca], [Na] and [K] gradients across the sarcolemma. In addition, since cytosolic Mg is strongly buffered by ATP, the decline in [ATP] also results in an increase in free [Mg]$_i$ (Murphy *et al.*, 1989b). The higher [Mg]$_i$ (along with the lower pH$_i$) will also affect numerous Ca-dependent systems and ion channels. For example elevated [Mg]$_i$ itself depresses myofilament Ca sensitivity, Ca-ATPases, ryanodine receptor gating and outward current carried by inwardly rectifying K channels (such as I_{K1} and $I_{K(ATP)}$, see chapters 2, 4 & 7). These effects can contribute to both contractile and electrophysiological dysfunction during ischemia.

As high energy phosphates are depleted, [ATP]$_i$ declines and [ADP]$_i$ rises, both of which contribute to the activation of ATP-sensitive K current ($I_{K(ATP)}$, Noma, 1983, see pg 82). $I_{K(ATP)}$ is inhibited by μM ATP (K_i for ATP=20 μM, Nichols & Lederer, 1990) and appears to be preferentially inhibited by ATP produced by glycolysis (Weiss & Lamp, 1987, 1989). The ATP sensitivity of $I_{K(ATP)}$ is shifted by increasing ADP in the context of ischemia (to K_i 100-300 μM, Weiss *et al.*, 1992; Deutsch & Weiss, 1993). So, perhaps appropriately, this channel responds

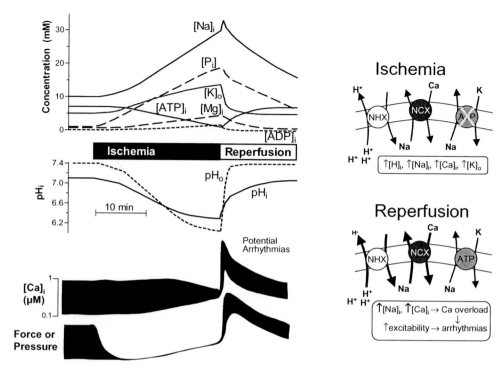

Figure 173. Schematic diagram of some changes which occur during ischemia and reperfusion. Points were extrapolated from a wide variety of sources and are not intended to be an accurate quantitative description for any specific ischemic condition.

more directly to ΔG_{ATP} (i.e. [ATP]/[ADP]) rather than just [ATP]. Moreover, these channels are numerous in heart cells and they have high unitary conductance. This means that activation of less than 1% of maximal $I_{K(ATP)}$ can shorten AP duration by 50%, and this can happen with only a small change in [ATP] (Nichols *et al.*, 1991; Weiss *et al.*, 1992). Put simply, [ATP] declining from 10 to 9 mM would not change $I_{K(ATP)}$, but if ADP shifts the K_i from 20 to 100 μM, that would produce 1% of maximal $I_{K(ATP)}$. There is experimental evidence that $I_{K(ATP)}$ activation shortens AP duration during the early contractile failure and then prevents the AP altogether in rat ventricular myocytes under complete metabolic blockade (Lederer *et al.*, 1989). Thus, $I_{K(ATP)}$ may protect energetically compromised cells by preventing depolarization and Ca transients. This allows the cell to conserve energy, since the myofilaments and Ca pumps should have minimal energy consumption in this state. However, this could create islands of non-excitable cells, and alter the normal conduction pathway in the heart. This might then contribute to setting the stage for reentrant arrhythmias.

During early ischemia and hypoxia there is also a large increase in [42]K efflux which elevates [K]$_o$ during ischemia (to as high as 20 mM), and could be partially prevented by glibenclamide, a selective $I_{K(ATP)}$ blocker (Weiss & Lamp, 1989). While $I_{K(ATP)}$ activation seemed an initially plausible explanation of the K loss in hypoxia and ischemia, the same group demonstrated that this is not the case (Shivkumar *et al.*, 1997). One concern was that K loss via $I_{K(ATP)}$ would be self-limiting. That is, increasing K conductance drives E_m toward E_K, and that would limit the driving force for K efflux ($E_m - E_K$). Moreover, when they activated $I_{K(ATP)}$ with cromakalim, they found AP duration shortening comparable to that in hypoxia, but there was no significant [42]K loss.   They found that if they prevented the Na gain in hypoxia, they could also prevent the K loss. They concluded that the K loss is largely a passive consequence of Na gain. Thus, Na gain is centrally involved in pH regulation, Ca gain and also elevated $[K]_o$ in ischemia.

During severe hypoxia (associated with ischemia) there is a large rise in $[Na]_i$ which can reach 40 mM in prolonged anoxia.   An elegant study by Eigel & Hadley (1999) evaluated the cellular basis of the Na gain.   While the two main pathways for normal Na influx are I_{Na} and inward $I_{Na/Ca}$ (~10 and 30 µmol/L cytosol/beat respectively), the main mechanisms of net Na gain during anoxia are via TTX sensitive Na channels and HOE-642-sensitive Na/H exchange. TTX and HOE-642 each blocked ~50% of the Na gain during simple anoxia. For anoxia with acidosis the Na gain was blocked by TTX, but not by HOE-642.   However, when anoxia was coupled with high $[K]_o$ (10 mM) or high $[K]_o$ plus acidosis (pH_o 6.85 to simulate ischemia), the Na gain was suppressed almost completely by HOE-642, but not appreciably altered by TTX. This may be most relevant to ischemia and accounts for the dramatic protective effect of Na/H exchange blockers in ischemia and reperfusion (below). It is not clear why TTX-sensitive Na influx would occur in the two cases with normal $[K]_o$ (while cells are quiescent), but anoxia and ischemic metabolites have been shown to produce persistent Na channel opening in ventricular myocytes (Ju *et al.*, 1996; Undrovinas *et al.*, 1992).   Since 10 mM $[K]_o$ prevented the TTX-sensitive Na gain, it is possible that anoxia allows a tiny window I_{Na} at resting E_m, but inactivation prevails upon depolarization in high $[K]_o$. Thus, during ischemia, the large rise in $[Na]_i$ may be mediated mainly by Na/H exchange, but TTX sensitive Na entry may also occur (Xiao & Allen, 1999).

Reperfusion-Acute effects.   Ischemia or metabolic blockade produces acidosis and progressive gain in cellular Na and Ca (Fig 173, as discussed above for acidosis, but now with additional energetic limitations and extracellular effects).   In ischemia, the increase in $[Na]_i$ via Na/H exchange is limited by low pH_o (Bountra & Vaughan-Jones, 1989).   Indeed, Yan & Kléber (1992) showed that pH_o declines more than pH_i during ischemia (presumably because the cell is struggling to maintain normal pH_i). Upon reperfusion, pH_o is quickly restored, creating a large outward $[H^+]$ gradient. This causes rapid Na gain via Na/H exchange, which in turn induces rapid Ca gain via Na/Ca exchange (which becomes more active as pH_i recovers). Indeed, this large bolus of Ca entry upon reperfusion can produce Ca overload, and with the variable recovery of excitability and the electrophysiological substrate, there is an enhanced propensity for arrhythmias. This mechanistic scenario (Fig 173) now has overwhelming experimental support (reviewed by Karmazyn *et al.*, 1999). Moreover, Na/H exchange inhibitors, including amiloride, ethylisopropylamiloride (EIPA), HOE-642 (cariporide), HOE-694 and EMD-85131, all prevent (or limit) hypercontracture and arrhythmias associated with reperfusion after ischemia (Karmazyn, 1988, Murphy *et al.*, 1991; Scholz *et al.*, 1993, 1995; Hendrikx *et al.*, 1994; Yasutake *et al.*, 1994; Xue *et al.*, 1996; Gumina *et al.*, 1998; Karmazyn *et al.*, 1999; Strömer *et al.*, 2000). Inhibition of Ca entry via Na/Ca exchange (KB-R7943) also limited post-ischemic arrhythmias and improved mechanical recovery (Mukai *et al.*, 2000).

It is worth considering the quantity of protons that are extruded upon reperfusion. If pH_i must recover ~0.5 pH units, this would require extrusion of ~23 mmol protons/L cytosol from the cell (based on pH buffering, pg 304) and for a 1:1 Na/H exchange this would require 23 mM Na influx. If all of this were to exchange for extracellular Ca via Na/Ca exchange, the total Ca gain would be 7-8 mM! Clearly this is an extreme upper limit, because the Na/K-ATPase will be expected to deal with most of Na extrusion, but this takes time. Even if the Na/Ca exchange brings in only 5% of this Ca (350 μmol/L cytosol) is a large Ca bolus for the cell to deal with. This is especially the case while [Na]$_i$ is high, which limits the ability of the Na/Ca exchanger to extrude Ca. Moreover, this explains the large, potentially lethal rise in [Ca]$_i$ during reperfusion.

Another major problem which occurs upon reperfusion (or reoxygenation after hypoxia) is a burst of free oxygen radical generation (Goldhaber, 1997). This is partly because of a decrease in free radical scavengers (e.g. glutathione peroxidase and superoxide dismutase, SOD), but it is also due to infiltration of activated neutrophils which produce superoxide, hydrogen peroxide and hypochlorous anion (Ferrari *et al.*, 1985; Shlafer *et al.*, 1987; McCord, 1974; Rowe *et al.*1984). These neutrophils can also produce cytokines (e.g. interleukins and TNF-α) that can further stimulate nitric oxide and free radical production, and may also exert direct effects on myocytes. Several studies have shown that post-ischemic recovery can be improved when free radical production and/or neutrophil effects are inhibited (Werns *et al.*, 1985, Ambrosio *et al.*, 1986; Hearse & Tosaki, 1987; Puett *et al.*, 1987; Mak & Weglicki, 1988; Przyklenk & Kloner, 1989; Lefer *et al.*, 1990; Flaherty *et al.*, 1994).

While details of how free radicals and cytokines worsen recovery are complex and not entirely understood, cellular Ca mismanagement appears to be a common endpoint. For example, oxygen free radical production can cause myocyte Ca overload, transient inward currents (I$_{ti}$) and triggered action potentials (Barrington *et al.*1988; Matsuura & Shattock, 1991; Josephson *et al.*, 1991). Indeed, many Ca transporters appear to be affected by free radicals, including the SR Ca-ATPase (Hess *et al.*, 1983,1984b; Goldhaber & Liu, 1994), RyR (Boraso & Williams, 1994), Na/Ca exchanger (Reeves *et al.*, 1986; Coetzee *et al.*, 1994; Goldhaber, 1996), mitochondria (Harris *et al.*, 1982) and sarcolemmal Ca-ATPase (Kaneko *et al.*, 1989). Na/K-ATPase is also inhibited by free radicals (Kim & Akera, 1987; Shattock & Matsuura, 1993), which would contribute to Na gain. Since Ca leak and Na window current may also be increased by free radicals (Wang *et al.*, 1995b; Bhatnagar *et al.*, 1990), cellular Na and Ca gain may mediate Ca overload as discussed earlier. Moreover, the activation of Na/Ca exchange by free radicals may worsen the Ca overload in response to increased [Na]$_i$ (especially during reperfusion, see Fig 173). Thus, it appears that this free radical pathway may exacerbate the Na/H exchange-Na/Ca exchange problem with respect to reperfusion after ischemia.

Hibernation.   Hibernating myocardium is a term used to describe temporary depressed contractile function upon reduction of regional blood flow (Feigl, 1983; Braunwald & Ruterford, 1986; Marbán, 1991). This decrease is completely and reversible upon resumption of perfusion pressure and occurs without change in pH$_i$, [P$_i$] or high energy phosphates. It had been supposed that this might be due to the "garden hose effect" where local vascular stretch increased sarcomere length and increased contractility via Starling's law (Fig 19). However, Kitakaze & Marbán (1989) showed that higher perfusion pressure increased contraction, even though end-diastolic length was already optimal. Moreover, they found reversible changes in Ca transients that may explain the altered contraction with altered coronary perfusion. Heusch (1998) noted that reduction of ΔG_{ATP} or Ca responsiveness might also be involved, but the mechanism remains unclear. While such hypoperfusion and function can be chronic, key features of hibernation are that there is no necrosis and function is promptly restored when flow is restored. Of course, during prolonged hypoperfusion secondary changes can occur which complicates things further.

Stunning. Myocardial stunning is quite distinct from hibernation (Braunwald & Kloner, 1982; Bolli, 1990; Marbán, 1991; Bolli & Marbán, 1999). Stunning is post-ischemic contractile dysfunction which persists for hours or days after restoration of perfusion, but is not associated with either reduced coronary flow or irreversible damage (i.e. no necrosis). Bolli & Marbán (1999) consider that there are two plausible contributing pathways to myocardial stunning and they are not mutually exclusive: 1) oxygen free radicals and 2) Ca-overload/myofilament dysfunction. Indeed, the contractile dysfunction can persist when energetic status is completely restored and even with normal action potentials and Ca transients (Hanich *et al.*, 1993; Gao *et al.*, 1995). It is now clear that myofilament maximal force and/or Ca sensitivity are reduced in the stunned heart (Westfall & Solaro, 1992; Hoffman *et al.*, 1993; McDonald *et al.*, 1995b; Gao *et al.*, 1995). Troponin I (TnI) appears to be selectively degraded in stunned heart, although α-actinin and other myofilament proteins may also degraded after longer ischemic episodes (Westfall & Solaro, 1992; Gao *et al.*, 1995, 1997d; Van Eyk *et al.*, 1998). These studies also showed that reperfusion is required for both TnI degradation and for the myofilament dysfunction (Miller *et al.*, 1996). Replacing endogenous troponin with troponin from stunned hearts also reduces myofilament Ca sensitivity (McDonald *et al.*, 1998). Murphy *et al.* (2000) created transgenic mice overexpressing a truncated TnI (1-193, which matches the major degradation product in stunned hearts). This truncated TnI replaced 9-17% of the endogenous TnI and caused a similar decrease in contractile function and myofilament responsiveness to Ca, without altered cellular Ca transients. Moreover, these transgenic hearts were hypocontractile and developed ventricular dilatation. Thus TnI degradation during reperfusion is likely to be a major factor in contractile dysfunction in myocardial stunning. The slow functional recovery (hours-days) may reflect the time required to synthesize replacement TnI.

So how does reperfusion cause TnI degradation? The leading theory is that Ca-activated proteases (calpains) activated by high $[Ca]_i$ during reperfusion are responsible (Bolli & Marbán, 1999). I have already discussed the basis of Ca overload upon reperfusion, and calpain I (present in the ventricle) is activated by [Ca] in the 1-20 μM range in vitro (Suzuki, 1990) and by ischemia/reperfusion (Yoshida *et al.*, 1995). TnI has also been shown to be a substrate for Calpain I (DeLisa *et al.* 1995). This also brings us back to the role of oxygen free radicals in the genesis of stunning. As described above, the production of these free radicals upon reperfusion can exacerbate Na and Ca overload and this can add to the likelihood of both TnI degradation as well as other potentially reversible dysfunction. Thus, while stunning is complex and there will surely be additional explanations identified for its many etiologies, some first steps in molecular understanding are becoming clearer.

Preconditioning.   Ischemic preconditioning is an intriguing aspect of the ischemic response. Preconditioning refers to the result that brief periods (e.g. 5-10 min) of ischemia, which do not create any dysfunction after reperfusion *per se,* can protect the heart from damage during a subsequent prolonged ischemic episode (Murry *et al.*, 1986; Bolli, 2000; Cohen *et al.*, 2000). There is an initial acute phase of preconditioning (<3 hr after the initial ischemic episode) and also a delayed or late phase (developing over 24 hr) sometimes called the second window of protection (see reviews by Okubo *et al.*, 1999; Bolli, 2000; O'Rourke, 2000). Several factors may contribute to ischemic preconditioning, including adenosine, nitric oxide, protein kinase C, $I_{K(ATP)}$ and heat shock proteins.

Adenosine is produced during ischemia and administration of adenosine receptor agonists can simulate preconditioning, while blocking adenosine (A_1) receptors can inhibit preconditioning (Van Wylen *et al.*, 1990; Baxter *et al.*, 1994). Some other G-protein coupled receptors such as bradykinin and endothelin can also activate this pathway. Blocking nitric oxide synthase (eNOS) can inhibit the protective effects of brief ischemic episodes, while exogenous nitric oxide can reproduce the effects of preconditioning (Bolli *et al.*, 1997; Takano *et al.*, 1998; Banerjee *et al.*, 1999). The effect of nitric oxide is not blocked by guanylyl cyclase inhibitors (suggesting that cGMP and PKG are not involved; Kodani *et al.*, 2000), but is blocked by antioxidants (suggesting peroxynitrite or hydroxyl free radical involvement, Takano *et al.*, 1998). Protein kinase C isoforms PKCε and PKCη are activated by ischemia, but only PKCε activation is required to simulate preconditioning (Qiu *et al.*, 1998; Ping *et al.*, 1999a). The PKCε activation can be blocked by blocking nitric oxide production, linking these pathways (Ping *et al.*, 1999b). Moreover, transgenic mice expressing a constitutively active PKCε recapitulate the preconditioning phenotype (Ping *et al.*, 2000). PKCε may also work through a downstream activation of the mitogen activated protein kinase (MAPK) known as ERK1/ERK2 or p38 (Ping *et al.*, 1999c; Nakano *et al.*, 2000).

$I_{K(ATP)}$ has also been implicated in ischemic preconditioning (O'Rourke, 2000; Grover & Garlid, 2000). The sarcolemmal K_{ATP} channel may contribute to action potential shortening and abortion during ischemia, and was thought to play a role in preconditioning. $I_{K(ATP)}$ activators (pinacidil & cromakalim) could simulate preconditioning, while $I_{K(ATP)}$ blockers (glibenclamide) inhibited the protective effect (Grover *et al.*, 1989, 1990). However, it became clear that there were discrepancies between effects on sarcolemmal $I_{K(ATP)}$ or AP duration and protective effects of these K-channel openers (Yao & Gross, 1994; Grover *et al.*, 1995a,b). There was early evidence of a novel K_{ATP} channel on the inner mitochondrial membrane (mito-K_{ATP}, Inoue *et al.*, 1991), but characterization of mito-$I_{K(ATP)}$ has developed slowly, because it is not as amenable to patch clamp studies as are sarcolemmal channels (see reviews by O'Rourke, 2000 and Grover & Garlid, 2000). Garlid *et al.* (1997) showed that diazoxide opened mito-$I_{K(ATP)}$ with a K_m of ~0.5 µM, (*vs.* 840 µM for sarcolemmal $I_{K(ATP)}$) and that 5-hydroxydecanoate (5-HD) could selectively block mito-$I_{K(ATP)}$ (K_i ~50 µM). They went on to show that selective activation of mito-$I_{K(ATP)}$ protected hearts from ischemic contracture and that this could be blocked by a mito-$I_{K(ATP)}$-selective concentration of 5-HD. Note that pinacidil & cromakalim activate both sarcolemmal and mitochondrial $I_{K(ATP)}$ and glibenclamide is also a non-selective blocker. Another group (Liu *et al.*, 1998; Sato *et al.*, 2000a) found parallel results with different methods, and both groups concluded that the protective effect of $I_{K(ATP)}$ activation was attributable to mitochondrial, rather than sarcolemmal K_{ATP} channels. Sato *et al.* (1998a, 2000b) and Takashi *et al.* (1999) have gone on to show that both adenosine and PKC activation are upstream modulators of mito-$I_{K(ATP)}$ activation, and Sasaki *et al.* (2000) showed that nitric oxide facilitates activation by diazoxide. This connects the mito-$I_{K(ATP)}$ pathway to the aforementioned roles of adenosine, NO and PKC in ischemic preconditioning. What is less clear at this stage is why opening mito-K_{ATP} channels elicits protection. Indeed, opening a K channel may be expected to dissipate the mitochondrial membrane potential (E_{mito}) and proton gradient. This would waste the energy required to rebuild the mitochondrial [H] gradient and E_{mito}. Three possible mechanistic hypotheses discussed by O'Rourke (2000) are that mito-$I_{K(ATP)}$ activation: 1) causes mitochondrial swelling and a consequent higher rate of energy production (Halestrap, 1989). 2) lowers E_{mito} which might limit mitochondrial Ca overload (Holmuhamedov *et al.*, 1999). 3) alters mitochondrial production of oxygen free radicals, somehow conferring protection. At this point it is too early to speculate as to which pathway (if any of these) is important in the mito-$I_{K(ATP)}$ induced cardioprotection.

Finally, there is evidence that heat shock proteins (HSP) may be involved in ischemic preconditioning (Benjamin & McMillan, 1998). These stress-activated proteins are molecular chaperones, and they can facilitate protein folding and translocation. HSPs can confer cross-tolerance to different stressors, and their function may be to aid refolding of proteins damaged by these noxious stimuli (e.g. hyperthermia or ischemia). HSP-70 is rapidly induced during ischemia (Knowlton *et al.*, 1991), and HSP-70, HSP-27 and HSP-22 (αB-crystallin) all exhibit cardioprotective effects (Marber *et al.*, 1995; Mestril *et al.*, 1996; Martin *et al.*, 1997). How these HSP effects interdigitate with the other mechanisms above is not clear at present. Thus, there may be several factors involved in ischemic preconditioning and additional work will be required to clarify which mechanisms are most dominant. However, it would not be surprising to find that these systems constitute an array of partially redundant protective mechanisms.

Ischemic preconditioning and Na/H exchange inhibition are generally similar with respect to cardioprotection during ischemia and reperfusion (Shipolini *et al.*, 1997; Gumina *et al.*,1999; Avkiran, 1999; Xiao & Allen, 1999; Mosca & Cingolani, 2000). However, with longer ischemia (>60 min) Na/H exchange inhibition may be even more protective (Gumina *et al.*, 1999). Na/H exchange inhibition and preconditioning are also additive and provide greater protection when combined. It is controversial whether preconditioning works partly by inhibiting Na/H exchange (Shipolini *et al.*, 1997; Xiao & Allen, 1999). In conclusion, ischemia and reperfusion are very complex. While much work is needed to clarify the basis of post-ischemic dysfunction and how it might be improved, clearly multiple mechanisms are involved.

Hypertrophy

Ventricular hypertrophy occurs in response to numerous physiological and patho-physiological stimuli. In all cases the increase in ventricular mass is paralleled by myocyte hypertrophy (i.e. most investigators agree that myocyte hyperplasia does not occur; Soonpaa & Field, 1998, but see Anversa & Kajstura, 1998). The classic physiological hypertrophy example is where endurance training causes a "healthy" hypertrophy with increased cardiac function and stroke volume (and lower resting heart rate). Pathophysiological stimuli include hemodynamic load (pressure or volume) and neurohumoral stimuli (e.g. renin-angiotensin II, endothelin, adrenergic). In general then, hypertrophy can be viewed initially as an adaptive process, to help the heart deal with an increase in work load. To the extent that the hypertrophy allows the heart to meet the needs of the body, this can be considered compensatory hypertrophy. At some point, the hypertrophic response may be inadequate, and further changes can become decompensatory and contribute to the genesis of heart failure (HF). Thus the transition or progression from hypertrophy to HF is functionally quite important, but is not unidirectional (Lorell, 1997; Katz, 2000). Ventricular hypertrophy can be either concentric or eccentric. Concentric hypertrophy, where the walls & myocytes thicken, but the chamber does not dilate, is especially common with pressure overload (i.e. when the heart cannot generate sufficient pressure to adequately overcome elevated afterload). Eccentric hypertrophy, where the chamber becomes dilated and myocytes become elongated, is most common in volume overload (e.g. valvular insufficiencies).

The heart and myocytes seem somehow tuned to produce optimal function, a variety of factors can disturb this balance. In addition to hemodynamic load and neurohumoral factors, hypertrophy is induced by many transgenic or gene knockouts that may unbalance the tuning of excitation and contraction processes in the heart, or in more overt ways undermine cardiac function. An example is familial hypertrophic cardiomyopathy (FHC) caused by congenital defects in myofilament proteins (Seidman & Seidman, 1998).   This somewhat generalized response has led some investigators to suggest a relatively stereotypical pathway to hypertrophy. In addition, some gene expression changes commonly observed in hypertrophy seem to recapitulate a neonatal or fetal phenotype (e.g. switches from α-MHC to β-MHC reexpression of skeletal α-actin, reduced SERCA2 and increased Na/Ca exchange). These 2 points support the idea that hypertrophy is a programmed reversion toward a more fetal phenotype. While there is surely truth in this, it is increasingly clear that multiple and complexly interacting pathways and phenotypes are involved in the etiology of hypertrophy (see Fig 174). Moreover, the pathways which cause changes in gene expression (Fig 174) are not yet well connected to the resulting molecular and functional phenotypes, especially with respect to contractile proteins, Ca transporters, ion channels and modulators (e.g. kinases & phosphatases).

The signaling pathways in hypertrophic remodeling are very complex (for references see reviews by Sadoshima & Izumo, 1997; Hefti *et al.*, 1997; Sugden, 1999; Molkentin & Dorn, 2001).   The most detailed analysis of the central molecular signaling cascades has been from work in primary cultures of neonatal rat ventricular myocytes (NRVM).   One important set of pathways are the mitogen-activated protein kinase (MAPK) pathways, illustrated in Fig 174 (Sugden & Clerk, 1998, 2000; Sugden, 1999). There are three main MAPKs (Ser-Thr kinases): 1) ERK1 and ERK2 (extracellular regulated protein kinase, also known as p44-MAPK and p42-MAPK), 2) JNKs (the c-*Jun* N-terminal kinases) and 3) the p38-MAPK. The MAPKs are focal points of this complex cascade and they phosphorylation numerous substrates, including nuclear transcription factors (which activate expression of different groups of genes, Fig 174). Some of the early response genes used as indicators of hypertrophic gene expression are c-*Jun*, c-*Fos*, c-*Myc*, *Egr-1*, ANP (atrial natriuretic peptide) and BNP (brain natriuretic peptide).

The MAPK cascades are activated by several G_q-protein coupled receptors, such as the α_1-AR, endothelin (ET$_A$), and angiotensin II receptor (AT$_1$). Indeed, ET-1 and to a less complete degree phenylephrine and angiotensin II have been shown to activate all 3 MAPKs and be a potent stimulator of cellular hypertrophy (see Sugden, 1999 for references). The receptors above all activate a G_q to release its $\beta\gamma$ subunit, activating phospholipase C to produce diacylglycerol (DAG) and IP$_3$. DAG activates PKC, and PKCδ and PKCϵ seem to be the key isoforms in hypertrophic signaling. PKC and several other signals can activate Ras a small G-protein (21 kDa) and other related members of this group (Rac, Rho). These other Ras-activating pathways include receptor tyrosine kinases activated by growth factors (e.g. fibroblast growth factor {FGF}, insulin-like growth factor-1 {IGF-1} and platelet-derived growth factor {PDGF}) and mechanical stretch (via activation of the focal adhesion kinase FAK, and also via an autocrine/ paracrine release of ET-1 or angiotensin-II). Ras activates Raf and some other upstream kinases which are collectively referred to as MKKKs (MAPK kinase kinases) because they phosphorylate MKKs (MAPK kinases) which in turn phosphorylate the MAPKs themselves. While some key elements and interactions in this cascade are well worked out, there are constantly new players and interactions being uncovered in this very active field. These pathways studied in NRVM undoubtedly contribute to hypertrophic signaling in the intact animal and man, but this obviously adds additional layers of complexity.

Stretch is an important physiological hypertrophic stimulus that may work independently or in concert with neurohumoral factors above. Mechanical stretch of isolated myocytes can rapidly activate all three MAPK cascade at multiple sites from phospholipase C to ERK1/2, JNKs and c-*fos* (Komuro *et al.*, 1991; Sadoshima & Izumo, 1993, 1997). Candidates for the mechanosensor have included stretch-activated ion channels (e.g. letting Ca in), integrins (via activation of FAK, a tyrosine kinase) and other tyrosine kinases. Blocking some stretch-activated channels by Gadolinium or some integrin signaling by an RGD peptide does not block stretch-induced c-*fos* expression, while tyrosine kinase blockade can (Sadoshima *et al.*, 1992, 1993). However, this does not rule out other stretch-activated channels or integrin signaling. Indeed, FAK and mechanical stretch appear to be important in ET-1 induced hypertrophy (Eble *et al.*, 2000). Thus, all three of these pathways might contribute to hypertrophic signaling.

Mechanical stretch can also cause autocrine/paracrine release of angiotensin II and ET-1 (Sadoshima *et al.*, 1993; Lin *et al.*, 1995; Yamazaki *et al.*, 1996; Cingolani *et al.*, 1998). In this case stretch can induce release of angiotensin II and/or ET-1 from ventricular myocytes as well as nonmyocyte cells. Thus, angiotensin II (and ET-1) may work both globally (e.g. in reno-vascular hypertrophy) and locally via this autocrine/paracrine pathway. Indeed, angiotensin converting enzyme (ACE) inhibitors and AT_1 receptor blockers can prevent or revert ventricular hypertrophy induced by pressure overload (Baker *et al.*, 1990, 1992; Kojima *et al.*, 1994). The mechanisms by which stretch causes angiotensin II or ET-1 secretion is still unknown.

Elevation of cellular Ca has been implicated in cardiac hypertrophic signaling, and Ramirez *et al.* (1997) showed that activation of cardiac nuclear CaMKII-δ_B was important in hypertrophic gene expression. The next year it became clear that calcineurin (a Ca-calmodulin activated phosphatase, phosphatase 2b) may also be involved in cardiac hypertrophy (Molkentin *et al.*, 1998; Sussman *et al.*, 1998; Olson & Molkentin, 1998; reviewed by Molkentin, 2000). Calcineurin binds to the nuclear transcription factor NF-AT3, which is basally phosphorylated and cytoplasmic. When calcineurin is activated by Ca-CaM it dephosphorylates NF-AT3, which is then translocated to the nucleus where it promotes gene expression. Transgenic over-expression of calcineurin or NF-AT3 in mice caused hypertrophy and HF. Furthermore, inhibitors of calcineurin (cyclosporin and FK-506) could ameliorate the hypertrophy induced by overexpression of either calcineurin or 3 different sarcomeric protein mutants, or by pressure overload (but not that due to overexpression of the retinoic acid receptor). Molkentin & Dorn (2001) reviewed 7 other studies in different hypertrophic models which confirmed this effect, but also 4 studies that did not find significant prevention of hypertrophy with calcineurin blockers. More recently cardiac myocyte-targeted expression of 3 different calcineurin inhibitory proteins was shown to attenuate hypertrophy in vivo (DeWindt *et al.*, 2001; Rothermel *et al.*, 2001). The latter study showed that the myocyte-enriched calcineurin interacting protein (MCIP1) resulted in a 5-10% smaller heart and inhibited exercise-induced hypertrophy as well. This means that it

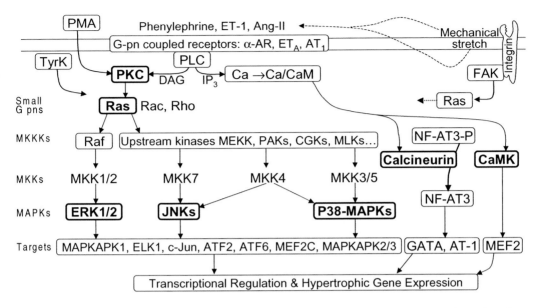

Figure 174. Hypertrophic signaling cascades. G_q-protein (G-pn) coupled receptors bind agonists above, activating phospholipase C to produce diacylglycerides (DAG) that activate PKC, which can also be activated by membrane permeant phorbol esters like PMA. Mechanical stretch induced activation of focal adhesion kinase (FAK) and receptor- and nonreceptor tyorine kinases (TyrK) along with PKC can activate the small G-protein Ras or its relatives (Rac, Rho). This stimulates the three MAPK cascades (see text and Sugden, 1999, Molkentin & Dorn, 2001 for abbreviations). Two Ca/calmodulin (CaM) activated pathways are also indicated. These work via calcineurin which dephosphorylates a nuclear factor of activated T cells (NF-AT3), and via Ca-Calmodulin dependent protein kinase (CaMK). All of these pathways converge on various targets which are mostly nuclear transcription factors that alter gene expression. Diagram is based on related ones by Sugden (1999), Passier *et al.* (2000) and Molkentin & Dorn (2001).

may be hard, at this point in the pathway, to selectively inhibit pathophysiological *vs.* physiological hypertrophy. Thus, while Ca/CaM and calcineurin may not be a unique pathway to hypertrophy, it seems clear that it is an important one.

An interesting side point in the calcineurin story (from the E-C coupling standpoint) is that the FK-506 receptor which blocks calcineurin activation is the same FKBP (12 & 12.6) that binds to the ryanodine receptor and is thought to modulate E-C coupling (see pg 198-200). That is, the inhibition of calcineurin occurs when the FK-506-FKBP (or cyclosporin-cyclophilin) complex binds to calcineurin and prevents its activation by Ca-CaM.

Passier *et al.* (2000) showed that CaMK can activate a Ca-dependent hypertrophic pathway that is parallel to, and additive with, the calcineurin pathway in producing hypertrophy. Zhu *et al.* (2000) also showed that CaMKII activation may be critical in the hypertrophy induced by endothelin-1. Thus Ca-dependent signaling may play a prominent role in hypertrophy. An unanswered question is how these signaling systems can decipher the relevant Ca signal from the dynamically complex and modulated Ca transients associated with E-C coupling. Presumably this is via either some sort of integration of Ca signals or localized signaling (see pg 243 & 284).

PKC activation is directly involved in the MAPK cascade, but it can additionally activate Na/H exchange either directly (Wallert & Frölich, 1992) or via downstream ERK activation

(Snabaitis *et al.*, 2000). This Na/H exchange activation causes proton extrusion and intracellular alkalosis which can alter $[Na]_i$ and $[Ca]_i$ (see pg 284-285). However, alkalosis can be a hypertrophic stimulus itself. One possible explanation is that high pH_i may increase Ca binding to calmodulin just as it does for troponin C (a related Ca-binding protein) where high pH increases myofilament Ca sensitivity. This increased Ca affinity of CaM may enhance signaling through the Ca-CaM, CaMKII and calcineurin pathways.

An unusual Ca link to this story is that enhancing Ca transients and SR Ca-ATPase by SERCA2a gene transfer or phospholamban gene ablation can inhibit hypertrophy and HF due to aortic banding or hypertrophy/HF where the cause is an apparently unrelated structural gene (Miyamoto *et al.*, 2000; Minamisawa *et al.*, 1999). This emphasizes that while there are many pathways which lead to hypertrophy and HF, cellular Ca regulation and its ability to regulate contractility play a central and interactive role in determining the ultimate cardiac phenotype.

So what are the results of these hypertrophic changes in gene regulation on Ca transport proteins, Ca transients, contractions and APs? The extensive literature is really quite variable, and phenotype may depend on the stage of hypertrophy and progression to HF. Thus, while there are reports that may, in majority, suggest that SR Ca-ATPase is downregulated and Na/Ca exchange is upregulated in hypertrophy (Arai *et al.*, 1993; Kent *et al.*, 1993; Hasenfuss, 1998b), there is tremendous variation in the effects of hypertrophy on cellular Ca transients, ionic currents and contractions (increased, decreased & unaltered). This may reflect real biological differences in relative states of compensation-decompensation during hypertrophy, but it makes summarizing results complicated. Thus, I will reserve this type of discussion to the following section on HF (where there is somewhat broader, if still incomplete agreement).

Heart Failure (HF)

HF is an increasing health problem, affecting >2 million people in the U.S. alone. In the simplest terms HF means that the heart is unable to provide sufficient cardiac output to supply the metabolic demands of the organism. Thus the bottom line is that contractile function of the heart is depressed. The diagnosis of HF carries a very high 5-yr mortality rate (~50%), and there are two fatal pathways: 1) progressive decline in contractile function (pump failure) and 2) sudden cardiac death due to arrhythmias. While a certain component of mechanical dysfunction may be due to geometric factors, with respect to the law of LaPlace (Tension =Pressure × radius / (2 × wall thickness)), it is clear that intrinsic defects in contraction occur at the myocyte and trabecular level. For arrhythmias, there are also important tissue factors (e.g. pg 99-100) involved in propagation of arrhythmias, and the initiation of some. However, many arrhythmias also have their basis at the cellular level and may be related to both Ca handling and cellular ionic currents. Therefore, this section will focus on the cellular basis of contractile dysfunction and arrhythmogenesis.

So what is the basis of the contractile dysfunction? As for hypertrophy, there are a plethora of different HF model studies and some disagree about whether particular factors (e.g. I_{Ca}, SR Ca-ATPase, Na/Ca exchange, myofilament Ca sensitivity) are increased, decreased or unchanged (see reviews by Hasenfuss, 1998b; Richard *et al.*, 1998; Mukherjee & Spinale, 1998; Wickenden *et al.*, 1998; Näbauer & Kääb, 1998; Phillips *et al.*, 1998, de Tombe, 1998; Houser *et al.*, 2000). I will not try to review the entire area here, but Table 26 provides a summary of some results in human HF. I have tried to indicate the most usual findings, which are also largely consistent with animal HF models. Choosing one working phenotypic hypothesis is hazardous in that it unfairly discounts some discordant findings that are genuine, but it makes it much easier to integrate. The integration below will reflect my working hypothesis and some balance as well.

Twitch contraction, Ca transients and APD. Almost by definition, reduced twitch force and cell contraction in HF are expected, and this is seen in almost all HF models. However, at very low heart rates HF may have little effect on force (Pieske *et al.*, 1995). In general, there is a less positive (or even negative) force-frequency relationship in failing *vs.* nonfailing heart (see Fig 148B). Thus, the lower force in HF becomes increasingly apparent at physiological heart rates. These force changes are usually paralleled by changes in Ca transient amplitudes. In addition, there is a slowing of the rate of relaxation and $[Ca]_i$ decline in HF in most cases. This is related to changes in Ca transport discussed below. Another ubiquitous finding in HF is a prolongation of AP duration (Beuckelmann *et al.*, 1992, 1993; Kääb *et al.*, 1996, Näbauer & Kääb, 1998). This is particularly prominent at very low heart rates, but as frequency increases the AP duration shortens and there is a smaller difference between failing and nonfailing hearts (Vermeulen *et al.*, 1994; Pieske *et al.*, 1995).

Myofilament Ca sensitivity. Most studies have found unaltered myofilament Ca sensitivity in HF (Gwathmey & Hajjar, 1990; Perrault *et al.*, 1990; D'Agnolo *et al.*, 1992; Wolff *et al.*, 1995b, 1996; Hajjar *et al.*, 2000), although the Wolff papers found increased myofilament Ca sensitivity until they corrected for the lower phosphorylation state of the HF myofilaments. In two rat HF studies there was a reduction in maximal force and Ca sensitivity (Fan *et al.*, 1997; Pérez *et al.*, 1999). It should be noted that rats (and mice) shift from fast to slow myosin heavy chain (α to β-MHC) during hypertrophy and HF, whereas larger adult mammals (rabbit, dog and human) are predominantly β-MHC to begin with and don't change much. Even Miyata *et al.* (2000), whose data challenged the prevailing dogma that human ventricle is all β-MHC, found α-MHC to drop from only 7% to 0% of total MHC in human HF. There are also reports of changes in other myofilament proteins that could alter force development (TnT, TnI and myosin light chains, see deTombe, 1998 for review). However, there are clearly decreases in contraction in HF which are more likely to be ascribable to altered Ca transients. Indeed, many HF studies that have measured both contraction and $[Ca]_i$ have found roughly proportional decreases in both, consistent with unaltered myofilament Ca sensitivity in HF. Thus, while myofilament changes may occur in HF, it is probably not the most central factor in explaining reduced function.

Ca current. Many reports show no change in peak I_{Ca} density in HF, but decreases have also been reported (see Table 26 & Mukherjee & Spinale, 1998). There was no HF-associated change in I_{Ca} at any voltage in human (Beuckelmann & Erdmann *et al.*, 1992), rat (Gómez *et al.*, 1997), canine (Kääb *et al.*, 1996; O'Rourke *et al.*, 1999), rabbit (Pogwizd *et al.*, 1999) or guinea-pig ventricular myocytes (Ahmmed *et al.*, 2000), despite strong depression of both contractions and Ca transients. This demonstrates that reduced Ca transients occur in many HF models with unchanged I_{Ca}. Thus, while I_{Ca} may be reduced in some HF models, I conclude that I_{Ca} is not primarily responsible for the reduced Ca transient in HF. Indeed, it is remarkable that with nearly doubling of cell size, in HF the density of I_{Ca} (in A/F) can keep pace exactly with this cellular hypertrophy (Pogwizd *et al.*, 1999).

SR Ca-ATPase & phospholamban (PLB).   A tremendous number of studies have measured cardiac SR Ca-ATPase expression and function, since de la Bastie *et al.* (1990) first reported down-regulation of SERCA2 expression in pressure-overloaded rat heart. Feldman *et al.* (1993) showed data suggesting that down-regulation of SERCA2a expression may mark the transition from hypertrophy to HF. It seems clear that SR Ca-ATPase is functionally decreased in almost all HF models (despite a few reports to the contrary; Table 26). PLB also appears to be down-regulated in HF, roughly in proportion to SERCA2. This should not alter the [Ca]$_i$-dependence of SR Ca transport, but of course would decrease Ca transport at all [Ca]$_i$. There are also data to suggest that the phosphorylation state of PLB may be reduced in HF (Huang *et al.*, 1999; Schwinger *et al.*, 1999c, but see Currie & Smith, 1999). This would reduce the [Ca]-sensitivity of SR Ca uptake and further slow Ca transport at physiological [Ca]$_i$. Furthermore, if SERCA2 were down-regulated without altered PLB, the depressant effect on SR Ca transport could be disproportionately high (since more SR Ca-pumps would be PLB-inhibited, see pg 165). An example where this SERCA2:PLB ratio changes dramatically is in response to thyroid hormone state, which may decline in HF (Hamilton *et al.*, 1990; Kiss *et al.*, 1994; Ojamaa *et al.*, 2000). Increases in thyroid hormone increase SERCA2 expression and decrease PLB expression. This greatly increases the SERCA2:PLB ratio, and disproportionately stimulates SR Ca transport. The hypothyroid state results in the converse and the greatly reduced SERCA2:PLB ratio, profoundly depresses SR Ca transport.

Reduced SR Ca-ATPase function fits well with the characteristic slowed relaxation and [Ca]$_i$ decline of HF. Moreover, when SERCA2 expression in myocytes is increased by adenoviral gene transfer, relaxation and [Ca]$_i$ decline can be accelerated (del Monte *et al.*, 1999; Miyamoto *et al.*, 2000). Thus, it seems clear that reduced SERCA expression and function are important in the slowed relaxation and [Ca]$_i$ decline characteristic of HF.

RyR and SR Ca content.   RyR mRNA seems to be reduced in human HF, but Western blot and ryanodine binding indicate that RyR protein levels are unchanged (Go *et al.*, 1995; Schillinger *et al.*, 1996; Sainte Beuve *et al.*, 1997). In the pacing-induced dog HF model there seems to be down-regulation of RyR (Vatner *et al.*, 1994; Yano *et al.*, 2000), but not in spontaneous hypertensive HF rat (Gómez *et al.*, 1997). Thus, results are somewhat mixed for RyR number, but intriguing new results have also suggested that RyR regulation may be altered in HF. Marx *et al.* (2000) showed that in HF the RyR2 can be hyper-phosphorylated by PKA, causing displacement of FKBP12.6 from the RyR (see pg 189-190 & 199-200). The hyperphos-phorylation may be due to their finding of less phosphatase associated with the RyR complex, despite a generalized increase in phosphatase expression in HF (Neumann *et al.*, 1997). Without FKBP12.6 the RyR open probability is higher at rest, but shows less coordinated gating. This could increase diastolic SR Ca leak, as seen in intact cells treated with FK-506, which also displaces FKBP12.6 from the RyR (McCall *et al.*, 1996a). This may contribute to a lower SR Ca content in HF and might also alter how the RyR responds to I$_{Ca}$ during E-C coupling. Yano *et al.* (2000) also found reduced FKBP:RyR stoichiometry in HF and greater Ca leak from SR vesicles.

On the surface, the Marx *et al.* (2000) story seems consistent with an intrinsic depression of E-C coupling in hypertrophy or HF in rats (Gómez *et al.*, 1997; McCall *et al.*, 1998). In those studies there was reduced SR Ca release in hypertrophy or HF for the same I$_{Ca}$ and SR Ca content. On the other hand, removal of FKBP from RyR by FK-506 enhances (rather than depresses) fractional SR Ca release (McCall *et al.*, 1996a) and also sensitizes the RyR to activator Ca (Marx *et al.*, 2000). This would imply increased Ca transients in HF. Eisner *et al.* (1998, 2000) also argued that an alteration in RyR gating alone cannot produce long-lasting depression of Ca transients, because of the sort of autoregulation discussed on pg 266-267. Thus, it may be that the diastolic SR Ca leak induced by the PKA/FKBP effect in HF is the more functionally important aspect of this RyR modification in HF.

Table 26

Alterations of Expression and Function in Human Heart Failure.

	Change in HF*	Prevalence	Data type[‡] & Ref (*Counter-ref*)
Twitch Contraction	lower/slowed	~all	F-1,2,3
Twitch $\Delta[Ca]_i$	lower/slowed	~all	F-1,2,4,5
Force-frequency	from + to more −	~all	F-2,3,6,7; (see also Fig 148)
MF Ca sensitivity	unaltered (*higher*)	~all	F-8,9,10,11,12 *(13)*
I_{Ca} / DHPR	unaltered (*lower*)	most	F-4,16,17,18 *(19,20)*; R-14 *(15)*;
SR Ca ATPase	lower (*unaltered*)	most	F-1,2,30,31; R-15,21,22,23,24,25; P-26,27,28 *(22,25,29)*
SR Ca content	lower	~all	F-10,30,32
Phospholamban	lower (*unaltered*)	most	R-22,24,25,33; P-27 *(22,25,29)*
Calsequestrin	unaltered	~all	R-15,24; P-27,29
Calreticulin	unaltered	~all	P-27
RyR	unaltered (*lower*)	mixed	R-24 *(34,35)*; P-27,36,37; F-38 *(8,39)*
Na/Ca exchange	higher (*unaltered*)	~all	F-30,41,42; R-28,40; P-28,40,41,42 *(43)*;
Na/K-ATPase	lower	~all	P-43,44,45
AP duration	higher	~all	F-4,46,47
I_{to}	lower	~all	F-46,48,49
I_{K1}	lower	~all	F-46,47
G_i	higher	~all	F-53; R-50; P-51,52,53
G_s	unaltered (*higher*)	~all	R-50 *(54)*

*where groups disagree, I have weighed evidence in an attempt to provide more useful information. In cases of disagreement, there may be true differences in etiology or direct cause of dysfunction.
[‡] supporting data are from **F** (functional tests in cells, hearts or transport assays), **R** (mRNA measurements) or **P** (protein measurements; Western blot or ligand binding). Prepared with the help of L.S Maier.

1 Gwathmey *et al.*, 1987
2 Pieske *et al.*, 1995
3 Davies *et al.*, 1995
4 Beuckelmann *et al.*, 1992
5 Sipido *et al.*, 1998b
6 Mulieri *et al.*, 1992
7 Hasenfuss *et al.*, 1992
8 D'Agnolo *et al.*, 1992
9 Hajjar *et al.*, 1992
10 Denvir *et al.*, 1995
11 Gwathmey & Hajjar, 1990
12 Hajjar *et al.*, 2000
13 Wolff *et al.*, 1996
14 Schwinger *et al.*, 1999a
15 Takahashi *et al.*, 1992
16 Beuckelmann & Erdmann, 1992
17 Rasmussen *et al.*, 1990
18 Mewes & Ravens, 1994

19 Piot *et al.*, 1996
20 Ouadid *et al.*, 1995
21 Mercadier *et al.*, 1990
22 Schwinger *et al.*, 1995
23 Limas *et al.*, 1987
24 Arai *et al.*, 1993
25 Linck *et al.*, 1996
26 Hasenfuss *et al.*, 1994
27 Meyer *et al.*, 1995
28 Studer *et al.*, 1994
29 Movsesian *et al.*, 1994
30 Pieske *et al.*, 1999a
31 Schmidt *et al.*, 1998
32 Lindner *et al.*, 1998
33 Feldman *et al.*, 1991
34 Brillantes *et al.*, 1992
35 Go *et al.*, 1995
36 Schillinger *et al.*, 1996

37 Sainte Beuve *et al.*, 1997
38 Holmberg & Williams, 1989
39 Nimer *et al.*, 1995
40 Flesch *et al.*, 1996
41 Reinecke *et al.*, 1996
42 Hasenfuss *et al.*, 1999
43 Schwinger *et al.*, 1999b
44 Schmidt *et al.*, 1993
45 Nørgaard *et al.*, 1988
46 Beuckelmann *et al.*, 1993
47 Koumi *et al.*, 1995
48 Wettwer *et al.*, 1994
49 Näbauer *et al.*, 1996
50 Eschenhagen *et al.*, 1992
51 Neumann *et al.*, 1988
52 Feldman *et al.*, 1988
53 Böhm *et al.*, 1990
54 Feldman *et al.*, 1989

Intra-SR Ca buffering capacity is probably unchanged, since calsequestrin (and calreticulin) does not seem to be altered in HF (Hasenfuss, 1998b). This means that if SR Ca content is lower in HF, the free $[Ca]_{SR}$ is also lower. There are few measures of SR Ca under relatively physiological conditions. Nevertheless, in HF the SR Ca content does seems to be reduced in human (Lindner *et al.*, 1998), rabbit (Pogwizd *et al.*, 1999; 2001) and dog (Hobai & O'Rourke, 2001), based on caffeine-induced Ca transients. Moreover, the reduced SR Ca content is completely consistent with the reduced SR Ca-ATPase activity, the increased RyR leak above and also the upregulation of Na/Ca exchange (below). A reduced SR Ca content would also explain the reduced twitch $\Delta[Ca]_i$ and contractile function.

Na/Ca exchange.   Studer *et al.* (1994) first showed an increase in Na/Ca exchange mRNA in human HF. This seems to be a rather consistent finding in HF in human (Flesch *et al.*, 1996; Hasenfuss *et al.*, 1999) and most rabbit, guinea-pig and dog HF models (e.g. Pogwizd *et al.*, 1999; Hobai & O'Rourke, 2000; Sipido *et al.*, 2000; Ahmmed *et al.*, 2000), as well as in rabbit myocytes from the peri-infarct zone during post-infarct HF (Litwin & Bridge, 1997). Indeed, in our non-ischemic rabbit HF model, we find that Na/Ca exchange is consistently upregulated by ~100% at the level of mRNA, protein, $[Ca]_i$ decline of caffeine-induced contractures and $I_{Na/Ca}$ (with either $[Ca]_i$ clamped or dynamically changing, Pogwizd, 1999, 2001). To the extent that Na/Ca exchange is primarily engaged in Ca extrusion, higher Na/Ca exchange will be expected to compete better with the SR Ca-ATPase during relaxation (and diastole). This would tend to reduce SR Ca content (as above). This interpretation is supported by overexpression of Na/Ca exchange in rabbit ventricular myocytes, where the phenotype was depressed contractility, blunted force-frequency relationship and reduced SR Ca content (Schillinger, *et al.*, 2000).

As we have seen (pg 147-150 & 290-294), the effects of Na/Ca exchange are complicated by its bi-directional nature and its dependence on E_m and gradients for [Na] and [Ca]. Indeed, if Ca transients in HF are of low amplitude, greater Ca influx via Na/Ca exchange could occur, even early in the AP (see Figs 72 & 74). Also with low $[Ca]_i$ and long AP duration in HF, there can be an extended period of Ca influx via Na/Ca exchange during the AP (Dipla *et al.*, 1999), which would not be expected for large Ca transients and short AP duration. It seems that this Ca influx enhancement via Na/Ca exchange would be most likely at low frequency in HF, where AP duration is especially prolonged. This may also explain why the Ca transients and contractile force are less depressed compared to control at low heart rates. Thus it seems likely that Na/Ca exchange upregulation is an important factor in altered Ca handling in HF.

Na/K-ATPase and $[Na]_i$.   The way that Na/Ca exchange functions is critically dependent on the level of $[Na]_i$, which is in turn dependent on the activity of the Na/K-ATPase (see Chapter 6 and pg 286-294). There are several reports which indicate reduced Na/K-ATPase expression in HF (Dixon *et al.*, 1992; Semb *et al.*, 1998; Schwinger *et al.*, 1999b). This would be expected to elevate $[Na]_i$ and be inotropic. While only preliminary data are available, there does seem to be higher $[Na]_i$ in HF *vs.* control ventricle from human (Maier *et al.*, 1997b), dog (Verdonck *et al.*, 2001) and rabbit (S Despa, M Islam, SP Pogwizd & DM Bers, unpublished). It is premature to evaluate how this perturbs Ca regulation, but one would expect a shift toward less Ca extrusion and greater Ca influx via Na/Ca exchange (as in glycoside inotropy). It is possible that this elevated $[Na]_i$ partly offsets an even greater depression of Ca transients and contractile function that might otherwise be observed in HF.   While lower Na/K-ATPase could explain higher [Na]$_i$ in HF, there is also evidence to suggest a more prominent contribution of a very slowly inactivating I$_{Na}$ component (I$_{Na,Slow}$) in HF (Saint *et al.*, 1992; Maltsev *et al.*, 1998; Undrovinas *et al.*, 1999). I$_{Na,Slow}$ could also contribute significantly to the AP prolongation observed in HF.

Other ion currents.   Other ventricular ion currents may also be altered in HF.   The most consistent findings so far are reductions in I$_{to}$ and I$_{K1}$ in HF (Table 26, reviewed by Wickenden *et al.*, 1998 and Näbauer & Kääb, 1998). Reduction in I$_{to}$ can reduce the early repolarization during the AP (phase 1).   This notch in the AP may normally serve to enhance the driving force for Ca entry once Ca channels are activated.   Hence, in HF reduced I$_{to}$ could decrease early Ca influx and triggering of SR Ca release, but this has not been tested.   However, reducing I$_{to}$ is expected to have little effect on overall AP duration in human, dog, rabbit or guinea-pig ventricle (e.g. Priebe & Beuckelmann, 1998).   Exceptions to this are rat and mouse ventricle, where the very large I$_{to}$ is a predominant cause of repolarization of the very short AP that is observed in those species.   The decrease in I$_{K1}$ may contribute to AP prolongation, but this would be mainly in the very late phases of final repolarization, because of its inward rectification (see Figs 41 & 45). An even more important aspect of the 40-50% I$_{K1}$ reduction in human, dog and rabbit HF (Beuckelmann *et al.*, 1993; Kääb *et al.*, 1996; Pogwizd *et al.*, 2001) is that it destabilizes the diastolic E$_m$. This may increase the propensity for arrhythmogenesis (see pg 298-299 & below).

There is some data to suggest that delayed rectifier K currents (I$_{Kr}$, I$_{Ks}$, I$_{Kur}$) may also be reduced in HF (Volders *et al.*, 1999), but there is not enough data available to provide definitive conclusions about this.   This is partly because these currents vary among species and are also somewhat more tricky to dissect electrophysiologically.   On the other hand, changes in these delayed rectifier K currents can strongly alter AP duration (Priebe & Beuckelmann, 1998), so additional information on delayed rectifiers would be particularly valuable.

So which currents contribute to APD prolongation in HF?   Reductions in the outward currents I$_{to}$, I$_{K1}$ (and possibly other K currents) and Na/K-ATPase could all contribute.   In addition increases in inward currents (I$_{Ca}$, I$_{Na,Slow}$ & I$_{Na/Ca}$) could also contribute.   If peak I$_{Ca}$ is unchanged in HF, but SR Ca release is reduced, we might expect less Ca-dependent inactivation of I$_{Ca}$ and hence more integrated Ca influx (see Fig 60; Ahmmed *et al.*, 2000).   This would increase the total inward current during the AP.   It would also mean that there must be more overall inward I$_{Na/Ca}$ during the cardiac cycle to extrude all of the Ca which entered via I$_{Ca}$. Thus, greater inward I$_{Na/Ca}$ may result from upregulation of Na/Ca exchange expression and the slower [Ca]$_i$ decline in HF (which would drive more inward I$_{Na/Ca}$). Of course an elevated [Na]$_i$ would also tend to shift I$_{Na/Ca}$ in the outward direction, such that the exact mode of I$_{Na/Ca}$ during the AP is hard to predict.   Thus several factors probably contribute to the AP prolongation typically observed in HF.   In addition, it should be appreciated that the AP prolongation itself has a salutary effect on Ca transients (Kaprielian *et al.*, 1999), since it increases Ca influx (by I$_{Ca}$ and possibly by I$_{Na/Ca}$) and slows Ca extrusion via Na/Ca exchange.   Thus, the longer AP may partly offset other negative inotropic effects of HF.

The contractile dysfunction in HF (Fig 175) is probably largely due to a reduction of SR Ca content during steady state physiological conditions. Three factors may contribute to the lower SR Ca content: 1) reduced SR Ca-ATPase function, 2) increased Ca efflux via Na/Ca

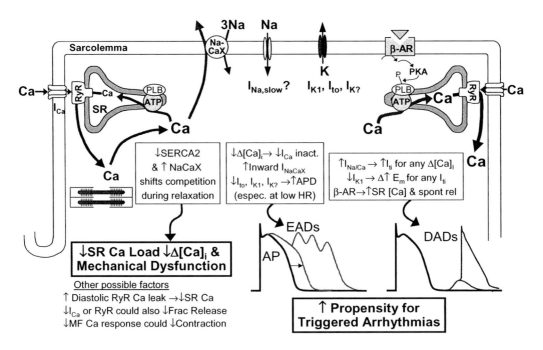

Figure 175. Contractile dysfunction and arrhythmogenesis in HF. The contractile dysfunction probably results from a reduction in SR Ca content (due to reduced SR Ca-ATPase, increased Na/Ca exchange, and increased diastolic SR Ca leak). Other possible contributors are indicated. Arrhythmogenesis may be triggered by either early or delayed afterdepolarizations (EADs or DADs). EADs are more likely at longer AP duration and factors which may contribute to this are shown. DADs are due to spontaneous SR Ca release and there may be three key factors which increase propensity for EADs in HF (see text).

exchange (by competing with the SR Ca-ATPase for Ca) and 3) possible diastolic Ca leak from the SR. Furthermore, a lower SR Ca content reduces SR Ca release both because there is less Ca available for release and also because fractional release is reduced for a given I_{Ca} trigger (pg 224-226). In some HF cases there might also be decreases in trigger I_{Ca}, reduced intrinsic RyR responsiveness during E-C coupling, or reduced myofilament Ca sensitivity. However, I find the reduced SR Ca content explanation a more simple and unifying working model right now.

Reduced SR Ca-ATPase and increased Na/Ca exchange can both tend to lower SR Ca content, but exert opposite effects on relaxation rate and $[Ca]_i$ decline. This combination can thus result in unchanged relaxation rate, as we found in our rabbit HF model where a doubling of Na/Ca exchange appeared to offset ~24% decrease in SR Ca-pump function (Pogwizd *et al.*, 1999). Hasenfuss *et al.* (1999) found this same situation in 44% of human HF (nearly doubled Na/Ca exchanger with modest SERCA reduction). These muscles did not show elevated diastolic force at 3 Hz (*vs.* 0.5 Hz). However, another group of HF muscles (25%) that showed slower relaxation and elevated diastolic force at 3 Hz, had a greater reduction in SERCA2 expression, but unaltered Na/Ca exchange. Thus, there may be a real heterogeneity of diastolic dysfunction in HF that depends on the balance of SR Ca-ATPase and Na/Ca exchange function.

With respect to arrhythmogenesis in HF, I will restrict discussion to triggered arrhythmias (i.e. DADs and EADs). Electrical reentry (pg 99-100) contributes to ventricular tachycardia (VT), but 3-dimensional mapping studies have shown that most VTs in HF initiate by a non-reentrant mechanism such as DADs and EADs (Pogwizd, 1994, 1995; Wit & Rosen, 1992). In human HF this is true for 100% of VT in nonischemic HF and 50% in post-ischemic HF (Pogwizd *et al.*, 1992, 1998). Figure 175 indicates possible reasons for the enhanced arrhythmogenesis observed in HF. EADs are more likely when AP duration is prolonged (as occurs in HF, especially at low heart rates). The same factors described above may prolong the AP and increase the likelihood that I_{Ca} has recovered sufficiently during the late plateau phase to induce the type of EAD discussed on pg 97-98. Thus, EADs may be most common in brady-arrhythmias. However, as noted above, AP duration is not always so prolonged in HF, especially at physiological frequencies, and tachyarrhythmias occur at short cycle lengths. DADs would initially seem unlikely in HF because spontaneous SR Ca release is less likely to occur at low SR Ca content (as seen in HF). However, as discussed on pg 299, bursts of β-AR activation can readily drive SR Ca content to the point where spontaneous SR Ca release occurs in HF (Pogwizd *et al.*, 1999, 2001). Moreover, any given SR Ca release causes greater I_{ti} in HF (because Na/Ca exchange is increased), and any given I_{ti} causes a greater DAD in HF (largely because I_{K1} is decreased). If, during very long APs, there is Ca loading occurring via Na/Ca exchange, one could even get a spontaneous SR Ca release, triggering what looks like an EAD, but is more mechanistically related to a DAD. Thus the key facets of HF that contribute to DAD-induced triggered arrhythmias are: 1) increased $I_{Na/Ca}$, 2) reduced I_{K1} and 3) residual β-AR activity (to cause SR Ca load to sufficiently for spontaneous Ca release). Indeed, with loss of β-AR responsiveness in very late stage HF, arrhythmias are less common (see pg 299).

In hypertrophy and HF there can also be energetic limitations. This may not be apparent under low work conditions, but may manifest as a limited cardiac reserve, when cells, muscles or hearts are challenged with higher work loads (Neubauer *et al.*, 1995; Tian *et al.*, 1997; Brandes *et al.*, 1998; Ito *et al.*, 2000). This may also contribute somewhat to the blunted force-frequency relationship seen in human HF (Pieske *et al.*, 1995). The limiting factor could be the alteration in ΔG_{ATP} as discussed above for ischemia (which could alter SR Ca transport, Na/K-ATPase and myofilament function). This may also result, in part from a reduction in the ratio of cell volume occupied mitochondria *vs.* myofilaments (Lund & Tomaneck, 1978; Anversa *et al.*, 1979). This value is 16-37% higher in control than hypertrophied rat hearts.

In conclusion, there are several interdependent factors that may contribute to both the mechanical dysfunction and the propensity for arrhythmias in the failing heart. There is much still to clarify in this area, but a tremendous amount of research effort is targeted in this direction. The coming years should make this complex HF story increasingly clear.

SITES FOR INDUCTION OF CARDIAC INOTROPY

Since contractility is depressed during HF, it is important to consider mechanisms that can improve contractility. The two main inotropic mechanisms are: 1) increasing the amplitude or time course of the Ca transient, so that more Ca is supplied to the myofilaments, and 2) enhancing myofilament Ca sensitivity, by either increasing the Ca affinity of troponin C (TnC) or increasing force for a given degree of Ca occupancy of TnC. I will focus below on some of the

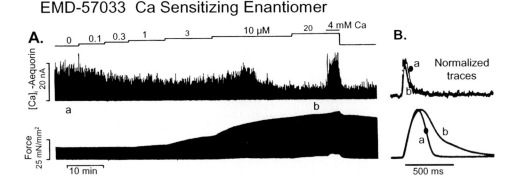

Figure 176. The effect of EMD-57033 on contractions and Ca transients (assessed by aequorin luminescence, a non-linear [Ca]$_i$ indicator) in ferret ventricle at 30°C, 0.33 Hz. **A.** [EMD-57033] was progressively increased and [Ca]$_o$ was raised from 1 to 4 mM as indicated to verify that [Ca]$_i$ and force could still be increased. **B.** Normalized traces from points a and b are superimposed to compare the kinetics of Ca transients and contractions. Figure is modified from White *et al.*, 1993, with permission).

advantages and disadvantages of specific inotropic strategies or targets, rather than review results with many individual agents. While there are certainly many ways to increase myofilament Ca sensitivity and Ca transients, one must always be mindful of key limitations, such as energetics, diastolic force and arrhythmogenesis. Anything we do to increase Ca transients and myofilament ATPase will consume more energy, and the heart (especially in pathophysiological conditions) may have trouble matching increased energy demands with oxygen/energy supply. Increased myofilament Ca sensitivity may result in elevated diastolic force, which can require more diastolic ATP consumption, and also mechanically limit ventricular filling and coronary blood flow during diastole. If we bring more Ca into the cell, the necessary Ca transport will use ATP, and can also lead to diastolic dysfunction and arrhythmias, as discussed above. Thus, there are very practical limitations that overlay this entire discussion of inotropic mechanisms.

Modulation of Myofilament Ca Sensitivity

Several agents can increase the myofilament Ca sensitivity (e.g. caffeine, theophylline, pimobendan, sulmazole, isomazole, adibendan, perhexiline, bepridil, CGP-48506, EMD-57033, MCI-154, levosimendan, see pg 35). This is a rather direct strategy to increase contractility. That is, increasing myofilament Ca sensitivity will lead to greater force for the same amount of activating Ca (SR Ca release + Ca influx). If the sensitization works by increasing Ca affinity of TnC, then peak [Ca]$_i$ during the contraction is expected to be lower. This is a consequence of TnC being a major [Ca]$_i$ buffer and the fact that >95% of the activating Ca is buffered during the Ca transient (pg 41-47). Thus the peak [Ca]$_i$ is determined by both the amount of activating Ca and the amount of intracellular Ca buffering. Sulmazole (AR-L 115BS) is a fairly typical early drug which increases myofilament Ca binding and sensitivity and showed these characteristics (Solaro & Rüegg, 1982; Blinks & Endoh, 1984). However, sulmazole, like many other inotropic drugs, is not a pure Ca sensitizer. It also inhibits a cyclic nucleotide phosphodiesterase (PDE-III) which raises cAMP levels and increases PKA activity (Endoh *et al.*, 1985). Sulmazole also has a caffeine-like action to open SR Ca release channels (Williams & Holmberg, 1990).

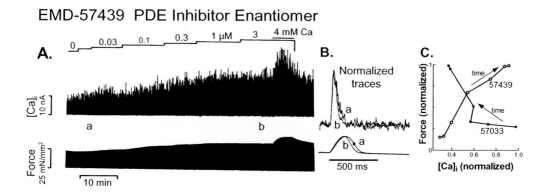

Figure 177. The effect of EMD-57439 on contractions and Ca transients (assessed by aequorin) in ferret ventricle at 30°C, 0.33 Hz. **A**. [EMD-57439] was progressively increased and [Ca]$_o$ was raised from 1 to 4 mM as indicated. **B**. Normalized traces from points a and b. **C**. [Ca]$_i$-dependence of force (peak values) for data in A and Fig 176A, showing that with EMD-57033 force increases as peak [Ca]$_i$ declines, while for EMD-57439 they increase in parallel. Figure is modified from White *et al.*, 1993, with permission).

EMD-53998 is another cardiotonic agent which shows both Ca sensitizing effects and PDE inhibition (Allen & Lee, 1989; Beier *et al.*, 1991). An intriguing aspect of this drug is that the two effects seem to be separately attributable to the two optical stereoisomers of the compound ((+)EMD-57033 & (–)EMD-57439, Lues *et al.*, 1993; Solaro *et al.*, 1993; White *et al.*, 1993). Figure 176 shows the effect of the pure Ca sensitizer (EMD-57033). There is a progressive increase in force and decrease in the peak of Ca transients (as expected due to increased Ca binding by TnC, see Fig 177C). In Fig 176A there is only a slight increase in diastolic force at 10-20 μM EMD-57033, although Solaro *et al.* (1993) found greater diastolic contracture at lower [EMD-57033]. The normalized traces show that Ca transient kinetics were little changed, but that relaxation was slowed. This is an intrinsic limitation of the myofilament sensitization approach, where relaxation is slowed and diastolic filling is reduced (Hgashiyama *et al.*, 1995; Hajjar *et al.*, 1997). On the other hand, *in vivo* studies have shown that EMD-57033 can produce strong inotropic effects (at relatively lower energy cost), without slowing ventricular relaxation or filling (Senzaki *et al.*, 2000). EMD-57033 and CGP-48506 (Neumann *et al.*, 1996; Wolska *et al.*, 1996a) seem to be Ca sensitizers which most clearly lack PDE inhibitory activity, although CGP-48506 may increase I$_{Ca}$, (Herzig, 1996).

Figure 177 shows the effects of the other EMD-53998 isomer (EMD-57439) which exhibits primarily PDE inhibitory effects (White *et al.*, 1993). In this case Ca transients and contractions increase roughly in parallel, and there is faster relaxation and [Ca]$_i$ decline. These effects mainly reflect PDE inhibition, which can increase cAMP levels and thereby activate the same cascade of effects as β-AR activation (pg 275-282). The net results expected are: 1) increased I$_{Ca}$, 2) more rapid SR Ca-ATPase and [Ca]$_i$ decline, 3) increased SR Ca release (due to higher trigger and load) and 4) an a decrease in myofilament Ca sensitivity. For drugs which are both Ca sensitizers and PDE inhibitors, the net effect on myofilament Ca sensitivity will be a compromise between the direct increase and the decrease due to the PKA-dependent TnI phosphorylation. Indeed, for these mixed Ca sensitizer-PDE inhibitors, the PKA-dependent

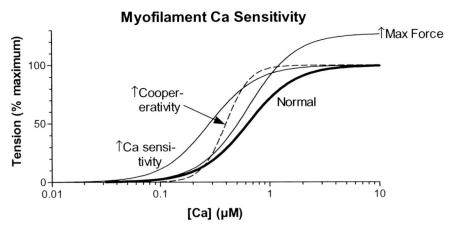

Figure 178. Increasing myofilament Ca sensitivity can limit relaxation. For Normal, a Hill curve was used with K_m=630 nM [Ca] and n=2. Increased maximal force used 127% of Normal, but the same other parameters. A parallel shift of myofilament Ca sensitivity is assumed to change K_m to 280 nM [Ca] (with n=2). Increased myofilament cooperativity used K_m= 400 nM [Ca] and an Hill slope n=4.

stimulation of SR Ca uptake may offset the problem of slower relaxation caused by increased myofilament Ca sensitivity. Thus, while both Ca sensitization and PDE inhibition have pluses and minuses, they may synergize. There may even be an optimal balance in the combination of these two attributes.

The rate of Ca binding to TnC is fast (nearly diffusion-limited, Table 11). If this is correct, then changes in Ca affinity would depend primarily on changes in the rate of dissociation of Ca from TnC. Smith & England (1990) found that the rate of Ca dissociation from the bovine cardiac troponin-tropomyosin complex was unaffected by sulmazole or pimobendan, but reduced by isomazole, perhexiline and bepridil. These results are consistent with an increased Ca binding with isomazole, perhexiline and bepridil (Solaro *et al.*, 1986), but not with results which showed that Ca binding to dog myofilaments was also increased by sulmazole and pimobendan (Solaro & Rüegg, 1982; Jaquet & Heilmeyer, 1987). It should also be noted that myofilament Ca sensitivity can be increased without a change in Ca binding (as with caffeine, Powers & Solaro, 1995). For example, alterations in cross-bridge cycling or the coupling between contractile proteins downstream from Ca binding could increase the Hill coefficient of activation by Ca (see pg 23-25 and Solaro, 2001). Along these lines, peptides derived from the myosin head can alter TnI-actin interaction and thereby increase myofilament Ca sensitivity (Rüegg *et al.*, 1989).

A pure increase in myofilament Ca sensitivity can increase the amount of force for a given amount of activating Ca. A key advantage is that the balance of transsarcolemmal Ca fluxes need not be altered. Thus, the cells are not subject to additional Ca load (and the potential negative inotropic, energetic and arrhythmogenic consequences). Figure 178 shows a key disadvantage of Ca sensitizers which produce parallel shifts of the [Ca]-force relationship (typical of many Ca sensitizers). At diastolic $[Ca]_i$ (~150 nM) there can be incomplete relaxation, and this may be of particular concern in pathological conditions where diastolic $[Ca]_i$ is elevated or $[Ca]_i$ decline is slowed. Thus, it is crucial to know what diastolic $[Ca]_i$ is with respect to the threshold for contractile activation (and this may change with conditions). The dotted curve in

Fig 178 shows an increase in the steepness of the [Ca]-force relationship (with a smaller shift in $K_{1/2}$). This type of change could be especially beneficial, because the threshold for contractile activation is not shifted to lower $[Ca]_i$, but myofilament Ca sensitivity is greatly increased. However, as a practical matter it should be kept in mind that >95% of the Ca released from the SR or entering the cell is bound (for a $\Delta[Ca]_i$ of 1 µM a total flux of ~60 µmol/L cytosol is required, Chapter 3). The steeper [Ca]-force relationship may allow a greater fraction of activating Ca to bind to TnC (*vs.* other Ca buffers), but the absolute amount of activating Ca may still be limiting. That is, if most of the activating Ca is already bound to TnC, there may be little Ca available for further saturation of TnC (without increasing the amount of activating Ca). The other inotropic mechanisms discussed below all deal with changing the amount of activating Ca.

On balance, enhancing myofilament Ca sensitivity seems an appropriate inotropic target. This is because it does not require additional Ca transport, does not have intrinsic electrophysiological complications, and the main extra energy can go directly toward the work output of the heart. The key challenges may be to obtain sufficient selectivity and avoid diastolic dysfunction.

Phosphodiesterase Inhibition

Many inotropic agents are PDE inhibitors. These include caffeine, theophylline, amrinone, milrinone, enoximone, piroximone, saterinone, pimobendan, adibendan, sulmazole, EMD-5998, MCI-154 and levosimendan (Butcher & Sutherland, 1962; Alousi *et al.*, 1983; Endoh *et al.*, 1985; Weishaar *et al.*, 1988; von der Leyen *et al.*, 1988). There are at least 11 classes of PDE, with 6 expressed in the heart (I-V and VII, see Table 27, Beavo, 1988; Beavo & Reifsnyder, 1990; Schmitz *et al.*, 1989; Francis *et al.*, 2000). Caffeine, theophylline, isobutyl-lmethylxanthine (IBMX) and other methylxanthines are relatively non-selective PDE inhibitors. Most of the inotropic drugs above are relatively selective inhibitors of PDE III, whereas agents which inhibit PDE-I, II & IV do not appear to be particularly good inotropes. Bode *et al.* (1991) showed that the most abundant PDE in heart (PDE-I) was absent in isolated cardiac myocytes, suggesting that PDE-I is restricted to other cells in the heart.

These PDE-III inhibitors prevent the breakdown of cAMP to 5'-AMP and can thereby increase cellular cAMP levels. This, of course, activates the same cascade as β-AR agonists (see pages 275-282). An advantage over β-AR agonists is that these agents can still inhibit PDE-III, when β-ARs are down-regulated and cells are unresponsive to catecholamines. However, if the

Table 27

Classification of Cardiac Phosphodiesterases and Inhibitors

Class	Substrates	Key Regulator	Inhibitors
I	cAMP, cGMP	Ca-CaM-stimulated	KS-505
II	cAMP, cGMP	cGMP-stimulated	EHNA
III	cAMP> cGMP	cGMP-inhibited	Milrinone, amrinone, pimobendan, sulmazole...
IV	cAMP	cAMP-specific cGMP-insensitive	Rolipram, RO 201724
V	cGMP		Zaprinast, sildenafil (Viagra)
VII	cAMP		??

rate of cAMP production by adenylyl cyclase is too low, PDE inhibition may not greatly elevate [cAMP]$_i$. This limitation can occur in human HF, where reduced β-AR numbers and elevated G$_i$ levels may limit cAMP formation (Schmitz *et al.*, 1989; Bristow *et al.*, 1982, 1986). While one could circumvent this by direct activation of adenylyl cyclase with forskolin, the side effects of forskolin (including excessive vasodilation) are prohibitive.

When cAMP is increased by PDE-III inhibition, we expect an increase in I$_{Ca}$, an increase of SR Ca pumping, and a decrease in myofilament Ca sensitivity. While in some cases these effects have been reported, there are again multiple effects of most of these agents (e.g. myofilament Ca sensitization or ion channel effects). The myofilament sensitizing effect might more than offset the Ca desensitizing effect expected from cAMP-dependent phosphorylation of TnI. Ohte *et al.* (1997) found that in HF the response to a simple PDE-III inhibitor (amrinone) was blunted, while pimobendan (a Ca sensitizer with some PDE-III inhibitory activity) was still robust. Sulmazole and milrinone also exhibit caffeine-like actions on the SR Ca release channel, which may offset the PKA-dependent phosphorylation of phospholamban and stimulation of the SR Ca-pump (Rapundalo *et al.*, 1986; Holmberg *et al.*, 1990; Williams & Holmberg, 1990). Thus the net results on Ca fluxes and contractile force can be rather complicated.

A major advantage with PDE-III inhibitors compared to Ca channel activators (and catecholamines) is that the inotropy is accompanied by vasodilation. This effect is a consequence of the relaxant effect of cAMP in vascular smooth muscle (Somlyo & Himpens, 1989). This combination of effects is desirable in a cardiac inotrope and the emphasis on development of PDE-III inhibitors as inotropic agents seems justified. Disadvantages with PDE-III inhibitors are side effects, that they are not effective if the cAMP pool is low, and importantly, that they increase Ca cycling and overall energy consumption just as β-AR activation does. This makes PDE-III inhibitors expensive inotropes energetically, and the β-AR-like effects may also increase the propensity for arrhythmogenesis (as discussed on pg 299 & 323).

Ca Current Modulation

Dihydropyridine Ca channel agonists such as Bay K 8644 can increase I$_{Ca}$ and produce dramatic positive inotropic effects (Schramm *et al.*, 1983). The potential advantage with Ca channel activators is that Ca influx is increased precisely when it can best contribute to inotropy. That is, Ca influx is increased during the AP, when it can increase: 1) the fraction of SR Ca release (via CICR), 2) the amount of Ca supplied directly to the myofilaments and 3) SR Ca loading. During diastole, Ca extrusion via Na/Ca exchange should not be compromised (as it is with Na-pump inhibition). Thus, during diastole the cell may be able to extrude the larger amount of Ca which enters during a steady state AP in the presence of Bay K 8644. This interpretation is consistent with measurements of net Ca fluxes in rabbit ventricle using extracellular Ca selective microelectrodes (Bers & MacLeod, 1986). Bay K 8644 did not increase the net Ca uptake nearly as much as did increased frequency (where Ca efflux may be compromised). Thus, Ca channel activators may produce a large inotropic effect, with less of the Ca overload problems which limit cardiac glycoside action.

The main disadvantage with Ca channel activators is the major effects of these agents on other tissues (e.g. causing smooth muscle vasoconstriction and central nervous system effects). Modulating Ca channels in this way might also increase the likelihood of EADs, caused by reopening of Ca channels.   Nevertheless, if a highly cardiac-muscle-selective Ca channel activator could be found, it might be a good inotropic agent, but this goal has so far been elusive. Compared to Bay K 8644, Sandoz 202-791 has less vasoconstricting action for a given cardiac inotropic effect (Bechem *et al.*, 1988; Hof *et al.*, 1985) and the Lilly compound (LY249933) produced modest cardiac inotropy and vasodilation (Holland *et al.*, 1989), but these drugs are not nearly selective enough.   Bay Y 5959 appeared to have particular initial promise, and increased cardiac efficiency in dogs and cardiac function in patients (Bechem *et al.*, 1997; Sato *et al.*, 1997; Rousseau *et al.*, 1997), but CNS side effects may have been too great.   Given the molecular and functional diversity of Ca channels (Chapter 5), there is certainly reason to hope that a highly cardiac muscle selective compound can be found.   As we learn more about the molecular structure of Ca channels and how they differ, progress in this area could accelerate.

Na/Ca Exchange and [Na]ᵢ Modulation

Cardioactive steroids were prototypical inotropes which function via Na/Ca exchange, where the Ca movements are secondary to $[Na]_i$ elevation (see pg 286-294).   I will simply point out that any agent which elevates $[Na]_i$ (or reduces the transsarcolemmal [Na] gradient) will have the same consequences.   This includes Na-ionophores (e.g. monensin), or agents which increase Na channel open time (e.g. veratridine, batrachotoxin, grayanotoxin, DPI 201-106, SDZ 210-921, see Scholtysik *et al.*, 1989).   Direct inhibitors of Na/Ca exchange may also be expected to produce the same type of effects (e.g. benzamil, dichlorobenzamil).   Unfortunately, all of the Na/Ca exchange inhibitors identified so far are not particularly selective (see Chapter 6).   DPI 201-106 is a Na channel activator which has been extensively studied as an inotropic agent.   It does increase contractility and prolong AP duration (Buggisch *et al.*, 1985; Scholtysik *et al.*, 1985; Kihara *et al.*, 1989), and this AP prolongation will limit Ca extrusion via Na/Ca exchange. Like many other inotropes, DPI 201-106 has multiple effects.   It also increases myofilament Ca sensitivity, and may also have Ca channel blocking effects (Scholtysik *et al.*, 1985; Siegl *et al.*, 1988; Kihara *et al.*, 1989).

Na channel activation might have some functional advantage over Na-pump inhibition. If Na entry via I_{Na} can activate Ca entry via Na/Ca exchange, due to the higher $[Na]_i$ near the sarcolemma. (as suggested by Leblanc & Hume, 1990; see pg 232-234), then this might be a way to boost SR Ca release right when it matters, but without loading the cells with Na and Ca.   That is, Ca influx via Na/Ca exchange may increase phasically during contraction, but the cell may be able to extrude much of the extra Na and Ca gain during diastole.   Anything that increases AP duration would tend to reduce Ca extrusion and possibly favor Ca influx.   This was discussed in the context of HF (pg 320), where the contractile dysfunction could be even worse without this Ca loading effect.   Again, this is still shifting Ca into the cell in a relatively general way.

As discussed earlier, Ca overload and the negative inotropic and arrhythmogenic consequences are a general disadvantage for digitalis or any inotropic strategy which shifts the Na/Ca exchange system to be less effective at Ca extrusion.   Since Na/Ca exchange seems to be the main means by which Ca is extruded from the cell (see Chapter 5), prevention of Ca extrusion can increase cellular Ca load and force.   Indeed, from a historical perspective, this has clearly been the most successful type of inotropic agent.   However, the consequences of Ca overload are a serious limitation (see pg 294-300).   KB-R7943 is the novel Na/Ca exchange blocker which seems to preferentially inhibit Ca influx *vs.* efflux (see pg 144 & 294). This might help to limit Ca overload associated with Na-pump inhibition and reperfusion, but precisely how this drug works is not known (although it may compete with $[Ca]_o$). The lack of specificity of KB-R7943 is also likely to limit its overall usefulness.

SR Ca Uptake and Release

Ryanodine receptors may not be an ideal inotropic target, at least from the perspective that their systolic function is subject to autoregulatory influences (pg 267, Eisner *et al.*, 2000). That is, increasing SR Ca release would increase Ca extrusion via Na/Ca exchange, tending to lower SR Ca content, and thereby reducing SR Ca release at subsequent beats. This may limit how much intrinsic gain-of-function might be obtainable by manipulating RyR gating. On the other hand, diastolic Ca leak from the SR via Ca sparks may limit the SR Ca content, both under normal conditions and in HF (pg 175, 192, 199 & 318). If this is the case, then reducing this diastolic leak may raise SR Ca content and enhance Ca transients (due to both increased SR Ca availability and fractional release). If this could be accomplished by a shift to slightly lower Ca-sensitivity (such that fewer diastolic Ca sparks and waves occur), but so that normal E-C coupling still occurred with a good margin for safety (e.g. analogous to the dashed curve for myofilament Ca sensitivity in Fig 178), then this might increase systolic cardiac function, without being arrhythmogenic. This may be a role that FKBP normally serves (pg 199 & 318). Thus, enhancing this effect of FKBP might be beneficial, as suggested by FKBP-12.6 overexpression in rabbit myocytes (Prestle *et al.*, 2001). It is also important that the RyR turns off promptly during the cellular Ca transient. While late RyR openings would prolong the active state, they would also delay relaxation and increase futile Ca cycling during pump-release fluxes (thereby using more ATP). Indeed, desynchronized SR Ca release and late Ca sparks during twitches have been reported in myocytes from the peri-infarct zone in post-infarction HF rabbit hearts (Litwin *et al.*, 2000). Overall goals with the RyR would be to 1) minimize leak during diastole (to maximize SR Ca load and not waste ATP in futile Ca cycling), and 2) ensure that RyRs open and close with high fidelity, synchrony and Ca flux during systole.

The SR Ca-ATPase and phospholamban (PLB) are also important inotropic targets. Results with the PLB knockout (KO) mouse, where PLB cannot inhibit the SR Ca-ATPase, directly attest to this (Luo *et al.*, 1994; Hoit *et al.*, 1995; Wolska *et al.*, 1996b; Li *et al.*, 1998; reviewed by Kiriazis & Kranias, 2000). The PLB-KO mouse exhibits hyperdynamic cardiac function, with larger Ca transients, and SR Ca content. Surprisingly, there is little down side, since the PLB-KO mice do not seem to develop cardiovascular disease, exercise as well as wild type mice and do not die prematurely. That is, there is neither evidence of detrimental effects of higher energy consumption by the heart, nor of arrhythmias which might have been expected based on the high SR Ca content. While there are more Ca sparks and waves in isolated myocytes from PLB-KO mice (Santana *et al.*, 1997; Hüser *et al.*, 1998b) this does not appear to translate into triggered or fatal arrhythmias in the mice. In general, these sorts of Ca overload and spontaneous SR Ca release events (pg 294-300) are the principal potential disadvantage of strategies which increase SR Ca-pump function.

Transgenic overexpression of SERCA2a can produce similar, but less dramatic effects compared to the PLB-KO (He *et al.*, 1997; Baker *et al.*, 1998). Notably, the increase in SERCA2 protein expression is only 20-50%, despite mRNA increases of 160-700%. It has been speculated that, because the SR membrane is already crowded with Ca-ATPase molecules, there may be little room to incorporate more of the protein. Nevertheless, SERCA2 overexpression can enhance cardiac contraction and relaxation (del Monte *et al.*, 1999; Miyamoto *et al.*, 2000).

A particular advantage of the PLB-KO compared to β-AR activation is that the effect is isolated to the SR Ca-pump function. None of the other PKA-mediated effects should occur. These include the decrease in myofilament Ca sensitivity (due to TnI phosphorylation) and the disproportionate increase in oxygen consumption *vs.* cardiac output. If PLB also decreases the energetic efficiency of the SR Ca-ATPase (Frank *et al.*, 2000; Shannon *et al.*, 2001), PLB inhibition could have direct energetic benefits, in terms of either the amount of ATP needed for a given SR Ca load or the maximal $[Ca]_{SR}$ that can be attained for a given $[Ca]_i$. Some other novel agent which interferes specifically with the PLB-SERCA interaction could have the same remarkable benefits that are observed in the PLB-KO.

CONCLUSION

In the end, the normal ventricular myocyte (and heart) is a remarkably well tuned system, which can rapidly vary its contractile output by changing ion currents, Ca handling and myofilament properties in response to a wide variety of physiological stimuli. On one hand there is a dynamic, yet delicate balance of Ca fluxes, electrophysiological & mechanical properties. On the other hand, this system is extremely robust in short- and long-term adaptation. In this context there are some redundancies to assure this robustness. For example, β-AR activation is still inotropic in the absence of phospholamban and there are multiple overlapping hypertrophic signaling systems. Nevertheless, if there are major perturbations in any system, it may throw off the normal tuning of the system (and its ability to respond to stress). Moreover, when there are major problems in one aspect with little redundancy (e.g. key myosin mutations in FHC or drastic reductions in SR function), it is not surprising that a generalized hypertrophic signal results. That is, if the short term cellular regulation can't cope with the mechanical demands on the heart, the logical next line of defense would be to make more muscle mass to deal with that load. Somewhat surprisingly, even changes which appear to be unrelated to the causative nature of mechanical dysfunction, but which enhance Ca transients and function (e.g. phospholamban knockout) can take the heart out of this maladaptive mode. Clearly there is much more to learn about how the heart cell modulates Ca and contraction. A clear understanding of how the cellular and molecular processes regulate Ca movements and contractile force should help make it possible to design inotropic agents to act specifically at strategic locations in the heart. I hope that this chapter and book help the reader develop a greater understanding of the dynamic regulation of Ca in cardiac muscle cells, particularly as it relates to the control of contraction.

REFERENCES

[Chapter where citation occurs]

Aass H, Skomedal T, Osnes JB: Demonstration of an α adrenoceptor-mediated inotropic effect of norepinephrine in rabbit papillary muscle. *J Pharmacol Exp Ther.* 226:572-578, **1983**. *[10]*

Abramson JJ: Regulation of the sarcoplasmic reticulum calcium permeability by sulfhydryl oxidation and reduction. *J Memb Sci.* 33:241-248, **1987**. *[8]*

Abramson JJ, Trimm JL, Weden L, Salama G: Heavy metals induce rapid calcium release from sarcoplasmic reticulum vesicles isolated from skeletal muscle. *Proc Natl Acad Sci USA.* 80:1526-1530, **1983**. *[8]*

Adachi-Akahane S, Cleemann L, Morad M: Cross-signaling between L-type Ca^{2+} channels and ryanodine receptors in rat ventricular myocytes. *J Gen Physiol.* 108:435-454, **1996**. *[5]*

Adachi-Akahane S, Lu LY, Li ZP, Frank JS, Philipson KD, Morad M: Calcium signaling in transgenic mice overexpressing cardiac Na^+-Ca^{2+} exchanger. *J Gen Physiol.* 109:717-729, **1997**. *[6]*

Adachi-Akahane S, Cleemann L, Morad M: BAY K 8644 modifies Ca^{2+} cross signaling between DHP and ryanodine receptors in rat ventricular myocytes. *Am J Physiol.* 276:H1178-H1189, **1999**. *[8]*

Adams BA, Beam KG: Muscular dysgenesis in mice: A model system for studying excitation-contraction coupling. *FASEB J.* 4:2809-2816, **1990**. *[8]*

Adams SR, Kao JPY, Grynkiewicz G, Minta A, Tsien RY: Biologically useful chelators that release Ca^{2+} upon illumination. *J Am Chem Soc.* 110:3212-3220, **1988**. *[8]*

Adams BA, Tanabe T, Mikami A, Numa S, Beam KG: Intramembrane charge movement restored in dysgenic skeletal muscle by injection of dihydropyridine receptor cDNAs. *Nature.* 346:569-572, **1990**. *[8]*

Aggarwal SK, MacKinnon R: Contribution of the S4 segment to gating charge in the *Shaker* K^+ channel. *Neuron.* 16:1169-1177, **1996**. *[4]*

Aggarwal R, Shorofsky SR, Goldman L, Balke CW: Tetrodotoxin-blockable calcium currents in rat ventricular myocytes; a third type of cardiac cell sodium current. *J Physiol.* 505:353-369, **1997**. *[4,8]*

Aguilar-Bryan L, Clement JP, Gonzalez G, Kunjilwar K, Babenko A, Bryan J: Toward understanding the assembly and structure of K_{ATP} channels. *Physiol Rev.* 78:227-245, **1998**. *[4]*

Ahern GP, Junankar PR, Dulhunty AF: Single channel activity of the ryanodine receptor calcium release channel is modulated by FK-506. *FEBS Lett.* 352:369-374, **1994**. *[7]*

Ahmad Z, Green FJ, Subuhi HS, Watanabe AM: Autonomic regulation of type 1 protein phosphatase in cardiac muscle. *J Biol Chem.* 264:3859-3863, **1989**. *[7]*

Ahmmed GU, Dong PH, Song GJ, Ball NA, Xu YF, Walsh RA, Chiamvimonvat N: Changes in Ca^{2+} cycling proteins underlie cardiac action potential prolongation in a pressure-overloaded guinea pig model with cardiac hypertrophy and failure. *Circ Res.* 86:558-570, **2000**. *[10]*

Akera T: Pharmacological agents and myocardial calcium, in Calcium and the Heart. Langer GA (ed). *New York, NY, Raven Press.* 299-331, **1990**. *[10]*

Akera T, Bennet RT, Olgaard MK, Brody TM: Cardiac Na^+, K^+-adenosine triphosphate inhibition by ouabain and myocardial sodium: A computer simulation. *J Pharmacol Exp Ther.* 199:287-297, **1976**. *[3,8]*

Akita T, Joyner RW, Lu C, Kumar R, Hartzell HC: Developmental changes in modulation of calcium currents of rabbit ventricular cells by phosphodiesterase inhibitors. *Circulation.* 90:469-478, **1994**. *[9]*

Aksoy M, Williams D, Sharkey E, Hartshorne D: A relationship between Ca^{2+} sensitivity and phosphorylation of gizzard myosin. *Biochem Biophys Res Commun.* 69:35-41, **1976**. *[2]*

Alderson BH, Feher JJ: The interaction of calcium and ryanodine with cardiac sarcoplasmic reticulum. *Biochim Biophys Acta.* 900:221-229, **1987**. *[7]*

Allen DG, Kurihara S: The effects of muscle length on intracellular calcium transients in mammalian cardiac muscle. *J Physiol.* 327:79-94, **1982**. *[2]*

Allen DG, Lee JA: EMD 53998 increases tension with little effect on the amplitude of calcium transients in isolated ferret ventricular muscle. *J Physiol.* 416:43P, **1989**. *[10]*

Allen DG, Orchard CH: The effects of changes of pH on intracellular calcium transients in mammalian cardiac muscle. *J Physiol.* 335:555-567, **1983**. *[10]*

Allen DG, Orchard CH: Myocardial contractile function during ischemia and hypoxia. *Circ Res.* 60:153-168, **1987**. *[2,10]*

Allen DG, Jewell BR, Murray JW: The contribution of activation processes to the length-tension relation of cardiac muscle. *Nature.* 248:606-607, **1974**. *[2]*

Allen DG, Jewell BR, Wood EH: Studies of the contractility of mammalian myocardium at low rates of stimulation. *J Physiol.* 254:1-17, **1976**. *[3,9]*

Allen DG, Eisner DA, Orchard CH: Factors influencing free intracellular calcium concentration in quiescent ferret ventricular muscle. *J Physiol.* 350:615-630, **1984a**. *[10]*

Allen DG, Eisner DA, Orchard CH: Characterization of oscillations of intracellular calcium concentration in ferret ventricular muscle. *J Physiol.* 352:113-128, **1984b**. *[8]*

Allen DG, Morris PG, Orchard CH, Pirolo JS: A nuclear magnetic resonance study of metabolism in the ferret heart during hypoxia and inhibition of glycolysis. *J Physiol.* 361:185-204, **1985a**. *[7]*

Allen DG, Eisner DA, Pirolo JS, Smith GL: The relationship between intracellular calcium and contraction in calcium-overloaded ferret papillary muscles. *J Physiol.* 364:169-182, **1985b**. *[10]*

Allen IS, Cohen NM, Gaa ST, Lederer WJ, Rogers TB: Angiotensin II increases spontaneous contractile frequency and stimulates calcium current in cultured neonatal rat heart myocytes: Insights into the underlying biochemical mechanisms. *Circ Res.* 62:524-534, **1988**. *[5]*

Allen DG, Lee JA, Smith GL: The consequences of simulated ischaemia on intracellular Ca^{2+} and tension in isolated ferret ventricular muscle. *J Physiol.* 410:297-323, **1989**. *[10]*

Almers W, McCleskey EW: Non-selective conductance in calcium channels of frog muscle: Calcium selectivity in a single-file pore. *J Physiol.* 353:585-608, **1984**. *[5]*

Almers W, Palade PT: Slow calcium and potassium currents across frog muscle membrane: Measurements with a vaseline-gap technique. *J Physiol.* 312:159-176, **1981**. *[5]*

Almers W, Stirling C: Distribution of transport proteins over animal cell membranes. *J Memb Biol.* 77:169-186, **1984**. *[1]*

Almers W, Fink R, Palade PT: Calcium depletion in frog muscle tubules: The decline of calcium current under maintained depolarization. *J Physiol.* 312:177-207, **1981**. *[1]*

Al-Nasser I, Crompton M: The reversible Ca^{2+}-induced permeabilization of rat liver mitochondria. *Biochem J.* 239:19-29, **1986**. *[3]*

Alousi AA, Canter JM, Montenaro MJ, Fort DJ, Ferrari RA: Cardiotonic activity of milrinone, a new and potent cardiac bipyridine, on the normal and failing heart of experimental animals. *J Cardiovasc Pharmacol.* 5:792-803, **1983**. *[10]*

Altamirano J, DeSantiago J, Bers DM: The inotropic effect of acetylstrophantidin and digoxin in ferret ventricular myocytes requires Na/Ca exchanger function. *Biophys J.* 76:A300, **1999**. *[8,10]*

Ambrosio G, Becker LC, Hutchins GM, Weisman HF, Weisfeldt ML: Reduction in experimental infarct size by recombinant human superoxide dismutase: insights into the pathophysiology of reperfusion injury. *Circulation.* 74:1424-1433, **1986**. *[10]*

Anand-Srivastava MB, Cantin M: Atrial natriuretic factors are negatively coupled to adenylate cyclase in cultured atrial and ventricular cardiocytes. *Biochem Biophys Res Commun.* 138:427-436, **1986**. *[5]*

Andersen JP, Vilsen B: Structure-function relationships of the calcium binding sites of the sarcoplasmic reticulum Ca^{2+}-ATPase. *Acta Physiol Scand Suppl.* 643:45-54, **1998**. *[7]*

Anderson RGW: Caveolae: Where incoming and outgoing messengers meet. *Proc Natl Acad Sci USA.* 90:10909-10913, **1993**. *[1]*

Anderson PAW, Moore GE, Nassar RN: Developmental changes in the expression of rabbit left ventricular troponin T. *Circ Res.* 63:742-747, **1988**. *[2]*

Anderson PAW, Malouf NN, Oakeley AE, Pagani ED, Allen PD: Troponin T isoform expression in humans. A comparison among normal and failing adult heart, fetal heart, and adult and fetal skeletal muscle. *Circ Res.* 69:1226-1233, **1991**. *[2]*

Anderson ME, Braun AP, Schulman H, Premack BA: Multifunctional Ca^{2+}/calmodulin-dependent protein kinase mediates Ca^{2+}-induced enhancement of the L-type Ca^{2+} current in rabbit ventricular myocytes. *Circ Res.* 75:854-861, **1994a**. *[5]*

Anderson K, Cohn AH, Meissner G: High-affinity [^{3}H]PN200-110 and [^{3}H]ryanodine binding to rabbit and frog skeletal muscle. *Am J Physiol.* 266:C462-C466, **1994b**. *[8]*

Anderson PAW, Greig A, Mark TM, Malouf NN, Oakeley AE, Ungerleider RM, Allen PD, Kay BK: Molecular basis of human cardiac troponin T isoforms expressed in the developing, adult, and failing heart. *Circ Res.* 76:681-686, **1995**. *[2]*

Angelotti T, Hofmann F: Tissue-specific expression of splice variants of the mouse voltage-gated calcium channel $\alpha_2\delta$ subunit. *FEBS Lett.* 397:331-337, **1996**. *[5]*

Anthonio RL, Brodde OE, van Veldhuisen DJ, Scholtens E, Crijns HJ, van Gilst WH: β-Adrenoceptor density in chronic infarcted myocardium: a subtype specific decrease of β_1-adrenoceptor density. *Int J Cardiol.* 72:137-141, **2000**. *[10]*

Antipenko AY, Spielman AI, Kirchberger MA: Comparison of the effects of phospholamban and jasmone on the calcium pump of cardiac sarcoplasmic reticulum. Evidence for modulation by phospholamban of both Ca^{2+} affinity and $V_{max(Ca)}$ of calcium transport. *J Biol Chem.* 272:2852-2860, **1997a**. *[7]*

Antipenko AY, Spielman AI, Sassaroli M, Kirchberger MA: Comparison of the kinetic effects of phospholamban phosphorylation and anti-phospholamban monoclonal antibody on the calcium pump in purified cardiac sarcoplasmic reticulum membranes. *Biochemistry.* 36:12903-12910, **1997b**. *[7]*

Antoniu B, Kim DH, Morii M, Ikemoto N: Inhibitors of Ca^{2+} release from the isolated sarcoplasmic reticulum. I. Ca^{2+} channel blockers. *Biochim Biophys Acta.* 816:9-17, **1985**. *[7]*

Antzelevitch C, Sicouri S, Litovsky SH, Lukas A, Krishnan SC, Di DJ, Gintant GA, Liu DW: Heterogeneity within the ventricular wall. Electrophysiology and pharmacology of epicardial, endocardial, and M cells. *Circ Res.* 69:1427-1449, **1991**. *[4]*

Anumonwo JMB, Jalife J: Cellular and subcellular mechanisms of pacemaker activity initiation and synchronization in heart, in Cardiac Electrophysiology: From Cell to Bedside. Zipes DP, Jalife J (eds). *Philadelphia, PA, W.B. Saunders.* 151-164, **1995**. *[4]*

Anumonwo JMB, Freeman LC, Kwok WM, Kass RS: Delayed rectification in single cells isolated from guinea pig sinoatrial node. *Am J Physiol.* 262:H921-H925, **1992**. *[4]*

Anversa P, Kajstura J: Ventricular myocytes are not terminally differentiated in the adult mammalian heart. *Circ Res.* 83:1-14, **1998**. *[10]*

Anversa P, Olivetti G, Melissari M, Loud AV: Morphometric study of myocardial hypertrophy induced by abdominal aortic stenosis. *Lab Invest.* 40:341-349, **1979**. *[10]*

Apkon M, Nerbonne JM: α_1-Adrenergic agonists selectively suppress voltage-dependent K^+ current in rat ventricular myocytes. *Proc Natl Acad Sci USA.* 85:8756-8760, **1988**. *[4,10]*

Arai M, Alpert NR, MacLennan DH, Barton P, Periasamy M: Alterations in sarcoplasmic reticulum gene expression in human heart failure: A possible mechanism for alterations in systolic and diastolic properties of the failing myocardium. *Circ Res.* 72:463-469, **1993**. *[10]*

Argibay JA, Fischmeister R, Hartzell HD: Inactivation, reactivation and pacing dependence of calcium current in frog cardiocytes: Correlation with current density. *J Physiol.* 401:201-226, **1988**. *[5,8]*

Armstrong CM: Interaction of tetraethylammonium ion derivatives with the potassium channels of giant axons. *J Gen Physiol.* 58:413-437, **1971**. *[4]*

Armstrong CM: Ionic pores, gates, and gating currents. *Q Rev Biophys.* 7:179-210, **1974**. *[4]*

Armstrong CM, Bezanilla F: Currents related to movement of the gating particles of the sodium channels. *Nature.* 242:459-461, **1973**. *[4]*

Armstrong CM, Bezanilla F: Inactivation of the sodium channel. II. Gating current experiments. *J Gen Physiol.* 70:567-590, **1977**. *[4]*

Armstrong CM, Neyton J: Ion permeation through calcium channels. A one-site model. *Ann NY Acad Sci.* 635:18-25, **1991**. *[5]*

Armstrong CM, Benzanilla FM, Horowicz P: Twitches in the presence of ethylene glycol bis(β-aminoethyl ether)-N,N'-tetraacetic acid. *Biochim Biophys Acta.* 267:605-608, **1972**. *[8]*

Armstrong CM, Bezanilla F, Rojas E: Destruction of sodium conductance inactivation in squid axons perfused with pronase. *J Gen Physiol.* 62:375-391, **1973**. *[4]*

Arnon A, Hamlyn JM, Blaustein MP: Ouabain augments Ca^{2+} transients in arterial smooth muscle without raising cytosolic Na^+. *Am J Physiol.* 279:H679-H691, **2000**. *[10]*

Artalejo CR, Ariano MA, Perlman RL, Fox AP: Activation of facilitation calcium channels in chromaffin cells by D1 dopamine receptors through a cAMP/protein kinase A-dependent mechanism. *Nature.* 348:239-242, **1990**. *[5]*

Artalejo CR, Rossie S, Perlman RL, Fox AP: Voltage-dependent phosphorylation may recruit Ca^{2+} current facilitation in chromaffin cells. *Nature.* 358:63-66, **1992**. *[5]*

Artman M: Developmental Changes in Myocardial Inotropic Responsiveness. *Austin, TX, Medical Intelligence Unit, R.G. Landes Company.* 1-121, **1994**. *[6]*

Artman M, Ichikawa H, Avkiran M, Coetzee WA: Na^+/Ca^{2+} exchange current density in cardiac myocytes from rabbits and guinea pigs during postnatal development. *Am J Physiol.* 268:H1714-H1722, **1995**. *[9]*

Asahi M, McKenna E, Kurzydlowski K, Tada M, MacLennan DH: Physical interactions between phospholamban and sarco(endo)plasmic reticulum Ca^{2+}-ATPases are dissociated by elevated Ca^{2+}, but not by phospholamban phosphorylation, vanadate, or thapsigargin, and are enhanced by ATP. *J Biol Chem.* 275:15034-15038, **2000**. *[7]*

Ashcroft SJ, Ashcroft FM: Properties and functions of ATP-sensitive K-channels. *Cell Signal.* 2:197-214, **1990**. *[4]*

Ashida T, Schaeffer J, Goldman WF, Wade JB, Blaustein MP: Role of sarcoplasmic reticulum in arterial contraction; comparison of ryanodine's effect in a conduit and a muscular artery. *Circ Res.* 67:854-863, **1988**. *[8]*

Atkison P, Joubert G, Barron A, Grant D, Paradis K, Seidman E, Wall W, Rosenberg H, Howard J, Williams S: Hypertrophic cardiomyopathy associated with tacrolimus in paediatric transplant patients. *Lancet.* 345:894-896, **1995**. *[7]*

Austin C, Wray S: Interactions between Ca^{2+} and H^+ and functional consequences in vascular smooth muscle. *Circ Res.* 86:355-363, **2000**. *[8]*

Autry JM, Jones LR: Functional co-expression of the canine cardiac Ca^{2+} pump and phospholamban in *Spodoptera frugiperda* (Sf21) cells reveals new insights on ATPase regulation. *J Biol Chem.* 272:15872-15880, **1997**. *[7]*

Avkiran M: Protection of the myocardium during ischemia and reperfusion: Na^+/H^+ exchange inhibition versus ischemic preconditioning. *Circulation.* 100:2469-2472, **1999**. *[10]*

Baartscheer A, Schumacher CA, Opthof T, Fiolet JWT: The origin of increased cytoplasmic calcium upon reversal of the Na^+/Ca^{2+} exchanger in isolated rat ventricular myocytes. *J Mol Cell Cardiol.* 28:1963-1973, **1996**. *[8]*

Babcock DF, Herrington J, Goodwin PC, Park YB, Hille B: Mitochondrial participation in the intracellular Ca^{2+} network. *J Cell Biol.* 136:833-844, **1997**. *[3]*

Babu A, Sonnenblick E, Gulati J: Molecular basis for the influence of muscle length on myocardial performance. *Science.* 240:74-76, **1988**. *[2]*

Backx PH, Marbán E: Background potassium current active during the plateau of the action potential in guinea pig ventricular myocytes. *Circ Res.* 72:890-900, **1993**. *[4]*

Backx PH, de Tombe PP, van Deen JHK, Mulder BJ, ter Keurs HEDJ: A model of propagating calcium-induced calcium release mediated by calcium diffusion. *J Gen Physiol.* 93:963-977, **1989**. *[8,10]*

Backx PH, Yue DT, Lawrence JH, Marbán E, Tomaselli GF: Molecular localization of an ion-binding site within the pore of mammalian sodium channels. *Science.* 257:248-251, **1992**. *[4]*

Backx PH, Gao WD, Azan-Backx MD, Marbán E: The relationship between contractile force and intracellular [Ca^{2+}] in intact rat cardiac trabeculae. *J Gen Physiol.* 105:1-19, **1995**. *[2,3]*

Baker PF, Blaustein MP, Hodgkin AL, Steinhardt RA: The influence of calcium on sodium efflux in squid axons. *J Physiol.* 200:431-458, **1969**. *[6,10]*

Baker KM, Chernin MI, Wixson SK, Aceto JF: Renin-angiotensin system involvement in pressure-overload cardiac hyper-trophy in rats. *Am J Physiol.* 259:H324-H332, **1990**. *[10]*

Baker KM, Booz GW, Dostal DE: Cardiac actions of angiotensin II: Role of an intracardiac renin-angiotensin system. *Annu Rev Physiol.* 54:227-241, **1992**. *[10]*

Baker DL, Hashimoto K, Grupp IL, Ji Y, Reed T, Loukianov E, Grupp G, Bhagwhat A, Hoit B, Walsh R, Marbán E, Periasamy M: Targeted overexpression of the sarcoplasmic reticulum Ca^{2+}-ATPase increases cardiac contractility in transgenic mouse hearts. *Circ Res.* 83:1205-1214, **1998**. *[10]*

Balaguru D, Haddock PS, Puglisi JL, Bers DM, Coetzee WA, Artman M: Role of the sarcoplasmic reticulum in contraction and relaxation of immature rabbit ventricular myocytes. *J Mol Cell Cardiol.* 29:2747-2757, **1997**. *[9]*

Balke CW, Egan TM, Wier WG: Processes that remove calcium from the cytoplasm during excitation-contraction coupling in intact rat heart cells. *J Physiol.* 474:447-462, **1994**. *[3,7]*

Balke CW, Goldman L, Aggarwal R, Shorofsky SR: Whether "slip-mode conductance" occurs - Technical Comments. *Science.* 284:711a, **1999**. *[4]*

Ball KL, Johnson MD, Solaro RJ: Isoform specific interactions of troponin I and troponin C determine pH sensitivity of myofibrillar Ca^{2+} activation. *Biochemistry.* 33:8464-8471, **1994**. *[2]*

Ballard C, Schaffer S: Stimulation of the Na^+/Ca^{2+} exchanger by phenylephrine, angiotensin II and endothelin 1. *J Mol Cell Cardiol.* 28:11-17, **1996**. *[6]*

Balligand JL, Kelly RA, Marsden PA, Smith TW, Michel T: Control of cardiac muscle cell function by an endogenous nitric oxide signaling system. *Proc Natl Acad Sci USA.* 90:347-351, **1993**. *[5]*

Balnave CD, Vaughan-Jones RD: Effect of intracellular pH on spontaneous Ca^{2+} sparks in rat ventricular myocytes. *J Physiol.* 528:25-37, **2000**. *[10]*

Balshaw D, Gao L, Meissner G: Luminal loop of the ryanodine receptor: A pore-forming segment? *Proc Natl Acad Sci USA.* 96:3345-3347, **1999**. *[7]*

Banerjee S, Tang XL, Qiu Y, Takano H, Manchikalapudi S, Dawn B, Shirk G, Bolli R: Nitroglycerin induces late pre-conditioning against myocardial stunning via a PKC-dependent pathway. *Am J Physiol.* 277:H2488-H2494, **1999**. *[10]*

Bangalore R, Mehrke G, Gingrich K, Hofmann F, Kass RS: Influence of L-type Ca channel α_2/δ-subunit on ionic and gating current in transiently transfected HEK 293 cells. *Am J Physiol.* 270:H1521-H1528, **1996**. *[5]*

Banijamali HS, Gao WD, MacIntosh BR, ter Keurs HEDJ: Force-interval relations of twitches and cold contractures in rat cardiac trabeculae: Effect of ryanodine. *Circ Res.* 69:937-948, **1991**. *[9]*

Barcenas-Ruiz L, Beuckelmann DJ, Wier WG: Sodium-calcium exchange in heart: Membrane currents and changes in $[Ca^{2+}]_i$. *Science.* 238:1720-1722, **1987**. *[6]*

Barg S, Copello JA, Fleischer S: Different interactions of cardiac and skeletal muscle ryanodine receptors with FK-506 binding protein isoforms. *Am J Physiol.* 272:C1726-C1733, **1997**. *[7]*

Barhanin J, Lesage F, Guillemare E, Fink M, Lazdunski M, Romey G: K_VLQT1 and IsK (minK) proteins associate to form the I_{Ks} cardiac potassium current. *Nature.* 384:78-80, **1996**. *[4]*

Baró I, Eisner DA: The effects of thapsigargin on $[Ca^{2+}]_i$ in isolated rat mesenteric artery vascular smooth muscle cells. *Pflügers Arch.* 420:115-117, **1992**. *[8]*

Barrington PL, Meier CF, Weglicki WB: Abnormal electrical activity induced by free radical generating systems in isolated cardiocytes. *J Mol Cell Cardiol.* 20:1163-1178, **1988**. *[10]*

Barry WH, Smith TW: Movements of Ca across the sarcolemma: Effects of abrupt exposure to zero external Na concentration. *J Mol Cell Cardiol.* 16:155-164, **1984**. *[6]*

Barry WH, Rasmussen CAF Jr, Ishida H, Bridge JHB: External Na-independent Ca extrusion in cultured ventricular cells. *J Gen Physiol.* 88:393-411, **1986**. *[6]*

Barry DM, Trimmer JS, Merlie JP, Nerbonne JM: Differential expression of voltage-gated K^+ channel subunits in adult rat heart: Relation to functional K^+ channels. *Circ Res.* 77:361-369, **1995**. *[4]*

Bartel S, Willenbrock R, Haase H, Karczewski P, Wallukat G, Dietz R, Krause EG: Cyclic GMP-mediated phospholamban phosphorylation in intact cardiomyocytes. *Biochem Biophys Res Commun.* 214:75-80, **1995**. *[7]*

Barth E, Stammler G, Speiser B, Schaper J: Ultrastructural quantitation of mitochondria and myofilaments in cardiac muscle from 10 different animal species including man. *J Mol Cell Cardiol.* 24:669-681, **1992**. *[1,3]*

Barzalai A, Spanier R, Rahamimoff H: Isolation, purification and reconstitution of the Na^+ gradient dependent Ca^{2+} transporter (Na^+-Ca^{2+} exchanger) from brain synaptic plasma membranes. *Proc Natl Acad Sci USA.* 81:6521-6525, **1984**. *[6]*

Barzalai A, Spanier R, Rahamimoff H: Immunological identification of the synaptic plasma membrane Na^+-Ca^{2+} exchanger. *J Biol Chem.* 262:10315-10320, **1987**. *[6]*

Baskin RJ, Deamer DW: Comparative ultrastructure and calcium transport in heart and skeletal muscle microsomes. *J Cell Biol.* 43:610-617, **1969**. *[1]*

Bassani RA, Bers DM: Na-Ca exchange is required for rest-decay but not for rest-potentiation of twitches in rabbit and rat ventricular myocytes. *J Mol Cell Cardiol.* 26:1335-1347, **1994**. *[6,9]*

Bassani RA, Bers DM: Rate of diastolic Ca release from the sarcoplasmic reticulum of intact rabbit and rat ventricular myocytes. *Biophys J.* 68:2015-2022, **1995**. *[3,7,9]*

Bassani RA, Bassani JWM, Bers DM: Mitochondrial and sarcolemmal Ca transport can reduce $[Ca]_i$ during caffeine contractures in rabbit cardiac myocytes. *J Physiol.* 453:591-608, **1992**. *[3]*

Bassani JWM, Bassani RA, Bers DM: Ca^{2+} cycling between sarcoplasmic reticulum and mitochondria in rabbit cardiac myocytes. *J Physiol.* 460:603-621, **1993a**. *[3]*

Bassani JWM, Bassani RA, Bers DM: Twitch-dependent SR Ca accumulation and release in rabbit ventricular myocytes. *Am J Physiol.* 265:C533-C540, **1993b**. *[3,7,8,9]*

Bassani JWM, Bassani RA, Bers DM: Relaxation in rabbit and rat cardiac cells: Species-dependent differences in cellular mechanisms. *J Physiol.* 476:279-293, **1994a**. *[3,6,7,9]*

Bassani RA, Bassani JWM, Bers DM: Relaxation in ferret ventricular myocytes: Unusual interplay among calcium transport systems. *J Physiol.* 476:295-308, **1994b**. *[3,6,9]*

Bassani RA, Bassani JWM, Bers DM: Relaxation in ferret ventricular myocytes: Role of the sarcolemmal Ca ATPase. *Pflügers Arch.* 430:573-578, **1995a**. *[3,6,7,9]*

Bassani JWM, Yuan W, Bers DM: Fractional SR Ca release is regulated by trigger Ca and SR Ca content in cardiac myocytes. *Am J Physiol.* 268:C1313-C1319, **1995b**. *[7,8]*

Bassani RA, Mattiazzi A, Bers DM: CaMKII is responsible for activity-dependent acceleration of relaxation in rat ventricular myocytes. *Am J Physiol.* 268:H703-H712, **1995c**. *[7,9]*

Bassani JWM, Bassani RA, Bers DM: Calibration of indo-1 and resting intracellular $[Ca]_i$ in intact rabbit cardiac myocytes. *Biophys J.* 68:1453-1460, **1995d**. *[3]*

Bassani RA, Shannon TR, Bers DM: Passive Ca^{2+} binding in ventricular myocardium of neonatal and adult rats. *Cell Calcium.* 23:433-442, **1998**. *[3,9]*

Baudet S, Shaoulian R, Bers DM. Effects of thapsigargin and cyclopiazonic acid on twitch force and SR Ca content of rabbit ventricular muscle. *Circ Res.* 73:813-819, **1993**. *[7,9]*

Baxter GF, Marber MS, Patel VC, Yellon DM: Adenosine receptor involvement in a delayed phase of myocardial protection 24 hours after ischemic preconditioning. *Circulation.* 90:2993-3000, **1994**. *[10]*

Baylor SM, Chandler WK: Optical indications of excitation-contraction coupling in striated muscle, in Biophysical Aspects of Cardiac Muscle. Morad M (ed). *New York, NY, Adacemic Press.* 207-228, **1978**. *[7]*

Baylor SM, Chandler WK, Marshall MW: Sarcoplasmic reticulum calcium release in frog skeletal muscle fibres estimated from Arsenazo III calcium transients. *J Physiol.* 344:625-666, **1983**. *[8]*

Beam KG, Adams BA: Reduced intramembrane charge movement in dysgenic skeletal muscle myotubes. *Biophys J.* 57:177a, **1990**. *[8]*

Beam KG, Knudson CM, Powell JA: A lethal mutation in mice eliminates the slow calcium current in skeletal muscle cells. *Nature.* 320:168-170, **1986**. *[8]*

Bean BP: Nitrendipine block of cardiac calcium channels: High-affinity binding to the inactivated state. *Proc Natl Acad Sci USA.* 81:6388-6392, **1984**. *[5]*

Bean BP: Two kinds of calcium channels in canine atrial cells. Differences in kinetics, selectivity, and pharmacology. *J Gen Physiol.* 86:1-30, **1985**. *[5]*

Bean BP: Classes of calcium channels in vertebrate cells. *Annu Rev Physiol.* 51:367-384, **1989**. *[5]*

Bean BP: β-Adrenergic regulation of cardiac calcium channels: Ionic current and gating current. *Biophys J.* 57:23a, **1990**. *[5]*

Bean BP, Ríos E: Nonlinear charge movement in mammalian cardiac ventricular cells. *J Gen Physiol.* 94:65-93, **1989**. *[5,8]*

Bean BP, Nowycky MG, Tsien RW: β-Adrenergic modulation of calcium channels in frog ventricular heart cells. *Nature.* 307:371-375, **1984**. *[5]*

Beavo JA: Multiple isozymes of cyclic nucleotide phosphodiesterase. *Adv Second Messenger Phosphoprotein Res.* 22:1-38, **1988**. *[10]*

Beavo JA, Reifsnyder DH: Primary sequence of cyclic nucleotide phosphodiesterase isozymes and the design of selective inhibitors. *Trends Pharmacol Sci.* 11:150-155, **1990**. *[10]*

Bechem M, Hebisch S, Schramm M: Ca^{2+} agonists: New sensitive probes for Ca^{2+} channels. *Trends Pharmacol Sci.* 9:257-261, **1988**. *[10]*

Bechem M, Goldmann S, Gross R, Hallermann S, Hebisch S, Hütter J, Rounding HP, Schramm M, Stoltefuss J, Straub A: A new type of Ca-channel modulation by a novel class of 1,4-dihydropyridines. *Life Sci.* 60:107-118, **1997**. *[5,10]*

Beeler GW Jr, Reuter H: The relation between membrane potential, membrane currents and activation of contraction in ventricular myocardial fibres. *J Physiol.* 207:211-229, **1970**. *[5]*

Beier N, Harting J, Jonas R, Klockow M, Lues I, Haeusler G: The novel cardiotonic agent EMD 53 998 is a potent "calcium sensitizer". *J Cardiovasc Pharmacol.* 18:17-27, **1991**. *[10]*

Belardinelli L, Isenberg G: Actions of adenosine and isoproterenol on isolated mammalian ventricular myocytes. *Circ Res.* 53:287-297, **1983a**. *[4]*

Belardinelli L, Isenberg G: Isolated atrial myocytes: Adenosine and acetylcholine increase potassium conductance. *Am J Physiol.* 244:H734-H737, **1983b**. *[4]*

Bellemann P, Ferry D, Lubbecke F, Glossmann H: [^{3}H]-nitrendipine, a potent calcium antagonist binds with high affinity to cardiac membranes. *Arzneimittelforsch.* 31:2064-2067, **1981**. *[5]*

Benfey BG: Function of myocardial α-adrenoceptors. *Life Sci.* 46:743-757, **1990**. *[10]*

Benham CD, Bolton TB: Spontaneous transient outward currents in single visceral and vascular smooth muscle cells of the rabbit. *J Physiol.* 381:385-406, **1986**. *[8]*

Benitah JP, Gómez AM, Bailly P, Da PJ, Berson G, Delgado C, Lorente P: Heterogeneity of the early outward current in ventricular cells isolated from normal and hypertrophied rat hearts. *J Physiol.* 469:111-138, **1993**. *[4]*

Benjamin IJ, McMillan DR: Stress (heat shock) proteins: Molecular chaperones in cardiovascular biology and disease. *Circ Res.* 83:117-132, **1998**. *[10]*

Bennett HS: Morphological aspects of extracellular polysaccharides. *J Histochem Cytochem.* 11:14, **1963**. *[1]*

Bennett PB, McKinney LC, Begenisich T, Kass RS: Adrenergic modulation of the delayed rectifier potassium channel in calf cardiac Purkinje fibers. *Biophys J.* 49:839-848, **1986**. *[10]*

Bennett PB, Yazawa K, Makita N, George AL Jr: Molecular mechanism for an inherited cardiac arrhythmia. *Nature.* 376:683-685, **1995**. *[4]*

Beresewicz A, Reuter H: The effects of adrenaline and theophylline on action potential and contraction of mammalian ventricular muscle under "rested-state" and "steady-state" stimulation. *Arch Pharmacol.* 301:99-107, **1977**. *[9]*

Berlin JR: Spatiotemporal changes of Ca^{2+} during electrically evoked contractions in atrial and ventricular cells. *Am J Physiol.* 269:H1165-H1170, **1995**. *[9]*

Berlin JR, Bassani JWM, Bers DM: Intrinsic cytosolic calcium buffering properties of single rat cardiac myocytes. *Biophys J.* 67:1775-1787, **1994**. *[3]*

Berridge MJ: Inositol triphosphate and diacylglycerol: Two interacting second messengers. *Annu Rev Biochem.* 56:159-193, **1987**. *[7,8]*

Berridge MJ: Inositol trisphosphate and calcium signalling. *Nature.* 361:315-325, **1993**. *[8]*

Berridge MJ: Capacitative calcium entry. *Biochem J.* 312:1-11, **1995**. *[8]*

Berridge MJ: Elementary and global aspects of calcium signalling. *J Physiol.* 499:291-306, **1997**. *[8]*

Berridge MJ, Galione A: Cytosolic calcium oscillators. *FASEB J.* 2:3074-3082, **1988**. *[7,8]*

Berridge MJ, Irvine RF: Inositol phosphates and cell signalling. *Nature.* 341:197-205, **1989**. *[7,8]*

Bers DM: A simple method for the accurate determination of free [Ca] in Ca-EGTA solutions. *Am J Physiol.* 242:C404-C408, **1982**. *[2]*

Bers DM: Early transient depletion of extracellular [Ca] during individual cardiac muscle contractions. *Am J Physiol.* 244:H462-H468, **1983**. *[7,9]*

Bers DM: Ca influx and sarcoplasmic reticulum Ca release in cardiac muscle activation during post-rest recovery. *Am J Physiol.* 248:H366-H381, **1985**. *[1,3,7,9]*

Bers DM: Ryanodine and Ca content of cardiac SR assessed by caffeine and rapid cooling contractures. *Am J Physiol.* 253:C408-C415, **1987a**. *[7]*

Bers DM: Mechanisms contributing to the cardiac inotropic effect of Na pump inhibition and reduction of extracellular Na. *J Gen Physiol.* 90:479-504, **1987b**. *[6,7,9,10]*

Bers DM: SR Ca loading in cardiac muscle preparations based on rapid-cooling contractures. *Am J Physiol.* 256:C109-C120, **1989**. *[9]*

Bers DM: <u>Excitation-Contraction Coupling and Cardiac Contractile Force.</u> 1st ed. *Dordrecht, Netherlands, Kluwer Academic Publishers,* **1991**. *[1,3]*

Bers DM, Berlin JR: Kinetics of [Ca]$_i$ decline in cardiac myocytes depend on peak [Ca]$_i$. *Am J Physiol.* 268:C271-C277, **1995**. *[9]*

Bers DM, Bridge JHB: The effect of acetylstrophanthidin on twitches, microscopic tension fluctuations and cooling contractures in rabbit ventricular muscle. *J Physiol.* 404:53-69, **1988**. *[7,10]*

Bers DM, Bridge JHB: Relaxation of rabbit ventricular muscle by Na-Ca exchange and sarcoplasmic reticulum Ca-pump: Ryanodine and voltage sensitivity. *Circ Res.* 65:334-342, **1989**. *[3,6,7]*

Bers DM, Christensen DM: Functional interconversion of rest decay and ryanodine effects in rabbit or rat ventricle depends on Na/Ca exchange. *J Mol Cell Cardiol.* 22:715-723, **1990**. *[9,10]*

Bers DM, Ellis D: Intracellular calcium and sodium activity in sheep heart Purkinje fibers: Effect of changes of external sodium and intracellular pH. *Pflügers Arch.* 393:171-178, **1982.** *[3,10]*

Bers DM, Fill M: Coordinated feet and the dance of ryanodine receptors. *Science.* 281:790-791, **1998.** *[7,8]*

Bers DM, MacLeod KT: Cumulative extracellular Ca depletions in rabbit ventricular muscle monitored with Ca selective microelectrodes. *Circ Res.* 58:769-782, **1986.** *[7,9,10]*

Bers DM, Perez-Reyes E: Ca channels in cardiac myocytes: Structure and function in Ca influx and intracellular Ca release. *Cardiovasc Res.* 42:339-360, **1999.** *[5]*

Bers DM, Peskoff A: Diffusion around a cardiac calcium channel and the role of surface bound calcium. *Biophys J.* 59:703-721, **1991.** *[5,8]*

Bers DM, Stiffel VM: Ratio of ryanodine to dihydropyridine receptors in cardiac and skeletal muscle and implications for E-C coupling. *Am J Physiol.* 264:C1587-C1593, **1993.** *[1,3,5,7,8,10]*

Bers DM, Philipson KD, Nishimoto AY: Sodium-calcium exchange and sidedness of isolated cardiac sarcolemmal vesicles. *Biochim Biophys Acta.* 601:358-371, **1980.** *[6]*

Bers DM, Philipson KD, Langer GA: Cardiac contractility and sarcolemmal calcium binding in several cardiac preparations. *Am J Physiol.* 240:H576-H583, **1981.** *[1]*

Bers DM, Philipson KD, Peskoff A: Calcium at the surface of cardiac plasma membrane vesicles: Cation binding, surface charge screening and Na-Ca exchange. *J Memb Biol.* 85:251-261, **1985.** *[5,6]*

Bers DM, Allen LA, Kim Y: Calcium binding to cardiac sarcolemma isolated from rabbit ventricular muscle: It's possible role in modifying contractile force. *Am J Physiol.* 251:C861-C871, **1986.** *[3]*

Bers DM, Bridge JHB, MacLeod KT: The mechanism of ryanodine action in cardiac muscle assessed with Ca selective microelectrodes and rapid cooling contractures. *Can J Physiol Pharmacol.* 65:610-618, **1987.** *[7,8,9]*

Bers DM, Christensen DM, Nguyen TX: Can Ca entry via Na-Ca exchange directly activate cardiac muscle contraction? *J Mol Cell Cardiol.* 20:405-414, **1988.** *[6,8,10]*

Bers DM, Bridge JHB, Spitzer KW: Intracellular Ca transients during rapid cooling contractures in guinea-pig ventricular myocytes. *J Physiol.* 417:537-553, **1989.** *[6,7,9]*

Bers DM, Lederer WJ, Berlin JR: Intracellular Ca transients in rat cardiac myocytes: Role of Na/Ca exchange in excitation-contraction coupling. *Am J Physiol.* 258:C944-C954, **1990.** *[6,8]*

Bers DM, Hryshko LV, Harrison SM, Dawson DD: Citrate decreases contraction and Ca current in cardiac muscle independent of its buffering action. *Am J Physiol.* 260:C900-C909, **1991.** *[9]*

Bers DM, Bassani RA, Bassani JWM, Baudet S, Hryshko LV: Paradoxical twitch potentiation after rest in cardiac muscle: Increased fractional release of SR calcium. *J Mol Cell Cardiol.* 25:1047-1057, **1993.** *[9]*

Bers DM, Patton CW, Nuccitelli R: A practical guide to the preparation of Ca²⁺ buffers. *Methods Cell Biol.* 40:3-29, **1994.** *[2]*

Bersohn MM, Philipson KD, Fukushima JY: Sodium-calcium exchange and sarcolemmal enzymes in ischemic rabbit hearts. *Am J Physiol.* 242:C288-C295, **1982.** *[6]*

Best PM, Donaldson SKB, Kerrick WGL: Tension in mechanically disrupted mammalian cardiac cells: Effects of magnesium adenosine triphosphate. *J Physiol.* 265:1-17, **1977.** *[2]*

Beuckelmann DJ, Erdmann E: Ca²⁺-currents and intracellular [Ca²⁺]-transients in single ventricular myocytes isolated from terminally failing human myocardium. *Basic Res Cardiol.* 87:I235-I243, **1992.** *[10]*

Beuckelmann DJ, Wier WG: Mechanism of release of calcium from sarcoplasmic reticulum of guinea-pig cardiac cells. *J Physiol.* 405:233-255, **1988.** *[8]*

Beuckelmann DJ, Wier WG: Sodium-calcium exchange in guinea-pig cardiac cells: Exchange current and changes in intracellular Ca²⁺. *J Physiol.* 414:499-520, **1989.** *[6]*

Beuckelmann DJ, Näbauer M, Erdmann E: Intracellular calcium handling in isolated ventricular myocytes from patients with terminal heart failure. *Circulation.* 85:1046-1055, **1992.** *[10]*

Beuckelmann DJ, Näbauer M, Erdmann E: Alterations of K⁺ currents in isolated human ventricular myocytes from patients with terminal heart failure. *Circ Res.* 73:379-385, **1993.** *[4,10]*

Beurg M, Sukhareva M, Strube C, Powers PA, Gregg RG, Coronado R: Recovery of Ca²⁺ current, charge movements, and Ca²⁺ transients in myotubes deficient in dihydropyridine receptor β₁ subunit transfected with β₁ cDNA. *Biophys J.* 73:807-818, **1997.** *[8]*

Beurg M, Sukhareva M, Ahern CA, Conklin MW, Perez-Reyes E, Powers PA, Gregg RG, Coronado R: Differential regulation of skeletal muscle L-type Ca²⁺ current and excitation-contraction coupling by the dihydropyridine receptor β subunit. *Biophys J.* 76:1744-1756, **1999a.** *[8]*

Beurg M, Ahern CA, Vallejo P, Conklin MW, Powers PA, Gregg RG, Coronado R: Involvement of the carboxy-terminus region of the dihydropyridine receptor β₁ₐ subunit in excitation-contraction coupling of skeletal muscle. *Biophys J.* 77:2953-2967, **1999b.** *[8]*

Beyer ED, Paul D, Goodenough DA: Connexin43: A protein from rat heart homologous to a gap junction protein from liver. *J Cell Biol.* 105:2621-2629, **1987.** *[1]*

Beyer EC, Kistler J, Paul DL, Goodenough DA: Antisera directed against connexin43 peptides react with a 43-kD protein localized to gap junctions in myocardium and other tissues. *J Cell Biol.* 108:595-605, **1989.** *[1]*

Bezprozvanny I, Ehrlich BE: ATP modulates the function of inositol 1,4,5-trisphosphate-gated channels at two sites. *Neuron.* 10:1175-1184, **1993.** *[7]*

Bezprozvanny I, Ehrlich BE: Inositol (1,4,5)-trisphosphate (InsP3)-gated Ca channels from cerebellum: Conduction properties for divalent cations and regulation by intraluminal calcium. *J Gen Physiol.* 104:821-856, **1994.** *[7]*

Bezprozvanny I, Ehrlich BE: The inositol 1,4,5-trisphosphate (InsP3) receptor. *J Membr Biol.* 145:205-216, **1995.** *[7]*

Bezprozvanny I, Watras J, Ehrlich BE: Bell-shaped calcium-response curves of Ins(1,4,5)P3- and calcium-gated channels from endoplasmic reticulum of cerebellum. *Nature.* 351:751-754, **1991.** *[7]*

Bhatnagar A, Srivastava SK, Szabo G: Oxidative stress alters specific membrane currents in isolated cardiac myocytes. *Circ Res.* 67:535-549, **1990.** *[10]*

Bhojani IH, Chapman RA: The effects of bathing sodium ions upon the intracellular sodium activity in calcium-free media and the calcium paradox of isolated ferret ventricular muscle. *J Mol Cell Cardiol.* 22:507-522, **1990**. *[1]*

Bielefeld DR, Hadley RW, Vassilev PM, Hume JR: Membrane electrical properties of vesicular sodium-calcium exchange inhibitors in single atrial myocytes. *Circ Res.* 59:381-389, **1986**. *[6]*

Bielen FV, Glitsch HG, Verdonck F: Na+ pump current-voltage relationships of rabbit cardiac Purkinje cells in Na+-free solution. *J Physiol.* 465:699-714, **1993**. *[4]*

Biermans G, Vereecke J, Carmeliet E: The mechanism of the inactivation of the inward-rectifying K current during hyperpolarizing steps in guinea-pig ventricular myocytes. *Pflügers Arch.* 410:604-613, **1987**. *[4]*

Blanchard EM, Solaro RJ: Inhibition of the activation of troponin calcium binding of dog cardiac myofibrils by acidic pH. *Circ Res.* 55:382-391, **1984**. *[2,10]*

Blanco G, Mercer RW: Isozymes of the Na-K-ATPase: Heterogeneity in structure, diversity in function. *Am J Physiol.* 275:F633-F650, **1998**. *[4]*

Blatter LA: Depletion and filling of intracellular calcium stores in vascular smooth muscle. *Am J Physiol.* 268:C503-C512, **1995**. *[8]*

Blatter LA, McGuigan JA: Free intracellular magnesium concentration in ferret ventricular muscle measured with ion selective micro-electrodes. *Q J Exp Physiol.* 71:467-473, **1986**. *[3]*

Blatter LA, Niggli E: Confocal near-membrane detection of calcium in cardiac myocytes. *Cell Calcium.* 23:269-279, **1998**. *[1]*

Blatter LA, Hüser J, Ríos E: Sarcoplasmic reticulum Ca²⁺ release flux underlying Ca²⁺ sparks in cardiac muscle. *Proc Natl Acad Sci USA.* 94:4176-4181, **1997**. *[7]*

Blaustein MP: Sodium-calcium exchange in mammalian smooth muscles, in Sodium-Calcium Exchange. Allen TJA, Noble D, Reuter H (eds). *New York, NY, Oxford University Press.* 208-232, **1989**. *[6]*

Blaustein MP, Lederer WJ: Sodium/calcium exchange: Its physiological implications. *Physiol Rev.* 79:763-854, **1999**. *[6]*

Blinks JR: Intracellular [Ca] measurements, in The Heart and Cardiovascular System. Fozzard HA (ed). *New York, NY, Raven Press.* 671-701, **1986**. *[3]*

Blinks JR, Endoh M: Sulmazol (AR-L 115 BS) alters the relation between [Ca²⁺] and tension in living canine ventricular muscle. *J Physiol.* 353:63P, **1984**. *[10]*

Blinks JR, Koch-Weser J: Analysis of the effects of changes in rate and rhythm upon myocardial contractility. *J Pharmacol Exp Ther.* 134:373-389, **1961**. *[9]*

Blinks JR, Koch-Weser J: Physical factors in the analysis of the actions of drugs on myocardial contractility. *Pharmacol Rev.* 15:531-599, **1963**. *[10]*

Blinks JR, Cai YD, Lee NKM: Inositol 1,4,5-trisphosphate causes calcium release in frog skeletal muscle only when transverse tubules have been interrupted. *J Physiol.* 394:23P, **1987**. *[8]*

Bloch RJ: The membrane-asociated cytoskeleton and exoskeleton, in Molecular Biology of Membrane Transport Disorders. Schultz SG (ed). *New York, NY, Plenum Press.* **1996**. *[1]*

Block BA, Imagawa T, Campbell KP, Franzini-Armstrong C: Structural evidence for direct interaction between the molecular components of the transverse tubule/sarcoplasmic reticulum junction in skeletal muscle. *J Cell Biol.* 107:2587-2600, **1988**. *[1,8]*

Blondel O, Takeda J, Janssen H, Seino S, Bell GI: Sequence and functional characterization of a third inositol trisphosphate receptor subtype, IP3R-3, expressed in pancreatic islets, kidney, gastrointestinal tract, and other tissues. *J Biol Chem.* 268:11356-11363, **1993**. *[7]*

Blood BE: The influences of low doses of ouabain and potassium ions on sheep Purkinje fibre contractility. *J Physiol.* 266:76-77, **1975**. *[10]*

Bluhm WF, Kranias EG, Dillmann WH, Meyer M: Phospholamban: A major determinant of the cardiac force-frequency relationship . *Am J Physiol.* 278:H249-H255, **2000**. *[9]*

Bode DC, Brunton LL: Post-receptor modulation of the effects of cyclic AMP in isolated cardiac myocytes. *Mol Cell Biochem.* 82:13-18, **1988**. *[10]*

Bode DC, Kanter J, Brunton LL: Cellular distribution of phosphodiesterase isoforms in rat cardiac tissue. *Circ Res.* 68:1070-1079, **1991**. *[10]*

Boerth SR, Zimmer DB, Artman M: Steady-state mRNA levels of the sarcolemmal Na+-Ca²⁺ exchanger peak near birth in developing rabbit and rat hearts. *Circ Res.* 74:354-359, **1994**. *[9]*

Bogdanov KY, Zakharov SI, Rosenshtraukh LV: The origin of two components in contraction of guinea-pig papillary muscle in the presence of noradrenaline. *Can J Physiol Pharmacol.* 57:866-872, **1979**. *[10]*

Böhm M, Gierschik P, Jakobs KH, Pieske B, Schnabel P, Ungerer M, Erdmann E: Increase of Giα in human hearts with dilated but not ischemic cardiomyopathy. *Circulation.* 82:1249-1265, **1990**. *[10]*

Bolli R: Mechanism of myocardial "stunning". *Circulation.* 82:723-738, **1990**. *[10]*

Bolli R: The late phase of preconditioning. *Circ Res.* 87:972-983, **2000**. *[10]*

Bolli R, Marbán E: Molecular and cellular mechanisms of myocardial stunning. *Physiol Rev.* 79:609-634, **1999**. *[10]*

Bolli R, Bhatti ZA, Tang XL, Qiu Y, Zhang Q, Guo Y, Jadoon AK: Evidence that late preconditioning against myocardial stunning in conscious rabbits is triggered by the generation of nitric oxide. *Circ Res.* 81:42-52, **1997**. *[10]*

Bolton TB, Prestwich SA, Zholos AV, Gordienko DV: Excitation-contraction coupling in gastrointestinal and other smooth muscles. *Annu Rev Physiol.* 61:85-115, **1999**. *[8]*

Bond RA, Leff P, Johnson TD, Milano CA, Rockman HA, McMinn TR, Apparsundaram S, Hyek MF, Kenakin TP, Allen LF, Lefkowitz RJ: Physiological effects of inverse agonists in transgenic mice with myocardial overexpression of the β₂-adrenoceptor. *Nature.* 374:272-276, **1995**. *[10]*

Boraso A, Williams AJ: Modification of the gating of the cardiac sarcoplasmic reticulum Ca²⁺-release channel by H₂O₂ and dithiothreitol. *Am J Physiol.* 267:H1010-H1016, **1994**. *[10]*

Bosse E, Regulla S, Biel M, Ruth P, Meyer HE, Flockerzi V, Hofmann F: The cDNA and deduced amino acid sequence of the γ subunit of the L-type calcium channel from rabbit skeletal muscle. *FEBS Lett.* 267:153-156, **1990**. *[5]*

Bossen EH, Sommer JR: Comparative stereology of the lizard and frog myocardium. *Tissue Cell.* 16:173-178, **1984**. *[1]*

Bossen EH, Sommer JR, Waugh RA: Comparative stereology of the mouse and finch left ventricle. *Tissue Cell.* 10:773-784, **1978**. *[1]*

Bossen EH, Sommer JR, Waugh RA: Comparative stereology of mouse atria. *Tissue Cell.* 13:71-77, **1981**. *[1]*

Bou-Abboud E, Nerbonne JM: Molecular correlates of the calcium-independent, depolarization-activated K^+ currents in rat atrial myocytes. *J Physiol.* 517:407-420, **1999**. *[4]*

Bouchard RA, Bose D: Analysis of the interval-force relationship in rat and canine ventricular myocardium. *Am J Physiol.* 257:H2036-H2047, **1989**. *[9]*

Bouchard RA, Clark RB, Giles WR: Role of sodium-calcium exchange in activation of contraction in rat ventricle. *J Physiol.* 472:391-413, **1993**. *[8]*

Bountra C, Vaughan-Jones RD: Effect of intracellular and extracellular pH on contraction in isolated mammalian cardiac tissue. *J Physiol.* 418:163-187, **1989**. *[10]*

Bountra C, Powell T, Vaughan-Jones RD: Comparison of intracellular pH transients in single ventricular myocytes and isolated ventricular muscle of guinea-pig. *J Physiol.* 424:343-365, **1990**. *[3]*

Bowditch HP: Über die Eigenthümlichkeiten der Reizbarkeit, welche die Muskelfasern des Herzens zeigen. *Ber Sachs Ges Wiss.* 23:652-689, **1871**. *[9]*

Boyett MR, Fedida D: The effect of heart rate on the membrane currents of isolated sheep Purkinje fibres. *J Physiol.* 399:467-491, **1988**. *[5]*

Boyett MR, Jewell BR: A study of the factors responsible for rate-dependent shortening of the action potential in mammalian ventricular muscle. *J Physiol.* 285:359-380, **1978**. *[8]*

Boyett MR, Jewell BR: Analysis of the effects of changes in rate and rhythm upon electrical activity of the heart. *Prog Biophys Molec Biol.* 36:1-52, **1980**. *[8]*

Boyett MR, Hart G, Levi AJ, Roberts A: Effects of repetitive activity on developed force and intracellular sodium in isolated sheep and dog Purkinje fibres. *J Physiol.* 388:295-322, **1987**. *[9]*

Boyle WA, Nerbonne JM: A novel type of depolarization-activated K^+ current in isolated adult rat atrial myocytes. *Am J Physiol.* 260:H1236-H1247, **1991**. *[4]*

Brady AJ: Length dependence of passive stiffness in single cardiac myocytes. *Am J Physiol.* 260:H1062-H1071, **1991**. *[1]*

Brahmajothi MV, Campbell DL, Rasmusson RL, Morales MJ, Trimmer JS, Nerbonne JM, Strauss HC: Distinct transient outward potassium current (I_{to}) phenotypes and distribution of fast-inactivating potassium channel α subunits in ferret left ventricular myocytes. *J Gen Physiol.* 113:581-600, **1999**. *[4]*

Brandes R, Bers DM: Intracellular Ca^{2+} increases the mitochondrial NADH concentration during elevated work in intact cardiac muscle. *Circ Res.* 80:82-87, **1997**. *[3]*

Brandes R, Maier LS, Bers DM: Regulation of mitochondrial [NADH] by cytosolic $[Ca^{2+}]$ and work in trabeculae from hypertrophic and normal rat hearts. *Circ Res.* 82:1189-1198, **1998**. *[10]*

Brandl CJ, Green NM, Korczak B, MacLennan DH: Two Ca^{2+} ATPase genes: Homologies and mechanistic implications of deduced amino acid sequences. *Cell.* 44:597-607, **1986**. *[7]*

Brandl CJ, deLeon S, Martin DR, MacLennan DH: Adult forms of the Ca^{2+} ATPase of sarcoplasmic reticulum. *J Biol Chem.* 262:3768-3774, **1987**. *[7]*

Brandt N: Identification of two populations of cardiac microsomes with nitrendipine receptors: Correlation of the distribution of dihydropyridine receptors with organelle specific markers. *Archiv Biochem Biophys.* 242:306-319, **1985**. *[1]*

Brandt NR, Caswell AN, Wen SR, Talvenheimo JA: Molecular interactions of the junctional foot protein and dihydropyridine receptor in skeletal muscle triads. *J Memb Biol.* 113:237-251, **1990**. *[8]*

Braun AP, Schulman H: The multifunctional calcium/calmodulin-dependent protein kinase: From form to function. *Annu Rev Physiol.* 57:417-445, **1995**. *[9,10]*

Braunwald E, Kloner RA: The stunned myocardium: Prolonged, postischemic ventricular dysfunction. *Circulation.* 66:1146-1149, **1982**. *[10]*

Braunwald E, Rutherford JD: Reversible ischemic left ventricular dysfunction: evidence for the "hibernating myocardium". *J Am Coll Cardiol.* 8:1467-1470, **1986**. *[10]*

Braveny P, Kruta V: Dissociation de deux facteurs: Restitution et potentiatoin dens l'action de l'intervalle sur l'amplitude de la contraction du myocarde. *Arch Int Physiol Biochim.* 66:633-652, **1958**. *[9]*

Braveny P, Sumbera J: Electromechanical correlations in the mammalian heart muscle. *Pflügers Arch.* 319:36-48, **1970**. *[9]*

Brenner B: Mechanical and structural approaches to correlation of cross-bridge action in muscle with actomyosin ATPase in solution. *Annu Rev Physiol.* 49:655-672, **1987**. *[2]*

Brenner B, Eisenberg E: Rate of force generation in muscle: Correlation with actomyosin ATPase activity in solution. *Proc Natl Acad Sci USA.* 83:3542-3546, **1986**. *[2]*

Bridge JHB: Relationships between the sarcoplasmic reticulum and transarcolemmal Ca transport revealed by rapidly cooling rabbit ventricular muscle. *J Gen Physiol.* 88:437-473, **1986**. *[7,9]*

Bridge JHB, Bersohn MM, Gonzalez F, Bassingthwaighte JB: Synthesis and use of radio cobaltic EDTA as an extracellular marker in rabbit heart. *Am J Physiol.* 242:H671-H676, **1982**. *[1]*

Bridge JHB, Spitzer KW, Ershler PR: Relaxation of isolated ventricular cardiomyocytes by a voltage-sensitive process. *Science.* 241:823-825, **1988**. *[6]*

Bridge JHB, Smolley JR, Spitzer KW: Isolation of the sodium-calcium exchange current underlying sodium-dependent relaxation in heart muscle. *Science.* 248:376-378, **1990**. *[6]*

Bridge JHB, Ershler PR, Cannell MB: Properties of Ca^{2+} sparks evoked by action potentials in mouse ventricular myocytes. *J Physiol.* 518:469-478, **1999**. *[7,8]*

Briggs FN, Lee KF, Wechsler AW, Jones LR: Phospholamban expressed in slow-twitch and chronically stimulated fast-twitch muscles minimally affects calcium affinity of sarcoplasmic reticulum Ca^{2+}-ATPase. *J Biol Chem.* 267:26056-26061, **1992**. *[7]*

Brillantes AM, Allen P, Takahashi T, Izumo S, Marks AR: Differences in cardiac calcium release channel (ryanodine receptor) expression in myocardium from patients with end-stage heart failure caused by ischemic versus dilated cardiomyopathy. *Circ Res.* 71:18-26, **1992**. *[10]*

Brillantes AM, Ondrias K, Scott A, Kobrinsky E, Ondriasová E, Moschella MC, Jayaraman T, Landers M, Ehrlich BE, Marks AR: Stabilization of calcium release channel (ryanodine receptor) function by FK506-binding protein. *Cell.* 77:513-523, **1994**. *[7]*

Bristow MR, Ginsburg R, Minobe W, Cubicciotti RS, Sageman WS, Lurie K, Billingham ME, Harrison DC, Stinson EB: Decreased catecholamine sensitivity and β-adrenergic receptor density in failing human hearts. *N Engl J Med.* 307:205-211, **1982**. *[10]*

Bristow MR, Ginsburg R, Umans V, Fowler M, Minobe W, Stinson EB: β₁- and β₂-adrenergic receptor subpopulations in nonfailing and failing human ventricular myocardium: Coupling of both receptor subtypes to muscle contraction and selective β₁-receptor downregulation in heart failure. *Circ Res.* 59:297-309, **1986**. *[10]*

Bristow MR, Hershberger RE, Port JD, Minobe W, Rasmussen R: β₁-and β₂-adrenergic receptor-mediated adenylate cyclase stimulation in nonfailing and failing human ventricular muscle. *Mol Pharmacol.* 35:295-303, **1989**. *[10]*

Brodde OE: β-Adrenoceptors in cardiac disease. *Pharmacol Ther.* 60:405-430, **1993**. *[10]*

Brodde OE: β-adrenergic receptors in failing human myocardium. *Basic Res Cardiol.* 91:II35-II40, **1996**. *[10]*

Brodde OE, Michel MC: Adrenergic and muscarinic receptors in the human heart. *Pharmacol Rev.* 51:651-689, **1999**. *[10]*

Brodde OE, Vogelsang M, Broede A, Michel-Reher M, Beisenbusch-Schafer E, Hakim K, Zerkowski HR: Diminished responsiveness of Gs-coupled receptors in severely failing human hearts: No difference in dilated versus ischemic cardiomyopathy. *J Cardiovasc Pharmacol.* 31:585-594, **1998**. *[10]*

Brown JH, Jones LG: Phosphoinositide metabolism in the heart, in Phosphoinositides and Receptor Mechanisms. Putney JW Jr (ed). *New York, NY, Alan R. Liss, Inc.* 245-270, **1986**. *[7,10]*

Brown AM, Kunze DL, Yatani A: The agonist effect of dihydropyridines on Ca channels. *Nature.* 311:570-572, **1984**. *[5]*

Brown AM, Kunze DL, Yatani A: Dual effects of dihydropyridines on whole cell and unitary calcium currents in single ventricular cells of guinea-pig. *J Physiol.* 379:495-514, **1986**. *[5]*

Brückner R, Scholz H: Effects of α-adrenoceptor stimulation with phenylephrine in the presence of propranolol on force of contraction, slow inward current and cyclic AMP content in the bovine heart. *Br J Pharmacol.* 82:223-232, **1984**. *[10]*

Brum G, Flockerzi V, Hofmann F, Osterrieder W, Trautwein W: Injection of catalytic subunit of cAMP-dependent protein kinase into isolated cardiac myocytes. *Pflügers Arch.* 398:147-154, **1983**. *[5]*

Brum G, Osterrieder W, Trautwein W: β-adrenergic increase in the calcium conductance of cardiac myocytes studied with the patch clamp. *Pflügers Arch.* 401:111-118, **1984**. *[5]*

Brum G, Ríos E, Stefani E: Effects of extracellular calcium on calcium movements of excitation-contraction coupling in frog skeletal muscle fibres. *J Physiol.* 398:441-473, **1988a**. *[8]*

Brum G, Fitts R, Pizarró G, Ríos E: Voltage sensors of the frog skeletal muscle membrane require calcium to function in excitation-contraction coupling. *J Physiol.* 398:475-505, **1988b**. *[8]*

Buggisch D, Isenberg G, Ravens U, Scholtysik G: The role of sodium channels in the effects of the cardiotonic compound DPI 201-106 on contractility and membrane potentials in isolated mammalian heart preparations. *Eur J Pharmacol.* 118:303-311, **1985**. *[10]*

Bünemann M, Gerhardstein BL, Gao TY, Hosey MM: Functional regulation of L-type calcium channels via protein kinase A-mediated phosphorylation of the β₂ subunit. *J Biol Chem.* 274:33851-33854, **1999**. *[5]*

Buntinas L, Gunter KK, Sparagna GC, Gunter TE: Further characteristics of the rapid mechanism of mitochondrial calcium uptake in heart mitochondria. *Biophys J.* 72:A409, **1997**. *[3]*

Burgess GM, Bird GS, Obie JF, Putney JW Jr: The mechanism for synergism between phospholipa. *J Biol Chem.* 266:4772-4781, **1991**. *[7]*

Burt JM: Block of intercellular communication: Interaction of intracellular H⁺ and Ca²⁺. *Am J Physiol.* 253:C607-C612, **1987**. *[1]*

Busch AE, Malloy K, Groh WJ, Varnum MD, Adelman JP, Maylie J: The novel class III antiarrhythmics NE-10064 and NE-10133 inhibit IsK channels expressed in *Xenopus* oocytes and IKS in guinea pig cardiac myocytes. *Biochem Biophys Res Commun.* 202:265-270, **1994**. *[4]*

Butcher RW, Sutherland EW: Adenosine 3',5'-phosphate in biological materials. I. Purification and properties of cyclic 3',5'-nucleotide phosphodiesterase and the use of this enzyme to characterize adenosine 3',5'-phosphate in human urine. *J Biol Chem.* 237:1244-1250, **1962**. *[7,9,10]*

Buxton ILO, Brunton LL: Action of the cardiac α₁-adrenergic receptor activation of cyclic AMP degradation. *J Biol Chem.* 26:6733-6737, **1985**. *[10]*

Cachelin AB, DePeyer JE, Kokubun S, Reuter H: Ca²⁺ channel modulation by 8-bromocyclic AMP in cultured heart cells. *Nature.* 304:462-464, **1983**. *[5]*

Cahalan MD, Almers W: Block of sodium conductance and gating current in squid giant axons poisoned with quaternary strychnine. *Biophys J.* 27:57-73, **1979**. *[4]*

Cahill MA, Janknecht R, Nordheim A: Signalling pathways: Jack of all cascades. *Curr Biol.* 6:16-19, **1996**. *[8]*

Caillé J, Ildefonse M, Rougier O: Evidence of an action of sodium ions in the activation of contraction of twitch muscle fibre. *Pflügers Arch.* 379:117-119, **1979**. *[8]*

Caldwell JJS, Caswell AH: Identification of a constituent of the junctional feet linking the terminal cisternae to transverse tubules in skeletal muscle. *J Cell Biol.* 93:543-550, **1982**. *[1]*

Callewaert G, Cleemann L, Morad M: Epinephrine enhances Ca²⁺ current-regulated Ca²⁺ release and Ca²⁺ reuptake in rat ventricular myocytes. *Proc Natl Acad Sci USA.* 85:2009-2013, **1988**. *[8]*

Callewaert G, Cleemann L, Morad M: Caffeine-induced Ca²⁺ release activates Ca²⁺ extrusion via Na⁺-Ca²⁺ exchanger in cardiac myocytes. *Am J Physiol.* 257:C147-C152, **1989**. *[7]*

Cameron AM, Steiner JP, Sabatini DM, Kaplin AI, Walensky LD, Snyder SH: Immunophilin FK506 binding protein associated with inositol 1,4,5-trisphosphate receptor modulates calcium flux. *Proc Natl Acad Sci USA.* 92:1784-1788, **1995**. *[7]*

Cameron AM, Nucifora FC Jr, Fung ET, Livingston DJ, Aldape RA, Ross CA, Snyder SH: FKBP12 binds the inositol 1,4,5-

trisphosphate receptor at leucine-proline (1400-1401) and anchors calcineurin to this FK506-like domain. *J Biol Chem.* 272:27582-27588, **1997**. *[7]*

Campbell KP: Protein components and their roles in sarcoplasmic reticulum function, in <u>Sarcoplasmic Reticulum in Muscle Physiology</u>. Entman ML, Van Winkle WB (eds). *Boca Raton, FL, CRC Press, Inc.* 65-99, **1986**. *[7]*

Campbell KP: Three muscular dystrophies: Loss of cytoskeleton-extracellular matrix linkage. *Cell.* 80:675-679, **1995**. *[1]*

Campbell KP, Franzini-Armstrong C, Shamoo AE: Further characterization of light and heavy sarcoplasmic reticulum vesicles. Identification of the "sarcoplasmic reticulum feet" associated with heavy sarcoplasmic reticulum vesicles. *Biochim Biophys Acta.* 602:97-116, **1980**. *[7]*

Campbell KP, MacLennan DH, Jorgensen AO, Mintzer MC: Purification and characterization of calsequestrin from canine cardiac sarcoplasmic reticulum and identification of the 53,000 Dalton glycoprotein. *J Biol Chem.* 258:1197-1204, **1983**. *[7]*

Campbell KP, Imagawa T, Smith JS, Coronado R: Purified ryanodine receptor from skeletal muscle sarcoplasmic reticulum is the Ca^{2+}-permeable pore of the calcium release channel. *J Biol Chem.* 262:16636-16643, **1987**. *[7]*

Campbell DL, Rasmusson RL, Strauss HC: Theoretical study of the voltage and concentration dependence of the anomalous mole fraction effect in single calcium channels. New insights into the characterization of multi-ion channels. *Biophys J.* 54:945-954, **1988**. *[4]*

Cannell MB, Lederer WJ: The arrhythmogenic current I_{TI} in the absence of electrogenic sodium-calcium exchange in sheep cardiac Purkinje fibres. *J Physiol.* 374:201-219, **1986**. *[10]*

Cannell MB, Soeller C: Numerical analysis of ryanodine receptor activation by L-type channel activity in the cardiac muscle diad. *Biophys J.* 73:112-122, **1997**. *[8]*

Cannell MB, Eisner DA, Lederer WJ, Valdeolmillos M: Effects of membrane potential on intracellular calcium concentration in sheep Purkinje fibres in sodium-free solutions. *J Physiol.* 381:193-203, **1986**. *[6]*

Cannell MB, Berlin JR, Lederer WJ: Effect of membrane potential changes on the calcium transient in single rat cardiac muscle cells. *Science.* 238:1419-1423, **1987**. *[6,8]*

Cannell MB, Cheng H, Lederer WJ: Spatial non-uniformities in $[Ca^{2+}]_i$ during excitation- contraction coupling in cardiac myocytes. *Biophys J.* 67:1942-1956, **1994**. *[7,8]*

Cannell MB, Cheng H, Lederer WJ: The control of calcium release in heart muscle. *Science.* 268:1045-1049, **1995**. *[7,8]*

Capogrossi MC, Lakatta EG: Frequency modulation and synchronization of spontaneous oscillations in cardiac cells. *Am J Physiol.* 248:H412-H418, **1985**. *[10]*

Capogrossi MC, Kort AA, Spurgeon HA, Lakatta EG: Single adult rabbit and rat cardiac myocytes retain the Ca^{2+}-and species-dependent systolic and diastolic contractile properties of intact muscle. *J Gen Physiol.* 88:589-613, **1986a**. *[8,10]*

Capogrossi MC, Suarez-Isla BA, Lakatta EG: The interaction of electrically stimulated twitches and spontaneous contractile waves in single cardiac myocytes. *J Gen Physiol.* 88:615-633, **1986b**. *[8,10]*

Capogrossi MC, Houser SR, Bahinski A, Lakatta EG: Synchronous occurrence of spontaneous localized calcium release from the sarcoplasmic reticulum generates action potentials in rat cardiac ventricular myocytes at normal resting membrane potential. *Circ Res.* 61:498-503, **1987**. *[10]*

Caputo C, Benzanilla F, Horowicz P: Depolarization-contraction coupling in short frog muscle fibers. *J Gen Physiol.* 84:133-154, **1984**. *[8]*

Carafoli E: Mitochondria, Ca^{2+} transport and the regulation of heart contraction and metabolism. *J Mol Cell Cardiol.* 7:83-89, **1975**. *[3]*

Carafoli E: Intracellular calcium homeostasis. *Annu Rev Biochem.* 56:395-433, **1987**. *[3]*

Carafoli E: Biogenesis - Plasma membrane calcium ATPase: 15 years of work on the purified enzyme. *FASEB J.* 8:993-1002, **1994**. *[6]*

Carafoli E, Lehninger AL: A survey of the interaction of calcium ions with mitochondria from different tissues and species. *Biochem J.* 122:618-690, **1971**. *[3]*

Carafoli E, Stauffer T: The plasma membrane calcium pump: Functional domains, regulation of the activity, and tissue specificity of isoform expression. *J Neurobiol.* 25:312-324, **1994**. *[6]*

Carl SL, Felix K, Caswell AH, Brandt NR, Ball WJJ, Vaghy PL, Meissner G, Ferguson DG: Immunolocalization of sarcolemmal dihydropyridine receptor and sarcoplasmic reticular triadin and ryanodine receptor in rabbit ventricle and atrium. *J Cell Biol.* 129:672-682, **1995**. *[1]*

Carmeliet E: Use-dependent block and use-dependent unblock of the delayed rectifier K^+ current by almokalant in rabbit ventricular myocytes. *Circ Res.* 73:857-868, **1993**. *[4]*

Carmeliet E: Cardiac ionic currents and acute ischemia: From channels to arrhythmias. *Physiol Rev.* 79:917-1017, **1999**. *[4]*

Caroni P, Carafoli E: An ATP-dependent Ca^{2+}-pumping system in dog heart sarcolemma. *Nature.* 283:765-767, **1980**. *[6]*

Caroni P, Carafoli E: The Ca^{2+}-pumping ATPase of heart sarcolemma. *J Biol Chem.* 256:3263-3270, **1981a**. *[6]*

Caroni P, Carafoli E: Regulation of Ca^{2+}-pumping ATPase of heart sarcolemma by a phosphoylation-dephosphorylation process. *J Biol Chem.* 256:9371-9373, **1981b**. *[6]*

Caroni P, Carafoli E: The regulation of the Na^+-Ca^{2+} exchanger of heart sarcolemma. *Eur J Biochem.* 132:451-460, **1983**. *[6]*

Caroni P, Reinlib L, Carafoli E: Charge movements during the Na^+-Ca^{2+} exchange in heart sarcolemmal vesicles. *Proc Natl Acad Sci USA.* 77:6354-6358, **1980**. *[6]*

Caroni P, Villani F, Carafoli E: The cardiotoxic antibiotic doxorubicin inhibits the Na^+/Ca^{2+} exchange of dog heart sarcolemmal vesicles. *FEBS Lett.* 130:184-186, **1981**. *[6]*

Carsten M, Miller J: Ca^{2+} release by inositol trisphosphate from Ca^{2+}-transporting microsomes derived from uterine sarcoplasmic reticulum. *Biochem Biophys Res Commun.* 130:1027-1031, **1985**. *[8]*

Caswell AH, Corbett AM: Interaction of glyceraldehyde-3-phosphate dehydrogenase with isolated muscle subfractions of skeletal muscle. *J Biol Chem.* 269:6892-6898, **1985**. *[8]*

Caswell AH, Lau YH, Garcia M, Brunschwig JP: Recognition and junction formation by isolated transverse tubules and terminal cisternae of skeletal muscle. *J Biol Chem.* 254:202-208, **1979**. *[8]*

Caswell AH, Brandt NR, Brunschwig JP, Purkerson S: Localization and partial characterization of the oligomeric disulfide-linked molecular weight 95,000 protein (triadin) which binds the ryanodine and dihydropyridine receptors in skeletal muscle triadic vesicles. *Biochemistry.* 30:7507-7513, **1991.** *[7]*

Catterall WA: Structure and function of voltage-gated ion channels. *Annu Rev Biochem.* 64:493-531, **1995.** *[4]*

Cavalié A, McDonald TF, Pelzer D, Trautwein W: Temperature-induced transitory and steady-state changes in the calcium current of guinea-pig ventricular myocytes. *Pflügers Arch.* 405:294-296, **1985.** *[10]*

Chacon E, Ohata H, Harper IS, Trollinger DR, Herman B, Lemasters JJ: Mitochondrial free calcium transients during excitation-contraction coupling in rabbit cardiac myocytes. *FEBS Lett.* 382:31-36, **1996.** *[3]*

Chadwick CC, Saito A, Fleischer S: Isolation and characterization of the inositol triphosphate receptor from smooth muscle. *Proc Natl Acad Sci USA.* 87:2132-2136, **1990.** *[7]*

Chalovich JM, Chock PB, Eisenberg E: Mechanism of action of troponin-tropomyosin. *J Biol Chem.* 256:557-578, **1981.** *[2]*

Chandler WK, Rakowski RF, Schneider MF: A non-linear voltage dependent charge movement in frog skeletal muscle. *J Physiol.* 254:245-283, **1976a.** *[8]*

Chandler WK, Rakowski RF, Schneider MF: Effects of glycerol treatment and maintained depolarization on charge movement in skeletal muscle. *J Physiol.* 254:285-316, **1976b.** *[8]*

Chandra R, Chauhan VS, Starmer CF, Grant AO: β-adrenergic action on wild-type and KPQ mutant human cardiac Na^+ channels: Shift in gating but no change in Ca^{2+}:Na^+ selectivity. *Cardiovasc Res.* 42:490-502, **1999.** *[8]*

Chapman RA: Control of cardiac contractility at the cellular level. *Am J Physiol.* 245:H535-H552, **1983.** *[9]*

Chapman RA: Sodium/calcium exchange and intracellular calcium buffering in ferret myocardium: An ion-sensitive microelectrode study. *J Physiol.* 373:163-179, **1986.** *[10]*

Chapman RA, Léoty C: The time-dependent and dose-dependent effects of caffeine on the contraction of the ferret heart. *J Physiol.* 256:287-314, **1976.** *[7]*

Chapman RA, Tunstall J: The interaction of sodium and calcium ions at the cell membrane and the control of contractile strength in frog atrial muscle. *J Physiol.* 305:109-123, **1980.** *[6]*

Chapman RA, Tunstall J: The tension-depolarization relationship of frog atrial trabeculae as determined by potassium contractures. *J Physiol.* 310:97-115, **1981.** *[9]*

Chapman RA, Tunstall J: The calcium paradox of the heart. *Prog Biophys Molec Biol.* 50:57-96, **1987.** *[1]*

Chen XH, Tsien RW: Aspartate substitutions establish the concerted action of P-region glutamates in repeats *I* and *III* in forming the protonation site of L-type Ca^{2+} channels. *J Biol Chem.* 272:30002-30008, **1997.** *[5]*

Chen L, Goings GE, Upshaw-Earley J, Page E: Cardiac gap junctions and gap junction-associated vesicles: Ultrastructural comparison of *in situ* negative staining with conventional positive staining. *Circ Res.* 64:501-514, **1989.** *[1]*

Chen SRW, Zhang L, MacLennan DH: Asymmetrical blockade of the Ca^{2+} release channel (ryanodine receptor) by 12-kDa

FK506 binding protein. *Proc Natl Acad Sci USA.* 91:11953-11957, **1994.** *[7]*

Chen XH, Bezprozvanny I, Tsien RW: Molecular basis of proton block of L-type Ca^{2+} channels. *J Gen Physiol.* 108:363-374, **1996a.** *[5]*

Chen W, Steenbergen C, Levy LA, Vance J, London RE, Murphy E: Measurement of free Ca^{2+} in sarcoplasmic reticulum in perfused rabbit heart loaded with 1,2-bis(2-amino-5,6-difluorophenoxy)ethane-N,N,N',N'-tetraacetic acid by ^{19}F NMR. *J Biol Chem.* 271:7398-7403, **1996b.** *[7]*

Chen WN, London R, Murphy E, Steenbergen C: Regulation of the Ca^{2+} gradient across the sarcoplasmic reticulum in perfused rabbit heart: A ^{19}F nuclear magnetic resonance study. *Circ Res.* 83:898-907, **1998.** *[7]*

Chen JY, Capdevila JH, Zeldin DC, Rosenberg RL: Inhibition of cardiac L-type calcium channels by epoxyeicosatrienoic acids. *Mol Pharmacol.* 55:288-295, **1999a.** *[5]*

Chen L, Molinski TF, Pessah IN: Bastadin 10 stabilizes the open conformation of the ryanodine-sensitive Ca^{2+} channel in an FKBP12-dependent manner. *J Biol Chem.* 274:32603-32612, **1999b.** *[7]*

Cheng H, Lederer WJ, Cannell MB: Calcium sparks: Elementary events underlying excitation-contraction coupling in heart muscle. *Science.* 262:740-744, **1993.** *[7,8]*

Cheng H, Cannell MB, Lederer WJ: Partial inhibition of Ca^{2+} current by methoxyverapamil (D600) reveals spatial nonuniformities in $[Ca^{2+}]_i$ during excitation-contraction coupling in cardiac myocytes. *Circ Res.* 76:236-241, **1995.** *[8]*

Cheng H, Lederer MR, Lederer WJ, Cannell MB: Calcium sparks and $[Ca^{2+}]_i$ waves in cardiac myocytes. *Am J Physiol.* 270:C148-C159, **1996.** *[7,8]*

Chen-Izu Y, Xiao RP, Izu LT, Cheng H, Kuschel M, Spurgeon H, Lakatta EG: G_i-dependent localization of $β_2$-adrenergic receptor signaling to L-type Ca^{2+} channels. *Biophys J.* 79:2547-2556, **2000.** *[10]*

Cheon J, Reeves JP: Site density of the sodium-calcium exchange carrier in reconstituted vesicles from bovine cardiac sarcolemma. *J Biol Chem.* 263:2309-2315, **1988.** *[10]*

Chien KR, Han A, Sen A, Buja M, Willerson JT: Accumulation of unesterified arachidonic acid in ischemic canine myocardium. *Circ Res.* 54:313-322, **1984.** *[6]*

Chien AJ, Carr KM, Shirokov RE, Ríos E, Hosey MM: Identification of palmitoylation sites within the L-type calcium channel $β_{2a}$ subunit and effects on channel function. *J Biol Chem.* 271:26465-26468, **1996.** *[5]*

Chin TK, Spitzer KW, Philipson KD, Bridge JHB: The effect of exchanger inhibitory peptide (XIP) on sodium-calcium exchange current in guinea pig ventricular cells. *Circ Res.* 72:497-503, **1993.** *[6]*

Ching LL, Williams AJ, Sitsapesan R: Evidence for Ca^{2+} activation and inactivation sites on the luminal side of the cardiac ryanodine receptor complex. *Circ Res.* 87:201-206, **2000.** *[7]*

Choi HS, Eisner DA: The role of sarcolemmal Ca^{2+}-ATPase in the regulation of resting calcium concentration in rat ventricular myocytes. *J Physiol.* 515:109-118, **1999.** *[6]*

Choi HS, Trafford AW, Orchard CH, Eisner DA: The effect of acidosis on systolic Ca^{2+} and sarcoplasmic reticulum calcium content in isolated rat ventricular myocytes. *J Physiol.* 529:661-668, **2000**. *[10]*

Chu G, Dorn GW, Luo W, Harrer JM, Kadambi VJ, Walsh RA, Kranias EG: Monomeric phospholamban overexpression in transgenic mouse hearts. *Circ Res.* 81:485-492, **1997**. *[7]*

Cifuentes ME, Ronjat M, Ikemoto N: Polylysine induces a rapid Ca^{2+} release from sarcoplasmic reticulum vesicles by mediation of its binding to the foot protein. *Arch Biochem Biophys.* 273:554-561, **1989**. *[7]*

Cingolani HE, Alvarez BV, Ennis IL, de Hurtado MC: Stretch-induced alkalinization of feline papillary muscle. An autocrine-paracrine system. *Circ Res.* 83:775-780, **1998**. *[10]*

Clapham DE: Not so funny anymore: Pacing channels are cloned. *Neuron.* 21:5-7, **1998**. *[4]*

Clarke DM, Mauryama K, Loo TW, Leberer E, Inesi G, MacLennan DH: Functional consequences of glutamate, aspartate, glutamine, and asparagine mutations in the stalk sector of the Ca^{2+}-ATPase of sarcoplasmic reticulum. *J Biol Chem.* 264:11246-11251, **1989a**. *[7]*

Clarke DM, Loo TW, Inesi G, MacLennan DH: Location of high affinity Ca^{2+}-binding sites within the predicted transmembrane domain of the sarcoplasmic reticulum Ca^{2+}-ATPase. *Nature.* 339:476-478, **1989b**. *[6,7]*

Cleemann L, Morad M: Analysis of role of Ca^{2+} in cardiac excitation-contraction coupling: Evidence from simultaneous measurements of intracellular Ca^{2+} contraction and Ca^{2+} current. *J Physiol.* 432:283-312, **1991**. *[8]*

Cleemann L, Wang W, Morad M: Two-dimensional confocal images of organization, density, and gating of focal Ca^{2+} release sites in rat cardiac myocytes. *Proc Natl Acad Sci USA.* 95:10984-10989, **1998**. *[8]*

Clemo HF, Baumgarten CM: Swelling-activated Gd^{3+}-sensitive cation current and cell volume regulation in rabbit ventricular myocytes. *J Gen Physiol.* 110:297-312, **1997**. *[4]*

Clemo HF, Stambler BS, Baumgarten CM: Swelling-activated chloride current is persistently activated in ventricular myocytes from dogs with tachycardia-induced congestive heart failure. *Circ Res.* 84:157-165, **1999**. *[4]*

Clusin WT, Fischmeister R, DeHaan RL: Caffeine-induced current in embryonic heart cells: Time course and voltage dependence. *Am J Physiol.* 245:H528-H532, **1983**. *[6]*

Coetzee WA, Ichikawa H, Hearse DJ: Oxidant stress inhibits Na-Ca-exchange current in cardiac myocytes: Mediation by sulfhydryl groups. *Am J Physiol.* 266:H909-H919, **1994**. *[10]*

Cohen NM, Lederer WJ: Changes in the calcium current of rat heart ventricular myocytes during development. *J Physiol.* 406:115-146, **1988**. *[5]*

Cohen I, Daut J, Noble D: An analysis of the actions of low concentrations of ouabain on membrane currents in Purkinje fibers. *J Physiol.* 260:75-103, **1976**. *[10]*

Cohen CJ, Fozzard HA, Sheu SS: Increase in intracellular sodium ion activity during stimulation in mammalian cardiac muscle. *Circ Res.* 50:651-662, **1982**. *[9]*

Cohen MV, Baines CP, Downey JM: Ischemic preconditioning: From adenosine receptor of K$_{ATP}$ channel. *Annu Rev Physiol.* 62:79-109, **2000**. *[10]*

Cole WC, Chartier D, Martin F, Leblanc N: Ca^{2+} permeation through Na$^+$ channels in guinea pig ventricular myocytes. *Am J Physiol.* 273:H128-H137, **1997**. *[4]*

Collier ML, Levesque PC, Kenyon JL, Hume JR: Unitary Cl$^-$ channels activated by cytoplasmic Ca^{2+} in canine ventricular myocytes. *Circ Res.* 78:936-944, **1996**. *[4]*

Collier ML, Thomas AP, Berlin JR: Relationship between L-type Ca^{2+} current and unitary sarcoplasmic reticulum Ca^{2+} release events in rat ventricular myocytes. *J Physiol.* 516:117-128, **1999**. *[8]*

Collin T, Wang JJ, Nargeot J, Schwartz A: Molecular cloning of three isoforms of the L-type voltage- dependent calcium channel β subunit from normal human heart. *Circ Res.* 72:1337-1344, **1993**. *[5]*

Collins A, Somlyo AV, Hilgemann DW: The giant cardiac membrane patch method: Stimulation of outward Na$^+$-Ca^{2+} exchange current by MgATP. *J Physiol.* 454:27-57, **1992**. *[6]*

Colquhoun D, Neher E, Reuter H, Stevens CF: Inward current channels activated by intracellular Ca in cultured cardiac cells. *Nature.* 294:752-754, **1981**. *[4,10]*

Colvin RA, Ashavaid TF, Herbette LG: Structure-functions studies of canine cardiac sarcolemmal membranes. I. Estimation of receptor site densities. *Biochim Biophys Acta.* 812:601-608, **1985**. *[6,10]*

Colyer J, Wang JH: Dependence of cardiac sarcoplasmic reticulum calcium pump activity on the phosphorylation status of phospholamban. *J Biol Chem.* 266:17486-17493, **1991**. *[7]*

Conklin MW, Barone V, Sorrentino V, Coronado R: Contribution of ryanodine receptor type 3 to Ca^{2+} sparks in embryonic mouse skeletal muscle. *Biophys J.* 77:1394-1403, **1999**. *[8]*

Connors SP, Terrar DA: The effect of forskolin on activation and de-activation of time-dependent potassium current in ventricular cells isolated from guinea-pig heart. *J Physiol. (Lond.)* 429:109, **1990**. *[10]*

Constantin LL, Podolsky RJ: Depolarization of the internal membrane system in the activation of frog skeletal muscle. *J Gen Physiol.* 50:1101-1124, **1967**. *[8]*

Conti A, Gorza L, Sorrentino V: Differential distribution of ryanodine receptor type 3 (RyR3) gene product in mammalian skeletal muscles. *Biochem J.* 316:19-23, **1996**. *[8]*

Cooke R: Actomyosin interaction in striated muscle. *Physiol Rev.* 77:671-697, **1997**. *[2]*

Coraboeuf E: Membrane electrical activity and double component contraction in cardiac tissue. *J Mol Cell Cardiol.* 6:215-225, **1974**. *[9]*

Coraboeuf E, Deroubaix E, Hoerter J: Control of ionic permeabilities in normal and ischemic heart. *Circ Res.* 38:I92-I98, **1976**. *[10]*

Corbett AM, Caswell AH, Brandt NR, Brunschwig JP: Determinants of triad junction reformation: Identification and isolation of an endogenous promoter for junction reformation in muscle. *J Memb Biol.* 86:267-276, **1985**. *[8]*

Cordeiro JM, Spitzer KW, Giles WR: Repolarizing K$^+$ currents in rabbit heart Purkinje cells. *J Physiol.* 508:811-823, **1998**. *[4]*

Cornea RL, Jones LR, Autry JM, Thomas DD: Mutation and phosphorylation change the oligomeric structure of phospholamban in lipid bilayers. *Biochemistry.* 36:2960-2967, **1997**. *[7]*

Coronado R, Affolter H: Insulation of the conduction pathway of muscle transverse tubule calcium channels from the surface charge of bilayer phospholipid. *J Gen Physiol.* 87:933-953, **1986**. *[5]*

Coronado R, Miller C: Voltage-dependent caesium blockade of a cation channel from fragmented sarcoplasmic reticulum. *Nature.* 280:807-819, **1979**. *[7]*

Coronado R, Miller C: Decamethonium and hexamethonium block K+ channels of sarcoplasmic reticulum. *Nature.* 288:495-497, **1980**. *[7]*

Coronado R, Rosenberg RL, Miller C: Ionic selectivity, saturation, and block in a K+ channel from sarcoplasmic reticulum. *J Gen Physiol.* 76:425-446, **1980**. *[7]*

Coronado R, Morrissette J, Sukhareva M, Vaughan DM: Structure and function of ryanodine receptors. *Am J Physiol.* 266:C1485-C1504, **1994**. *[7]*

Costantin J, Noceti F, Qin N, Wei XY, Birnbaumer L, Stefani E: Facilitation by the β_{2a} subunit of pore openings in cardiac Ca^{2+} channels. *J Physiol.* 507:93-103, **1998**. *[5]*

Cozens B, Reithmeier RAF: Size and shape of rabbit skeletal muscle calsequestrin. *J Biol Chem.* 259:6248-6252, **1984**. *[7]*

Cramb G, Banks R, Rugg EL, Aiton JF: Actions of atrial natriuretic peptide (ANF) on cyclic nucleotide concentrations and phosphatidylinositol turnover in ventricular myocytes. *Biochem Biophys Res Commun.* 148:962-970, **1987**. *[5]*

Cranefield PF, Aronson RS: Cardiac Arrhythmias: The Role of Triggered Activity and other Mechanisms. *Mount Kisco, NY, Futura.* **1988**. *[4]*

Crank J: The Mathematics of Diffusion. 2nd ed. *Bristol, UK, Oxford University Press.* **1975**. *[7]*

Crespo LM, Grantham CJ, Cannell MB: Kinetics, stoichiometry and role of the Na-Ca exchange mechanism in isolated cardiac myocytes. *Nature.* 345:618-621, **1990**. *[6]*

Cribbs LL, Lee JH, Yang J, Satin J, Zhang Y, Daud A, Barclay J, Williamson MP, Fox M, Rees M, Perez-Reyes E: Cloning and characterization of $\alpha 1H$ from human heart, a member of the T-type Ca^{2+} channel gene family. *Circ Res.* 83:103-109, **1998**. *[5]*

Crompton M: The regulation of mitochondrial calcium transport in heart. *Curr Top Membr Transp.* 25:231-276, **1985**. *[3]*

Crompton M: The role of Ca^{2+} in the function and dysfunction of heart mitochondria, in Calcium and the Heart. Langer GA (ed). *New York, NY, Raven Press.* 167-198, **1990**. *[3]*

Crompton M: The mitochondrial permeability transition pore and its role in cell death. *Biochem J.* 341:233-249, **1999**. *[3]*

Crompton M, Capana M, Carafoli E: The sodium-induced efflux of calcium from heart mitochondria. A possible mechanism for the regulation of mitochondrial calcium. *Eur J Biochem.* 69:453-462, **1976**. *[3]*

Crush KG: Carnosine and related substances in animal tissues. *Comp Biochem Physiol.* 34:3-30, **1970**. *[2]*

Cruz JDS, Santana LF, Frederick CA, Isom LL, Malhotra JD, Mattei LN, Kass RS, Xia J, An RH, Lederer WJ: Whether "slip-mode conductance" occurs - Technical Comments. *Science.* 284:711a, **1999**. *[4,8]*

Cukierman S: Regulation of voltage-dependent sodium channels. *J Membr Biol.* 151:203-214, **1996**. *[4]*

Currie S, Smith GL: Enhanced phosphorylation of phospholamban and downregulation of sarco/endoplasmic reticulum Ca^{2+} ATPase type 2 (SERCA 2) in cardiac sarcoplasmic reticulum from rabbits with heart failure. *Cardiovasc Res.* 41:135-146, **1999**. *[10]*

Curtis BM, Catterall WA: Purification of the calcium antagonist receptor of the voltage-sensitive calcium channel from skeletal muscle transverse tubules. *Biochem.* 23:2113-2118, **1984**. *[5]*

Curtis BM, Catterall WA: Phosphorylation of the calcium antagonist receptor of the voltage-sensitive calcium channel by cAMP-dependent protein kinase. *Proc Natl Acad Sci USA.* 82:2528-2532, **1985**. *[5]*

D'Agnolo A, Luciani GB, Mazzucco A, Gallucci V, Salviati G: Contractile properties and Ca^{2+} release activity of the sarcoplasmic reticulum in dilated cardiomyopathy. *Circulation.* 85:518-525, **1992**. *[10]*

Dang TX, McCleskey EW: Ion channel selectivity through stepwise changes in binding affinity. *J Gen Physiol.* 111:185-193, **1998**. *[5]*

Dani AM, Cittadini A, Inesi G: Calcium transport and contractile activity in dissociated mammalian heart cells. *Am J Physiol.* 237:C147-C155, **1979**. *[7]*

Danilczyk UG, Cohen-Doyle MF, Williams DB: Functional relationship between calreticulin, calnexin, and the endoplasmic reticulum luminal domain of calnexin. *J Biol Chem.* 275:13089-13097, **2000**. *[7]*

Danko S, Kim DH, Sreter FA, Ikemoto N: Inhibitors of Ca^{2+} release from the isolated sarcoplasmic reticulum. II. The effects of dantrolene on Ca^{2+} release induced by caffeine, Ca^{2+} and depolarization. *Biochim Biophys Acta.* 816:18-24, **1985**. *[7]*

Davidenko JM, Pertsov AV, Salomonsz R, Baxter W, Jalife J: Stationary and drifting spiral waves of excitation in isolated cardiac muscle. *Nature.* 355:349-351, **1992**. *[4]*

Davidson GA, Varhol RJ: Kinetics of thapsigargin-Ca^{2+}-ATPase (sarcoplasmic reticulum) interaction reveals a two-step binding mechanism and picomolar inhibition. *J Biol Chem.* 270:11731-11734, **1995**. *[7]*

Davies CH, Davia K, Bennett JG, Pepper JR, Poole-Wilson PA, Harding SE: Reduced contraction and altered frequency response of isolated ventricular myocytes from patients with heart failure. *Circulation.* 92:2540-2549, **1995**. *[10]*

de Koninck P, Schulman H: Sensitivity of CaM kinase II to the frequency of Ca^{2+} oscillations. *Science.* 279:227-230, **1998**. *[9,10]*

de la Bastie D, Levitsky D, Rappapport L, Mercadier JJ, Marotte F, Wisnewsky C, Brovkovich V, Schwartz K, Lompré A-M: Function of the sarcoplasmic reticulum and expression of its Ca^{2+}-ATPase gene in pressure overload-induced cardiac hypertrophy in the rat. *Circ Res.* 66:554-564, **1990**. *[10]*

de la Peña P, Reeves JP: Inhibition and activation of sodium-calcium exchange activity in cardiac sarcolemmal vesicles by quinacrine. *Am J Physiol.* 252:C24-C29, **1987**. *[6]*

de Leon M, Wang Y, Jones L, Perez-Reyes E, Wei XY, Soong TW, Snutch TP, Yue DT: Essential Ca^{2+}-binding motif for Ca^{2+}-sensitive inactivation of L-type Ca^{2+} channels. *Science.* 270:1502-1506, **1995**. *[5]*

de Tombe PP: Altered contractile function in heart failure. *Cardiovasc Res.* 37:367-380, **1998**. *[10]*

de Waard M, Pragnell M, Campbell KP: Ca^{2+} channel regulation by a conserved β subunit domain. *Neuron.* 13:495-503, **1994**. *[5]*

de Windt LJ, Lim HW, Bueno OF, Liang Q, Delling U, Braz JC, Glascock BJ, Kimball TF, del Monte F, Hajjar RJ, Molkentin JD: Targeted inhibition of calcineurin attenuates cardiac hypertrophy invivo. *Proc Natl Acad Sci USA.* 98:3322-3327, **2001**. *[10]*

Deitmer JW, Ellis D: Interactions between the regulation of the intracellular pH and sodium activity of sheep cardiac Purkinje fibres. *J Physiol.* 304:471-488, **1980**. *[10]*

del Monte F, Harding SE, Schmidt U, Matsui T, Kang ZB, Dec W, Gwathmey JK, Rosenzweig A, Hajjar RJ: Restoration of contractile function in isolated cardiomyocytes from failing human hearts by gene transfer of SERCA2a. *Circulation.* 100:2308-2311, **1999**. *[10]*

Delbridge LM, Bassani JWM, Bers DM: Steady-state twitch Ca^{2+} fluxes and cytosolic Ca^{2+} buffering in rabbit ventricular myocytes. *Am J Physiol.* 270:C192-C199, **1996**. *[3,7,9,10]*

Delbridge LM, Satoh H, Yuan W, Bassani JWM, Qi M, Ginsburg KS, Samarel AM, Bers DM: Cardiac myocyte volume, Ca^{2+} fluxes, and sarcoplasmic reticulum loading in pressure-overload hypertrophy. *Am J Physiol.* 272:H2425-H2435, **1997**. *[8,9]*

Delgado C, Artiles A, Gómez AM, Vassort G: Frequency-dependent increase in cardiac Ca^{2+} current is due to reduced Ca^{2+} release by the sarcoplasmic reticulum. *J Mol Cell Cardiol.* 31:1783-1793, **1999**. *[5]*

DelPrincipe F, Egger M, Niggli E: Calcium signalling in cardiac muscle: Refractoriness revealed by coherent activation. *Nat Cell Biol.* 1:323-329, **1999**. *[8]*

DelPrincipe F, Egger M, Niggli E: L-type Ca^{2+} current as the predominant pathway of Ca^{2+} entry during I_{Na} activation in β-stimulated cardiac myocytes. *J Physiol.* 527:455-466, **2000**. *[8]*

DeMeis L, Vianna AL: Energy interconversion by the Ca^{2+}-dependent ATPase of the sarcoplasmic reticulum. *Annu Rev Biochem.* 48:275-292, **1979**. *[7]*

DeMello WC: Effect of intracellular injection of calcium and strontium on cell communication in heart. *J Physiol.* 250:231-245, **1975**. *[1]*

Demir SS, Clark JW, Murphey CR, Giles WR: A mathematical model of a rabbit sinoatrial node cell. *Am J Physiol.* 266:C832-C852, **1994**. *[4]*

Demir SS, Clark JW, Giles WR: Parasympathetic modulation of sinoatrial node pacemaker activity in rabbit heart: A unifying model. *Am J Physiol.* 276:H2221-H2244, **1999**. *[4]*

Deng XF, Chemtob S, Varma DR: Characterization of $α_{1D}$-adrenoceptor subtype in rat myocardium, aorta and other tissues. *Br J Pharmacol.* 119:269-276, **1996**. *[10]*

Denton RM, McCormack JG: On the role of the calcium transport cycle in heart and other mammalian mitochondria. *FEBS Lett.* 119:1-8, **1980**. *[3]*

Denton RM, McCormack JG: Ca^{2+} transport by mammalian mitochondria and its role in hormone action. *Am J Physiol.* 249:E543-E554, **1985**. *[3]*

Denton RM, McCormack JG: Ca^{2+} as a second messenger within mitochondria of the heart and other tissues. *Annu Rev Physiol.* 52:451-466, **1990**. *[3]*

Denvir MA, MacFarlane NG, Cobbe SM, Miller DJ: Sarcoplasmic reticulum and myofilament function in chemically-treated ventricular trabeculae from patients with heart failure. *Cardiovasc Res.* 30:377-385, **1995**. *[10]*

DeSantiago J, Bers, DM: CaMKII inhibitor prevents the frequency-dependent acceleration of relaxation (FDAR) in cardiac muscle of phospholamban knock-out mice. *Biophys J.* 78:375A, **2000**. *[9]*

DeSantiago J, Li Y, Schlotthauer K, Bers DM: Phenylephrine induced inotropy is not associated with IP_3 induced Ca release in ventricular myocytes. *Biophys J.* 74:A57, **1998**. *[10]*

Désilets M, Baumgarten CM: Isoproterenol directly stimulates the Na^+-K^+ pump in isolated cardiac myocytes. *Am J Physiol.* 251:H218-H225, **1986**. *[4,10]*

Dettbarn C, Palade P: Effects of three sarcoplasmic/endoplasmic reticulum Ca^{2+} pump inhibitors on release channels of intracellular stores. *J Pharmacol Exp Ther.* 285:739-745, **1998**. *[7]*

Deutsch N, Weiss JN: ATP-sensitive K^+ channel modification by metabolic inhibition in isolated guinea-pig ventricular myocytes. *J Physiol.* 465:163-179, **1993**. *[10]*

Di Lisa F, De Tullio R, Salamino F, Barbato R, Melloni E, Siliprandi N, Schiaffino S, Pontremoli S: Specific degradation of troponin T and I by mu-calpain and its modulation by substrate phosphorylation. *Biochem J.* 308:57-61, **1995**. *[10]*

Díaz ME, Cook SJ, Chamunorwa JP, Trafford AW, Lancaster MK, O'Neill SC, Eisner DA: Variability of spontaneous Ca^{2+} release between different rat ventricular myocytes is correlated with Na^+-Ca^{2+} exchange and $[Na^+]_i$. *Circ Res.* 78:857-862, **1996**. *[10]*

Díaz ME, Trafford AW, O'Neill SC, Eisner DA: Measurement of sarcoplasmic reticulum Ca^{2+} content and sarcolemmal Ca^{2+} fluxes in isolated rat ventricular myocytes during spontaneous Ca^{2+} release. *J Physiol.* 501:3-16, **1997a**. *[6,8,10]*

Díaz ME, Trafford AW, O'Neill SC, Eisner DA: A measurable reduction of s.r. Ca content follows spontaneous Ca release in rat ventricular myocytes. *Pflügers Arch.* 434:852-854, **1997b**. *[8]*

DiFrancesco D: A new interpretation of the pacemaker current in calf Purkinje fibres. *J Physiol.* 314:359-376, **1981a**. *[4]*

DiFrancesco D: A study of the ionic nature of the pacemaker current in calf Purkinje fibres. *J Physiol.* 314:377-393, **1981b**. *[4]*

DiFrancesco D: Block and activation of the pace-maker channel in calf purkinje fibres: Effects of potassium, caesium and rubidium. *J Physiol.* 329:485-507, **1982**. *[4]*

DiFrancesco D: The cardiac hyperpolarizing-activated current, I_f. Origins and developments. *Prog Biophys Mol Biol.* 46:163-183, **1985**. *[4]*

DiFrancesco D: Characterization of single pacemaker channels in cardiac sino-atrial node cells. *Nature.* 324:470-473, **1986**. *[4,10]*

DiFrancesco D, Noble D: A model of cardiac electrical activity incorporating ionic pumps and concentration changes. *Phil Trans Roy Soc London.* B 307:353-409, **1985**. *[6]*

DiFrancesco D, Tortora P: Direct activation of cardiac pacemaker channels by intracellular cyclic AMP. *Nature.* 351:145-147, **1991**. *[4]*

DiFrancesco D, Tromba C: Inhibition of the hyperpolarization-activated current (I_f) induced by acetylcholine in rabbit sino-atrial node myocytes. *J Physiol.* 405:477-491, **1988**. *[4]*

DiFrancesco D, Ferroni A, Mazzanti M, Tromba C: Properties of the hyperpolarizing-activated current (I_f) in cells isolated from the rabbit sino-atrial node. *J Physiol.* 377:61-88, **1986**. *[10]*

DiFrancesco D, Mangoni M, Maccaferri G: The pacemaker current in cardiac cells, in Cardiac Electrophysiology: From Bench to Bedside. Zipes DP, Jalife J (eds). 2nd ed. *Philadelphia, PA, W.B. Saunders.* 96-103, **1995**. *[4]*

Ding XL, Akella AB, Gulati J: Contributions of troponin I and troponin C to the acidic pH-induced depression of contractile Ca^{2+} sensitivity in cardiotrabeculae. *Biochemistry.* 34:2309-2316, **1995**. *[2]*

Dipla K, Mattiello JA, Margulies KB, Jeevanandam V, Houser SR: The sarcoplasmic reticulum and the Na^+/Ca^{2+} exchanger both contribute to the Ca^{2+} transient of failing human ventricular myocytes. *Circ Res.* 84:435-444, **1999**. *[10]*

DiPolo R, Beaugé L: Characterization of the reverse Na/Ca exchange in squid axons and its modulation by Ca_i and ATP. *J Gen Physiol.* 90:505-525, **1987**. *[6]*

DiPolo R, Beaugé L: Ca^{2+} transport in nerve fibers. *Biochim Biophys Acta.* 927:549-569, **1988**. *[6]*

DiPolo R, Beaugé L: Regulation of Na-Ca exchange. An overview. *Ann NY Acad Sci.* 639:100-111, **1991**. *[6]*

DiPolo R, Beaugé L: Cardiac sarcolemmal Na/Ca-inhibiting peptides XIP and FMRF-amide also inhibit Na/Ca exchange in squid axons. *Am J Physiol.* 267:C307-C311, **1994**. *[6]*

Dirksen RT, Beam KG: Role of calcium permeation in dihydropyridine receptor function. Insights into channel gating and excitation-contraction coupling. *J Gen Physiol.* 114:393-403, **1999**. *[8]*

Dirksen RT, Sheu SS: Modulation of ventricular action potential by α_1-adrenoceptors and protein kinase C. *Am J Physiol.* 258:H907-H911, **1990**. *[10]*

Dixon DA, Haynes DH: Kinetic characterization of the Ca^{2+}-pumping ATPase of cardiac sarcolemma in four states of activation. *J Biol Chem.* 264:13612-13622, **1989**. *[6]*

Dixon IM, Hata T, Dhalla NS: Sarcolemmal Na^+-K^+-ATPase activity in congestive heart failure due to myocardial infarction. *Am J Physiol.* 262:C664-C671, **1992**. *[10]*

Dode L, Wuytack F, Kools PF, Baba-Aissa F, Raeymaekers L, Brike F, van de Ven WJ, Casteels R, Brik F: cDNA cloning, expression and chromosomal localization of the human sarco/endoplasmic reticulum Ca^{2+}-ATPase 3 gene. *Biochem J.* 318:689-699, **1996**. *[7]*

Doering AE, Lederer WJ: The mechanism by which cytoplasmic protons inhibit the sodium-calcium exchanger in guinea-pig heart cells. *J Physiol.* 466:481-499, **1993**. *[6,10]*

Doering AE, Lederer WJ: The action of Na^+ as a cofactor in the inhibition by cytoplasmic protons of the cardiac Na^+-Ca^{2+} exchanger in the guinea-pig. *J Physiol.* 480:9-20, **1994**. *[6]*

Doering AE, Nicoll DA, Lu YJ, Lu LY, Weiss JN, Philipson KD: Topology of a functionally important region of the cardiac Na^+/Ca^{2+} exchanger. *J Biol Chem.* 273:778-783, **1998**. *[6]*

Doerr T, Denger R, Doerr A, Trautwein W: Ionic currents contributing to the action potential in single ventricular myocytes of the guinea pig studied with action potential clamp. *Pflügers Arch.* 416:230-237, **1990**. *[5]*

Dolber PC, Sommer JR: Corbular sarcoplasmic reticulum of rabbit cardiac muscle. *J Ultrastruct Res.* 87:190-196, **1984**. *[1]*

Dolphin AC: Mechanisms of modulation of voltage-dependent calcium channels by G proteins. *J Physiol.* 506:3-11, **1998**. *[5]*

Donaldson SKB: Peeled mammalian skeletal muscle fibers. Possible stimulation of Ca^{2+} release via a transverse tubule-sarcoplasmic reticulum mechanism. *J Gen Physiol.* 86:501-525, **1985**. *[8]*

Donaldson SKB, Hermansen L: Differential, direct effects of H^+ on Ca^{2+}-activated force of skinned fibers from the soleus,
cardiac and adductor magnus muscles of rabbit. *Pflügers Arch.* 376:55-65, **1978**. *[10]*

Donaldson SKB, Goldberg ND, Walserth TF, Huetteman DA: Inositol triphosphate stimulates calcium release from peeled skeletal muscle fibers. *Biochim Biophys Acta.* 927:92-99, **1987**. *[8]*

Donaldson SKB, Goldberg ND, Walserth TF, Huetteman DA: Voltage-dependence of inositol 1,4,5-trisphosphate-induced Ca^{2+} release in peeled skeletal muscle fibers. *Proc Natl Acad Sci USA.* 85:5749-5753, **1988**. *[8]*

Donoso P, Hidalgo C: Sodium-calcium exchange in transverse tubules isolated from frog skeletal muscle. *Biochim Biophys Acta.* 978:8-16, **1989**. *[6]*

Dosemeci A, Dhallan RS, Cohen NM, Lederer WJ, Rogers TB: Phorbol ester increases calcium current and simulates the effects of angiotensin II on cultured neonatal rat heart myocytes. *Circ Res.* 62:347-357, **1988**. *[5]*

Downey JM: Free radicals and their involvement during long-term myocardial ischemia and reperfusion. *Annu Rev Physiol.* 52:487-504, **1990**. *[10]*

Doyle DD, Brill DM, Wasserstrom JA, Karrison T, Page E: Saxitoxin binding and "fast" sodium channel inhibition in sheep heart plasma membrane. *Am J Physiol.* 249:H328-H336, **1985**. *[10]*

Doyle DD, Kamp TJ, Palfrey HC, Miller RJ, Page E: Separation of cardiac plasmalemma into cell surface and T-tubular components. *J Biol Chem.* 261:6556-6563, **1986**. *[1]*

Doyle DA, Cabral JM, Pfuetzner RA, Kuo AL, Gulbis JM, Cohen SL, Chait BT, MacKinnon R: The structure of the potassium channel: Molecular basis of K^+ conduction and selectivity. *Science.* 280:69-77, **1998**. *[4]*

Dresdner KP, Kline RP: Extracellular calcium ion depletion in frog cardiac ventricular muscle. *Biophys J.* 48:33-45, **1985**. *[7]*

Duan D, Winter C, Cowley S, Hume JR, Horowitz B: Molecular identification of a volume-regulated chloride channel. *Nature.* 390:417-421, **1997a**. *[4]*

Duan D, Hume JR, Nattel S: Evidence that outwardly rectifying Cl^- channels are volume-regulated Cl^- currents in heart. *Circ Res.* 80:103-113, **1997b**. *[4]*

duBell WH, Houser SR: A comparison of cytosylic free Ca^{2+} in resting feline and rat ventricular myocytes. *Cell Calcium.* 8:259-268, **1987**. *[9]*

duBell WH, Houser SR: Voltage and beat dependence of the Ca^{2+} transient in feline ventricular myocytes. *Am J Physiol.* 257:H746-H759, **1989**. *[8]*

duBell WH, Lederer WJ, Rogers TB: Dynamic modulation of excitation-contraction coupling by protein phosphatases in rat ventricular myocytes. *J Physiol.* 493:793-800, **1996**. *[7]*

Dulhunty AF, Laver DR, Gallant EM, Casarotto MG, Pace SM, Curtis S: Activation and inhibition of skeletal RyR channels by a part of the skeletal DHPR II-III loop: Effects of DHPR Ser^{687} and FKBP12. *Biophys J.* 77:189-203, **1999**. *[8]*

Dumaine R, Wang Q, Keating MT, Hartmann HA, Schwartz PJ, Brown AM, Kirsch GE: Multiple mechanisms of Na^+ channel-linked long-QT syndrome. *Circ Res.* 78:916-924, **1996**. *[4]*

DuPont Y: Kinetics and regulation of sarcoplasmic reticulum ATPase. *Eur J Biochem.* 72:185-190, **1977**. *[7]*

Durell SR, Hao YL, Guy HR: Structural models of the transmembrane region of voltage-gated and other K^+

channels in open, closed, and inactivated conformations. *J Struct Biol*. 121:263-284, **1998**. *[4]*

Durkin JT, Ahrens DC, Pan YC, Reeves JP: Purification and amino-terminal sequence of the bovine cardiac sodium-calcium exchanger: Evidence for the presence of a signal sequence. *Arch Biochem Biophys*. 290:369-375, **1991**. *[6]*

Dyck C, Maxwell K, Buchko J, Trac M, Omelchenko A, Hnatowich M, Hryshko LV: Structure-function analysis of CALX1.1, a Na^+-Ca^2 exchanger from *Drosophila*. Mutagenesis of ionic regulatory sites. *J Biol Chem*. 273:12981-12987, **1998**. *[6]*

Ebashi S: Calcium binding activity of vesicular relaxing factor. *J Biochem*. 50:236-244, **1961**. *[7]*

Ebashi S, Lipmann F: Adenosine triphosphate-linked concentration of calcium ions in a particulate fraction of rabbit muscle. *J Cell Biol*. 14:389-400, **1962**. *[7]*

Eble DM, Strait JB, Govindarajan G, Lou J, Byron KL, Samarel AM: Endothelin-induced cardiac myocyte hypertrophy: Role for focal adhesion kinase. *Am J Physiol*. 278:H1695-H1707, **2000**. *[10]*

Edes I, Kiss E, Kitada Y, Powers FM, Papp JG, Kranias EG, Solaro RJ: Effects of Levosimendan, a cardiotonic agent targeted to troponin C, on cardiac function and on phosphorylation and Ca^{2+} sensitivity of cardiac myofibrils and sarcoplasmic reticulum in guinea pig heart. *Circ Res*. 77:107-113, **1995**. *[2]*

Edman KAP, Johannsson M: The contractile state of rabbit papillary muscle in relation to stimulation frequency. *J Physiol*. 254:565-581, **1976**. *[8,9]*

Egan TM, Noble D, Noble SJ, Powell T, Spindler AJ, Twist VW: Sodium-calcium exchange during the action potential in guinea-pig ventricular cells. *J Physiol*. 411:639-661, **1989**. *[6]*

Egdell RM, MacLeod KT: Calcium extrusion during aftercontractions in cardiac myocytes: the role of the sodium-calcium exchanger in the generation of the transient inward current. *J Mol Cell Cardiol*. 32:85-93, **2000**. *[10]*

Egdell RM, De Souza AI, MacLeod KT: Relative importance of SR load and cytoplasmic calcium concentration in the genesis of aftercontractions in cardiac myocytes. *Cardiovasc Res*. 47:769-777, **2000**. *[8]*

Egger M, Niggli E: Regulatory function of Na-Ca exchange in the heart: Milestones and outlook. *J Membr Biol*. 168:107-130, **1999**. *[6]*

Egger M, Niggli E: Paradoxical block of the Na^+-Ca^{2+} exchanger by extracellular protons in guinea-pig ventricular myocytes. *J Physiol*. 523:353-366, **2000**. *[6]*

Egger M, Ruknudin A, Niggli E, Lederer WJ, Schulze DH: Ni^{2+} transport by the human Na^+/Ca^{2+} exchanger expressed in Sf9 cells. *Am J Physiol*. 276 :C1184-C1192, **1999**. *[6]*

Ehara T, Matsuura H: Single-channel study of the cyclic AMP-regulated chloride current in guinea-pig ventricular myocytes. *J Physiol*. 464:307-320, **1993**. *[4]*

Ehara T, Noma A, Ono K: Calcium-activated non-selective cation channel in ventricular cells isolated from adult guinea-pig hearts. *J Physiol*. 403:117-133, **1988**. *[4]*

Ehrlich BE, Watras J: Inositol 1,4,5-triphosphate activates a channel from smooth muscle sarcoplasmic reticulum. *Nature*. 336:583-586, **1988**. *[8]*

Eigel BN, Hadley RW: Contribution of the Na^+ channel and Na^+/H^+ exchanger to the anoxic rise of $[Na^+]$ in ventricular myocytes. *Am J Physiol*. 277:H1817-H1822, **1999**. *[10]*

Eisenberg BR: Quantitative ultrastructure of mammalian skeletal muscle, in Handbook of Physiology. Section 10. Skeletal Muscle. Peachey LD (ed). *Bethesda, MD, Am Physiol Soc*. 73-112, **1983**. *[1]*

Eisenberg BR, Kuda AM: Stereological analysis of mammalian skeletal muscle. II. White vastus muscle of the adult guinea-pig. *J Ultrastruct Res*. 51:176-187, **1975**. *[1]*

Eisenberg BR, Kuda AM: Discrimination between fiber populations in mammalian skeletal muscle by using ultrastructural parameters. *J Ultrastruct Res*. 54:76-88, **1976**. *[1]*

Eisenberg BR, Cohen IS: The ultrastructure of the cardiac Purkinje strand in the dog: A morphometric analysis. *Proc Roy Soc Lond*. B 217:191-213, **1983**. *[1]*

Eisenberg BR, Kuda AM, Peter JB: Stereological analysis of mammalian skeletal muscle. I. Soleus muscle of the adult guinea-pig. *J Cell Biol*. 60:732-754, **1974**. *[1]*

Eisenberg RS, McCarthy RT, Milton RL: Paralysis of frog skeletal muscle fibres by the calcium antagonist D-600. *J Physiol*. 341:495-505, **1983**. *[8]*

Eisner DA, Lederer WJ: Inotropic and arrhythmogenic effects of potassium-depleted solutions on mammalian cardiac muscle. *J Physiol*. 294:255-277, **1979**. *[6]*

Eisner DA, Lederer WJ: Characterization of the electrogenic sodium pump in cardiac Purkinje fibres. *J Physiol*. 303:441-474, **1980**. *[10]*

Eisner DA, Valdeolmillos M: The mechanism of the increase of tonic tension produced by caffeine in sheep in cardiac Purkinje fibres. *J Physiol*. 364:313-326, **1985**. *[7]*

Eisner DA, Lederer WJ, Vaughan-Jones RD: The control of tonic tension by membrane potential and intracellular sodium activity in the sheep cardiac Purkinje fibre. *J Physiol*. 335:723-743, **1983**. *[6,9]*

Eisner DA, Lederer WJ, Vaughan-Jones RD: The quantitative relationship between twitch tension and intracellular sodium activity in sheep cardiac Purkinje fibres. *J Physiol*. 355:251-266, **1984**. *[10]*

Eisner DA, Trafford AW, Díaz ME, Overend CL, O'Neill SC: The control of Ca release from the cardiac sarcoplasmic reticulum: Regulation versus autoregulation. *Cardiovasc Res*. 38:589-604, **1998**. *[9,10]*

Eisner DA, Choi HS, Díaz ME, O'Neill SC, Trafford AW: Integrative analysis of calcium cycling in cardiac muscle. *Circ Res*. 87:1087-1094, **2000**. *[9,10]*

el-Hayek R, Ikemoto N: Identification of the minimum essential region in the II-III loop of the dihydropyridine receptor α_1 subunit required for activation of skeletal muscle-type excitation-contraction coupling. *Biochemistry*. 37:7015-7020, **1998**. *[8]*

el-Hayek R, Antoniu B, Wang JP, Hamilton SL, Ikemoto N: Identification of calcium release-triggering and blocking regions of the II-III loop of the skeletal muscle dihydropyridine receptor. *J Biol Chem*. 270:22116-22118, **1995**. *[8]*

Ellinor PT, Yang J, Sather WA, Zhang JF, Tsien RW: Ca^{2+} channel selectivity at a single locus for high-affinity Ca^{2+} interactions. *Neuron*. 15:1121-1132, **1995**. *[5]*

Ellis D: Effects of stimulation and diphenylhydantoin on the intracellular sodium activity in Purkinje fibres of sheep heart. *J Physiol*. 362:331-348, **1985**. *[9]*

Ellis D, MacLeod KT: Sodium-dependent control of intracellular pH in Purkinje fibers of sheep heart. *J Physiol.* 359:81-105, **1985**. *[10]*

Ellis D, Thomas RC: Direct measurement of the intracellular pH of mammalian cardiac muscle. *J Physiol.* 262:755-771, **1976**. *[3]*

Ellis KO, Wessels JLFL, Carpenter JF: A comparison of skeletal, cardiac and smooth muscle actions of dantrolene sodium: A skeletal muscle relaxant. *Arch Int Pharmacodyn.* 224:118-132, **1976**. *[7]*

Ellis SB, Williams ME, Ways NR, Brenner R, Sharp AH, Leung AT, Campbell KP, McKenna E, Koch WJ, Hui A, Schwartz A, Harpold MM: Sequence and expression of mRNAs encoding the α_1 and α_2 subunits of a DHP-sensitive calcium channel. *Science.* 241:1661-1664, **1988**. *[5]*

el-Saleh SC, Solaro RJ: Troponin I enhances pH-induced depression of Ca^{2+} binding to the regulatory sites in skeletal troponin C. *J Biol Chem.* 263:3274-3278, **1988**. *[10]*

el-Sayed MF, Gesser H: Sarcoplasmic reticulum, potassium, and cardiac force in rainbow trout and plaice. *Am J Physiol.* 257:R599-R604, **1989**. *[9]*

Endo M: Conditions required for calcium-induced release of calcium from the sarcoplasmic reticulum. *Proc Japan Acad.* 51:467-472, **1975a**. *[8]*

Endo M: Mechanism of action of caffeine on the sarcoplasmic reticulum of skeletal muscle. *Proc Japan Acad.* 51:479-484, **1975b**. *[7,8]*

Endo M: Calcium release from the sarcoplasmic reticulum. *Physiol Rev.* 57:71-108, **1977**. *[8]*

Endo M: Calcium release from sarcoplasmic reticulum. *Curr Top Membr Transp.* 25:181-230, **1985**. *[8]*

Endo M, Kitazawa T: E-C coupling on skinned cardiac fibers, in *Biophysical Aspects of Cardiac Muscle.* Morad M (ed). *New York, NY, Academic Press.* 307-327, **1977**. *[2]*

Endo M, Tanaka M, Ogawa Y: Calcium induced release of calcium from the sarcoplasmic reticulum of skinned skeletal muscle fibres. *Nature.* 228:34-36, **1970**. *[8]*

Endo M, Yagi S, Ishizuka T, Koriuti H, Koga K, Amaha K: Changes in the Ca-induced Ca release mechanism in the sarcoplasmic reticulum of the muscle from a patient with malignant hyperthermia. *Biomed Res.* 4:83-92, **1983**. *[7]*

Endoh M: Cardiac α_1-adrenoceptors that regulate contractile function: Subtypes and subcellular signal transduction mechanisms. *Neurochem Res.* 21:217-229, **1996**. *[8,10]*

Endoh M: Changes in intracellular Ca^{2+} mobilization and Ca^{2+} sensitization as mechanisms of action of physiological interventions and inotropic agents in intact myocardial cells. *Jpn Heart J.* 39:1-44, **1998**. *[2]*

Endoh M, Blinks JR: Actions of sympathomimetic amines of the Ca^{2+} transients and contractions of rabbit myocardium: Reciprocal changes in myofibrillar responsiveness to Ca^{2+} mediated through α-and β-adrenoceptors. *Circ Res.* 62:247-265, **1988**. *[10]*

Endoh M, Iijima T, Motomura S: Inhibition by theophylline of the early component of canine ventricular contraction. *Am J Physiol.* 11:H349-H358, **1982**. *[9]*

Endoh M, Yanagisawa T, Morita T, Taira N: Differential effects of sulmazole (AR-L 115 BS) on contractile force and cyclic AMP levels in canine ventricular muscle: Comparison with MDL 17,043. *J Pharmacol Exp Ther.* 234:267, **1985**. *[10]*

Endoh M, Hiramoto T, Ishihata A, Takanashi M, Inui J: Myocardial α_1-adrenoceptors mediate positive inotropic effect and changes in phosphatidylinositol metabolism. Species differences in receptor distribution and the intracellular coupling process in mammalian ventricular myocardium. *Circ Res.* 68:1179-1190, **1991**. *[10]*

England PJ: The significance of phosphorylation of myosin light chains in heart. *J Mol Cell Cardiol.* 16:591-595, **1984**. *[2]*

Entman ML, Van Winkle WB: Sarcoplasmic Reticulum in Muscle Physiology. Vol 1, *Boca Raton, FL, CRC Press, Inc.* **1986**. *[7]*

Enyedi A, Penniston JT: Autoinhibitory domains of various Ca^{2+} transporters cross-react. *J Biol Chem.* 268:17120-17125, **1993**. *[6]*

Eriksson A, Thornell LE: Intermediate (skeletin) filaments in heart Purkinje fibers. A correlative morphological and biochemical identification with evidence of a cytoskeletal function. *J Cell Biol.* 80:231-247, **1979**. *[1]*

Ertl R, Jahnel U, Nawrath H, Carmeliet E, Vereecke J: Differential electrophysiologic and inotropic effects of phenylephrine in atrial and ventricular heart muscle preparations from rats. *Naunyn Schmiedebergs Arch Pharmacol.* 344:574-581, **1991**. *[5]*

Ervasti JM, Campbell KP: Dystrophin and the membrane skeleton. *Curr Opin Cell Biol.* 5:82-87, **1993**. *[1]*

Eschenhagen T, Mende U, Nose M, Schmitz W, Scholz H, Haverich A, Hirt S, Doring V, Kalmar P, Hoppner W: Increased messenger RNA level of the inhibitory G protein α subunit $G_{i\alpha2}$ in human end-stage heart failure. *Circ Res.* 70:688-696, **1992**. *[10]*

Fabiato A: Sarcomere length dependence of calcium release from the sarcoplasmic reticulum of skinned cardiac cells demonstrated by differential microspectrophotometry with arsenazo III. *J Gen Physiol.* 76:15a, **1980**. *[7]*

Fabiato A: Myoplasmic free calcium concentration reached during the twitch of an intact isolated cardiac cell and during calcium-induced release of calcium from the sarcoplasmic reticulum of a skinned cardiac cell from the adult rat or rabbit ventricle. *J Gen Physiol.* 78:457-497, **1981a**. *[2,8]*

Fabiato A: Effects of cyclic AMP and phosphodiesterase inhibitors on the contractile activation and the Ca^{2+} transient detected with aequorin in skinned cardiac cells from rat and rabbit ventricles. *J Gen Physiol.* 78:15a-16a, **1981b**. *[2,7]*

Fabiato A: Calcium release in skinned cardiac cells: Variations with species, tissues, and development. *Fed Proc.* 41:2238-2244, **1982**. *[1,2,9]*

Fabiato A: Calcium-induced release of calcium from the cardiac sarcoplasmic reticulum. *Am J Physiol.* 245:C1-C14, **1983**. *[3,7,8]*

Fabiato A: Dependence of the Ca^{2+}-induced release from the sarcoplasmic reticulum of skinned skeletal muscle fibres from the frog semitendinosus on the rate of change of free Ca^{2+} concentration at the outer surface of the sarcoplasmic reticulum. *J Physiol.* 353:56P, **1984**. *[8]*

Fabiato A: Rapid ionic modifications during the aequorin-detected calcium transient in a skinned canine cardiac Purkinje cell. *J Gen Physiol.* 85:189-246, **1985a**. *[8]*

Fabiato A: Time and calcium dependence of activation and inactivation of calcium-induced release of calcium from the sarcoplasmic reticulum of a skinned canine cardiac Purkinje cell. *J Gen Physiol.* 85:247-290, **1985b**. *[2,7,8]*

Fabiato A: Simulated calcium current can both cause calcium loading in and trigger calcium release from the sarcoplasmic reticulum of a skinned canine cardiac Purkinje cell. *J Gen Physiol.* 85:291-320, **1985c**. *[8]*

Fabiato A: Effects of ryanodine in skinned cardiac cells. *Fed Proc.* 44:2970-2976, **1985d**. *[7]*

Fabiato A: Use of aequorin for the appraisal of the hypothesis of the release of calcium from the sarcoplasmic reticulum induced by a change of pH in skinned cardiac cells. *Cell Calcium.* 6:95-108, **1985e**. *[7,8,10]*

Fabiato A: Appraisal of the hypothesis of the "depolarization-induced" release of calcium from the sarcoplasmic reticulum in skinned cardiac cells from the rat or pigeon ventricle, in Structure and Function of Sarcoplasmic Reticulum. Fleischer S, Tonomura Y (eds). *New York, NY, Academic Press.* 479-519, **1985f**. *[7]*

Fabiato A: Ca-induced release of Ca from the sarcoplasmic reticulum of skinned fibers from the frog semitendinosus. *Biophys J.* 47:195a, **1985g**. *[8]*

Fabiato A: Inositol (1,4,5)-trisphosphate induced release of Ca^{2+} from the sarcoplasmic reticulum of skinned cardiac cells. *Biophys J.* 49:190a, **1986a**. *[8]*

Fabiato A: Inositol (1,4,5)-triphosphate-induced versus Ca^{2+}-induced release of Ca^{2+} from the cardiac sarcoplasmic reticulum. *Proc Int Union Physiol Sci.* 16:350, **1986b**. *[8]*

Fabiato A: Appraisal of the hypothesis of the sodium-induced release of calcium from the sarcoplasmic reticulum or the mitochondria in skinned cardiac cells from the rat ventricle and the canine Purkinje tissue, in Sarcoplasmic Reticulum in Muscle Physiology. Vol. II. Entman ML, van Winkle WB (eds). *Boca Raton, FL, CRC Press, Inc.* 51-72, **1986c**. *[7]*

Fabiato A: Computer programs for calculating total from specified free or free from specified total ionic concentrations in aqueous solutions containing multiple metals and ligands. *Methods Enzymol.* 157:378-417, **1988**. *[2]*

Fabiato A: Comparison and relation between inositol (1,4,5)-triphosphate-induced release and calcium-induced release of calcium from the sarcoplasmic reticulum, in Recent Advances in Calcium Channels and Calcium Antagonists. Yamada K, Shibata S (eds). *Elmsford, NY, Pergamon Press, Inc.* 35-39, **1990**. *[7,8]*

Fabiato A, Fabiato F: Excitation-contraction coupling of isolated cardiac fibers with disrupted or closed sarcolemmas. Calcium-dependent cyclic and tonic contractions. *Circ Res.* 31:293-307, **1972**. *[8,10]*

Fabiato A, Fabiato F: Activation of skinned cardiac cells: Subcellular effects of cardioactive drugs. *Eur J Cardiol.* 1/2:143-155, **1973**. *[8]*

Fabiato A, Fabiato F: Contractions induced by a calcium-triggered release of calcium from the sarcoplasmic reticulum of single skinned cardiac cells. *J Physiol.* 249:469-495, **1975a**. *[2,7,8]*

Fabiato A, Fabiato F: Effects of magnesium on contractile activation of skinned cardiac cells. *J Physiol.* 249:497-517, **1975b**. *[2,8]*

Fabiato A, Fabiato F: Effects of pH on the myofilaments and the sarcoplasmic reticulum of skinned cells from cardiac and skeletal muscles. *J Physiol.* 276:233-255, **1978a**. *[2,7,8,9,10]*

Fabiato A, Fabiato F: Calcium induced release of calcium from the sarcoplasmic reticulum and skinned cells from adult human, dog, cat, rabbit, rat and frog hearts and from fetal and newborn rat ventriclues. *Ann NY Acad Sci.* 307:491-522, **1978b**. *[1,2,8,10]*

Fabiato A, Fabiato F: Use of chlorotetracycline fluorescence to demonstrate Ca $^{2+}$-induced release of Ca^{2+} from the sarcoplasmic reticulum of skinned cardiac cells. *Nature.* 281:146-148, **1979**. *[8]*

Fairhurst AS, Hasselbach W: Calcium efflux from a heavy sarcotubular fraction. Effects of ryanodine, caffeine and magnesium. *Eur J Biochem.* 13:504-509, **1970**. *[7]*

Fan JS, Palade P: One calcium ion may suffice to open the tetrameric cardiac ryanodine receptor in rat ventricular myocytes. *J Physiol.* 516:769-780, **1999**. *[8]*

Fan HR, Brandt NR, Peng M, Schwartz A, Caswell AH: Binding sites of monoclonal antibodies and dihydropyridine receptor α_1 subunit cytoplasmic II-III loop on skeletal muscle triadin fusion peptides. *Biochemistry.* 34:14893-14901, **1995**. *[8]*

Fan J, Shuba YM, Morad M: Regulation of cardiac sodium-calcium exchanger by β-adrenergic agonists. *Proc Natl Acad Sci USA.* 93:5527-5532, **1996**. *[6]*

Fan DS, Wannenburg T, de Tombe PP: Decreased myocyte tension development and calcium responsiveness in rat right ventricular pressure overload. *Circulation.* 95:2312-2317, **1997**. *[10]*

Fawcett DW, McNurr NS: The ultrastructure of the cat myocardium. I. Ventricular papillary muscle. *J Cell Biol.* 42:1-45, **1969**. *[1]*

Fedida D, Giles WR: Regional variations in action potentials and transient outward current in myocytes isolated from rabbit left ventricle. *J Physiol.* 442:191-209, **1991**. *[4]*

Fedida D, Noble D, Shimoni Y, Spindler AJ: Inward current related to contraction in guinea-pig ventricular myocytes. *J Physiol.* 385:565-589, **1987a**. *[8]*

Fedida D, Noble D, Rankin AC, Spindler AJ: The arrhythmogenic transient inward current I_{ti} and related contraction in isolated guinea-pig ventricular myocytes. *J Physiol.* 392:523-542, **1987b**. *[4,10]*

Fedida D, Noble D, Spindler AJ: Use-dependent reduction and facilitation of Ca^{2+} current in guinea-pig myocytes. *J Physiol.* 405:439-460, **1988a**. *[5]*

Fedida D, Noble D, Spindler AJ: Mechanism of the use-dependence of Ca^{2+} current in guinea-pig myocytes. *J Physiol.* 405:461-475, **1988b**. *[5]*

Fedida D, Shimoni Y, Giles WR: α-Adrenergic modulation of the transient outward current in rabbit atrial myocytes. *J Physiol.* 423:257-277, **1990**. *[10]*

Fedida D, Braun AP, Giles WR: α_1-adrenoceptors reduce background K^+ current in rabbit ventricular myocytes. *J Physiol.* 441:673-684, **1991**. *[10]*

Fedida D, Wible B, Wang Z, Fermini B, Faust F, Nattel S, Brown AM: Identity of a novel delayed rectifier current from human heart with a cloned K^+ channel current. *Circ Res.* 73:210-216, **1993**. *[4]*

Feher JJ, Briggs FN: The effect of calcium load on the calcium permeability of sarcoplasmic reticulum. *J Biol Chem.* 257:10191-10199, **1982**. *[7]*

Feher JJ, Briggs FN: Undirectional calcium and nucleotide fluxes in cardiac sarcoplasmic reticulum. II. Experimental results. *Biophys J.* 45:1135-1144, **1984**. *[7]*

Feigl EO: Coronary physiology. *Physiol Rev.* 63:1-205, **1983**. *[10]*

Feldman AM, Cates AE, Veazey WB, Hershberger RE, Bristow MR, Baughman KL, Baumgartner WA, van Dop C: Increase of the 40,000-mol wt Pertussis Toxin substrate (G protein) in the failing human heart. *J Clin Invest.* 82:189-197, **1988**. *[10]*

Feldman AM, Cates AE, Bristow MR, van Dop C: Altered expression of α-subunits of G proteins in failing human hearts. *J Mol Cell Cardiol.* 21:359-365, **1989**. *[10]*

Feldman AM, Ray PE, Silan CM, Mercer JA, Minobe W, Bristow MR: Selective gene expression in failing human heart. Quantification of steady-state levels of messenger RNA in endomyocardial biopsies using the polymerase chain reaction. *Circulation.* 83:1866-1872, **1991**. *[10]*

Feldman AM, Weinberg EO, Ray PE, Lorell BH: Selective changes in cardiac gene expression during compensated hypertrophy and the transition to cardiac decompensation in rats with chronic aortic banding . *Circ Res.* 73:184-192, **1993**. *[10]*

Felix R: Voltage-dependent Ca^{2+} channel $\alpha_2\delta$ auxiliary subunit: Structure, function and regulation. *Receptors Channels.* 6:351-362, **1999**. *[5]*

Felix R, Gurnett CA, de Waard M, Campbell KP: Dissection of functional domains of the voltage-dependent Ca^{2+} channel $\alpha_2\delta$ subunit. *J Neurosci.* 17:6884-6891, **1997**. *[5]*

Feng J, Wible B, Li GR, Wang Z, Nattel S: Antisense oligodeoxynucleotides directed against Kv1.5 mRNA specifically inhibit ultrarapid delayed rectifier K^+ current in cultured adult human atrial myocytes. *Circ Res.* 80:572-579, **1997**. *[4]*

Fentzke RC, Buck SH, Patel JR, Lin H, Wolska BM, Stojanovic MO, Martin AF, Solaro RJ, Moss RL, Leiden JM: Impaired cardiomyocyte relaxation and diastolic function in transgenic mice expressing slow skeletal troponin I in the heart. *J Physiol.* 517:143-157, **1999**. *[2]*

Ferguson SS, Downey WE, Colapietro AM, Barak LS, Menard L, Caron MG: Role of β-arrestin in mediating agonist-promoted G protein-coupled receptor internalization. *Science.* 271:363-366, **1996**. *[10]*

Feron O, Belhassen L, Kobzik L, Smith TW, Kelly RA, Michel T: Endothelial nitric oxide synthase targeting to caveolae. Specific interactions with caveolin isoforms in cardiac myocytes and endothelial cells. *J Biol Chem.* 271:22810-22814, **1996**. *[1]*

Ferrari R, Ceconi C, Curello S, Guarnieri C, Caldarera CM, Albertini A, Visioli O: Oxygen-mediated myocardial damage during ischaemia and reperfusion: Role of the cellular defences against oxygen toxicity. *J Mol Cell Cardiol.* 17:937-945, **1985**. *[10]*

Ferreira G, Yi JX, Ríos E, Shirokov R: Ion-dependent inactivation of barium current through L-type calcium channels. *J Gen Physiol.* 109:449-461, **1997**. *[5]*

Ferrier GR: Digitalis arrhythmias: Role of oscillatory afterpotentials. *Prog Cardiovasc Dis.* 19:459-474, **1977**. *[10]*

Ferrier GR, Howlett SE: Contractions in guinea-pig ventricular myocytes triggered by a calcium-release mechanism separate from Na^+ and L-currents. *J Physiol.* 484:107-122, **1995**. *[8]*

Ferrier GR, Moe GK: Effect of calcium on acetyl-strophanthidin-induced transient depolarizations in canine Purkinje tissue. *Circ Res.* 33:508-515, **1973**. *[4,10]*

Ferrier GR, Zhu JQ, Redondo IM, Howlett SE: Role of cAMP-dependent protein kinase A in activation of a voltage-

sensitive release mechanism for cardiac contraction in guinea-pig myocytes. *J Physiol.* 513:185-201, **1998**. *[8]*

Ferrier GR, Redondo IM, Mason CA, Mapplebeck C, Howlett SE: Regulation of contraction and relaxation by membrane potential in cardiac ventricular myocytes. *Am J Physiol.* 278:H1618-H1626, **2000**. *[8]*

Ferris CD, Huganir RL, Snyder SH: Calcium flux mediated by purified inositol 1,4,5-triphosphate receptor in reconstituted lipid vesicles is allosterically regulated by adenine nucleotides. *Proc Natl Acad Sci USA.* 87:2147-2151, **1990**. *[7]*

Ferris CD, Cameron AM, Bredt DS, Huganir RL, Snyder SH: Inositol 1,4,5-trisphosphate receptor is phosphorylated by cyclic AMP-dependent protein kinase at serines 1755 and 1589. *Biochem Biophys Res Commun.* 175:192-198, **1991a**. *[7]*

Ferris CD, Huganir RL, Bredt DS, Cameron AM, Snyder SH: Inositol trisphosphate receptor: Phosphorylation by protein kinase C and calcium calmodulin-dependent protein kinases in reconstituted lipid vesicles. *Proc Natl Acad Sci USA.* 88:2232-2235, **1991b**. *[7]*

Ferris CD, Cameron AM, Bredt DS, Huganir RL, Snyder SH: Autophosphorylation of inositol 1,4,5-trisphosphate receptors. *J Biol Chem.* 267:7036-7041, **1992**. *[7]*

Ficker E, Taglialatela M, Wible BA, Henley CM, Brown AM: Spermine and spermidine as gating molecules for inward rectifier K^+ channels. *Science.* 266:1068-1072, **1994**. *[4]*

Field AC, Hill C, Lamb GD: Asymmetric charge movement and calcium currents in ventricular myocytes of neonatal rat. *J Physiol.* 406:277-297, **1988**. *[5,8]*

Fill M, Coronado R, Mickelson JR, Vilven J, Ma J, Jacobson BA, Louis CF: Abnormal ryanodine receptor channels in malignant hyperthermia. *Biophys J.* 57:471-475, **1990**. *[7]*

Fill M, Stefani E, Nelson TE: Abnormal human sarcoplasmic reticulum Ca^{2+} release channels in malignant hyperthermic skeletal muscle. *Biophys J.* 59:1085-1090, **1991**. *[7]*

Fischmeister R, Hartzell HC: Mechanism of action of acetylcholine on calcium current in single cells from frog ventricle. *J Physiol.* 376:183-202, **1986**. *[5,8]*

Fischmeister R, Hartzell HC: Cyclic guanosine 3',5'-monophosphate regulates the calcium current in single cells from frog ventricle. *J Physiol.* 387:453-472, **1987**. *[5]*

Flagg-Newton JL, Simpson I, Loewenstein WR: Permeability of the cell-to-cell membrane channels in mammalian cell junction. *Science.* 205:404-407, **1979**. *[1]*

Flaherty JT, Pitt B, Gruber JW, Heuser RR, Rothbaum DA, Burwell LR, George BS, Kereiakes DJ, Deitchman D, Gustafson N: Recombinant human superoxide dismutase (h-SOD) fails to improve recovery of ventricular function in patients undergoing coronary angioplasty for acute myocardial infarction. *Circulation.* 89:1982-1991, **1994**. *[10]*

Fleischer S, Tonomura Y: <u>Structure and Function of Sarcoplasmic Reticulum.</u> New York, NY, Academic Press, **1985**. *[7]*

Fleischer S, Inui M: Biochemistry and biophysics of excitation-contraction coupling. *Ann Rev Biophys Chem.* 18:333-364, **1989**. *[1,7]*

Fleischer S, Ogunbunmi EM, Dixon MC, Fleer EAM: Localization of Ca^{2+} release channels with ryanodine in junctional terminal cisternae of sarcoplasmic reticulum of fast skeletal muscle. *Proc Natl Acad Sci USA*. 82:7256-7259, **1985**. *[7]*

Flesch M, Schwinger RH, Schiffer F, Frank K, Südkamp M, Kuhn-Regnier F, Arnold G, Böhm M: Evidence for functional relevance of an enhanced Na+-Ca2+ exchanger in failing human myocardium. *Circulation*. 94:992-1002, **1996**. *[10]*

Flicker PF, Phillips GN Jr, Cohen C: Troponin and its interactions with tropomyosin. An electron microscope study. *J Mol Biol*. 162:495-501, **1982**. *[2]*

Fliegel L, Ohnishi M, Carpenter MR, Khanna VK, Reithmeier RAF, MacLennan DH: Amino acid sequence of rabbit fast-twitch skeletal muscle calsequestrin deduced from cDNA and peptide sequencing. *Proc Natl Acad Sci USA*. 84:1167-1171, **1987**. *[7]*

Fliegel L, Burns K, Opas M, Michalak M: The high affinity calcium binding protein of sarcoplasmic reticulum. Tissue distribution and homology with calregulin. *Biochim Biophys Acta*. 982:1-8, **1989a**. *[7]*

Fliegel L, Burns K, MacLennan DH, Reithmeier RAF, Michalak M: Molecular cloning of the high affinity calcium-binding protein (calreticulin) of skeletal muscle sarcoplasmic reticulum. *J Biol Chem*. 264:21522-21528, **1989b**. *[7]*

Flockerzi V, Oeken HJ, Hofmann F, Pelzer D, Cavalie A, Trautwein W: Purified dihydropyridine-binding site from skeletal muscle T-tubules is a functional calcium channel. *Nature*. 323:66-68, **1986**. *[5]*

Follmer CH, Colatsky TJ: Block of delayed rectifier potassium current, Ik, by flecainide and E-4031 in cat ventricular myocytes. *Circulation*. 82:289-293, **1990**. *[4]*

Forbes MS, Van Niel EE: Membrane systems of guinea-pig myocardium: Ultrastructure and morphometric studies. *Anat Rec*. 222:362-379, **1988**. *[1]*

Forbes MS, Sperelakis N: Ultrastructure of mammalian cardiac muscle, in Physiology and Pathophysiology of the Heart. Sperelakis N (ed). *Dordrecht, Netherlands, Kluwer Academic Publishers*. 1-35, **1995**. *[1]*

Ford LE, Podolsky RJ: Regenerative calcium release within muscle cells. *Science*. 167:58-59, **1970**. *[8]*

Forester GV, Mainwood GW: Interval dependent inotropic effects in the rat myocardium and the effect of calcium. *Pflügers Arch*. 352:189-196, **1974**. *[9]*

Frampton JE, Harrison SM, Boyett MR, Orchard CH: Ca2+ and Na+ in rat myocytes showing different force-frequency relationships. *Am J Physiol*. 261:C739-C750, **1991**. *[9]*

Francis SH, Turko IV, Corbin JD: Cyclic nucleotide phosphodiesterases: Relating structure and function. *Prog Nucleic Acid Res Mol Biol*. 65:1-52, **2000**. *[10]*

Franckowiak G, Bechem M, Schramm M, Thomas G: The optical isomers of the 1,4-dihydropyridine Bay K 8644 show opposite effects on Ca channels. *Eur J Pharmacol*. 114:223-226, **1985**. *[5]*

Frank GB: The current view of the source of trigger calcium in excitation-contraction coupling in vertebrate skeletal muscle. *Biochem Pharmacol*. 29:2399-2406, **1980**. *[8]*

Frank JS: Ultrastructure of the unfixed myocardial sarcolemma and cell surface, in Calcium and the Heart. Langer GA (ed). *New York, NY, Raven Press*. 1-25, **1990**. *[1]*

Frank JS, Langer GA: The myocardial interstitium: Its structure and its role in ionic exchange. *J Cell Biol*. 60:586-601, **1974**. *[1]*

Frank M, Albrecht I, Sleator WW, Robinson RB: Stereological measurements of atrial ultrastructures in the guinea-pig. *Experientia*. 31:578-579, **1975**. *[1]*

Frank JS, Langer GA, Nudd LM, Seraydarian K: The myocardial cell surface, its histochemistry, and the effect of sialic acid and calcium removal on its structure and cellular ionic exchange. *Circ Res*. 41:702-714, **1977**. *[1]*

Frank JS, Rich TL, Beydler S, Kreman M: Calcium depletion in rabbit myocardium. *Circ Res*. 51:117-130, **1982**. *[1,8]*

Frank JS, Mottino G, Reid D, Molday RS, Philipson KD: Distribution of the Na+-Ca2+ exchange protein in mammalian cardiac myocytes: An immunofluorescence and immunocolloidal gold-labeling study. *J Cell Biol*. 117:337-345, **1992**. *[6]*

Frank K, Tilgmann C, Kranias EG: Phospholamban ablation results in enhanced efficiency of sarcoplasmic reticulum Ca2+-transport. *Circulation*. 100:I-764, **1999**. *[7]*

Frank K, Tilgmann C, Shannon TR, Bers DM, Kranias EG: Regulatory role of phospholamban in the efficiency of cardiac sarcoplasmic reticulum Ca2+ transport. *Biochemistry*. 39:14176-14182, **2000**. *[10]*

Frankis MB, Lindenmayer GE: Sodium-sensitive calcium binding to sarcolemma-enriched preparations from canine ventricles. *Circ Res*. 55:676-688, **1984**. *[3]*

Franks K, Cooke R, Stull JT: Myosin phosphorylation decreases the ATPase activity of cardiac myofibrils. *J Mol Cell Cardiol*. 16:597-604, **1984**. *[2]*

Franzini-Armstrong C: Studies of the triad. I. Structure of the junction in frog twitch fibers. *J Cell Biol*. 47:488-499, **1970**. *[1]*

Franzini-Armstrong C: Membrane particles and transmission at the triad. *Fed Proc*. 34:1382-1389, **1975**. *[1]*

Franzini-Armstrong C, Protasi F: Ryanodine receptors of striated muscles: A complex channel capable of multiple interactions. *Physiol Rev*. 77:699-729, **1997**. *[1,7]*

Franzini-Armstrong C, Kenney LJ, Verriano-Marston E: The structure of calsequestrin in triads of vertebrate skeletal muscle: A deep etch study. *J Cell Biol*. 105:49-56, **1987**. *[7]*

Franzini-Armstrong C, Protasi F, Ramesh V: Shape, size, and distribution of Ca2+ release units and couplons in skeletal and cardiac muscles. *Biophys J*. 77:1528-1539, **1999**. *[1,7]*

Fraser ID, Tavalin SJ, Lester LB, Langeberg LK, Westphal AM, Dean RA, Marrion NV, Scott JD: A novel lipid-anchored A-kinase anchoring protein facilitates cAMP-responsive membrane events. *EMBO J*. 17:2261-2272, **1998**. *[5]*

Frazer MJ, Lynch C III: Halothane and isoflurane effects on Ca2+ fluxes of isolated myocardial sarcoplasmic reticulum. *Anesthesiology*. 77:316-323, **1992**. *[7]*

Freiburg A, Gautel M: A molecular map of the interactions between titin and myosin-binding protein C. Implications for sarcomeric assembly in familial hypertrophic cardiomyopathy. *Eur J Biochem*. 235:317-323, **1996**. *[1]*

Freund P, Moller BB, Strein K, Kling L, Roegg JC: Ca2+-sensitizing effect of BM 14.478 on skinned cardiac muscle fibres of guinea-pig papillary muscle. *Eur J Pharmacol*. 136:243-246, **1987**. *[2]*

Friel DD, Tsien RW: Voltage-gated calcium channels: Direct observation of the anomalous mole fraction effect at the single-channel level. *Proc Natl Acad Sci USA*. 86:5207-5211, **1989**. *[5]*

Friel DD, Tsien RW: An FCCP-sensitive Ca^{2+} store in bullfrog sympathetic neurons and its participation in stimulus-evoked changes in $[Ca^{2+}]_i$. *J Neurosci.* 14:4007-4024, **1994**. *[3]*

Fry CH, Poole-Wilson PA: Effects of acid-base changes on excitation-contraction coupling in guinea-pig and rabbit cardiac ventricular muscle. *J Physiol.* 313:141-160, **1981**. *[10]*

Fry CH, Powell T, Twist VW, Ward JPT: Net calcium exchange in adult rat ventricular myocytes: An assessment of mitochondrial calcium accumulating capacity. *Proc Roy Soc Lond.* 223:223-238, **1984a**. *[3]*

Fry CH, Powell T, Twist VW, Ward JPT: The effects of sodium, hydrogen and magnesium ions on mitochondrial calcium sequestration in adult rat ventricular myocytes. *Proc Roy Soc Lond.* 223:239-254, **1984b**. *[3]*

Fuchs F: Chemical properties of the calcium receptor site of troponin as determined from binding studies, in Calcium Binding Proteins. Drabikowski W, Strzelecka-Golaszewski H, Carafoli E (eds). *Amsterdam, Netherlands, Elsevier.* 1-27, **1974**. *[2]*

Fuchs F: Mechanical modulation of the Ca^{2+} regulatory protein complex in cardiac muscle. *NIPS.* 10:6-12, **1995**. *[2]*

Fuchs F, Wang YP: Force, length, and Ca^{2+}-troponin C affinity in skeletal muscle. *Am J Physiol.* 261:C787-C792, **1991**. *[2]*

Fuchs F, Wang YP: Sarcomere length versus interfilament spacing as determinants of cardiac myofilament Ca^{2+} sensitivity and Ca^{2+} binding. *J Mol Cell Cardiol.* 28:1375-1383, **1996**. *[2]*

Fuentes O, Valdivia C, Vaughan D, Coronado R, Valdivia HH: Calcium-dependent block of ryanodine receptor channel of swine skeletal muscle by direct binding of calmodulin. *Cell Calcium.* 15:305-316, **1994**. *[7]*

Fujii J, Ueno A, Kitano K, Tanaka S, Kadoma M, Tada M: Complete complementary DNA-derived amino acid sequence of canine cardiac phospholamban. *J Clin Invest.* 70:301-304, **1987**. *[7]*

Fujino K, Sperelakis N, Solaro RJ: Sensitization of dog and guinea-pig heart myofilaments to Ca^{2+} activation and the inotropic effect of pimobendan: Comparison with milrinone. *Circ Res.* 63:911-922, **1988**. *[2]*

Fujioka Y, Komeda M, Matsuoka S: Stoichiometry of Na^+-Ca^{2+} exchange in inside-out patches excised from guinea-pig ventricular myocytes. *J Physiol.* 523:339-351, **2000**. *[6]*

Furuichi T, Yoshikawa S, Miyawaki A, Wada K, Maeda N, Mikoshiba K: Primary structure and functional expression of the inositol 1,4,5-trisphosphate-binding protein P400. *Nature.* 342:32-38, **1989**. *[7]*

Furukawa T, Yamane T, Terai T, Katayama Y, Hiraoka M: Functional linkage of the cardiac ATP-sensitive K^+ channel to the actin cytoskeleton. *Pflügers Arch.* 431:504-512, **1996**. *[4]*

Gadsby DC: Adrenoceptor agonists increase membrane K^+ conductance in cardiac Purkinje fibres. *Nature.* 306:691-693, **1983**. *[10]*

Gadsby DC, Rakowski RF, De Weer P: Extracellular access to the Na,K pump: Pathway similar to ion channel. *Science.* 260:100-103, **1993**. *[4]*

Gadsby DC, Nagel G, Hwang TC: The CFTR chloride channel of mammalian heart. *Annu Rev Physiol.* 57:387-416, **1995**. *[4]*

Galione A, Lee HC, Busa WB: Ca^{2+}-induced Ca^{2+} release in sea urchin egg homogenates: Modulation by cyclic ADP-ribose. *Science.* 253:1143-1146, **1991**. *[7]*

Galione A, McDougall A, Busa WB, Willmott N, Gillot I, Whitaker M: Redundant mechanisms of calcium-induced calcium release underlying calcium waves during fertilization of sea urchin eggs. *Science.* 261:348-352, **1993**. *[7]*

Galizzi JP, Borsotto M, Barhanin J, Fosset M, Lazdunski M: Characterization and photoaffinity labeling of receptor sites for the Ca^{2+} channel inhibitors d-cis-diltiazem, (+)-bepridil, desmethoxyverapamil and (+)PN200-110 in skeletal muscle transverse tubule membranes. *J Biol Chem.* 261:1393-1397, **1986**. *[5]*

Galvan DL, Borrego-Díaz E, Perez PJ, Mignery GA: Subunit oligomerization, and topology of the inositol 1,4,5-trisphosphate receptor. *J Biol Chem.* 274:29483-29492, **1999**. *[7]*

Gambassi G, Blank PS, Spurgeon HA, Chung O, Lakatta EG, Capogrossi MC: An increase in cytosolic pH accompanies the positive inotropic effect of α-adrenergic stimulation. *Circulation.* 82:III-562, **1990**. *[10]*

Gambassi G, Spurgeon HA, Ziman BD, Lakatta EG, Capogrossi MC: Opposing effects of α_1-adrenergic receptor subtypes on Ca^{2+} and pH homeostasis in rat cardiac myocytes. *Am J Physiol.* 274:H1152-H1162, **1998**. *[8,10]*

Gao WD, Backx PH, Azan-Backx M, Marbán E: Myofilament Ca^{2+} sensitivity in intact versus skinned rat ventricular muscle. *Circ Res.* 74:408-415, **1994**. *[2,3]*

Gao WD, Atar D, Backx PH, Marbán E: Relationship between intracellular calcium and contractile force in stunned myocardium. Direct evidence for decreased myofilament Ca^{2+} responsiveness and altered diastolic function in intact ventricular muscle. *Circ Res.* 76:1036-1048, **1995**. *[10]*

Gao J, Mathias RT, Cohen IS, Shi J, Baldo GJ: The effects of β-stimulation on the Na^+-K^+ pump current-voltage relationship in guinea-pig ventricular myocytes. *J Physiol.* 494:697-708, **1996**. *[4,10]*

Gao TY, Yatani A, Dell'Acqua ML, Sako H, Green SA, Dascal N, Scott JD, Hosey MM: CAMP-dependent regulation of cardiac L-type Ca^{2+} channels requires membrane targeting of PKA and phosphorylation of channel subunits. *Neuron.* 19:185-196, **1997a**. *[5]*

Gao TY, Puri TS, Gerhardstein BL, Chien AJ, Green RD, Hosey MM: Identification and subcellular localization of the subunits of L-type calcium channels and adenylyl cyclase in cardiac myocytes. *J Biol Chem.* 272:19401-19407, **1997b**. *[5]*

Gao J, Mathias RT, Cohen IS, Baldo GJ: Comparison of Na^+/K^+ pump current measured by K^+ activation and DHO blockade methods in guinea pig and rat ventricular myocytes. *Biophys J.* 72:A51, **1997c**. *[4,10]*

Gao WD, Atar D, Liu YG, Perez NG, Murphy AM, Marbán E: Role of troponin I proteolysis in the pathogenesis of stunned myocardium. *Circ Res.* 80:393-399, **1997d**. *[10]*

Gao J, Cohen IS, Mathias RT, Baldo GJ: The inhibitory effect of β-stimulation on the Na/K pump current in guinea pig ventricular myocytes is mediated by a cAMP-dependent PKA pathway. *Pflügers Arch.* 435:479-484, **1998a**. *[4,10]*

Gao MH, Ping PP, Post S, Insel PA, Tang RY, Hammond HK: Increased expression of adenylylcyclase type VI proportionately increases β-adrenergic receptor-stimulated production of cAMP in neonatal rat cardiac myocytes. *Proc Natl Acad Sci USA.* 95:1038-1043, **1998b.** *[10]*

Gao TY, Chien AJ, Hosey MM: Complexes of the α_{1C} and β subunits generate the necessary signal for membrane targeting of class C L-type calcium channels. *J Biol Chem.* 274:2137-2144, **1999.** *[5]*

Gao L, Balshaw D, Xu L, Tripathy A, Xin CL, Meissner G: Evidence for a role of the lumenal M3-M4 loop in skeletal muscle Ca^{2+} release channel (ryanodine receptor) activity and conductance. *Biophys J.* 79:828-840, **2000.** *[7]*

Garcia ML, Slaughter RS, King VF, Kaczorowski GJ: Inhibition of sodium-calcium exchange in cardiac sarcolemmal membrane vesicles: II. Mechanism of inhibition by bepridil. *Biochemistry.* 27:2410-2415, **1988.** *[6]*

Garlid KD, Paucek P, Yarov-Yarovoy V, Sun X, Schindler PA: The mitochondrial KATP channel as a receptor for potassium channel openers. *J Biol Chem.* 271:8796-8799, **1996.** *[4]*

Garlid KD, Paucek P, Yarov-Yarovoy V, Murray HN, Darbenzio RB, D'Alonzo AJ, Lodge NJ, Smith MA, Grover GJ: Cardioprotective effect of diazoxide and its interaction with mitochondrial ATP-sensitive K^+ channels. Possible mechanism of cardioprotection. *Circ Res.* 81:1072-1082, **1997.** *[4,10]*

Gaskell WH: On the tonicity of the heart and blood vessels. *J Physiol.* 3:48-75, **1880.** *[10]*

Gatto C, Milanick MA: Inhibition of the red blood cell calcium pump by eosin and other fluorescein analogues. *Am J Physiol.* 264:C1577-C1586, **1993.** *[3,6]*

Gatto C, Hale CC, Xu W, Milanick MA: Eosin, a potent inhibitor of the plasma membrane Ca pump, does not inhibit the cardiac Na-Ca exchanger. *Biochemistry.* 34:965-972, **1995.** *[6]*

Gaughan JP, Hefner CA, Houser SR: Electrophysiological properties of neonatal rat ventricular myocytes with α_1-adrenergic-induced hypertrophy. *Am J Physiol.* 275:H577-H590, **1998.** *[5]*

Gauss R, Seifert R, Kaupp UB: Molecular identification of a hyperpolarization-activated channel in sea urchin sperm. *Nature.* 393:583-587, **1998.** *[4]*

Gautel M, Goulding D: A molecular map of titin/connectin elasticity reveals two different mechanisms acting in series. *FEBS Lett.* 385:11-14, **1996.** *[1]*

Gauthier C, Tavernier G, Charpentier F, Langin D, Le Marec H: Functional β_3-adrenoceptor in the human heart. *J Clin Invest.* 98:556-562, **1996.** *[10]*

Gauthier C, Leblais V, Kobzik L, Trochu JN, Khandoudi N, Bril A, Balligand JL, Le Marec H: The negative inotropic effect of β_3-adrenoceptor stimulation is mediated by activation of a nitric oxide synthase pathway in human ventricle. *J Clin Invest.* 102:1377-1384, **1998.** *[10]*

Gauthier C, Tavernier G, Trochu JN, Leblais V, Laurent K, Langin D, Escande D, Le Marec H: Interspecies differences in the cardiac negative inotropic effects of β_3-adrenoceptor agonists. *J Pharmacol Exp Ther.* 290:687-693, **1999.** *[10]*

Gauthier C, Langin D, Balligand JL: β_3-Adrenoceptors in the cardiovascular system. *Trends Pharmacol Sci.* 21:426-431, **2000.** *[10]*

Gee NS, Brown JP, Dissanayake VU, Offord J, Thurlow R, Woodruff GN: The novel anticonvulsant drug, gabapentin (Neurontin), binds to the $\alpha_2\delta$ subunit of a calcium channel. *J Biol Chem.* 271:5768-5776, **1996.** *[5]*

Gellens ME, George AL Jr, Chen L, Chahine M, Horn R, Barchi RL, Kallen RG: Primary structure and functional expression of the human cardiac tetrodotoxin-insensitive voltage-dependent sodium channel. *Proc Natl Acad Sci USA.* 89:554-558, **1992.** *[4]*

Gerster U, Neuhuber B, Groschner K, Striessnig J, Flucher BE: Current modulation and membrane targeting of the calcium channel α_{1C} subunit are independent functions of the β subunit. *J Physiol.* 517:353-368, **1999.** *[5]*

Gevers W: The unsolved problem of whether and when myosin light-chain phosphorylation is important in the heart. *J Mol Cell Cardiol.* 16:587-590, **1984.** *[2]*

Gibbons WR, Fozzard HA: Slow inward current and contraction of sheep cardiac Purkinje fibers. *J Gen Physiol.* 65:367-384, **1975.** *[8]*

Gilmour RF, Zipes DP: Positive inotropic effect of acetylcholine in canine cardiac Purkinje fibers. *Am J Physiol.* 249:H735-H740, **1985.** *[8]*

Ginsburg KS, Bers DM: Isoproterenol does not increase the intrinsic gain of cardiac E-C coupling (ECC). *Biophys J.* 80:590A, **2001.** *[10]*

Ginsburg KS, Weber CR, Bers DM: Control of maximum sarcoplasmic reticulum Ca load in intact ferret ventricular myocytes. Effects of thapsigargin and isoproterenol. *J Gen Physiol.* 111:491-504, **1998.** *[7]*

Gisbert MP, Fischmeister R: Atrial natriuretic factor regulates the calcium current in frog isolated cardiac cells. *Circ Res.* 62:660-667, **1988.** *[5]*

Glitsch HG, Tappe A: The Na^+/K^+ pump of cardiac Purkinje cells is preferentially fuelled by glycolytic ATP production. *Pflügers Arch.* 422:380-385, **1993.** *[4]*

Glitsch HG, Tappe A: Change of Na^+ pump current reversal potential in sheep cardiac Purkinje cells with varying free energy of ATP hydrolysis. *J Physiol.* 484:605-616, **1995.** *[4]*

Glitsch HG, Krahn T, Pusch H, Suleymanian M: Effect of isoprenaline on active Na transport in sheep cardiac Purkinje fibres. *Pflügers Arch.* 415:88-94, **1989.** *[4]*

Glossmann H, Ferry DR, Goll A: Molecular pharmacology of the calcium channel. *Proc UIPHAR Internat Congress Pharmacol.* 2:329-336, **1984.** *[5]*

Glossmann H, Ferry DR, Goll A, Striessnig J, Zernig G: Calcium channels: Introduction into their molecular pharmacology, in <u>Cardiovascular Effects of Dihydropyridine-Type Calcium Antagonists and Agonists</u>. Fleckenstein A, van Breemen C, Groö R, Hoffmeister F (eds). *Berlin, Germany, Springer-Verlag.* 113-194, **1985.** *[5]*

Glynn IM: The action of cardiac glycosides on ion movements. *Pharmacol Rev.* 16:381-407, **1964.** *[10]*

Go LO, Moschella MC, Watras J, Handa KK, Fyfe BS, Marks AR: Differential regulation of two types of intracellular calcium release channels during end-stage heart failure. *J Clin Invest.* 95:888-894, **1995.** *[10]*

Godfraind T, Ghysel-Burton J: Binding sites related to ouabain-induced stimulation or inhibition of the sodium pump. *Nature.* 265:165-166, **1977.** *[10]*

Godt RE, Lindley BD: Influence of temperature upon contractile activation and isometric force production in mechanically skinned muscle fibers of the frog. *J Gen Physiol.* 80:279-297, **1982.** *[2]*

Goeger DE, Riley RT, Dorner JW, Cole RJ: Cyclopiazonic acid inhibition of the Ca^{2+}-transport ATPase in rat skeletal muscle sarcoplasmic reticulum vesicles. *Biochem Pharmacol.* 37:978-981, **1988**. *[7]*

Goetz AS, King HK, Ward SD, True TA, Rimele TJ, Saussy DL: BMY 7378 is a selective antagonist of the D subtype of α_1-adrenoceptors. *Eur J Pharmacol.* 272:R5-R6, **1995**. *[10]*

Goldhaber JI: Free radicals enhance Na^+/Ca^{2+} exchange in ventricular myocytes. *Am J Physiol.* 271:H823-H833, **1996**. *[10]*

Goldhaber JI: Metabolism in normal and ischemic myocardium, in The Myocardium. Langer GA (ed). 2nd ed. *San Diego, CA, Academic Press.* 325-393, **1997**. *[10]*

Goldhaber JI, Liu E: Excitation-contraction coupling in single guinea-pig ventricular myocytes exposed to hydrogen peroxide. *J Physiol.* 477:135-147, **1994**. *[10]*

Goldhaber JI, Lamp ST, Walter DO, Garfinkel A, Fukumoto GH, Weiss JN: Local regulation of the threshold for calcium sparks in rat ventricular myocytes: role of sodium-calcium exchange. *J Physiol.* 520:431-438, **1999**. *[10]*

Goldman YE: Kinetics of the actomyosin ATPase in muscle fibers. *Annu Rev Physiol.* 49:637-654, **1987**. *[2]*

Goldstein MA, Traeger L: Ultrastructural changes in postnatal development of the cardiac myocytes, in The Developing Heart. Legato MJ (ed). *Boston, MD, Martinus Nijhoff Publishing.* 1-20, **1985**. *[6]*

Goldman YE, Brenner B: Special topic: Molecular mechanism of muscle contraction. *Annu Rev Physiol.* 49:629-636, **1987**. *[2]*

Goldman YE, Hibberd MG, Trentham DR: Relaxation of rabbit psoas muscle fibres from rigor by photochemical generation of adenosine-5'-triphosphate. *J Physiol.* 354:577-604, **1984**. *[2]*

Gómez AM, Cheng H, Lederer WJ, Bers DM: Ca^{2+} diffusion and sarcoplasmic reticulum transport both contribute to $[Ca^{2+}]_i$ decline during Ca^{2+} sparks in rat ventricular myocytes. *J Physiol.* 496:575-581, **1996**. *[7,8]*

Gómez AM, Valdivia HH, Cheng H, Lederer MR, Santana LF, Cannell MB, McCune SA, Altschuld RA, Lederer WJ: Defective excitation-contraction coupling in experimental cardiac hypertrophy and heart failure. *Science.* 276:800-806, **1997**. *[10]*

González A, Kirsch WG, Shirokova N, Pizarro G, Brum G, Pessah IN, Stern MD, Cheng H, Ríos E: Involvement of multiple intracellular release channels in calcium sparks of skeletal muscle. *Proc Natl Acad Sci USA.* 97:4380-4385, **2000**. *[8]*

Gonzalez-Serratos H, Valle-Aguilera R, Lathrop DA, Garcia MC: Slow inward calcium currents have no obvious role in muscle excitation-contraction coupling. *Nature.* 298:292-294, **1982**. *[8]*

Goodenough DA: Lens gap junctions: A structural hypothesis for nonregulated low-resistance intercellular pathways. *Invest Ophthalmol Vis Sci.* 18:1104-1122, **1979**. *[1]*

Goodman OB, Krupnick JG, Santini F, Gurevich VV, Penn RB: β-arrestin acts as a clathrin adaptor in endocytosis of the β_2-adrenergic receptor. *Nature.* 383:447-450, **1996**. *[10]*

Gordon AM, Huxley AF, Julian FJ: The variation in isometric tension with sarcomere length in vertebrate muscle fibres. *J Physiol.* 184:170-192, **1966**. *[2]*

Gorza L, Schiaffino S, Volpe P: Inositol 1,4,5-trisphosphate receptor in heart: Evidence for its concentration in Purkinje myocytes of the conduction system. *J Cell Biol.* 121:345-353, **1993**. *[7]*

Goto M, Kimoto Y, Kato Y: A study on the excitation-contraction coupling of the bullfrog ventricle with voltage clamp technique. *Jap J Physiol.* 21:159-173, **1971**. *[9]*

Gould RJ, Murphy KMM, Reynolds IJ, Snyder SH: Antischizophrenic drugs of the diphenylbutylpiperidine type act as calcium channel agonists. *Proc Natl Acad Sci USA.* 80:5122-5125, **1983**. *[5]*

Gourdie RG, Severs NJ, Green CR, Rothery S, Germroth P, Thompson RP: The spatial distribution and relative abundance of gap-junctional connexin40 and connexin43 correlate to functional properties of components of the cardiac atrioventricular conduction system. *J Cell Sci.* 105:985-991, **1993**. *[1]*

Grabner M, Wang ZY, Hering S, Striessnig J, Glossmann H: Transfer of 1,4-dihydropyridine sensitivity from L-type to class A (BI) calcium channels. *Neuron.* 16:207-218, **1996**. *[5]*

Grabner M, Dirksen RT, Suda N, Beam KG: The II-III loop of the skeletal muscle dihydropyridine receptor is responsible for the bi-directional coupling with the ryanodine receptor. *J Biol Chem.* 274:21913-21919, **1999**. *[7,8]*

Graf E, Penniston JT: Equimolar interaction between calmodulin and the Ca^{2+} ATPase from human erythrocyte membranes. *Arch Biochem Biophys.* 210:257-262, **1981**. *[6]*

Grahame DC: The electrical double layer and the theory of electrocapillarity. *Chem Rev.* 41:441-501, **1947**. *[5]*

Grantham CJ, Cannell MB: Ca^{2+} influx during the cardiac action potential in guinea pig ventricular myocytes. *Circ Res.* 79:194-200, **1996**. *[5,9]*

Green FJ, Farmer BB, Wiseman GL, Jose MJL, Watanabe AM: Effect of membrane depolarization on binding of [³H]nitrendipine to rat cardiac myocytes. *Circ Res.* 56:576-585, **1985**. *[5]*

Gregorio CC, Fowler VM: Mechanisms of thin filament assembly in embryonic chick cardiac myocytes: Tropomodulin requires tropomyosin for assembly. *J Cell Biol.* 129:683-695, **1995**. *[1]*

Gregorio CC, Weber A, Bondad M, Pennise CR, Fowler VM: Requirement of pointed-end capping by tropomodulin to maintain actin filament length in embryonic chick cardiac myocytes. *Nature.* 377:83-86, **1995**. *[1]*

Griffiths EJ, Stern MD, Silverman HS: Measurement of mitochondrial calcium in single living cardiomyocytes by selective removal of cytosolic indo 1. *Am J Physiol.* 273:C37-C44, **1997**. *[3]*

Gross GJ: ATP-sensitive potassium channels and myocardial preconditioning. *Basic Res Cardiol.* 90:85-88, **1995**. *[4]*

Gross G, Hanft G, Rugevics C: 5-Methyl-urapidil discriminates between subtypes of the α_1-adrenoceptor. *Eur J Pharmacol.* 151:333-335, **1988**. *[10]*

Grover GJ, Garlid KD: ATP-Sensitive potassium channels: A review of their cardioprotective pharmacology. *J Mol Cell Cardiol.* 32:677-695, **2000**. *[10]*

Grover GJ, McCullough JR, Henry DE, Conder ML, Sleph PG: Anti-ischemic effects of the potassium channel activators pinacidil and cromakalim and the reversal of these effects with the potassium channel blocker glyburide. *J Pharmacol Exp Ther.* 251:98-104, **1989**. *[10]*

Grover GJ, Dzwonczyk S, Parham CS, Sleph PG: The protective effects of cromakalim and pinacidil on reperfusion function and infarct size in isolated perfused rat hearts and anesthetized dogs. *Cardiovasc Drugs Ther.* 4:465-474, **1990**. *[10]*

Grover GJ, D'Alonzo AJ, Parham CS, Darbenzio RB: Cardioprotection with the K$_{ATP}$ opener cromakalim is not correlated with ischemic myocardial action potential duration. J Cardiovasc Pharmacol. 26:145-152, **1995a**. [10]

Grover GJ, D'Alonzo AJ, Hess T, Sleph PG, Darbenzio RB: Glyburide-reversible cardioprotective effect of BMS-180448 is independent of action potential shortening. Cardiovasc Res. 30:731-738, **1995b**. [10]

Grover GJ, D'Alonzo AJ, Dzwonczyk S, Parham CS, Darbenzio RB: Preconditioning is not abolished by the delayed rectifier K+ blocker dofetilide. Am J Physiol. 271:H1207-H1214, **1996**. [4]

Guerini D, Garcia-Martin E, Zecca A, Guidi F, Carafoli E: The calcium pump of the plasma membrane: Membrane targeting, calcium binding sites, tissue-specific isoform expression. Acta Physiol Scand. 163:265-273, **1998**. [6]

Gumina RJ, Mizumura T, Beier N, Schelling P, Schultz JJ, Gross GJ: A new sodium/hydrogen exchange inhibitor, EMD 85131, limits infarct size in dogs when administered before or after coronary artery occlusion. J Pharmacol Exp Ther. 286:175-183, **1998**. [10]

Gumina RJ, Buerger E, Eickmeier C, Moore J, Daemmgen J, Gross GJ: Inhibition of the Na+/H+ exchanger confers greater cardioprotection against 90 minutes of myocardial ischemia than ischemic preconditioning in dogs. Circulation. 100:2519-2526, **1999**. [10]

Gunter TE, Buntinas L, Sparagna GC, Gunter KK: The Ca^{2+} transport mechanisms of mitochondria and Ca^{2+} uptake from physiological-type Ca^{2+} transients. Biochim Biophys Acta. 1366:5-15, **1998**. [3]

Guo X, Wattanapermpool J, Palmiter KA, Murphy AM, Solaro RJ: Mutagenesis of cardiac troponin I. Role of the unique NH$_2$- terminal peptide in myofilament activation. J Biol Chem. 269:15210-15216, **1994**. [2]

Guo JQ, Ono KI, Noma AN: A sustained inward current activated at the diastolic potential range in rabbit sino-atrial node cells. J Physiol. 483:1-13, **1995**. [4]

Guo XQ, Laflamme MA, Becker PL: Cyclic ADP-ribose does not regulate sarcoplasmic reticulum Ca^{2+} release in intact cardiac myocytes. Circ Res. 79:147-151, **1996**. [7]

Gurnett CA, Felix R, Campbell KP: Extracellular interaction of the voltage-dependent Ca^{2+} channel $\alpha_2\delta$ and α_1 subunits. J Biol Chem. 272:18508-18512, **1997**. [5]

Gurney AM, Charnet P, Pye JM, Nargeot J: Augmentation of cardiac calcium current by flash photolysis of intracellular caged-Ca^{2+} molecules. Nature. 341:65-68, **1989**. [5]

Gurrola GB, Arévalo C, Sreekumar R, Lokuta AJ, Walker JW, Valdivia HH: Activation of ryanodine receptors by imperatoxin A and a peptide segment of the II-III loop of the dihydropyridine receptor. J Biol Chem. 274:7879-7886, **1999**. [7,8]

Gwathmey JK, Hajjar RJ: Relation betwe, n steady-state force and intracellular [Ca^{2+}] in intact human myocardium. Index of myofibrillar responsiveness to Ca^{2+}. Circulation. 82:1266-1278, **1990**. [10]

Gwathmey JK, Copelas L, MacKinnon R, Schoen FJ, Feldman MD, Grossman W, Morgan JP: Abnormal intracellular calcium handling in myocardium from patients with end-stage heart failure. Circ Res. 61:70-76, **1987**. [10]

Gwathmey JK, Hajjar RJ, Solaro RJ: Contractile deactivation and uncoupling of crossbridges. Effects of 2,3-butanedione

monoxime on mammalian myocardium. Circ Res. 69:1280-1292, **1991**. [2]

Györke S, Fill M: Ryanodine receptor adaptation: Control mechanism of Ca^{2+}-induced Ca^{2+} release in heart. Science. 260:807-809, **1993**. [7,8]

Györke I, Györke S: Regulation of the cardiac ryanodine receptor channel by luminal Ca^{2+} involves luminal Ca^{2+} sensing sites. Biophys J. 75:2801-2810, **1998**. [7]

Györke S, Palade P: Role of local Ca^{2+} domains in activation of Ca^{2+}-induced Ca^{2+} release in crayfish muscle fibers. Am J Physiol. 264:C1505-C1512, **1993**. [8]

Györke S, Palade P: Ca^{2+}-dependent negative control mechanism for Ca^{2+}-induced Ca^{2+} release in crayfish muscle. J Physiol. 476:315-322, **1994**. [8]

Györke S, Lukyanenko V, Györke I: Dual effects of tetracaine on spontaneous calcium release in rat ventricular myocytes. J Physiol. 500:297-309, **1997**. [7]

Haase H, Karczewski P, Beckert R, Krause EG: Phosphorylation of the L-type calcium channel β subunit is involved in β-adrenergic signal transduction in canine myocardium. FEBS Lett. 335:217-222, **1993**. [5]

Hadcock JR, Wang HY, Malbon CC: Agonist-induced destabilization of β-adrenergic receptor mRNA. Attenuation of glucocorticoid-induced up-regulation of β-adrenergic receptors. J Biol Chem. 264:19928-19933, **1989**. [10]

Haddock PS, Coetzee WA, Artman M: Na+/Ca^{2+} exchange current and contractions measured under Cl-free conditions in developing rabbit hearts. Am J Physiol. 273:H837-H846, **1997**. [9]

Haddock PS, Coetzee WA, Cho E, Porter L, Katoh H, Bers DM, Jafri MS, Artman M: Subcellular [Ca^{2+}]$_i$ gradients during excitation-contraction coupling in newborn rabbit ventricular myocytes. Circ Res. 85:415-427, **1999**. [9]

Hadley RW, Hume JR: An intrinsic potential-dependent inactivation mechanism associated with calcium channels in guinea-pig myocytes. J Physiol. 389:205-222, **1987**. [5,8]

Hadley RW, Lederer WJ: Intramembrane charge movement in guinea-pig and rat ventricular myocytes. J Physiol. 415:601-624, **1989**. [5,8]

Hadley RW, Lederer WJ: Properties of L-type calcium channel gating current in isolated guinea pig ventricular myocytes. J Gen Physiol. 98:265-285, **1991**. [8]

Hagar RE, Ehrlich BE: Regulation of the type III InsP$_3$ receptor by InsP$_3$ and ATP. Biophys J. 79:271-278, **2000**. [7]

Hagar RE, Burgstahler AD, Nathanson MH, Ehrlich BE: Type III InsP$_3$ receptor channel stays open in the presence of increased calcium. Nature. 396:81-84, **1998**. [7]

Hagemann D, Kuschel M, Kuramochi T, Zhu W, Cheng H, Xiao RP: Frequency-encoding Thr^{17} phospholamban phosphorylation is independent of Ser^{16} phosphorylation in cardiac myocytes. J Biol Chem. 275:22532-22536, **2000**. [7,9]

Hagiwara N, Irisawa H: Modulation by intracellular Ca^{2+} of the hyperpolarization-activated inward current in rabbit single sino-atrial node cells. J Physiol. 409:121-141, **1989**. [4]

Hagiwara S, Fukuda J, Eaton DC: Membrane currents carried by Ca, SR, and Ba in barnacle muscle fiber during voltage clamp. J Gen Physiol. 63:564-578, **1974**. [5]

Hagiwara S, Ozawa S, Sand O: Voltage clamp analysis of two inward current mechanisms in the egg cell membrane of a starfish. J Gen Physiol. 65:617-644, **1975**. [5]

Hagiwara N, Irisawa H, Kameyama M: Contribution of two types of calcium currents to the pacemaker potentials of rabbit sino-atrial node cells. *J Physiol.* 359:233-253, **1988**. *[4,5]*

Hagiwara N, Masuda H, Shoda M, Irisawa H: Stretch-activated anion currents of rabbit cardiac myocytes. *J Physiol.* 456:285-302, **1992**. *[4]*

Haiech J, Klee B, Demaille JG: Effects of cations on affinity of calmodulin for calcium: Ordered binding of calcium ions allows the specific activation of calmodulin-stimulated enzymes. *Biochemistry.* 20:3890-3897, **1981**. *[3]*

Hain J, Onoue H, Mayrleitner M, Fleischer S, Schindler H: Phosphorylation modulates the function of the calcium release channel of sarcoplasmic reticulum from cardiac muscle. *J Biol Chem.* 270:2074-2081, **1995**. *[7]*

Hajdu S, Leonard E: Action of ryanodine on mammalian cardiac muscle. Effects on contractility, and reversal of digitalis-induced ventricular arrhythmias. *Circ Res.* 9:1283-1291, **1961**. *[7,9]*

Hajjar RJ, Grossman W, Gwathmey JK: Responsiveness of the myofilaments to Ca^{2+} in human heart failure: Implications for Ca^{2+} and force regulation. *Basic Res Cardiol.* 87:I143-I159, **1992**. *[10]*

Hajjar RJ, Schmidt U, Helm P, Gwathmey JK: Ca^{2+} sensitizers impair cardiac relaxation in failing human myocardium. *J Pharmacol Exp Ther.* 280:247-254, **1997**. *[10]*

Hajjar RJ, Schwinger RH, Schmidt U, Kim CS, Lebeche D, Doye AA, Gwathmey JK: Myofilament calcium regulation in human myocardium. *Circulation.* 101:1679-1685, **2000**. *[10]*

Hakamata Y, Nakai J, Takeshima H, Imoto K: Primary structure and distribution of a novel ryanodine receptor/calcium release channel from rabbit brain. *FEBS Lett* . 312:229-235, **1992**. *[7]*

Hale CC, Bliler S, Quinn TP, Peletskaya EN: Localization of an exchange inhibitory peptide (XIP) binding site on the cardiac sodium-calcium exchanger. *Biochem Biophys Res Commun.* 236:113-117, **1997**. *[6]*

Halestrap AP: The regulation of the matrix volume of mammalian mitochondria in vivo and in vitro and its role in the control of mitochondrial metabolism. *Biochim Biophys Acta.* 973:355-382, **1989**. *[10]*

Hals GD, Stein Pg, Palade PT: Single channel characteristics of a high-conductance anion channel in sarcoballs. *J Gen Physiol.* 93:385-410, **1989**. *[7]*

Hamilton MA, Stevenson LW, Luu M, Walden JA: Altered thyroid hormone metabolism in advanced heart failure. *J Am Coll Cardiol.* 16:91-95, **1990**. *[10]*

Hamlyn JM, Blaustein MP, Bova S, DuCharme DW, Harris DW, Mandel F, Mathews WR, Ludens JH: Identification and characterization of a ouabain-like compound from human plasma. *Proc Natl Acad Sci USA.* 88:6259-6263, **1991**. *[10]*

Hamlyn JM, Hamilton BP, Manunta P: Endogenous ouabain, sodium balance and blood pressure: A review and a hypothesis. *J Hypertens.* 14:151-167, **1996**. *[10]*

Han X, Shimoni Y, Giles WR: An obligatory role for nitric oxide in autonomic control of mammalian heart rate. *J Physiol.* 476:309-314, **1994a**. *[5]*

Han S, Schiefer A, Isenberg G: Ca^{2+} load of guinea-pig ventricular myocytes determines efficacy of brief Ca^{2+} currents as trigger for Ca^{2+} release. *J Physiol.* 480:411-421, **1994b**. *[8]*

Hancock WO, Martyn DA, Huntsman LL, Gordon AM: Influence of Ca^{2+} on force redevelopment kinetics in skinned rat myocardium. *Biophys J.* 70:2819-2829, **1996**. *[2]*

Hanich RF, Levine JH, Prood C, Weiss JL, Callans DJ, Spear JF, Moore EN: Electrophysiologic recovery in postischemic, stunned myocardium despite persistent systolic dysfunction. *Am Heart J.* 125:23-32, **1993**. *[10]*

Hansford RG: Relation between mitochondrial calcium transport and control of energy metabolism. *Rev Physiol Biochem Pharmacol.* 102:1-72, **1985**. *[3]*

Hansford RG: Relation between cytosolic free Ca^{2+} concentration and the control of pyruvate dehydrogenase in isolated cardiac myocytes. *Biochem J.* 241:145-151, **1987**. *[3]*

Hardie RC, Minke B: Novel Ca^{2+} channels underlying transduction in Drosophila photoreceptors: Implications for phosphoinositide-mediated Ca^{2+} mobilization. *Trends Neurosci.* 16:371-376, **1993**. *[8]*

Harkins AB, Kurebayashi N, Baylor SM: Resting myoplasmic free calcium in frog skeletal muscle fibers estimated with fluo-3. *Biophys J.* 65:865-881, **1993**. *[3]*

Harris EJ, Booth R, Cooper MB: The effect of superoxide generation on the ability of mitochondria to take up and retain Ca^{2+}. *FEBS Lett.* 146:267-272, **1982**. *[10]*

Harrison SM, Bers DM: The effect of temperature and ionic strength on the apparent Ca-affinity of EGTA, BAPTA and di-bromo-BAPTA. *Biochim Biophys Acta.* 925:133-143, **1987**. *[2]*

Harrison SM, Bers DM: The influence of temperature on the calcium sensitivity of the myofilaments of skinned ventricular muscle from the rabbit. *J Gen Physiol.* 93:411-427, **1989a**. *[2,3,7,10]*

Harrison SM, Bers DM: Correction of absolute stability constants of EGTA for temperature and ionic strength. *Am J Physiol.* 256:C1250-C1256, **1989b**. *[2]*

Harrison SM, Bers DM: Temperature-dependence of myofilament Ca-sensitivity of rat, guinea-pig and frog ventricular muscle. *Am J Physiol.* 258:C274-C281, **1990a**. *[2]*

Harrison SM, Bers DM: Modification of temperature-dependence of myofilament Ca-sensitivity by troponin C replacement. *Am J Physiol.* 258:C282-C288, **1990b**. *[2]*

Harrison SM, Lamont C, Miller DJ: Carnosine and other natural imidazoles enhance muscle Ca-sensitivity and are mimicked by caffeine and AR-L 115BS. *J Physiol.* 371:197P, **1986**. *[2]*

Harrison SM, Lamont C, Miller DJ: Hysteresis and the length dependence of calcium sensitivity in chemically skinned rat cardiac muscle. *J Physiol.* 401:115-143, **1988**. *[2]*

Harrison SM, McCall E, Boyett MR: The relationship between contraction and intracellular sodium in rat and guinea-pig ventricular myocytes. *J Physiol.* 449:517-550, **1992a**. *[4]*

Harrison SM, Frampton JE, McCall E, Boyett MR, Orchard CH: Contraction and intracellular Ca^{2+}, Na^+, and H^+ during acidosis in rat ventricular myocytes. *Am J Physiol.* 262:C348-C357, **1992b**. *[10]*

Hartmann HA, Mazzocca NJ, Kleiman RB, Houser SR: Effects of phenylephrine on calcium current and contractility of feline ventricular myocytes. *Am J Physiol.* 255:H1173-H1180, **1988**. *[5,10]*

Hartzell HC: Regulation of cardiac ion channels by catecholamines, acetylcholine and second messenger systems. *Prog Biophys Molec Biol.* 52:165-247, **1988**. *[5]*

Harvey RD, Hume JR: Autonomic regulation of a chloride current in heart. *Science.* 244:983-985, **1989**. *[10]*

Haselgrove JC: X-ray evidence for a conformational change in the actin containing filaments of vertebrate striated muscle. *Cold Spring Harbor Symp Quant Biol.* 37:341-352, **1973**. *[2]*

Hasenfuss G: Animal models of human cardiovascular disease, heart failure and hypertrophy. *Cardiovasc Res.* 39:60-76, **1998a**. *[9]*

Hasenfuss G: Alterations of calcium-regulatory proteins in heart failure. *Cardiovasc Res.* 37:279-289, **1998b**. *[10]*

Hasenfuss G, Mulieri LA, Leavitt BJ, Allen PD, Haeberle JR, Alpert NR: Alteration of contractile function and excitation-contraction coupling in dilated cardiomyopathy. *Circ Res.* 70:1225-1232, **1992**. *[10]*

Hasenfuss G, Reinecke H, Studer R, Meyer M, Pieske B, Holtz J, Holubarsch C, Posival H, Just H, Drexler H: Relation between myocardial function and expression of sarcoplasmic reticulum Ca^{2+}-AT-Pase in failing and nonfailing human myocardium. *Circ Res.* 75:434-442, **1994**. *[10]*

Hasenfuss G, Schillinger W, Lehnart SE, Preuss M, Pieske B, Maier LS, Prestle J, Minami K, Just H: Relationship between Na$^+$-Ca^{2+}-exchanger protein levels and diastolic function of failing human myocardium. *Circulation.* 99:641-648, **1999**. *[10]*

Hasselbach W, Makinose M: Die Kalciumpumpe der 'Erschlaffungsgrund' des Muskels und ihre Abhängigkeit von der ATP-Spaltung. *Biochem Z.* 333:518-528, **1961**. *[7]*

Hayes JS, Mayer SE: Regulation of guinea pig heart phosphorylase kinase by cAMP, protein kinase, and calcium. *Am J Physiol.* 240:E340-E349, **1981**. *[10]*

He HP, Giordano FJ, Hilal-Dandan R, Choi DJ, Rockman HA, McDonough PM, Bluhm WF, Meyer M, Sayen MR, Swanson E, Dillmann WH: Overexpression of the rat sarcoplasmic reticulum Ca^{2+} ATPase gene in the heart of transgenic mice accelerates calcium transients and cardiac relaxation. *J Clin Invest.* 100:380-389, **1997**. *[10]*

He Z, Tong Q, Quednau BD, Philipson KD, Hilgemann DW: Cloning, expression, and characterization of the squid Na$^+$-Ca^{2+}exchanger (NCX-SQ1). *J Gen Physiol.* 111:857-873, **1998**. *[6]*

He Z, Feng S, Tong Q, Hilgemann DW, Philipson KD: Interaction of PIP$_2$ with the XIP region of the cardiac Na/Ca exchanger. *Am J Physiol.* 278:C661-C666, **2000**. *[6]*

Hearse DJ, Tosaki A: Free radicals and reperfusion-induced arrhythmias: Protection by spin trap agent PBN in the rat heart. *Circ Res.* 60:375-383, **1987**. *[10]*

Hefti MA, Harder BA, Eppenberger HM, Schaub MC: Signaling pathways in cardiac myocyte hypertrophy. *J Mol Cell Cardiol.* 29:2873-2892, **1997**. *[10]*

Heinemann SH, Terlau H, Stühmer W, Imoto K, Numa S: Calcium channel characteristics conferred on the sodium channel by single mutations. *Nature.* 356:441-443, **1992**. *[4]*

Henderson D, Eibl H, Weber K: Structure and biochemistry of mouse hepatic gap junctions. *J Mol Biol.* 132:192-218, **1979**. *[1]*

Hendrikx M, Mubagwa K, Verdonck F, Overloop K, van Hecke P, Vanstapel F, van Lommel A, Verbeken E, Lauweryns J, Flameng W: New Na$^+$-H$^+$ exchange inhibitor HOE 694 improves postischemic function and high-energy phosphate resynthesis and reduces Ca^{2+} overload in isolated perfused rabbit heart. *Circulation.* 89:2787-2798, **1994**. *[10]*

Henry PD: Positive staircase effect in the rat heart. *Am J Physiol.* 228:360-364, **1975**. *[9]*

Heppner TJ, Bonev AD, Nelson MT: Ca^{2+}-activated K$^+$ channels regulate action potential repolarization in urinary bladder smooth muscle. *Am J Physiol.* 273:C110-C117, **1997**. *[8]*

Herbette LG, Vant Erve YM, Rhodes DG: Interaction of 1,4 dihydropyridine calcium channel antagonists with biological membranes: Lipid bilayer partitioning could occur before drug binding to receptors. *J Mol Cell Cardiol.* 21:187-201, **1989**. *[5]*

Hering S, Hughes AD, Timin EN, Bolton TB: Modulation of calcium channels in arterial smooth muscle cells by dihydropyridine enantiomers. *J Gen Physiol.* 101:393-410, **1993a**. *[5]*

Hering S, Savchenko A, Strübing C, Lakitsch M, Striessnig J: Extracellular localization of the benzothiazepine binding domain of L-type Ca^{2+} channels. *Mol Pharmacol.* 43:820-826, **1993b**. *[5]*

Hering S, Aczél S, Grabner M, Döring F, Berjukow S, Mitterdorfer J, Sinnegger MJ, Striessnig J, Degtiar VE, Wang ZY, Glossmann H: Transfer of high sensitivity for benzothiazepines from L-type to class A (BI) calcium channels. *J Biol Chem.* 271:24471-24475, **1996**. *[5]*

Herrington J, Park YB, Babcock DF, Hille B: Dominant role of mitochondria in clearance of large Ca^{2+} loads from rat adrenal chromaffin cells. *Neuron.* 16:219-228, **1996**. *[3]*

Herrmann-Frank A, Richter M, Sárközi S, Mohr U, Lehmann-Horn F: 4-chloro-*m*-cresol, a potent and specific activator of the skeletal muscle ryanodine receptor. *Biochim Biophys Acta Gen Subj.* 1289:31-40, **1996**. *[7]*

Hertzberg EL, Gilula NB: Isolation and characterization of gap junctions from rat liver. *J Biol Chem.* 254:2138-2147, **1979**. *[1]*

Herzig S: Ca^{2+} channel activation by CGP 48506, a new positive inotropic benzodiazocine derivative. *Eur J Pharmacol.* 295:113-117, **1996**. *[10]*

Herzig JW, Rüegg JC: Myocardial cross-bridge activity and its regulation by Ca^{2+}, phosphate and stretch, in Myocardial Failure. Riecker G, Weber A, Goodwin J (eds). *International Boehringer Mannheim Symposium*, **1977**. *[10]*

Herzig JE, Köhler G, Pfitzer G, Rüegg JC, Wölffle G: Cyclic AMP inhibits contractility of detergent treated glycerol extracted cardiac muscle. *Pflügers Arch.* 391:208-212, **1981**. *[2]*

Herzig S, Meier A, Pfeiffer M, Neumann J: Stimulation of protein phosphatases as a mechanism of the muscarinic-receptor-mediated inhibition of cardiac L-type Ca^{2+} channels. *Pflügers Arch.* 429:531-538, **1995**. *[5]*

Hescheler J, Pelzer D, Trube G, Trautwein W: Does the organic calcium channel blocker D600 act from inside or outside on the cardiac cell membrane? *Pflügers Arch.* 393:287-291, **1982**. *[5]*

Hescheler J, Kameyama M, Trautwein W: On the mechanism of muscarinic inhibition of the cardiac Ca current. *Pflügers Arch.* 407:182-189, **1986**. *[5]*

Hescheler J, Kameyama M, Trautwein W, Mieskes G, Doling HD: Regulation of the cardiac calcium channel by protein phosphatases. *Eur J Biochem.* 165:261-266, **1987a**. *[5]*

Hescheler J, Tang M, Jastorff B, Trautwein W: On the mechanism of histamine induced enhancement of the cardiac Ca^{2+} current. *Pflügers Arch.* 419:23-29, **1987b**. *[5]*

Hescheler J, Nawrath H, Tang M, Trautwein W: Adrenoreceptor-mediated changes of excitation and contraction in ventricular heart muscle from guinea-pigs and rabbits. *J Physiol.* 397:657-670, **1988**. *[5,10]*

Hesketh TR, Smith GA, Houslay MD, McGill KA, Birdsall NJ, Metcalfe JC, Warren GB: Annular lipids determine the ATPase activity of a calcium transport protein complexed with dipalmitoyllecithin. *Biochemistry.* 15:4145-4151, **1976**. *[7]*

Hess P: Elementary properties of cardiac calcium channels: A brief review. *Can J Physiol Pharmacol.* 66:1218-1223, **1988**. *[5]*

Hess P, Tsien RW: Mechanism of ion permeation through calcium channels. *Nature.* 309:453-456, **1984**. *[5]*

Hess ML, Krause S, Kontos HA: Mediation of sarcoplasmic reticulum disruption in the ischemic myocardium: Proposed mechanism by the interaction of hydrogen ions and oxygen free radicals. *Adv Exp Med Biol.* 161:377-389, **1983**. *[10]*

Hess P, Lansman JB, Tsien RW: Different modes of Ca channel gating behavior favored by dihydropyridine Ca agonists and antagonists. *Nature.* 311:538-544, **1984a**. *[5]*

Hess ML, Okabe E, Ash P, Kontos HA: Free radical mediation of the effects of acidosis on calcium transport by cardiac sarcoplasmic reticulum in whole heart homogenates. *Cardiovasc Res.* 18:149-157, **1984b**. *[10]*

Hess P, Lansman JB, Tsien RW: Calcium channel selectivity for divalent and monovalent cations. Voltage and concentration dependence of single channel current in ventricular heart cells. *J Gen Physiol.* 88:293-319, **1986**. *[4,5,8]*

Heusch G: Hibernating myocardium. *Physiol Rev.* 78:1055-1085, **1998**. *[10]*

Higashiyama A, Watkins MW, Chen ZY, LeWinter MM: Effects of EMD 57033 on contraction and relaxation in isolated rabbit hearts. *Circulation.* 92:3094-3104, **1995**. *[10]*

Hibberd MG, Jewell BR: Length-dependence of the sensitivity of the contractile system to calcium in rat ventricular muscle. *J Physiol.* 290:30P-31P, **1979**. *[2]*

Hibberd MG, Jewell BR: Calcium-and length-dependent force production in rat ventricular muscle. *J Physiol.* 329:527-540, **1982**. *[2]*

Hicks MJ, Shigekawa M, Katz AM: Mechanism by which cyclic adenosine 3':5'-monophosphate-dependent protein kinase stimulates calcium transport in cardiac sarcoplasmic reticulum. *Circ Res.* 44:384-391, **1979**. *[7]*

Hidalgo C, Jaimovich E: Inositol trisphosphate and excitation-contraction coupling in skeletal muscle. *J Bioenerg Biomemb.* 21:267-281, **1989**. *[8]*

Hidalgo C, Ikemoto N, Gergely J: Role of phospholipids in the calcium-dependent ATPase of sarcoplasmic reticulum. Enzymatic and ESR studies with phospholipid-replaced membranes. *J Biol Chem.* 251:4224-4232, **1976**. *[7]*

Hidalgo C, Carrasco MA, Magendzo K, Jaimovich E: Phosphorylation of phosphatidylinositol by transverse tubule vesicles and its possible role in excitation-contraction coupling. *FEBS Lett.* 202:69-73, **1986**. *[8]*

Hilgemann DW: Extracellular calcium transients and action potential configuration changes related to post-stimulatory potentiation in rabbit atrium. *J Gen Physiol.* 87:675-706, **1986a**. *[7,9]*

Hilgemann DW: Extracellular calcium transients at single excitations in rabbit atrium measured with tetramethylmurexide. *J Gen Physiol.* 87:707-735, **1986b**. *[7,9]*

Hilgemann DW: Giant excised cardiac sarcolemmal membrane patches: Sodium and sodium-calcium exchange currents. *Pflügers Arch.* 415:247-249, **1989**. *[6]*

Hilgemann DW: Regulation and deregulation of cardiac Na+-Ca2+ exchange in giant excised sarcolemmal membrane patches. *Nature.* 344:242-245, **1990**. *[6]*

Hilgemann DW: Unitary cardiac Na+,Ca2+ exchange current magnitudes determined from channel-like noise and charge movements of ion transport. *Biophys J.* 71:759-768, **1996**. *[6]*

Hilgemann DW, Ball R: Regulation of cardiac Na+,Ca2+ exchange and KATP potassium channels by PIP2. *Science.* 273:956-959, **1996**. *[4,6]*

Hilgemann DW, Collins A: Mechanism of cardiac Na+-Ca2+ exchange current stimulation by MgATP: Possible involvement of aminophospholipid translocase. *J Physiol.* 454:59-82, **1992**. *[6]*

Hilgemann DW, Langer GA: Transsarcolemmal calcium movements in arterially perfused rabbit right ventricle measured with extracellular calcium-sensitive dyes. *Circ Res.* 54:461-467, **1984**. *[7]*

Hilgemann DW, Noble D: Excitation-contraction coupling and extracellular calcium transients in rabbit atrium: Reconstruction of basic cellular mechanisms. *Proc R Soc Lond B Biol Sci.* 230:163-205, **1987**. *[9]*

Hilgemann DW, Delay MJ, Langer GA: Activation-dependent cumulative depletions of extracellular free calcium in guinea pig atrium measured with antipyrylazo III and tetramethylmurexide. *Circ Res.* 53:779-793, **1983**. *[7]*

Hilgemann DW, Collins A, Cash DP, Nagel GA: Cardiac Na+-Ca2+ exchange system in giant membrane patches. *Ann NY Acad Sci.* 639:126-139, **1991**. *[6]*

Hilgemann DW, Collins A, Matsuoka S: Steady-state and dynamic properties of cardiac sodium-calcium exchange. Secondary modulation by cytoplasmic calcium and ATP. *J Gen Physiol.* 100:933-961, **1992a**. *[6]*

Hilgemann DW, Matsuoka S, Nagel GA, Collins A: Steady-state and dynamic properties of cardiac sodium-calcium exchange. Sodium-dependent inactivation. *J Gen Physiol.* 100:905-932, **1992b**. *[6]*

Hill AV: The heat of shortening and dynamic constants of muscle. *Proc Roy Soc Lond.* 126:136-195, **1938**. *[2]*

Hille B: Local anesthetics: Hydrophilic and hydrophobic pathways for the drug-receptor reaction. *J Gen Physiol.* 69:497-515, **1977**. *[5]*

Hille B: Ionic Channels of Excitable Membranes. *Sunderland, MA, Sinauer Associates, Inc.* 1992. *[4,5]*

Himpens B, Missiaen L, Casteels R: Ca2+ homeostasis in vascular smooth muscle. *J Vasc Res.* 32:207-219, **1995**. *[8]*

Hiramoto T, Kushida H, Endoh M: Further characterization of the myocardial α-adrenoceptors mediating positive inotropic effects in the rabbit myocardium. *Eur J Pharmacol.* 152:301-310, **1988**. *[10]*

Hirano Y, Hiraoka M: Dual modulation of unitary L-type Ca2+ channel currents by [Ca2+]i in fura-2-loaded guinea-pig ventricular myocytes. *J Physiol.* 480:449-463, **1994**. *[5]*

Hirano Y, Fozzard HA, January CT: Characteristics of L- and T-type Ca2+ currents in canine cardiac Purkinje cells. *Am J Physiol.* 256:H1478-H1492, **1989**. *[5]*

Hirata M, Suematsu E, Hashimoto T, Hamachi T, Koga T: Release of Ca^{2+} from a non-mitochondrial store site in peritoneal macrophages treated with saponin by inositol 1,4,5-triphosphate. Biochem J. 223:229-236, 1984. [8]

Hirschberg B, Rovner A, Lieberman M, Patlak J: Transfer of twelve charges is needed to open skeletal muscle Na^+ channels. J Gen Physiol. 106:1053-1068, 1995. [4]

Hobai IA, Bates JA, Howarth FC, Levi AJ: Inhibition by external Cd^{2+} of Na/Ca exchange and L-type Ca channel in rabbit ventricular myocytes. Am J Physiol. 272:H2164-H2172, 1997a. [6]

Hobai IA, Howarth FC, Pabbathi VK, Dalton GR, Hancox JC, Zhu JQ, Howlett SE, Ferrier GR, Levi AJ: "Voltage-activated Ca release" in rabbit, rat and guinea-pig cardiac myocytes, and modulation by internal cAMP. Pflügers Arch. 435:164-173, 1997b. [8]

Hobai IA, O'Rourke B: Enhanced Ca^{2+}-activated Na^+-Ca^{2+} exchange activity in canine pacing-induced heart failure. Circ Res. 87:690-698, 2000. [10]

Hobai IA, O'Rourke B: Decreased sarcoplasmic reticulum calcium content is responsible for defective excitation-contraction coupling in canine heart failure. Circulation. 103:1577-1584, 2001. [10]

Hockerman GH, Peterson BZ, Johnson BD, Catterall WA: Molecular determinants of drug binding and action on L-type calcium channels. Annu Rev Pharmacol Toxicol. 37:361-396, 1997. [5]

Hodgkin AL, Horowicz P: Potassium contractures in single muscle fibres. J Physiol. 153:386-403, 1960. [8]

Hoerter J, Mazet F, Vassort G: Perinatal growth of the rabbit cardiac cell: Possible implications for the mechanism of relaxation. J Mol Cell Cardiol. 13:725-740, 1981. [9]

Hof RP, Rüegg UT, Hof A, Vogel A: Stereoselectivity at the calcium channel: Opposite action of the enantiomers of a 1,4-dihydropyridine. J Cardiovasc Pharmacol. 7:689-693, 1985. [10]

Hofer GF, Hohenthanner K, Baumgartner W, Groschner K, Klugbauer N, Hofmann F, Romanin C: Intracellular Ca^{2+} inactivates L-type Ca^{2+} channels with a Hill coefficient of approximately 1 and an inhibition constant of approximately 4 microM by reducing channel's open probability. Biophys J. 73:1857-1865, 1997. [5]

Hoffman PA, Fuchs F: Bound calcium and force development in skinned cardiac muscle bundles: Effect of sarcomere length. J Mol Cell Cardiol. 20:667-677, 1988. [2]

Hoffman BF, Bindler E, Suckling EE: Postextrasystolic potentiation of contraction in cardiac muscle. Am J Physiol. 185:95-102, 1956. [9]

Hofmann SL, Goldstein JL, Orth K, Moomaw CR, Slaughter CA, Brown MS: Molecular cloning of a histidine-rich Ca^{2+}-binding protein of sarcoplasmic reticulum that contains highly conserved repeated elements. J Biol Chem. 264:18083-18090, 1989. [7]

Hofmann PA, Miller WP, Moss RL: Altered calcium sensitivity of isometric tension in myocyte-sized preparations of porcine postischemic stunned myocardium. Circ Res. 72:50-56, 1993. [10]

Hoh JFY, Rossmanith GH, Kwan LJ, Hamilton AM: Adrenaline increases the rate of cycling of crossbridges in rat cardiac muscle as measured by pseudo-random binary noise-modulated perturbation analysis. Circ Res. 62:452-461, 1988. [10]

Hoit BD, Houry SF, Kranias EG, Ball N, Walsh RA: In vivo echocardiographic detection of enhanced left ventricular function in gene-targeted mice with phospholamban deficiency. Circ Res. 77:632-637, 1995. [10]

Holland DR, Wikel JH, Kauffman RF, Smallwood JK, Zimmerman KM, Utterback BG, Turk JA, Steinberg MI: LY249933: A cardioselective 1,4-dihydropyridine with positive inotropic activity. J Cardiovasc Pharmacol. 14:483-491, 1989. [10]

Hollingworth S, Harkins AB, Kurebayashi N, Konishi M, Baylor SM: Excitation-contraction coupling in intact frog skeletal muscle fibers injected with mmolar concentrations of fura-2. Biophys J. 63:224-234, 1992. [8]

Holmberg SRM, Williams AJ: Single channel recordings from human cardiac sarcoplasmic reticulum. Circ Res. 65:1445-1459, 1989. [10]

Holmberg SRM, Poole-Wilson PA, Williams AJ: Differential effects of phosphodiesterase inhibitors on the cardiac sarcoplasmic reticulum calcium release channel. Circulation 82:III-519, 1990. [10]

Holmuhamedov EL, Wang LW, Terzic A: ATP-sensitive K^+ channel openers prevent Ca^{2+} overload in rat cardiac mitochondria. J Physiol. 519:347-360, 1999. [4,10]

Holroyde MJ, Howe E, Solaro RJ: Modification of calcium requirements for activation of cardiac myofibrillar ATPase by cyclic AMP dependent phosphorylation. Biochim Biophys Acta. 586:63-69, 1979. [2,3]

Holroyde MJ, Robertson SP, Johnson JD, Solaro RJ, Potter JD: The calcium and magnesium binding sites on cardiac troponin and their role in the regulation of myofibrillar adenosine triphosphatase. J Biol Chem. 255:11688-11693, 1980. [2,3]

Homma N, Hirasawa A, Shibata K, Hashimito K, Tsujimoto G: Both α_{1A}- and α_{1B}-adrenergic receptor subtypes couple to the transient outward current (I_{To}) in rat ventricular myocytes. Br J Pharmacol. 129:1113-1120, 2000. [10]

Hondeghem LM, Katzung BG: Time- and voltage-dependent interactions of antiarrhythmic drugs with cardiac sodium channels. Biochim Biophys Acta. 472:373-398, 1977. [5]

Honore E, Challice CE, Guilbault P, Dupuis B: Two components of contraction in guinea pig papillary muscle. Can J Physiol Pharmacol. 64:1153-1159, 1986. [9]

Honore E, Adamantidis MM, Dupuis BA, Challice CE, Guilbault P: Calcium channels and excitation-contraction coupling in cardiac cells. I. Two components of contraction in guinea-pig papillary muscle. Can J Physiol Pharmacol. 65:1821-1831, 1987. [9]

Hool LC, Harvey RD: Role of β_1- and β_2-adrenergic receptors in regulation of Cl^- and Ca^{2+} channels in guinea pig ventricular myocytes. Am J Physiol. 273:H1669-H1676, 1997. [5]

Hool LC, Middleton LM, Harvey RD: Genistein increases the sensitivity of cardiac ion channels to β-adrenergic receptor stimulation. Circ Res. 83:33-42, 1998. [5]

Horackova M, Vassort G: Calcium conductance in relation to contractility in frog myocardium. J Physiol. 259:597-616, 1976. [9]

Horackova M, Vassort G: Sodium-calcium exchange in regulation of cardiac contractility. Evidence for an electrogenic, voltage-dependent mechanism. *J Gen Physiol.* 73:403-424, **1979**. *[6,9]*

Horowits R, Winegrad S: Cholinergic regulation of calcium sensitivity in cardiac muscle. *J Mol Cell Cardiol.* 15:277-280, **1983**. *[2]*

Horowitz B, Tsung SS, Hart P, Levesque PC, Hume JR: Alternative splicing of CFTR Cl⁻ channels in heart. *Am J Physiol.* 264:H2214-H2220, **1993**. *[4]*

Hosey MM, Borsotto M, Lazdunski M: Phosphorylation and dephosphorylation of dihydropyridine-sensitive voltage-dependent Ca²⁺ channel in skeletal muscle membranes by cAMP- and Ca²⁺-dependent processes. *Proc Natl Acad Sci. USA.* 83:3733-3737, **1986**. *[5]*

Hosey MM, Barhanin J, Schmid A, Vandaele S, Ptasienski J, O'Callahan C, Cooper C, Lazdunski M: Photoaffinity labelling and phosphorylation of a 165-kilodalton peptide associated with dihydropyridine and phenylalkylamine-sensitive calcium channels. *Biochem Biophys Res Commun.* 147:1137-1145, **1987**. *[5]*

Hoshi T, Zagotta WN, Aldrich RW: Biophysical and molecular mechanisms of Shaker potassium channel inactivation. *Science.* 250:533-538, **1990**. *[4]*

Hoshi T, Zagotta WN, Aldrich RW: Two types of inactivation in Shaker K⁺ channels: Effects of alterations in the carboxy-terminal region. *Neuron.* 7:547-556, **1991**. *[4]*

Hoth M, Penner R: Depletion of intracellular calcium stores activates a calcium current in mast cells. *Nature.* 355:353-356, **1992**. *[8]*

Hoth M, Penner R: Calcium release-activated calcium current in rat mast cells. *J Physiol.* 465:359-386, **1993**. *[8]*

Hougen TJ, Spicer N, Smith TW: Stimulation of monovalent cation active transport by low concentrations of cardiac glycosides. *J Clin Invest.* 68:1207-1214, **1981**. *[10]*

Houser SR, Piacentino V III, Mattiello J, Weisser J, Gaughan JP: Functional properties of failing human ventricular myocytes. *Trends Cardiovasc Med.* 10:101-107, **2000**. *[10]*

Hove-Madsen L, Bers DM: Indo-1 binding to protein in permeabilized ventricular myocytes alters its spectral and Ca binding properties. *Biophys J.* 63:89-97, **1992**. *[3]*

Hove-Madsen L, Bers DM: Passive Ca buffering and SR Ca uptake in permeabilized rabbit ventricular myocytes. *Am J Physiol.* 264:C677-C686, **1993a**. *[3,7]*

Hove-Madsen L, Bers DM: Sarcoplasmic reticulum Ca²⁺ uptake and thapsigargin sensitivity in permeabilized rabbit and rat ventricular myocytes. *Circ Res.* 73:820-828, **1993b**. *[7]*

Howlett SE, Zhu JQ, Ferrier GR: Contribution of a voltage-sensitive calcium release mechanism to contraction in cardiac ventricular myocytes. *Am J Physiol.* 274:H155-H170, **1998**. *[8]*

Hryshko LV: The cardiac Na⁺-Ca²⁺ exchanger, in Handbook of Physiology. Page E, Fozzard HA, Solaro RJ (eds). *New York, NY, Oxford University Press.* In press. **2001**. *[6]*

Hryshko LV, Bers DM: Ca current facilitation during post-rest recovery depends on Ca entry. *Am J Physiol.* 259:H951-H961, **1990**. *[5,9]*

Hryshko LV, Bouchard R, Chau T, Bose D: Inhibition of rest potentiation in canine ventricular muscle by BAY K 8644: Comparison with caffeine. *Am J Physiol.* 257:H399-H406, **1989a**. *[8]*

Hryshko LV, Kobayashi T, Bose D: Possible inhibition of canine ventricular sarcoplasmic reticulum by BAY K 8644. *Am J Physiol.* 257:H407-H414, **1889b**. *[8]*

Hryshko LV, Stiffel VM, Bers DM: Rapid cooling contractures as an index of SR Ca content in rabbit ventricular myocyte. *Am J Physiol.* 257:H1369-H1377, **1989c**. *[6,7]*

Hryshko LV, Nicoll DA, Weiss JN, Philipson KD: Biosynthesis and initial processing of the cardiac sarcolemmal Na⁺-Ca²⁺ exchanger. *Biochim Biophys Acta.* 1151:35-42, **1993**. *[6]*

Hryshko LV, Matsuoka S, Nicoll DA, Weiss JN, Schwarz EM, Benzer S, Philipson KD: Anomalous regulation of the Drosophila Na⁺-Ca²⁺ exchanger by Ca²⁺. *J Gen Physiol.* 108:67-74, **1996**. *[6]*

Hu H, Sachs F: Mechanically activated currents in chick heart cells. *J Membr Biol.* 154:205-216, **1996**. *[4]*

Hu H, Sachs F: Stretch-activated ion channels in the heart. *J Mol Cell Cardiol.* 29:1511-1523, **1997**. *[4]*

Huang CL, Feng SY, Hilgemann DW: Direct activation of inward rectifier potassium channels by PIP₂ and its stabilization by Gβγ. *Nature.* 391:803-806, **1998**. *[4]*

Huang BY, Wang S, Qin DY, Boutjdir M, El-Sherif N: Diminished basal phosphorylation level of phospholamban in the postinfarction remodeled rat ventricle - Role of β-adrenergic pathway, Gᵢ protein, phosphodiesterase, and phosphatases. *Circ Res.* 85:848-855, **1999**. *[10]*

Huggins JP, Cook EA, Piggott JR, Mattinsley TJ, England PJ: Phospholamban is a good substrate for cyclic GMP-dependent protein kinase in vitro, but not in intact cardiac or smooth muscle. *Biochem J.* 260:829-835, **1989**. *[7]*

Hui CS: Differential properties of two charge components in frog skeletal muscle. *J Physiol.* 337:531-552, **1983**. *[8]*

Hui CS, Chandler WK: Intramembranous charge movement in frog cut twitch fibers mounted in a double vaseline-gap chamber. *J Gen Physiol.* 96:257-297, **1990**. *[8]*

Hui CS, Milton RL, Eisenberg RS: Charge movement in skeletal muscle fibers paralyzed by the calcium-entry blocker D600. *Proc Natl Acad Sci USA.* 81:2582-2585, **1984**. *[8]*

Hullin R, Singer-Lahat D, Freichel M, Biel M, Dascal N, Hofmann F, Flockerzi V: Calcium channel β subunit heterogeneity: Functional expression of cloned cDNA from heart, aorta and brain. *EMBO J.* 11:885-890, **1992**. *[5]*

Hulme JT, Orchard CH: Effect of acidosis on Ca²⁺ uptake and release by sarcoplasmic reticulum of intact rat ventricular myocytes. *Am J Physiol.* 275:H977-H987, **1998**. *[10]*

Humbert JP, Matter N, Artault JC, Köppler P, Malviya AN: Inositol 1,4,5-trisphosphate receptor is located to the inner nuclear membrane vindicating regulation of nuclear calcium signaling by inositol 1,4,5-trisphosphate - Discrete distribution of inositol phosphate receptors to inner and outer nuclear membranes. *J Biol Chem.* 271:478-485, **1996**. *[8]*

Hume JR: Components of whole cell Ca current due to electrogenic Na-Ca-exchange in cardiac myocytes. *Am J Physiol.* 252:H666-H670, **1987**. *[6]*

Hume JR, Uehara A: Properties of "creep currents" in single frog atrial cells. *J Gen Physiol.* 87:833-855, **1986a**. *[6]*

Hume JR, Uehara A: "Creep currents" in single frog atrial cells may be generated by electrogenic Na/Ca exchange. *J Gen Physiol.* 87:857-884, **1986b**. *[6]*

Hume JR, Duan D, Collier ML, Yamazaki J, Horowitz B: Anion transport in heart. *Physiol Rev.* 80:31-81, **2000**. *[4]*

Hunter DR, Haworth RA: The Ca^{2+}-induced membrane transition in mitochondria. I. The protective mechanisms. *Arch Biochem Biophys.* 195:453-459, **1979**. *[3]*

Hunter DR, Haworth RA, Berkoff HA: Measurement of rapidly exchangeable cellular calcium in the perfused beating rat heart. *Proc Natl Acad Sci USA.* 78:5665-5668, **1981**. *[3,7]*

Hüser J, Lipsius SL, Blatter LA: Calcium gradients during excitation-contraction coupling in cat atrial myocytes. *J Physiol.* 494:641-651, **1996**. *[9]*

Hüser J, Rechenmacher CE, Blatter LA: Imaging the permeability pore transition in single mitochondria. *Biophys J.* 74:2129-2137, **1998a**. *[3]*

Hüser J, Bers DM, Blatter LA: Subcellular properties of $[Ca^{2+}]_i$ transients in phospholamban-deficient mouse ventricular cells. *Am J Physiol.* 274:H1800-H1811, **1998b**. *[10]*

Hüser J, Blatter L, Lipsius SL: Intracellular Ca^{2+} release contributes to automaticity in cat atrial pacemaker cells. *J Physiol.* 524:415-422, **2000**. *[4]*

Hussain M, Orchard CH: Sarcoplasmic reticulum Ca^{2+} content, L-type Ca^{2+} current and the Ca^{2+} transient in rat myocytes during β-adrenergic stimulation. *J Physiol .* 505:385-402, **1997**. *[8]*

Hussain M, Drago GA, Colyer J, Orchard CH: Rate-dependent abbreviation of Ca^{2+} transient in rat heart is independent of phospholamban phosphorylation. *Am J Physiol.* 273:H695-H706, **1997**. *[9]*

Huxley HE: The mechanism of muscular contraction. *Science.* 164:1356-1366, **1969**. *[2]*

Huxley HE: Structural changes in the actin and myosin containing filaments during contraction. *Cold Spring Harbor Symp Quant Biol.* 37:361-376, **1973**. *[2]*

Huxley AF, Simmons RM: Proposed mechanism of force generation in striated muscle. *Nature.* 233:533-538, **1971**. *[2]*

Hwang KS, Van Breemen C: Ryanodine modulation of ^{45}Ca efflux and tension in rabbit aortic smooth muscle. *Pflügers Arch.* 408:343-350, **1987**. *[8]*

Iino M, Kobayashi T, Endo M: Use of ryanodine for functional removal of the calcium store in smooth muscle cells of the guinea-pig. *Biochem Biophys Res Commun.* 152:417-422, **1988**. *[8]*

Ikeda SR, Dunlap K: Voltage-dependent modulation of N-type calcium channels: Role of G protein subunits. *Adv Second Messenger Phosphoprotein Res.* 33:131-151, **1999**. *[5]*

Ikemoto N, Bhatnagar GM, Nagy B, Gergely J: Interaction of divalent cations with the 55,000-dalton protein component of the sarcoplasmic reticulum. Studies of fluorescence and circular dichroism. *J Biol Chem.* 247:7835-7837, **1972**. *[7]*

Ikemoto N, Nagy B, Bhatnagar GM, Gergely J: Studies on a metal-binding protein of the sarcoplasmic reticulum. *J Biol Chem.* 249:2357-2365, **1974**. *[7]*

Ikemoto N, Antoniu B, Kim DH: Rapid calcium release from the isolated sarcoplasmic reticulum is triggered via the attached transverse tubular system. *J Biol Chem.* 259:13151-13158, **1984**. *[8]*

Ikemoto N, Ronjat M, Meszaros LG, Koshita M: Postulated role of calsequestrin in the regulation of calcium release from sarcoplasmic reticulum. *Biochemistry.* 28:6764-6771, **1989**. *[7]*

Ikemoto N, Antoniu B, Kang JJ, Meszaros LG, Ronjat M: Intravesicular calcium transient during calcium release from sarcoplasmic reticulum. *Biochemistry.* 30:5230-5237, **1991**. *[7]*

Ikemoto T, Iino M, Endo M: Enhancing effect of calmodulin on Ca^{2+}-induced Ca^{2+} release in the sarcoplasmic reticulum of rabbit skeletal muscle fibres. *J Physiol.* 487:573-582, **1995**. *[7]*

Im WB, Lee CO: Quantitative relation of twitch and tonic tensions to intracellular Na^+ activity in cardiac Purkinje fibers. *Am J Physiol.* 247:C478-C487, **1984**. *[10]*

Imagawa T, Leung AT, Campbell KP: Phosphorylation of the 1,4-dihydropyridine receptor of the voltage-dependent Ca^{2+} channel by an intrinsic protein kinase in isolated triads from rabbit skeletal muscle. *J Biol Chem.* 262:8333-8339, **1987a**. *[5]*

Imagawa T, Smith JS, Coronado R, Campbell KP: Purified ryanodine receptor from skeletal muscle sarcoplasmic reticulum is the Ca^{2+}-permeable pore of the calcium release channel. *J Biol Chem.* 262:16636-16643, **1987b**. *[7]*

Inagaki N, Gonoi T, Clement JP, Namba N, Inazawa J, Gonzalez G, Aguilar-Bryan L, Seino S, Bryan J: Reconstitution of I_{KATP}: An inward rectifier subunit plus the sulfonylurea receptor. *Science.* 270:1166-1170, **1995**. *[4]*

Inagaki N, Gonoi T, Clement JP, Wang CZ, Aguilar-Bryan L, Bryan J, Seino S: A family of sulfonylurea receptors determines the pharmacological properties of ATP-sensitive K^+ channels. *Neuron.* 16:1011-1017, **1996**. *[4]*

Inanobe A, Ito H, Ito M, Hosoya Y, Kurachi Y: Immunological and physical characterization of the brain G protein-gated muscarinic potassium channel. *Biochem Biophys Res Commun.* 217:1238-1244, **1995**. *[4]*

Inesi G: Mechanism of calcium transport. *Annu Rev Physiol.* 47:573-601, **1985**. *[7]*

Inesi G: Characterization of partial reactions in the catalytic and transport cycle of sarcoplasmic reticulum ATPase, in Proteins of Excitable Membranes. Hille B, Franbrough DM (eds). *New York, NY, John Wiley & Sons, Inc.* 231-255, **1987**. *[7]*

Inoue Y, Oike M, Nakao K, Kitamura K, Kuriyama H: Endothelin augments unitary calcium channel currents on the smooth muscle cell membrane of guinea-pig portal vein. *J Physiol.* 423:171-191, **1990**. *[5]*

Inoue I, Nagase H, Kishi K, Higuti T: ATP-sensitive K^+ channel in the mitochondrial inner membrane. *Nature.* 352:244-247, **1991**. *[10]*

Inui M, Chamberlain BK, Saito A, Fleischer S: The nature of the modulation of Ca^{2+} transport as studied by reconstitution of cardiac sarcoplasmic reticulum. *J Biol Chem.* 261:1794-1800, **1986**. *[7]*

Inui M, Saito A, Fleischer S: Purification of the ryanodine receptor and identity with feet structures of junctional terminal cisternae of sarcoplasmic reticulum from fast skeletal muscle. *J Biol Chem.* 262:1740-1747, **1987a**. *[1,7]*

Inui M, Saito A, Fleischer S: Isolation of the ryanodine receptor from cardiac sarcoplasmic reticulum and identity with the feet structures. *J Biol Chem.* 262:15637-15642, **1987b**. *[1,7]*

Irisawa H, Sato R: Intra- and extracellular actions of proton on the calcium current of isolated guinea pig ventricular cells. *Circ Res.* 59:348-355, **1986**. *[10]*

Irisawa H, Brown HF, Giles W: Cardiac pacemaking in the sinoatrial node. *Physiol Rev.* 73:197-227, **1993**. *[4]*

Isacoff EY, Jan YN, Jan LY: Putative receptor for the cytoplasmic inactivation gate in the Shaker K+ channel. *Nature.* 353:86-90, **1991**. *[4]*

Isenberg G, Wendt-Gallitelli MF: Cellular mechanisms of excitation contraction coupling, in Isolated Adult Cardiomyocytes. Piper HM, Isenberg G (eds). *Boca Raton, FL, CRC Press, Inc.* 213-248, **1989**. *[6]*

Isenberg G, Spurgeon H, Talo A, Stern M, Capogrossi M, Lakatta E: The voltage dependence of the myoplasmic calcium transient in guinea pig ventricular myocytes is modulated by sodium loading, in Biology of Isolated Adult Cardiac Myocytes. Clark WA, Decker RS, Bork TK (eds). *New York, NY, Elsevier.* 254-257, **1988**. *[7]*

Ishide N, Urayama T, Inoue K, Komaru T, Takishima T: Propagation and collision characteristics of calcium waves in rat myocytes. *Am J Physiol.* 259:H940-H950, **1990**. *[10]*

Ishihata A, Endoh M: Species-related differences in inotropic effects of angiotensin II in mammalian ventricular muscle: Receptors, subtypes and phosphoinositide hydrolysis. *Br J Pharmacol.* 114:447-453, **1995**. *[10]*

Ishikawa Y, Sorota S, Kiuchi K, Shannon RP, Komamura K, Katsushika S, Vatner DE, Vatner SF, Homcy CJ: Downregulation of adenylylcyclase types V and VI mRNA levels in pacing-induced heart failure in dogs. *J Clin Invest.* 93:2224-2229, **1994**. *[10]*

Ishizuka N, Berlin JR: β-adrenergic stimulation does not regulate Na pump function in voltage-clamped ventricular myocytes of the rat heart. *Pflügers Arch.* 424:361-363, **1993**. *[4]*

Ito K, Takakura S, Sato K, Sutko JL: Ryanodine inhibits the release of calcium from intracellular stores in guinea-pig aortic smooth muscle. *Circ Res.* 58:730-734, **1986**. *[8]*

Ito K, Yan X, Tajima M, Su Z, Barry WH, Lorell BH: Contractile reserve and intracellular calcium regulation in mouse myocytes from normal and hypertrophied failing hearts. *Circ Res.* 87:588-595, **2000**. *[10]*

Iwamoto T, Shigekawa M: Differential inhibition of Na+/Ca2+ exchanger isoforms by divalent cations and isothiourea derivative. *Am J Physiol.* 275:C423-C430, **1998**. *[6]*

Iwamoto T, Wakabayashi S, Shigekawa M: Growth factor-induced phosphorylation and activation of aortic smooth muscle Na+/Ca2+ exchanger. *J Biol Chem.* 270:8996-9001, **1995**. *[6]*

Iwamoto T, Watano T, Shigekawa M: A novel isothiourea derivative selectively inhibits the reverse mode of Na+/Ca2+ exchange in cells expressing NCX1. *J Biol Chem.* 271:22391-22397, **1996a**. *[6]*

Iwamoto T, Pan Y, Wakabayashi S, Imagawa T, Yamanaka HI, Shigekawa M: Phosphorylation-dependent regulation of cardiac Na+/Ca2+ exchanger via protein kinase C. *J Biol Chem.* 271:13609-13615, **1996b**. *[6]*

Iwamoto T, Pan Y, Nakamura TY, Wakabayashi S, Shigekawa M: Protein kinase C-dependent regulation of Na+/Ca2+ exchanger isoforms NCX1 and NCX3 does not require their direct phosphorylation. *Biochemistry.* 37:17230-17238, **1998**. *[6]*

Iwamoto T, Nakamura TY, Pan Y, Uehara A, Imanaga I, Shigekawa M: Unique topology of the internal repeats in the cardiac Na+/Ca2+ exchanger. *FEBS Lett.* 446:264-268, **1999**. *[6]*

Iwasa Y, Hosey MM: Phosphorylation of cardiac sarcolemma proteins by the calcium-activated phospholipid-dependent protein kinase. *J Biol Chem.* 259:534-540, **1984**. *[7]*

Jacobus WE, Pores IH, Lucas SK, Weisfeldt ML, Flaherty JT: Intracellular acidosis and contractility in the normal and ischemic heart as examined by NMR. *J Mol Cell Cardiol.* 14:13-20, **1982**. *[2]*

Jacquemond V, Klein M, Csernoch L, Schneider MF: BAPTA selectively suppresses peak Ca release in frog skeletal muscle fibers. *Biophys J.* 59:542A, **1991**. *[8]*

Jafri MS, Rice JJ, Winslow RL: Cardiac Ca2+ dynamics: The roles of ryanodine receptor adaptation and sarcoplasmic reticulum load. *Biophys J.* 74:1149-1168, **1998**. *[4]*

Jaggar JH, Porter VA, Lederer WJ, Nelson MT: Calcium sparks in smooth muscle. *Am J Physiol.* 278:C235-C256, **2000**. *[8]*

Jaimovitch E, Venosa RA, Shrager P, Horowicz P: Density and distribution of tetrodotoxin receptors in normal and detubulated frog sartorius muscle. *J Gen Physiol.* 67:399-416, **1976**. *[1]*

Jaimovich E, Reyes R, Liberona JL, Powell JA: IP3 receptors, IP3 transients, and nucleus-associated Ca2+ signals in cultured skeletal muscle. *Am J Physiol.* 278:C998-C1010, **2000**. *[8]*

Jakob H, Nawrath H, Rupp J: Adrenoceptor-mediated changes of action potential and force of contraction in human isolated ventricular heart muscle. *Br J Pharmacol.* 94:584-590, **1988**. *[10]*

James P, Maeda M, Fischer R, Verma AK, Krebs J, Penniston JT, Carafoli E: Identification and primary structure of a calmodulin binding domain of the Ca2+ pump of human erythrocytes. *J Biol Chem.* 263:2905-2910, **1988**. *[6]*

James P, Inui M, Tada M, Chiesi M, Carafoli E: Nature and site of phospholamban regulation of the Ca2+ pump of sarcoplasmic reticulum. *Nature.* 342:90-92, **1989**. *[6,7]*

Jan LY, Jan YN: Structural elements involved in specific K+ channel functions. *Annu Rev Physiol.* 54:537-555, **1992**. *[4]*

Janczewski AM, Lakatta EG: Buffering of calcium influx by sarcoplasmic reticulum during the action potential in guinea-pig ventricular myocytes. *J Physiol.* 471:343-363, **1993**. *[9]*

January CT, Fozzard HA: The effects of membrane potential, extracellular potassium, and tetrodotoxin on the intracellular sodium ion activity of sheep cardiac muscle. *Circ Res.* 54:652-665, **1984**. *[9]*

January CT, Riddle JM: Early afterdepolarizations: Mechanism of induction and block. A role for L-type Ca2+ current. *Circ Res.* 64:977-990, **1989**. *[4,5]*

Jaquet K, Heilmeyer LMG: Influence of association and of positive inotropic drugs on calcium binding to cardiac troponin C. *Biochem Biophys Res Commun.* 145:652-665, **1984**. *[10]*

Jay SD, Ellis SB, McCue AF, Williams ME, Vedvick TS, Harpold MM, Campbell KP: Primary structure of the γ subunit of the DHP-sensitive calcium channel from skeletal muscle. *Science.* 248:490-492, **1990**. *[5]*

Jay SD, Sharp AH, Kahl SD, Vedvick TS, Harpold MM, Campbell KP: Structural characterization of the dihydropyridine-sensitive calcium channel α2-subunit and the associated δ peptides. *J Biol Chem.* 266:3287-3293, **1991**. *[5]*

Jayaraman T, Brillantes AM, Timerman AP, Fleischer S, Erdjument-Bromage H, Tempst P, Marks AR: FK506 binding protein associated with the calcium release channel (ryanodine receptor). *J Biol Chem.* 267:9474-9477, **1992**. *[7]*

Jayaraman T, Ondrias K, Ondriasova E, Marks AR: Regulation of the inositol 1,4,5-trisphosphate receptor by tyrosine phosphorylation. *Science.* 272:1492-1494, **1996**. *[7]*

Jenden DJ, Fairhurst AS: The pharmacology of ryanodine. *Pharmacol Rev.* 21:1-25, **1969**. *[7]*

Jennings RB, Steenbergen C, Reimer KA: Myocardial ischemia and reperfusion. *Monogr Pathol.* 37:47-80, **1995**. *[10]*

Jentsch TJ, Friedrich T, Schriever A, Yamada H: The CLC chloride channel family. *Pflügers Arch.* 437:783-795, **1999**. *[4]*

Jeong SW, Wurster RD: Calcium channel currents in acutely dissociated intracardiac neurons from adult rats. *J Neurophysiol.* 77:1769-1778, **1997**. *[5]*

Jewett PH, Sommer JR, Johnson EA: Cardiac muscle. Its ultrastructure in the finch and hummingbird with special reference to the sarcoplasmic reticulum. *J Cell Biol.* 49:50-65, **1971**. *[1]*

Jewett PH, Leonard SD, Sommer JR: Chicken cardiac muscle. Its elusive extended junctional sarcoplasmic reticulum and sarcoplasmic reticulum fenestrations. *J Cell Biol.* 56:595-600, **1973**. *[1]*

Ji S, John SA, Lu YJ, Weiss JN: Mechanosensitivity of the cardiac muscarinic potassium channel. A novel property conferred by Kir3.4 subunit. *J Biol Chem.* 273:1324-1328, **1998**. *[4]*

John LM, Lechleiter JD, Camacho P: Differential modulation of SERCA2 isoforms by calreticulin. *J Cell Biol.* 142:963-973, **1998**. *[7]*

Johns EC, Simnett SJ, Mulligan IP, Ashley CC: Troponin I phosphorylation does not increase the rate of relaxation following laser flash photolysis of diazo-2 in guinea-pig skinned trabeculae. *Pflügers Arch.* 433:842-844, **1997**. *[2]*

Johnson EA: Force-interval relationship of cardiac muscle, in Handbook of Physiology, Section 2: The Cardiovascular System. Vol. I. Berne RM (ed)., *Bethesda, MD, Am Physiol Soc.* 475-496, **1979**. *[9]*

Jones LR, Cala SE: Biochemical evidence for functional heterogeneity of cardiac sarcoplasmic reticulum vesicles. *J Biol Chem.* 259:11809-11818, **1981**. *[7]*

Jones LR, Besch HR, Watanabe AM: Monovalent cation stimulation of Ca²⁺-ATPase uptake by cardiac membrane vesicles. Correlation with stimulation of Ca²⁺-ATPase activity. *J Biol Chem.* 252:3315-3323, **1977**. *[8]*

Jones LR, Besch HR Jr, Sutko JL, Willerson JT: Ryanodine-induced stimulation of net Ca²⁺ uptake by cardiac sarcoplasmic reticulum vesicles. *J Pharmacol Exp Ther.* 209:48-55, **1979**. *[7]*

Jones LG, Goldstein D, Brown JH: Guanine nucleotide-dependent inositol trisphosphate formation in chick heart cells. *Circ Res.* 62:299-305, **1988**. *[8,10]*

Jones LR, Zhang L, Sanborn K, Jorgensen AO, Kelley J: Purification, primary structure, and immunological characterization of the 26-kDa calsequestrin binding protein (junctin) from cardiac junctional sarcoplasmic reticulum. *J Biol Chem.* 270:30787-30796, **1995**. *[7]*

Jones LR, Suzuki YJ, Wang W, Kobayashi YM, Ramesh V, Franzini-Armstrong C, Cleemann L, Morad M: Regulation of Ca²⁺ signaling in transgenic mouse cardiac myocytes overexpressing calsequestrin. *J Clin Invest.* 101:1385-1393, **1998**. *[7]*

Jorgensen AO, Campbell KP: Evidence for the presence of calsequestrin in two structurally different regions of myocardial sarcoplasmic reticulum. *J Cell Biol.* 98:1597-1602, **1984**. *[1,7]*

Jorgensen AO, Shen ACY, Campbell KP: Ultrastructural localization of calsequestrin in adult rat atrial and ventricular muscle cells. *J Cell Biol.* 101:257-268, **1985**. *[1]*

Jorgensen AO, Borderick R, Somlyo AP, Somlyo AV: Two structurally distinct calcium storage sites in rat cardiac sarcoplasmic reticulum: An electron microprobe analysis study. *Circ Res.* 63:1060-1069, **1988**. *[7]*

Jorgensen AO, Shen ACY, Arnold W, Leung AT, Campbell KP: Subcellular distribution of the 1,4-dihydropyridine receptor in rabbit skeletal muscle in situ: An immunofluorescence and immunocolloidal gold-labeling study. *J Cell Biol.* 109:135-147, **1989**. *[1]*

Jorgensen AO, Shen AC, Arnold W, McPherson PS, Campbell KP: The Ca²⁺-release channel/ryanodine receptor is localized in junctional and corbular sarcoplasmic reticulum in cardiac muscle. *J Cell Biol.* 120:969-980, **1993**. *[1]*

Josephson I, Sperelakis N: 5'-Guanylimidodiphosphate stimulation of slow Ca current in myocardial cells. *J Mol Cell Cardiol.* 10:1157-1166, **1978**. *[5]*

Josephson IR, Sanchez-Chapula J, Brown AM: A comparison of calcium currents in rat and guinea pig single ventricular cells. *Circ Res.* 54:144-156, **1984**. *[5,8]*

Josephson RA, Silverman HS, Lakatta EG, Stern MD, Zweier JL: Study of the mechanisms of hydrogen peroxide and hydroxyl free radical-induced cellular injury and calcium overload in cardiac myocytes. *J Biol Chem.* 266:2354-2361, **1991**. *[10]*

Ju YK, Saint DA, Gage PW: Hypoxia increases persistent sodium current in rat ventricular myocytes. *J Physiol.* 497:337-347, **1996**. *[4,10]*

Juhaszova M, Blaustein MP: Na⁺ pump low and high ouabain affinity α subunit isoforms are differently distributed in cells. *Proc Natl Acad Sci USA.* 94:1800-1805, **1997**. *[4,10]*

Jung DW, Baysal K, Brierley GP: The sodium-calcium antiport of heart mitochondria is not electroneutral. *J Biol Chem.* 270:672-678, **1995**. *[3]*

Kääb S, Nuss HB, Chiamvimonvat N, O'Rourke B, Pak PH, Kass DA, Marbán E, Tomaselli GF: Ionic mechanism of action potential prolongation in ventricular myocytes from dogs with pacing-induced heart failure. *Circ Res.* 78:262-273, **1996**. *[4,10]*

Kaczorowski GJ, Barros F, Dethmers JK, Trumble MJ, Cragoe EJ Jr: Inhibition of Na⁺/Ca²⁺ exchange in pituitary plasma membrane vesicles by analogues of amiloride. *Biochemistry.* 24:1394-1403, **1985**. *[6]*

Kaczorowski GJ, Slaughter RS, King VF, Garcia ML: Inhibitors of sodium-calcium exchange: Identification and development of probes of transport activity. *Biochim Biophys Acta.* 988:287-302, **1989**. *[6]*

Kadambi VJ, Ponniah S, Harrer JM, Hoit BD, Dorn GW, Walsh RA, Kranias EG: Cardiac-specific overexpression of phospholamban alters calcium kinetics and resultant cardiomyocyte mechanics in transgenic mice. *J Clin Invest.* 97:533-539, **1996**. *[7]*

Kaftan E, Marks AR, Ehrlich BE: Effects of rapamycin on ryanodine receptor Ca²⁺-release channels from cardiac muscle. *Circ Res.* 78:990-997, **1996**. *[7]*

Kaibara M, Kameyama M: Inhibition of the calcium channel by intracellular protons in single ventricular myocytes of the guinea-pig. *J Physiol.* 403:621-640, **1988**. *[10]*

Kameyama M, Kakei M, Sato R, Shibasaki T, Matsuda H, Irisawa H: Intracellular Na⁺ activates a K⁺ channel in mammalian cardiac cells. *Nature.* 309:354-356, **1984**. *[4]*

Kameyama M, Hofmann F, Trautwein W: On the mechanisms of β-adrenergic regulation of the Ca channel in the guinea-pig heart. *Pflügers Arch.* 405:285-293, **1985**. *[5]*

Kamm KE, Stull JT: Regulation of smooth muscle contractile elements by second messengers. *Annu Rev Physiol.* 51:299-313, **1989**. *[8]*

Kamp TJ, Sanguinetti MC, Miller RJ: Voltage- and use-dependent modulation of cardiac calcium channels by the dihydropyridine (+)-202-791. *Circ Res.* 64:338-351, **1989**. *[5]*

Kamp TJ, Hu H, Marbán E: Voltage-dependent facilitation of cardiac L-type Ca channels expressed in HEK-293 cells requires β-subunit. *Am J Physiol.* 278:H126-H136, **2000**. *[5]*

Kaneko M, Beamish RE, Dhalla NS: Depression of heart sarcolemmal Ca²⁺-pump activity by oxygen free radicals. *Am J Physiol.* 256:H368-H374, **1989**. *[10]*

Kaneko T, Tanaka H, Oyamada M, Kawata S, Takamatsu T: Three distinct types of Ca²⁺ waves in Langendorff-perfused rat heart revealed by real-time confocal microscopy. *Circ Res.* 86:1093-1099, **2000**. *[10]*

Kanmura Y, Missiaen L, Raeymaekers L, Casteels R: Ryanodine reduces the amount of calcium in intracellular stores of smooth muscle cells of the rabbit ear artery. *Pflügers Arch.* 413:153-159, **1988**. *[8]*

Kanter HL, Laing JG, Beau SL, Beyer EC, Saffitz JE: Distinct patterns of connexin expression in canine Purkinje fibers and ventricular muscle. *Circ Res.* 72:1124-1131, **1993**. *[1]*

Kaplan JH, Ellis-Davies GCR: Photolabile chelators for the rapid photorelease of divalent cations. *Proc Natl Acad Sci USA.* 85:6571-6575, **1988**. *[8]*

Kappl M, Hartung K: Rapid charge translocation by the cardiac Na⁺-Ca²⁺ exchanger after a Ca²⁺ concentration jump. *Biophys J.* 71:2473-2485, **1996**. *[6]*

Kaprielian R, Wickenden AD, Kassiri Z, Parker TG, Liu PP, Backx PH: Relationship between K⁺ channel down-regulation and [Ca²⁺]ᵢ in rat ventricular myocytes following myocardial infarction. *J Physiol.* 517:229-245, **1999**. *[10]*

Karczewski P, Bartel S, Krause EG: Differential sensitivity to isoprenaline of troponin I and phospholamban phosphorylation in isolated rat hearts. *Biochem J.* 266:115-122, **1990**. *[2]*

Karin M, Hunter T: Transcriptional control by protein phosphorylation: Signal transmission from the cell surface to the nucleus. *Curr Biol.* 5:747-757, **1995**. *[8]*

Karmazyn M: Amiloride enhances postischemic ventricular recovery: possible role of Na⁺-H⁺ exchange. *Am J Physiol.* 255:H608-H615, **1988**. *[10]*

Karmazyn M, Gan XH, Humphreys RA, Yoshida H, Kusumoto K: The myocardial Na⁺-H⁺ exchange - Structure, regulation, and its role in heart disease. *Circ Res.* 85:777-786, **1999**. *[10]*

Kass RS, Arena JP: Influence of pHₒ on calcium channel block by amlodipine, a charged dihydropyridine compound. *J Gen Physiol.* 93:1109-1127, **1989**. *[5]*

Kass RS, Krafte D: Negative surface charge density near heart calcium channels. *J Gen Physiol.* 89:629-644, **1987**. *[5]*

Kass RS, Sanguinetti MC: Inactivation of calcium channel current in the calf cardiac Purkinje fiber. Evidence for voltage- and calcium-mediated mechanisms. *J Gen Physiol.* 84:705-726, **1984**. *[5,8]*

Kass RS, Lederer WJ, Tsien RW, Weingart R: Role of calcium ions in transient inward currents and after contractions induced by strophanthidin in cardiac Purkinje fibers. *J Physiol.* 281:187-208, **1978**. *[4,8,10]*

Kass RS, Arena JP, Chin S: Block of L-type calcium channels by charged dihydropyridines. Sensitivity to side of application and calcium. *J Gen Physiol.* 98:63-75, **1991**. *[5]*

Kassiri Z, Myers R, Kaprielian R, Banijamali HS, Backx PH: Rate-dependent changes of twitch force duration in rat cardiac trabeculae: Property of the contractile system. *J Physiol.* 524:221-231, **2000**. *[9]*

Katoh H, Schlotthauer K, Bers DM: Transmission of information from cardiac dihydropyridine receptor to ryanodine receptor: Evidence from BayK 8644 effects on resting Ca²⁺ sparks. *Circ Res.* 87:106-111, **2000**. *[8]*

Katsube Y, Yokoshiki H, Nguyen L, Yamamoto M, Sperelakis N: Inhibition of Ca²⁺ current in neonatal and adult rat ventricular myocytes by the tyrosine kinase inhibitor, genistein. *Eur J Pharmacol.* 345:309-314, **1998**. *[5]*

Katz AM, Takenaka H, Watras J: The Sarcoplasmic Reticulum, in The Heart and Cardiovascular System. Fozzard HA (ed). New York, NY, Raven Press. 731-746, **1986**. *[1]*

Katz AM: Heart Failure: Pathophysiology, Molecular Biology and Clinical Management. *Philadelphia, PA, Lippincott Williams & Wilkins.* 1-381, **2000**. *[10]*

Kaumann AJ, Hall JA, Murray KJ, Wells FC, Brown MJ: A comparison of the effects of adrenaline and noradrenaline on human heart: the role of β₁- and β₂-adrenoceptors in the stimulation of adenylate cyclase and contractile force. *Eur Heart J.* 10 Suppl B:29-37, **1989**. *[10]*

Kawai M, Konishi M: Measurement of sarcoplasmic reticulum calcium content in skinned mammalian cardiac muscle. *Cell Calcium.* 16:123-136, **1994**. *[7]*

Kawai M, Hussain M, Orchard CH: Excitation-contraction coupling in rat ventricular myocytes after formamide-induced detubulation. *Am J Physiol.* 277:H603-H609, **1999**. *[1]*

Kawakami K, Noguchi S, Noda M, Takahashi H, Ohta T, Kawamura M, Nojima H, Nagano K, Hirose T, Inayama S: Primary structure of the α-subunit of Torpedo californica (Na⁺-K⁺)ATPase deduced from cDNA sequence. *Nature.* 316:733-736, **1985**. *[4]*

Kawano S, Hirayama Y, Hiraoka M: Activation mechanism of Ca²⁺-sensitive transient outward current in rabbit ventricular myocytes. *J Physiol.* 486:593-604, **1995**. *[4]*

Kaye DM, Wiviott SD, Kelly RA: Activation of nitric oxide synthase (NOS3) by mechanical activity alters contractile activity in a Ca²⁺-independent manner in cardiac myocytes: role of troponin I phosphorylation. *Biochem Biophys Res Commun.* 256:398-403, **1999**. *[10]*

Kensler RW, Goodenough DA: Isolation of mouse myocardial gap junctions. *J Cell Biol.* 86:755-764, **1980**. *[1]*

Kent RL, Rozich JD, McCollam PL, McDermott DE, Thacker UF, Menick DR, McDermott PJ, Cooper G: Rapid expression of the Na⁺-Ca²⁺ exchanger in response to cardiac pressure overload. *Am J Physiol.* 265:H1024-H1029, **1993**. *[10]*

Kentish JD: The inhibitory effects of monovalent ions on force development in detergent-skinned ventricular muscle from guinea-pig. *J Physiol.* 352:353-374, **1984**. *[2]*

Kentish JC: The effects of inorganic phosphate and creatine phosphate on force production in skinned muscles from rat ventricle. *J Physiol.* 370:585-604, **1986**. *[2,10]*

Kentish JC, Nayler WG: The influence of pH on the Ca^{2+}-regulated ATPase of cardiac and white skeletal myofibrils. *J Mol Cell Cardiol.* 11:611-617, **1979**. *[10]*

Kentish JC, Wrzosek A: Changes in force and cytosolic Ca^{2+} concentration after length changes in isolated rat ventricular trabeculae. *J Physiol.* 506:431-444, **1998**. *[2]*

Kentish JC, Xiang JZ: Ca^{2+}- and caffeine-induced Ca^{2+} release from the sarcoplasmic reticulum in rat skinned trabeculae: Effects of pH and P_i. *Cardiovasc Res.* 33:314-323, **1997**. *[10]*

Kentish JC, ter Keurs HEDJ, Ricciardi L, Bucx JJJ, Noble MIM: Comparison between the sarcomere length-force relations of intact and skinned trabeculae from rat right ventricle. *Circ Res.* 58:755-768, **1986**. *[2]*

Kentish JC, Barsotti RJ, Lea TJ, Mulligan IP, Patel JR, Ferenczi MA: Calcium release from cardiac sarcoplasmic reticulum induced by photorelease of calcium or Ins(1,4,5)P3. *Am J Physiol.* 258:H610-H615, **1990**. *[8]*

Kerrick WGL, Donaldson SKB: The comparative effects of $[Ca^{2+}]$ and $[Mg^{2+}]$ on tension generation in the fibers of skinned frog skeletal muscle and mechanically disrupted rat ventricular cardiac muscle. *Pflügers Arch.* 358:195-201, **1975**. *[2]*

Kerrick WGL, Malencik DA, Hoar PE, Potter JD, Coby RL, Pocinwong S, Fischer EH: Ca^{2+} and Sr^{2+} activation: Comparison of cardiac and skeletal muscle contraction models. *Pflügers Arch.* 386:207-213, **1980**. *[2]*

Khananshvili D: Distinction between the two basic mechanisms of cation transport in the cardiac Na^+-Ca^{2+} exchange system. *Biochemistry.* 29:2437-2442, **1990**. *[6]*

Khananshvili D: Structure, mechanism and regulation of the cardiac sarcolemma Na^+-Ca^{2+} exchanger. *Adv Mol Cell Biol.* 23:311-358, **1998**. *[6]*

Khananshvili D, Price DC, Greenberg MJ, Sarne Y: Phe-Met-Arg-Phe-NH_2 (FMRFa)-related peptides inhibit Na^+-Ca^{2+} exchange in cardiac sarcolemma vesicles. *J Biol Chem.* 268:200-205, **1993**. *[6]*

Khananshvili D, Shaulov G, Weil-Maslansky E, Baazov D: Positively charged cyclic hexapeptides, novel blockers for the cardiac sarcolemma Na^+-Ca^{2+} exchanger. *J Biol Chem.* 270:16182-16188, **1995**. *[6]*

Khananshvili D, Baazov D, Weil-Maslansky E, Shaulov G, Mester B: Rapid interaction of FRCRCFa with the cytosolic side of the cardiac sarcolemma Na^+-Ca^{2+} exchanger blocks the ion transport without preventing the binding of either sodium or calcium. *Biochemistry.* 35:15933-15940, **1996**. *[6]*

Kielley WW, Meyerhof O: A new magnesium-activated adenosinetriphosphatase from muscle. *J Biol Chem.* 174:387-388, **1948**. *[7]*

Kieval RS, Bloch RJ, Lindenmayer GE, Ambesi A, Lederer WJ: Immunofluorescence localization of the Na-Ca exchanger in heart cells. *Am J Physiol.* 263:C545-C550, **1992**. *[6,8]*

Kihara Y, Gwathmey JK, Grossman W, Morgan JP: Mechanisms of positive inotropic effects and delayed relaxation produced by DPI 201-106 in mammalian working myocardium: Effects on intracellular calcium handling. *Br J Pharmacol.* 96:927-939, **1989**. *[10]*

Kijima Y, Ogunbunmi E, Fleischer S: Drug action of thapsigargin on the Ca^{2+} pump protein of sarcoplasmic reticulum. *J Biol Chem.* 266:22912-22918, **1991**. *[3]*

Kijima Y, Saito A, Jetton TL, Magnuson MA, Fleischer S: Different intracellular localization of inositol 1,4,5-trisphosphate and ryanodine receptors in cardiomyocytes. *J Biol Chem.* 268:3499-3506, **1993**. *[8]*

Kim D: Calcitonin-gene-related peptide activates the muscarinic-gated K^+ current in atrial cells. *Pflügers Arch.* 418:338-345, **1991a**. *[4]*

Kim D: Endothelin activation of an inwardly rectifying K^+ current in atrial cells. *Circ Res.* 69:250-255, **1991b**. *[4]*

Kim D: Mechanism of rapid desensitization of muscarinic K^+ current in adult rat and guinea pig atrial cells. *Circ Res.* 73:89-97, **1993a**. *[4]*

Kim D: Novel cation-selective mechanosensitive ion channel in the atrial cell membrane. *Circ Res.* 72:225-231, **1993b**. *[4]*

Kim MS, Akera T: O_2 free radicals: Cause of ischemia-reperfusion injury to cardiac Na^+-K^+-ATPase. *Am J Physiol.* 252:H252-H257, **1987**. *[10]*

Kim D, Clapham DE: Potassium channels in cardiac cells activated by arachidonic acid and phospholipids. *Science.* 244:1174-1176, **1989**. *[4]*

Kim D, Fu C: Activation of a nonselective cation channel by swelling in atrial cells. *J Membr Biol.* 135:27-37, **1993**. *[4]*

Kim DH, Speter FA, Ohnishi ST, Ryan JF, Roberts J, Allen PD, Meszaros LG, Antoniu B, Ikemoto N: Kinetic studies of Ca^{2+} release from sarcoplasmic reticulum of normal and malignant hyperthermia susceptible pig muscles. *Biochim Biophys Acta.* 775:320-327, **1984**. *[7]*

Kim KC, Caswell AH, Talvenheimo JA, Brandt NR: Isolation of a terminal cisterna protein which may link the dihydropyridine receptor to the junctional foot protein in skeletal muscle. *Biochemistry.* 29:9281-9289, **1990**. *[8]*

Kim HL, Kim H, Lee P, King RG, Chin H: Rat brain expresses an alternatively spliced form of the dihydropyridine-sensitive L-type calcium channel α_2 subunit. *Proc Natl Acad Sci USA.* 89:3251-3255, **1992**. *[5]*

Kim MS, Morii T, Sun LX, Imoto K, Mori Y: Structural determinants of ion selectivity in brain calcium channel. *FEBS Lett.* 318:145-148, **1993**. *[4]*

Kim I, Koh GY, Lee CO: Identification of alternatively spliced Na^+-Ca^{2+} exchanger isoforms expressed in the heart. *Comp Biochem Physiol B Biochem Mol Biol.* 119:157-161, **1998**. *[6]*

Kimura J: Na-Ca exchange and Ca-sensitive non-selective cation current components of transient inward current in isolated cardiac ventricular cells of the guinea-pig. *J Physiol. (Lond.)* 407:79P, **1988**. *[4,10]*

Kimura J, Noma A, Irisawa H: Na-Ca exchange current in mammalian heart cells. *Nature.* 319:596-597, **1986**. *[6]*

Kimura J, Miyamae S, Noma A: Identification of sodium-calcium exchange current in single ventricular cells in guinea pig. *J Physiol.* 384:199-222, **1987**. *[6]*

Kimura Y, Kurzydlowski K, Tada M, MacLennan DH: Phospholamban regulates the Ca^{2+}-ATPase through intramembrane interactions. *J Biol Chem.* 271:21726-21731, **1996**. *[7]*

Kimura Y, Kurzydlowski K, Tada M, MacLennan DH: Phospholamban inhibitory function is activated by depolymerization. *J Biol Chem.* 272:15061-15064, **1997**. *[7]*

Kimura J, Watano T, Kawahara M, Sakai E, Yatabe J: Direction-independent block of bi-directional Na+/Ca²+ exchange current by KB-R7943 in guinea-pig cardiac myocytes. *Br J Pharmacol.* 128:969-974, **1999**. *[6]*

King BW, Bose D: Mechanism of biphasic contractions in strontium-treated ventricular muscle. *Circ Res.* 52:65-75, **1983**. *[9]*

Kirchberger MA, Tada M, Katz AM: Adenosine 3'-5'-monophosphate dependent protein kinase-catalyzed phosphorylation reaction and its relationship to calcium transport in cardiac sarcoplasmic reticulum. *J Biol Chem.* 249:6166-6173, **1974**. *[2,7]*

Kiriazis H, Kranias EG: Genetically engineered models with alterations in cardiac membrane calcium-handling proteins. *Annu Rev Physiol.* 62:321-351, **2000**. *[10]*

Kirino Y, Shimizu H: Ca²+-induced Ca²+ release from fragmented sarcoplasmic reticulum: A comparison with skinned muscle fiber studies. *J Biochem.* 92:1287-1296, **1982**. *[7]*

Kirsch GE, Nichols RA, Nakajima S: Delayed rectification in the transverse tubules. *J Gen Physiol.* 70:1-21, **1977**. *[1]*

Kirstein M, Rivet-Bastide M, Hatem S, Bénardeau A, Mercadier JJ, Fischmeister R: Nitric oxide regulates the calcium current in isolated human atrial myocytes. *J Clin Invest.* 95:794-802, **1995**. *[5]*

Kiselyov K, Xu X, Mozhayeva G, Kuo T, Pessah I, Mignery G, Zhu X, Birnbaumer L, Muallem S: Functional interaction between InsP3 receptors and store-operated Htrp3 channels. *Nature.* 396:478-482, **1998**. *[8]*

Kiselyov K, Mignery GA, Zhu MX, Muallem S: The N-terminal domain of the IP3 receptor gates store-operated hTrp3 channels. *Mol Cell.* 4:423-429, **1999**. *[8]*

Kiss E, Jakab G, Kranias EG, Edes I: Thyroid hormone-induced alterations in phospholamban protein expression: Regulatory effects on sarcoplasmic reticulum Ca²+ transport and myocardial relaxation. *Circ Res.* 75:245-251, **1994**. *[7,10]*

Kitada Y, Narimatsu A, Matsumura N, Endo M: Contractile proteins: Possible targets for the cardiotonic action of MCl-154, a novel cardiotonic agent. *Eur J Pharmacol.* 134:229-231, **1987**. *[2]*

Kitada Y, Kobayashi M, Narimatsu A, Ohizumi Y: Potent stimulation of myofilament force and adenosine triphosphatase activity of canine cardiac muscle through a direct enhancement of troponin C Ca²+ binding by MCl-154, a novel cardiotonic agent. *J Pharmacol Exp Ther.* 250:272-277, **1989**. *[2]*

Kitakaze M, Marbán E: Cellular mechanism of the modulation of contractile function by coronary perfusion pressure in ferret hearts. *J Physiol.* 414:455-472, **1989**. *[10]*

Kjekshus J: Arrhythmias and mortality in congestive heart failure. *Am J Cardiol.* 65:42I-48I, **1990**. *[10]*

Klaus MM, Scordilis SP, Rapalus JM, Briggs RT, Powell JA: Evidence for dysfunction in the regulation of cytosolic Ca²+ in excitation-contraction uncoupled dysgenic muscle. *Dev Biol.* 99:152-166, **1983**. *[8]*

Klein MG, Simon BJ, Schneider MF: Effects of caffeine on calcium release from the sarcoplasmic reticulum in frog skeletal muscle fibres. *J Physiol.* 425:599-626, **1990**. *[8]*

Klein MG, Cheng H, Santana LF, Jiang YH, Lederer WJ, Schneider MF: Two mechanisms of quantized calcium release in skeletal muscle. *Nature.* 379:455-458, **1996**. *[8]*

Klugbauer N, Lacinová L, Marais E, Hobom M, Hofmann F: Molecular diversity of the calcium channel α2δ subunit. *J Neurosci.* 19:684-691, **1999**. *[5]*

Knot HJ, Nelson MT: Regulation of arterial diameter and wall [Ca²+] in cerebral arteries of rat by membrane potential and intravascular pressure. *J Physiol.* 508:199-209, **1998**. *[8]*

Knot HJ, Standen NB, Nelson MT: Ryanodine receptors regulate arterial diameter and wall [Ca²+] in cerebral arteries of rat via Ca²+-dependent K+ channels. *J Physiol.* 508:211-221, **1998**. *[8]*

Knowlton AA, Brecher P, Apstein CS: Rapid expression of heat shock protein in the rabbit after brief cardiac ischemia. *J Clin Invest.* 87:139-147, **1991**. *[10]*

Knowlton KU, Michel MC, Itani M, Shubeita HE, Ishihara K, Brown JH, Chien KR: The α1A-adrenergic receptor subtype mediates biochemical, molecular, and morphologic features of cultured myocardial cell hypertrophy. *J Biol Chem.* 268:15374-15380, **1993**. *[10]*

Knudson CM, Chaudhari N, Sharp AH, Powell JA, Beam KG, Campbell KP: Specific absence of the α1 subunit of the dihydropyridine receptor in mice with muscular dysgenesis. *J Biol Chem.* 264:1345-1348, **1989**. *[8]*

Knudson CM, Stang KK, Jorgensen AO, Campbell KP: Biochemical characterization and ultrastructural localization of a major junctional sarcoplasmic reticulum glycoprotein (Triadin). *J Biol Chem.* 268:12637-12645, **1993a**. *[7]*

Knudson CM, Stang KK, Moomaw CR, Slaughter CA, Campbell KP: Primary structure and topological analysis of a skeletal muscle-specific junctional sarcoplasmic reticulum glycoprotein (Triadin). *J Biol Chem.* 268:12646-12654, **1993b**. *[7]*

Kobayashi S, Kitazawa T, Somlyo AV, Somlyo AP: Cytosolic heparin inhibits muscarinic and α-adrenergic Ca²+ release in smooth muscle: Physiological role of inositol 1,4,5'-trisphosphate-dependent, but not the independent, calcium release induced by guanine nucleotide in vascular smooth muscle. *Biochem Biophys Res Commun.* 153:625-631, **1988**. *[8]*

Kobayashi S, Kitazawa T, Somlyo AV, Somlyo AP: Cytosolic heparin inhibits muscarinic and α-adrenergic Ca²+ release in smooth muscle: Physiological role of inositol 1,4,5'-trisphosphate in pharmacomechanical coupling. *J Biol Chem.* 264:17997-18004, **1989**. *[8]*

Kobayashi T, Miyauchi T, Sakai S, Kobayashi M, Yamaguchi I, Goto K, Sugishita Y: Expression of endothelin-1, ETA and ETB receptors, and ECE and distribution of endothelin-1 in failing rat heart. *Am J Physiol.* 276:H1197-H1206, **1999**. *[10]*

Koch-Weser J, Blinks JR: The influence of the interval between beats on myocardial contractility. *Pharmacol Rev.* 15:601-652, **1963**. *[9]*

Kockskämper J, Erlenkamp S, Glitsch HG: Activation of the cAMP-protein kinase A pathway facilitates Na+ translocation by the Na+-K+ pump in guinea-pig ventricular myocytes. *J Physiol.* 523:561-574, **2000**. *[4,10]*

Kodama I, Nikmaram MR, Boyett MR, Suzuki R, Honjo H, Owen JM: Regional differences in the role of the Ca²+ and Na+ currents in pacemaker activity in the sinoatrial node. *Am J Physiol.* 272:H2793-H2806, **1997**. *[4]*

Kodani E, Tang XL, Takano H, Shinmura K, Hill M, Bolli R: The role of cyclic guanosine monophosphate (cGMP) in late preconditioning against myocardial stunning in conscious rabbits. *J Mol Cell Cardiol.* 32:A23, **2000**. *[10]*

Kohmoto O, Spitzler KW, Movesian MA, Barry WH: Effects of intracellular acidosis on [Ca^{2+}] transients, transsarcolemmal Ca^{2+} fluxes, and contraction in ventricular myocytes. *Circ Res.* 66:622-632, **1990**. *[10]*

Kojima M, Shiojima I, Yamazaki T, Komuro I, Yunzeng Z, Ying W, Mizuno T, Ueki K, Tobe K, Kadowaki T, Nagai R, Yazaki Y: Angiotensin II receptor antagonist TCV-116 induces regression of hypertensive left ventricular hypertrophy in vivo and inhibits the intracellular signaling pathway of stretch-mediated cardiomyocyte hypertrophy in vitro. *Circulation.* 89:2204-2211, **1994**. *[10]*

Kokubun S, Irisawa H: Effects of various intracellular Ca ion concentrations on the calcium current of guinea-pig single ventricular cells. *Jap J Physiol.* 24:599-611, **1984**. *[5]*

Kokubun S, Reuter H: Dihydropyridine derivatives prolong the open state of Ca channels in cultured cardiac cells. *Proc Natl Acad Sci USA.* 81:4824-4827, **1984**. *[5]*

Kokubun S, Prod'hom B, Becker C, Porzig H, Reuter H: Studies on Ca channels in intact cardiac cells: Voltage-dependent effects and cooperative interactions of dihydropyridine enantiomers. *Mol Pharmacol.* 30:571-584, **1986**. *[5]*

Komalavilas P, Lincoln TM: Phosphorylation of the inositol 1,4,5-trisphosphate receptor by cyclic GMP-dependent protein kinase. *J Biol Chem.* 269:8701-8707, **1994**. *[7]*

Kompa AR, Molenaar P, Summers RJ: β-Adrenoceptor regulation and functional responses in the guinea-pig following chronic administration of the long-acting β$_2$-adrenoceptor agonist formoterol. *Naunyn Schmiedebergs Arch Pharmacol.* 351:576-588, **1995**. *[10]*

Komuro I, Katoh Y, Kaida T, Shibazaki Y, Kurabayashi M, Hoh E, Takaku F, Yazaki Y: Mechanical loading stimulates cell hypertrophy and specific gene expression in cultured rat cardiac myocytes. Possible role of protein kinase C activation. *J Biol Chem.* 266:1265-1268, **1991**. *[10]*

Konarzewska H, Peeters GA, Sanguinetti MC: Repolarizing K$^+$ currents in nonfailing human hearts: Similarities between right septal subendocardial and left subepicardial ventricular myocytes. *Circulation.* 92:1179-1187, **1995**. *[4]*

Kondo N: Excitation-contraction coupling in myocardium of nonhibernating and hibernating chipmunks: Effects of isoprenaline, a high calcium medium, and ryanodine. *Circ Res.* 59:221-228, **1986**. *[9]*

Kondo N: Comparison between effects of caffeine and ryanodine on electromechanical coupling in myocardium of hibernating chipmunks: Role of internal Ca stores. *Br J Pharmacol.* 95:1287-1291, **1988**. *[9]*

Kondo N, Shibata S: Calcium source for excitation-contraction coupling in myocardium of nonhibernating and hibernating chipmunks. *Science.* 225:641-643, **1984**. *[9]*

Konev SV, Aksentsev SL, Okun' IM, Merezhinskaia NV, Rakovich AA, Orlov SN, Pokudin NI, Kravtsov GM, Khodorov BI: Calcium transport in brain synaptosomes during depolarization. The role of potential-dependent channels and Na$^+$/Ca^{2+} metabolism. *Biokhimiia.* 54:1150-1162, **1989**. *[6]*

Konishi M, Kurihara S, Sakai T: Changes in intracellular calcium concentration induced by caffeine and rapid cooling in frog skeletal muscle fibres. *J Physiol.* 365:131-146, **1985**. *[8]*

Konishi M, Olson A, Hollingworth S, Baylor SM: Myoplasmic binding of fura-2 investigated by steady-state fluorescence

and absorbance measurements. *Biophys J.* 54:1089-1104, **1988**. *[3]*

Kort AA, Lakatta EG: Calcium-dependent mechanical oscillations occur spontaneously in unstimulated mammalian cardiac tissues. *Circ Res.* 54:396-404, **1984**. *[8,10]*

Kort AA, Lakatta EG: Bimodal effect of stimulation on light fluctuation transients monitoring spontaneous sarcoplasmic reticulum calcium release in rat cardiac muscle. *Circ Res.* 63:960-968, **1988a**. *[10]*

Kort AA, Lakatta EG: Spontaneous sarcoplasmic reticulum calcium release in rat and rabbit cardiac muscle: Relationship to transient and rested state twitch tension. *Circ Res.* 63:969-979, **1988b**. *[10]*

Koss KL, Kranias EG: Phospholamban: A prominent regulator of myocardial contractility. *Circ Res.* 79:1059-1063, **1996**. *[7]*

Koster OF, Szigeti GP, Beuckelmann DJ: Characterization of a [Ca^{2+}]$_i$-dependent current in human atrial and ventricular cardiomyocytes in the absence of Na$^+$ and K$^+$. *Cardiovasc Res.* 41:175-187, **1999**. *[10]*

Koumi S, Backer CL, Arentzen CE: Characterization of inwardly rectifying K$^+$ channel in human cardiac myocytes. Alterations in channel behavior in myocytes isolated from patients with idiopathic dilated cardiomyopathy. *Circulation.* 92:164-174, **1995**. *[10]*

Kovacs RJ, Nelson RT, Simmerman HKB, Jones LR: Phospholamban forms Ca^{2+}-selective channels in lipid bilayers. *J Biol Chem.* 263:18364-18368, **1988**. *[7]*

Krafte DS, Kass RS: Hydrogen ion modulation of Ca channel current in cardiac ventricular cells. *J Gen Physiol.* 91:641-657, **1988**. *[10]*

Kranias EG: Regulation of Ca^{2+} transport by cyclic 3',5'-AMP-dependent and calcium-calmodulin-dependent phosphorylation of cardiac sarcoplasmic reticulum. *Biochim Biophys Acta.* 844:193-199, **1985**. *[7]*

Kranias EG, Solaro RJ: Phosphorylation of troponin I and phospholamban during catecholamine stimulation of rabbit heart. *Nature.* 298:182-184, **1982**. *[7]*

Krapivinsky G, Gordon EA, Wickman K, Velimirovic B, Krapivinsky L, Clapham DE: The G-protein-gated atrial K$^+$ channel I$_{KACh}$ is a heteromultimer of two inwardly rectifying K$^+$-channel proteins. *Nature.* 374:135-141, **1995**. *[4]*

Kraus R, Reichl B, Kimball SD, Grabner M, Murphy BJ, Catterall WA, Striessnig J: Identification of benzothiazepine-binding regions within L-type calcium channel α$_1$ subunits. *J Biol Chem.* 271:20113-20118, **1996**. *[5]*

Krueger K, Daaka Y, Pitcher J, Lefkowitz R: The role of sequestration in G protein-coupled receptor resensitization. Regulation of β$_2$-adrenergic receptor dephosphorylation by vesicular acidification. *J Biol Chem.* 272:5-8, **1997**. *[10]*

Kruta V: Sur l'activité rhythmique du muscle cardiaque I. Variations de la réponse méchanique en fonction du rhythme. *Arch Int Physiol.* 45:332-357, **1937**. *[9,10]*

Kruta V: Sur l'activité rhythmique du muscle cardiaque. II. Variations, en fonction de la température, des relations entre la réponse mécanique et le rhythme. *Arch Int Physiol.* 47:35-62, **1938**. *[10]*

Kubo Y, Baldwin TJ, Jan YN, Jan LY: Primary structure and functional expression of a mouse inward rectifier potassium channel. *Nature.* 362:127-133, **1993**. *[4]*

Kunze DL, Rampe D: Characterization of the effects of a new Ca²⁺ channel activator, FPL 64176, in GH₃ cells. *Mol Pharmacol.* 42:666-670, **1992**. *[5]*

Kurachi Y: The effects of intracellular protons on the electrical activity of single ventricular cells. *Pflügers Arch.* 394:264-270, **1982**. *[10]*

Kurachi Y, Ito H, Sugimoto T, Shimizu T, Miki I, Ui M: Alpha-adrenergic activation of the muscarinic K⁺ channel is mediated by arachidonic acid metabolites. *Pflügers Arch.* 414:102-104, **1989**. *[10]*

Kurihara S, Sakai T: Effects of rapid cooling on mechanical and electrical responses in ventricular muscle of guinea pig. *J Physiol.* 361:361-378, **1985**. *[7,9]*

Kuschel M, Karczewski P, Hempel P, Schlegel WP, Krause EG, Bartel S: Ser¹⁶ prevails over Thr¹⁷ phospholamban phosphorylation in the β–adrenergic regulation of cardiac relaxation. *Am J Physiol.* 276:H1625-H1633, **1999a**. *[7]*

Kuschel M, Zhou YY, Spurgeon HA, Bartel S, Karczewski P, Zhang SJ, Krause EG, Lakatta EG, Xiao RP: β₂-adrenergic cAMP signaling is uncoupled from phosphorylation of cytoplasmic proteins in canine heart. *Circulation.* 99:2458-2465, **1999b**. *[10]*

Kuyayama H: The membrane potential modulates the ATP-dependent Ca²⁺ pump of cardiac sarcolemma. *Biochim Biophys Acta.* 940:295-299, **1988**. *[6]*

Lacerda AE, Brown AM: Nonmodal gating of cardiac calcium channels as revealed by dihydropyridines. *J Gen Physiol.* 93:1243-1273, **1989**. *[5]*

Lacerda AE, Rampe D, Brown AM: Effects of protein kinase C on cardiac Ca²⁺ channels. *Nature.* 335:249-251, **1988**. *[5]*

Laflamme MA, Becker PL: Ca²⁺-induced current oscillations in rabbit ventricular myocytes. *Circ Res.* 78:707-716, **1996**. *[4,10]*

Laflamme MA, Becker PL: Do β₂-adrenergic receptors modulate Ca²⁺ in adult rat ventricular myocytes? *Am J Physiol.* 274:H1308-H1314, **1998**. *[10]*

Lafontan M: Differential recruitment and differential regulation by physiological amines of fat cell β₁-β₂-β₃-adrenergic receptors expressed in native fat cells and in transfected cell lines. *Cell Signal.* 6:363-392, **1994**. *[10]*

Lagos NAV: Phosphoinositides in frog skeletal muscle: A quantitative analysis. *Biochim Biophys Acta.* 1043:235-244, **1990**. *[8]*

Lai FA, Erickson HF, Block BA, Meissner G: Evidence for a junctional feet-ryanodine receptor complex from sarcoplasmic reticulum. *Biochem Biophys Res Commun.* 143:704-709, **1987**. *[1,7]*

Lai FA, Erickson HF, Rousseau E, Liu QY, Meissner G: Purification and reconstitution of the calcium release channel from skeletal muscle. *Nature.* 331:315-319, **1988a**. *[1,7]*

Lai FA, Anderson K, Rousseau E, Liu QY, Meissner G: Evidence for a Ca²⁺ channel within the ryanodine receptor complex from cardiac sarcoplasmic reticulum. *Biochem Biophys Res Commun.* 151:441-449, **1988b**. *[7]*

Lai FA, Misra M, Xu L, Smith HA, Meissner G: The ryanodine receptor-Ca²⁺ release channel complex of skeletal muscle sarcoplasmic reticulum. *J Biol Chem.* 264:16776-16785, **1989**. *[7]*

Lakatta EG, Lappé DL: Diastolic scattered light fluctuation, resting force and twich force in mammalian cardiac muscle. *J Physiol.* 315:369-394, **1981**. *[10]*

Lamb GD: Components of charge movement in rabbit skeletal muscle: The effect of tetracaine and nifedipine. *J Physiol.* 376:85-100, **1986**. *[8]*

Lamb GD: Excitation-contraction coupling in skeletal muscle: Comparisons with cardiac muscle. *Clin Exp Pharmacol Physiol.* 27:216-224, **2000**. *[8]*

Lamb GD, Stephenson DG: Calcium release in skinned muscle fibres of the toad by transverse tubule depolarization or by direct stimulation. *J Physiol.* 423:495-517, **1990**. *[8]*

Lamb GD, Stephenson DG: Effects of intracellular pH and [Mg²⁺] on excitation-contraction coupling in skeletal muscle fibres of the rat. *J Physiol.* 478:331-339, **1994**. *[8]*

Lamb GD, Walsh T: Calcium currents, charge movement and dihydropyridine binding in fast- and slow-twitch muscles of the rat and rabbit. *J Physiol.* 393:595-617, **1987**. *[8]*

Lamb GD, el-Hayek R, Ikemoto N, Stephenson DG: Effects of dihydropyridine receptor II-III loop peptides on Ca²⁺ release in skinned skeletal muscle fibers. *Am J Physiol.* 279:C891-C905, **2000**. *[8]*

Lamont C, Eisner DA: The sarcolemmal mechanisms involved in the control of diastolic intracellular calcium in isolated rat cardiac trabeculae. *Pflügers Arch.* 432:961-969, **1996**. *[6]*

Lamont C, Luther PW, Balke CW, Wier WG: Intercellular Ca²⁺ waves in rat heart muscle. *J Physiol.* 512:669-676, **1998**. *[10]*

Langer GA: Kinetic studies of calcium distribution in ventricular muscle of the dog. *Circ Res.* 15:393-405, **1964**. *[6]*

Langer GA: Calcium exchange in dog ventricular muscle. Relation to frequency of contraction and maintenance of contractility. *Circ Res.* 17:78-88, **1965**. *[10]*

Langer GA, Brady AJ: The effects of temperature upon contraction and ionic exchange in rabbit ventricular myocardium. Relation to control of active state. *J Gen Physiol.* 52:682-713, **1968**. *[10]*

Langer GA, Peskoff A: Calcium concentration and movement in the diadic cleft space of the cardiac ventricular cell. *Biophys J.* 70:1169-1182, **1996**. *[6,8]*

Langer GA, Rich TL: Further characterization of the Na-Ca exchange-dependent Ca compartment in rat ventricular cells. *Am J Physiol.* 265:C556-C561, **1993**. *[7]*

Langer GA, Serena SD: Effects of strophanthidin upon contraction and ionic exchange in rabbit ventricular myocardium, relative to control of active state. *J Mol Cell Cardiol.* 1:65-90, **1970**. *[10]*

Langer GA, Frank JS, Brady AJ: The Myocardium, in Cardiovascular Physiology II. Guyton AC, Cowley AW (eds). Baltimore, MD, University Park Press. Vol. 9. 191-237, **1976**. *[1]*

Langer GA, Frank JS, Philipson KD: Ultrastructure and calcium exchange of the sarcolemma, sarcoplasmic reticulum and mitochondria of the myocardium. *Pharmacol Ther.* 16:331-376, **1982**. *[1]*

Langer GA, Rich TL, Orner FB: Calcium exchange under non-perfusion limited conditions in rat ventricular cells: Identification of subcellular compartments. *Am J Physiol.* 259:H592-H602, **1990**. *[3,7]*

Lansman JB, Hess P, Tsien RW: Blockade of current through single calcium channels by Cd²⁺, Mg²⁺, and Ca²⁺. Voltage and concentration dependence of calcium entry into the pore. *J Gen Physiol.* 88:321-347, **1986**. *[5]*

Lappé DL, Lakatta EG: Intensity fluctuation spectroscopy monitors contractile activation in "resting" cardiac muscle. *Science.* 207:1369-1371, **1980**. *[10]*

Lattanzio FA Jr, Schlatterer RG, Nicar M, Campbell KP, Sutko JL: The effects of ryanodine on passive calcium fluxes across sarcoplasmic reticulum membranes. *J Biol Chem.* 262:2711-2718, **1987**. *[7]*

Lauer MR, Gunn MD, Clusin WT: Endothelin activates voltage-dependent Ca^{2+} current by a G protein-dependent mechanism in rabbit cardiac myocytes. *J Physiol.* 448:729-747, **1992**. *[5]*

Läuger P: Electrogenic Ion Pumps. *Sunderland, MA, Sinauer Associates, Inc.* **1991**. *[4]*

Laver DR, Curtis BA: Response of ryanodine receptor channels to Ca^{2+} steps produced by rapid solution. *Biophys J.* 71:732-741, **1996**. *[7]*

Lawrence C, Rodrigo GC: A Na^+-activated K^+ current ($I_{K,Na}$) is present in guinea-pig but not rat ventricular myocytes. *Pflügers Arch.* 437:831-838, **1999**. *[4]*

Layland J, Kentish JC: Positive force- and $[Ca^{2+}]_i$-frequency relationships in rat ventricular trabeculae at physiological frequencies. *Am J Physiol.* 276:H9-H18, **1999**. *[9]*

Lazarides E: Intermediate filaments as mechanical integrators of cellular space. *Nature.* 283:249-256, **1980**. *[1]*

Lazarides E: Biochemical and immunocytological characterization of intermediate filaments in muscle cells. *Methods Cell Biol.* 25:333-357, **1982**. *[1]*

Lazdunski M, Frelin C, Vigne P: The sodium/hydrogen exchange system in cardiac cells: Its biochemical and pharmacological properties and its role in regulating internal concentrations of sodium and internal pH. *J Mol Cell Cardiol.* 17:1029-1042, **1985**. *[10]*

Le Grand B, Deroubaix E, Coulombe A, Coraboeuf E: Stimulatory effect of ouabain on T- and L-type calcium currents in guinea pig cardiac myocytes. *Am J Physiol.* 258:H1620-H1623, **1990**. *[10]*

Le Grand B, Hatem S, Deroubaix E, Couetil JP, Coraboeuf E: Calcium current depression in isolated human atrial myocytes after cessation of chronic treatment with calcium antagonists. *Circ Res.* 69:292-300, **1991**. *[5]*

Le Grand B, Deroubaix E, Couetil JP, Coraboeuf E: Effects of atrionatriuretic factor on Ca^{2+} current and Ca_i-independent transient outward K^+ current in human atrial cells. *Pflügers Arch.* 421:486-491, **1992**. *[5]*

Lea TJ, Griffiths PJ, Tregear RT, Ashley CC: An examination of the ability of inositol 1,4,5-triphosphate to induce calcium release and tension development in skinned skeletal muscle fibres of frog and crustacea. *FEBS Lett.* 207:153-161, **1986**. *[8]*

Leberer E, Charuk JHM, Clarke DM, Green NM, Zubrzycka-Gaarn E, MacLennan DH: Molecular cloning and expression of cDNA encoding the 53,000-dalton glycoprotein of rabbit skeletal muscle sarcoplasmic reticulum. *J Biol Chem.* 264:3484-3492, **1989a**. *[7]*

Leberer E, Charuk JHM, Green NM, MacLennan DH: Molecular cloning and expression of cDNA encoding a lumenal calcium binding protein from sarcoplasmic reticulum. *Proc Natl Acad Sci USA.* 86:6047-6051, **1989b**. *[7]*

Leberer E, Timms BG, Campbell KP, MacLennan DH: Purification, calcium binding properties, and ultrastructural localization of the 52,000- and 160,000 (sarcalumenin)-dalton glycoproteins of the sarcoplasmic reticulum. *J Biol Chem.* 265:10118-10124, **1990**. *[7]*

Leblanc N, Hume JR: D 600 block of L-type Ca^{2+} channel in vascular smooth muscle cells: Comparison with permanently charged derivative, D 890. *Am J Physiol.* 257:C689-C695, **1989**. *[5]*

Leblanc N, Hume JR: Sodium current-induced release of calcium from cardiac sarcoplasmic reticulum. *Science.* 248:372-376, **1990**. *[3,6,8,10]*

Lechleiter J, Girard S, Peralta E, Clapham D: Spiral calcium wave propagation and annihilation in Xenopus laevis oocytes. *Science.* 252:123-126, **1991**. *[4]*

Lederer WJ, Tsien RW: Transient inward current underlying arrhythmogenic effects of cardiotonic steroids in Purkinje fibres. *J Physiol.* 263:73-100, **1976**. *[4,10]*

Lederer WJ, Nichols CG, Smith GL: The mechanism of early contractile failure of isolated rat ventricular myocytes subjected to complete metabolic blockade. *J Physiol.* 413:329-349, **1989**. *[10]*

Lederer WJ, Niggli E, Hadley RW: Sodium-calcium exchange in excitable cells: Fuzzy space. *Science.* 248:283, **1990**. *[8]*

Ledvora RF, Hegyvary C: Dependence of sodium-calcium exchange and calcium-calcium exchange on monovalent cations. *Biochim Biophys Acta.* 729:123-136, **1983**. *[6]*

Lee CO: 200 years of digitalis: The emerging central role of the sodium ion in the control of cardiac force. *Am J Physiol.* 249:C367-C378, **1985**. *[10]*

Lee KS: Potentiation of the calcium-channel currents of internally perfused mammalian heart cells by repetitive depolarization. *Proc Natl Acad Sci USA.* 84:3941-3945, **1987**. *[5]*

Lee HC: A unified mechanism of enzymatic synthesis of two calcium messengers: Cyclic ADP-ribose and NAADP. *Biological Chemistry.* 380:785-793, **1999**. *[7]*

Lee CO, Dagostino M: Effect of strophanthidin on intracellular Na ion activity and twitch tension of constantly driven canine cardiac Purkinje fibers. *Biophys J.* 40:185-198, **1982**. *[10]*

Lee CO, Fozzard HA: Activities of potassium and sodium ions in rabbit heart muscle. *J Gen Physiol.* 65:695-708, **1975**. *[1]*

Lee KS, Tsien RS: Mechanism of calcium channel blockade by verapamil, D600, diltiazem and nitrendipine in singel dialysed heart cells. *Nature.* 302:790-794, **1983**. *[5]*

Lee CO, Vassalle M: Modulation of intracellular Na^+ activity and cardiac force by norepinephrine and Ca^{2+}. *Am J Physiol.* 244:C110-C114, **1983**. *[10]*

Lee CO, Kang DH, Sokol JH, Lee KS: Relation between intracellular Na ion activity and tension of sheep cardiac Purkinje fibers exposed to dihydro-ouabain. *Biophys J.* 29:315-330, **1980**. *[10]*

Lee KS, Marbán E, Tsien RW: Inactivation of calcium channels in mammalian heart cells: Joint dependence on membrane potential and intracellular calcium. *J Physiol.* 364:395-411, **1985**. *[5,8]*

Lee HC, Mohabir R, Smith N, Franz MR, Clusin WT: Effect of ischemia on calcium-dependent fluorescence transients in rabbit hearts containing Indo 1. *Circulation.* 78:1047-1059, **1988**. *[10]*

Lee JH, Daud AN, Cribbs LL, Lacerda AE, Pereverzev A, Klöckner U, Schneider T, Perez-Reyes E: Cloning and expression of a novel member of the low voltage-activated T-type calcium channel family. *J Neurosci.* 19:1912-1921, **1999a**. *[5]*

Lee JH, Gomora JC, Cribbs LL, Perez-Reyes E: Nickel block of three cloned T-type calcium channels: Low concentrations selectively block α1H. *Biophys J.* 77:3034-3042, **1999b**. *[5]*

Leem CH, Vaughan-Jones RD: Sarcolemmal mechanisms for pHi recovery from alkalosis in the guinea-pig ventricular myocyte. *J Physiol.* 509:487-496, **1998**. *[10]*

Leem CH, Lagadic-Gossmann D, Vaughan-Jones RD: Characterization of intracellular pH regulation in the guinea-pig ventricular myocyte. *J Physiol.* 517:159-180, **1999**. *[10]*

Lefer AM, Tsao P, Aoki N, Palladino MA: Mediation of cardioprotection by transforming growth factor-beta. *Science.* 249:61-64, **1990**. *[10]*

Lefkowitz RJ: G protein-coupled receptor kinases. *Cell.* 74:409-412, **1993**. *[10]*

Legato M: Cellular mechanisms of normal growth in the mammalian heart. II. A quantitative and qualitative comparison between the right and left ventricular myocytes in the dog from birth to five months of age. *Circ Res.* 44:263-279, **1979**. *[9]*

Lehninger AL: Ca^{2+} transport by mitochondria and its possible role in the cardiac excitation-contraction-relaxation cycle. *Circ Res.* 35:III83-III90, **1974**. *[3]*

Lehninger AL, Carafoli E, Rossi CS: Energy linked ion movements in mitochondrial systems. *Adv Enzymol.* 29:259-320, **1967**. *[3]*

Lehrer SS, Golitsina NL, Geeves MA: Actin-tropomyosin activation of myosin subfragment 1 ATPase and thin filament cooperativity. The role of tropomyosin flexibility and end-to-end interactions. *Biochemistry.* 36:13449-13454, **1997**. *[2]*

Lemaire S, Piot C, Seguin J, Nargeot J, Richard S: Tetrodotoxin-sensitive Ca^{2+} and Ba^{2+} currents in human atrial cells. *Receptors Channels.* 3:71-81, **1995**. *[8]*

Leong P, MacLennan DH: A 37-amino acid sequence in the skeletal muscle ryanodine receptor interacts with the cytoplasmic loop between domains II and III in the skeletal muscle dihydropyridine receptor. *J Biol Chem.* 273:7791-7794, **1998a**. *[8]*

Leong P, MacLennan DH: The cytoplasmic loops between domains II and III and domains III and IV in the skeletal muscle dihydropyridine receptor bind to a contiguous site in the skeletal muscle ryanodine receptor. *J Biol Chem.* 273:29958-29964, **1998b**. *[8]*

Leoty C, Raymond G: Mechanical activity and ionic currents in frog atrial trabeculae. *Pflügers Arch.* 334:114-128, **1972**. *[9]*

LePeuch CJ, Haiech J, Demaille JG: Concerted regulations of cardiac sarcoplasmic reticulum calcium transport by cyclic adenosine monophosphate dependent and calcium-calmodulin-dependent phosphorylation. *Biochemistry.* 18:5150-5157, **1979**. *[7]*

LePeuch CJ, LePeuch DAM, Demaille JG: Phospholamban activation of the cardiac sarcoplasmic reticulum calcium pump. Physicochemical properties and diagonal purification. *Biochemistry.* 19:3368-3373, **1980**. *[7]*

Lerche C, Seebohm G, Wagner CI, Scherer CR, Dehmelt L, Abitbol I, Gerlach U, Brendel J, Attali B, Busch AE: Molecular impact of MinK on the enantiospecific block of IKs by chromanols. *Br J Pharmacol.* 131:1503-1506, **2000**. *[10]*

Lesh RE, Nixon GF, Fleischer S, Airey JA, Somlyo AP, Somlyo AV: Localization of ryanodine receptors in smooth muscle. *Circ Res.* 82:175-185, **1998**. *[8]*

Letts VA, Felix R, Biddlecome GH, Arikkath J, Mahaffey CL, Valenzuela A, Bartlett FS II, Mori Y, Campbell KP, Frankel WN: The mouse stargazer gene encodes a neuronal Ca^{2+}-channel gamma subunit. *Nature Genet.* 19:340-347, **1998**. *[5]*

Levesque PC, Hume JR: ATP$_0$ but not cAMP$_i$ activates a chloride conductance in mouse ventricular myocytes. *Cardiovasc Res.* 29:336-343, **1995**. *[4]*

Levesque PC, Leblanc N, Hume JR: Release of calcium from guinea pig cardiac sarcoplasmic reticulum induced by sodium-calcium exchange. *Cardiovasc Res.* 28:370-378, **1994**. *[8]*

Levi RC, Alloatti G: Histamine modulates calcium current in guinea pig ventricular myocytes. *J Pharmacol Exp Ther.* 246:377-383, **1988**. *[5]*

Levi AJ, Spitzer KW, Kohmoto O, Bridge JHB: Depolarization-induced Ca entry via Na-Ca exchange triggers SR release in guinea pig cardiac myocytes. *Am J Physiol.* 266:H1422-H1433, **1994**. *[8]*

Levin KR, Page E: Quantitative studies on plasmalemmal folds and caveolae of rabbit ventricular myocardial cells. *Circ Res.* 46:244-255, **1980**. *[1]*

Levitsky DO, Benevolensky DS, Levchenko LS, Smirnov VN, Chazov EI: Calcium-binding rate and capacity of cardiac sarcoplasmic reticulum. *J Mol Cell Cardiol.* 13:785-796, **1981**. *[3,7,10]*

Levitsky DO, Nicoll DA, Philipson KD: Identification of the high affinity Ca^{2+}-binding domain of the cardiac Na$^+$-Ca^{2+} exchanger. *J Biol Chem.* 269:22847-22852, **1994**. *[6]*

Lew WYW, Hryshko LV, Bers DM: Dihydropyridine receptors are primarily functional L-type Ca channels in rabbit cardiac myocytes. *Circ Res.* 69:1139-1145, **1991**. *[5,7]*

Lewartowski B, Pytkowski B: Cellular mechanism of the relationship between myocardial force and frequency of contractions. *Prog Biophys Molec Biol.* 50:97-120, **1987**. *[7,9]*

Lewartowski B, Zdanowski K: Net Ca^{2+} influx and sarcoplasmic reticulum Ca^{2+} uptake in resting single myocytes of the rat heart: Comparison with guinea-pig. *J Mol Cell Cardiol.* 22:1221-1229, **1990**. *[9]*

Lewartowski B, Pytkowski B, Janczewski A: Calcium fraction correlating with contractile force of ventricular muscle of guinea-pig heart. *Pflügers Arch.* 401:198-203, **1984**. *[7]*

Lewartowski B, Hansford RG, Langer GA, Lakatta EG: Contraction and sarcoplasmic reticulum Ca^{2+} content in single myocytes of guinea pig heart: Effect of ryanodine. *Am J Physiol.* 259:H1222-H1229, **1990**. *[9]*

Lewis DL, Clapham DE: Somatostatin activates an inwardly rectifying K$^+$ channel in neonatal rat atrial cells. *Pflügers Arch.* 414:492-494, **1989**. *[4]*

Li J, Kimura J: Translocation mechanism of Na-Ca exchange in single cardiac cells of guinea pig. *J Gen Physiol.* 96:777-788, **1990**. *[6]*

Li ZP, Nicoll DA, Collins A, Hilgemann DW, Filoteo AG, Penniston JT, Weiss JN, Tomich JM, Philipson KD: Identification of a peptide inhibitor of the cardiac sarcolemmal Na$^+$-Ca^{2+} exchanger. *J Biol Chem.* 266:1014-1020, **1991**. *[6]*

Li ZP, Burke EP, Frank JS, Bennett V, Philipson KD: The cardiac Na+-Ca2+ exchanger binds to the cytoskeletal protein ankyrin. *J Biol Chem.* 268:11489-11491, **1993**. *[1]*

Li ZP, Matsuoka S, Hryshko LV, Nicoll DA, Bersohn MM, Burke EP, Lifton RP, Philipson KD: Cloning of the NCX2 isoform of the plasma membrane Na+-Ca2+ exchanger. *J Biol Chem.* 269:17434-17439, **1994**. *[6]*

Li J, Qu JH, Nathan RD: Ionic basis of ryanodine's negative chronotropic effect on pacemaker cells isolated from the sinoatrial node. *Am J Physiol.* 273:H2481-H2489, **1997a**. *[4]*

Li L, Satoh H, Ginsburg KS, Bers DM: The effect of Ca2+-calmodulin-dependent protein kinase II on cardiac excitation-contraction coupling in ferret ventricular myocytes. *J Physiol.* 501:17-31, **1997b**. *[5,7,9,10]*

Li L, Chu G, Kranias EG, Bers DM: Cardiac myocyte calcium transport in phospholamban knockout mouse: Relaxation and endogenous CaMKII effects. *Am J Physiol.* 274:H1335-H1347, **1998**. *[7,9,10]*

Li Y, Marx SO, Marks AR, Bers DM: Cardiac Ca channel II-III loop peptide reduces open probability of isolated SR Ca release channels and Ca spark frequency in ferret ventricular myocytes. *Biophys J.* 76:A463, **1999**. *[8]*

Li L, DeSantiago J, Chu G, Kranias EG, Bers DM: Phosphorylation of phospholamban and troponin I in β-adrenergic-induced acceleration of cardiac relaxation. *Am J Physiol.* 278:H769-H779, **2000**. *[7,10]*

Limas CJ, Olivari M, Goldenberg IF, Levine TB, Benditt DG, Simon A: Calcium uptake by cardiac sarcoplasmic reticulum in human dilated myocardium. *Cardiovasc Res.* 21:601-605, **1987**. *[10]*

Lin C, Baker KM, Thekkumkara TJ, Dostal DE: Sensitive bioassay for the detection and quantification of angiotensin II in tissue culture medium. *Biotechniques.* 18:1014-1020, **1995**. *[10]*

Linck B, Boknik P, Eschenhagen T, Müller FU, Neumann J, Nose M, Jones LR, Schmitz W, Scholz H: Messenger RNA expression and immunological quantification of phospholamban and SR-Ca2+-ATPase in failing and nonfailing human hearts. *Cardiovasc Res.* 31:625-632, **1996**. *[10]*

Linck B, Qiu ZY, He ZP, Tong QS, Hilgemann DW, Philipson KD: Functional comparison of the three isoforms of the Na+/Ca2+ exchanger (NCX1, NCX2, NCX3). *Am J Physiol.* 274:C415-C423, **1998**. *[6]*

Lincoln TM, Corbin JD: Purified cyclic GMP-dependent protein kinase catalyzes the phosphorylation of cardiac troponin inhibitory subunit (TN-1). *J Biol Chem.* 253:337-339, **1978**. *[10]*

Lindblad DS, Murphey CR, Clark JW, Giles WR: A model of the action potential and underlying membrane currents in a rabbit atrial cell. *Am J Physiol.* 271:H1666-H1696, **1996**. *[4]*

Lindemann JP, Watanabe AM: Muscarinic cholinergic inhibition of β-adrenergic stimulation of phospholamban phosphorylation and Ca2+ transport in guinea pig ventricles. *J Biol Chem.* 260:13122-13129, **1985a**. *[2]*

Lindemann JP, Watanabe AM: Phosphorylation of phospholamban in intact myocardium. Role of Ca2+-calmodulin-dependent mechanisms. *J Biol Chem.* 260:4516-4525, **1985b**. *[7]*

Lindemann JP, Watanabe AM: Mechanisms of adrenergic and cholinergic regulation of myocardial contractility, in *Physiology and Pathophysiology of the Heart.* Sperelakis N (ed). *Boston, MD, Kluwer Academic Publishers.* 423-452, **1989**. *[5]*

Lindemann JP, Jones LR, Hathaway DR, Henry BG, Watanabe A: β-Adrenergic stimulation of phospholamban phosphorylation and Ca2+ ATPase activity in guinea pig ventricles. *J Biol Chem.* 258:464-471, **1983**. *[7]*

Lindner M, Erdmann E, Beuckelmann DJ: Calcium content of the sarcoplasmic reticulum in isolated ventricular myocytes from patients with terminal heart failure. *J Mol Cell Cardiol.* 30:743-749, **1998**. *[10]*

Lingrel JB, Arguello JM, Van HJ, Kuntzweiler TA: Cation and cardiac glycoside binding sites of the Na,K-ATPase. *Ann NY Acad Sci.* 834:194-206, **1997**. *[4]*

Linz KW, Meyer R: Control of L-type calcium current during the action potential of guinea-pig ventricular myocytes. *J Physiol.* 513:425-442, **1998**. *[5]*

Lipp P, Niggli E: Microscopic spiral waves reveal positive feedback in subcellular calcium signaling. *Biophys J.* 65:2272-2276, **1993**. *[4,8]*

Lipp P, Niggli E: Sodium current-induced calcium signals in isolated guinea- pig ventricular myocytes. *J Physiol.* 474:439-446, **1994**. *[8]*

Lipp P, Niggli E: Submicroscopic calcium signals as fundamental events of excitation-contraction coupling in guinea-pig cardiac myocytes. *J Physiol.* 492:31-38, **1996**. *[8]*

Lipp P, Niggli E: Fundamental calcium release events revealed by two-photon excitation photolysis of caged calcium in guinea-pig cardiac myocytes. *J Physiol.* 508:801-809, **1998**. *[8]*

Lipp P, Schwaller B, Niggli E: Specific inhibition of Na-Ca exchange function by antisense oligodeoxynucleotides. *FEBS Lett.* 364:198-202, **1995**. *[6]*

Lipp P, Laine M, Tovey SC, Burrell KM, Berridge MJ, Li WH, Bootman MD: Functional InsP3 receptors that may modulate excitation-contraction coupling in the heart. *Curr Biol.* 10:939-942, **2000**. *[8]*

Lipsius SL, Fozzard HA, Gibbons WR: Voltage and time dependence of restitution in heart. *Am J Physiol.* 243:H68-H76, **1982**. *[8]*

Litwin SE, Bridge JHB: Enhanced Na+-Ca2+ exchange in the infarcted heart - Implications for excitation-contraction coupling. *Circ Res.* 81:1083-1093, **1997**. *[10]*

Litwin SE, Li J, Bridge JHB: Na-Ca exchange and the trigger for sarcoplasmic reticulum Ca release: Studies in adult rabbit ventricular myocytes. *Biophys J.* 75:359-371, **1998**. *[8]*

Litwin SE, Zhang DF, Bridge JHB: Dyssynchronous Ca2+ sparks in myocytes from infarcted hearts. *Circ Res.* 87:1040-1047, **2000**. *[10]*

Liu DW, Antzelevitch C: Characteristics of the delayed rectifier current (IKr and IKs) in canine ventricular epicardial, midmyocardial, and endocardial myocytes: A weaker IKs contributes to the longer action potential of the M cell. *Circ Res.* 76:351-365, **1995**. *[4]*

Liu SJ, Kennedy RH: α1-adrenergic activation of L-type Ca current in rat ventricular myocytes: Perforated patch-clamp recordings *Am J Physiol.* 274:H2203-H2207, **1998**. *[5]*

Liu W, Meissner G: Structure-activity relationship of xanthines and skeletal muscle ryanodine receptor/Ca2+ release channel. *Pharmacology.* 54:135-143, **1997**. *[7]*

Liu DW, Gintant GA, Antzelevitch C: Ionic bases for electrophysiological distinctions among epicardial, midmyocardial, and endocardial myocytes from the free wall of the canine left ventricle. *Circ Res.* 72:671-687, **1993**. *[4]*

Liu YG, Sato T, O'Rourke B, Marbán E: Mitochondrial ATP-dependent potassium channels - Novel effectors of cardioprotection? *Circulation.* 97:2463-2469, **1998**. *[4,10]*

Imers W, McCleskey EW, Palade PT: A non-selective cation conductance in frog muscle membrane blocked by micromolar extracellular calcium ions. *J Physiol.* 355:565-583, **1984**. *[5]*

Löffelholz K, Pappano AJ: The parasympathetic neuroeffector junction of the heart. *Pharmacol Rev.* 37:1-24, **1985**. *[10]*

Loke J, MacLennan DH: Malignant hyperthermia and central core disease: Disorders of Ca^{2+} release channels. *Am J Med.* 104:470-486, **1998**. *[7]*

Lokuta AJ, Rogers TB, Lederer WJ, Valdivia HH: Modulation of cardiac ryanodine receptors of swine and rabbit by a phosphorylation-dephosphorylation mechanism. *J Physiol.* 487:609-622, **1995**. *[7]*

Lokuta AJ, Meyers MB, Sander PR, Fishman GI, Valdivia HH: Modulation of cardiac ryanodine receptors by sorcin. *J Biol Chem.* 272:25333-25338, **1997**. *[7]*

London B, Krueger JW: Contraction in voltage-clamped, internally perfused single heart cells. *J Gen Physiol.* 88:475-505, **1986**. *[8]*

Lopatin AN, Makhina EN, Nichols CG: Potassium channel block by cytoplasmic polyamines as the mechanism of intrinsic rectification. *Nature.* 372:366-369, **1994**. *[4]*

López-López JR, Shacklock PS, Balke CW, Wier WG: Local, stochastic release of Ca^{2+} in voltage-clamped rat heart cells: Visualization with confocal microscopy. *J Physiol.* 480:21-29, **1994**. *[7,8]*

López-López JR, Shacklock PS, Balke CW, Wier WG: Local calcium transients triggered by single L-type calcium channel currents in cardiac cells. *Science.* 268:1042-1045, **1995**. *[7,8]*

Lorell BH: Transition from hypertrophy to failure. *Circulation.* 96:3824-3827, **1997**. *[10]*

Lorenz M, Poole KJ, Popp D, Rosenbaum G, Holmes KC: An atomic model of the unregulated thin filament obtained by X-ray fiber diffraction on oriented actin-tropomyosin gels. *J Mol Biol.* 246:108-119, **1995**. *[2]*

Louis CF, Turnquist J, Jarvis B: Phospholamban stoichiometry in canine cardiac muscle sarcoplasmic reticulum. *Neurochem Res.* 12:937-941, **1987**. *[7]*

Lu YZ, Kirchberger MA: Effects of a nonionic detergent on calcium uptake by cardiac microsomes. *Biochemistry.* 33:5056-5062, **1994**. *[7]*

Lu X, Xu L, Meissner G: Activation of the skeletal muscle calcium release channel by a cytoplasmic loop of the dihydropyridine receptor. *J Biol Chem.* 269:6511-6516, **1994**. *[8]*

Lucchesi PA, Sweadner KJ: Postnatal changes in Na,K-ATPase isoform expression in rat cardiac ventricle. Conservation of biphasic ouabain affinity. *J Biol Chem.* 266:9327-9331, **1991**. *[4]*

Lückhoff A: Measuring free calcium concentration in endothelial cells with indo-1: The pitfalls of using two fluorescence intensities recorded at different wavelengths. *Cell Calcium.* 7:233-248, **1986**. *[3]*

Ludwig A, Zong XG, Jeglitsch M, Hofmann F, Biel M: A family of hyperpolarization-activated mammalian cation channels. *Nature.* 393:587-591, **1998**. *[4]*

Ludwig A, Zong XG, Stieber J, Hullin R, Hofmann F, Biel M: Two pacemaker channels from human heart with profoundly different activation kinetics. *EMBO J.* 18:2323-2329, **1999**. *[4]*

Lues I, Siegel R, Harting J: Effect of isomazole on the responsiveness to calcium of the contractile elements in skinned cardiac muscle fibres of various species. *Eur J Pharmacol.* 146:145-153, **1988**. *[2]*

Lues I, Beier N, Jonas R, Klockow M, Haeusler G: The two mechanisms of action of racemic cardiotonic EMD 53998, calcium sensitization and phosphodiesterase inhibition, reside in different enantiomers. *J Cardiovasc Pharmacol.* 21:883-892, **1993**. *[10]*

Luk HN, Carmeliet E: Na^+-activated K^+ current in cardiac cells: Rectification, open probability, block and role in digitalis toxicity. *Pflügers Arch.* 416:766-768, **1990**. *[4]*

Lukyanenko V, Györke I, Györke S: Regulation of calcium release by calcium inside the sarcoplasmic reticulum in ventricular myocytes. *Pflügers Arch.* 432:1047-1054, **1996**. *[7]*

Lukyanenko V, Wiesner TF, Györke S: Termination of Ca^{2+} release during Ca^{2+} sparks in rat ventricular myocytes. *J Physiol.* 507:667-677, **1998**. *[8]*

Lukyanenko V, Subramanian S, Györke I, Wiesner TF, Györke S: The role of luminal Ca^{2+} in the generation of Ca^{2+} waves in rat ventricular myocytes. *J Physiol.* 518:173-186, **1999**. *[8,10]*

Lukyanenko V, Györke I, Subramanian S, Smirnov A, Wiesner TF, Györke S: Inhibition of Ca^{2+} sparks by ruthenium red in permeabilized rat ventricular myocytes. *Biophys J.* 79:1273-1284, **2000**. *[7]*

Lüllmann H, Peters T: Plasmalemmal calcium in cardiac excitation contraction coupling. *Clin Exp Pharmacol Physiol.* 4:49-57, **1977**. *[3]*

Lüllmann H, Peters T: Action of cardiac glycosides on the excitation-contraction coupling in heart muscle. *Prog Pharmacol.* 2:3-58, **1979**. *[3]*

Lund DD, Tomanek RJ: Myocardial morphology in spontaneously hypertensive and aortic-constricted rats. *Am J Anat.* 152:141-151, **1978**. *[10]*

Luo CH, Rudy Y: A model of the ventricular cardiac action potential. Depolarization, repolarization, and their interaction. *Circ Res.* 68:1501-1526, **1991**. *[4]*

Luo CH, Rudy Y: A dynamic model of the cardiac ventricular action potential: I. Simulations of ionic currents and concentration changes. *Circ Res.* 74:1071-1096, **1994a**. *[4,6]*

Luo CH, Rudy Y: A dynamic model of the cardiac ventricular action potential: II. Afterdepolarizations, triggered activity, and potentiation. *Circ Res.* 74:1097-1113, **1994b**. *[4]*

Luo W, Grupp IL, Harrer J, Ponniah S, Grupp G, Duffy JJ, Doetschman T, Kranias EG: Targeted ablation of the phospholamban gene is associated with markedly enhanced myocardial contractility and loss of β-agonist stimulation. *Circ Res.* 75:401-409, **1994**. *[7,10]*

Lüttgau HC, Niedergerke R: The antagonism between Ca and Na ions on the frog's heart. *J Physiol.* 143:466-505, **1958**. *[6]*

Lynch PJ, Tong JF, Lehane M, Mallet A, Giblin L, Heffron JA, Vaughan P, Zafra G, MacLennan DH, McCarthy TV: A mutation in the transmembrane/luminal domain of the ryanodine receptor is associated with abnormal Ca²⁺ release channel function and severe central core disease. *Proc Natl Acad Sci USA.* 96:4164-4169, **1999**. *[7]*

Lytton J, Westlin M, Burk SE, Shull GE, MacLennan DH: Functional comparisons between isoforms of the sarcoplasmic or endoplasmic reticulum family of calcium pumps. *J Biol Chem.* 267:14483-14489, **1992**. *[7]*

Ma J, Fill M, Knudson CM, Campbell KP, Coronado R: Ryanodine receptor of skeletal muscle is a gap junction-type channel. *Science.* 242:99-102, **1988**. *[7,8,10]*

MacKinnon R, Aldrich RW, Lee AW: Functional stoichiometry of Shaker potassium channel inactivation. *Science.* 262:757-759, **1993**. *[4]*

MacLennan DH, Green NM: Pumping Ions. *Nature.* 405:633-634, **2000**. *[7]*

MacLennan DH, Wong PTS: Isolation of a calcium-sequestering protein from sarcoplasmic reticulum. *Proc Natl Acad Sci USA.* 68:1231-1235, **1971**. *[7]*

MacLennan DH, Yip CC, Iles GH, Seeman P: Isolation of sarcoplasmic reticulum proteins. *Cold Spring Harbor Symp Quant Biol.* 37:469-478, **1972**. *[7]*

MacLennan DH, Brandl CJ, Bozena K, Green M: Amino-acid sequence of Ca²⁺+Mg²⁺-dependent ATPase from rabbit muscle sarcoplasmic reticulum, deduced from its complementary DNA sequence. *Nature.* 316:696-700, **1985**. *[7]*

MacLennan DH, Brandl CJ, Korczak B, Green NM: Calcium ATPases: Contribution of molecular genetics to our understanding of structure and function, in Proteins of Excitable Membranes. Hille B, Frambrough DM (eds). *New York, NY, John Wiley & Sons, Inc.* 287-300, **1987**. *[7]*

MacLennan DH, Clarke DM, Loo TW, Skerjanc IS: Site-directed mutagenesis of the Ca²⁺ ATPase of sarcoplasmic reticulum. *Acta Physiol Scand.* 607:141-150, **1992**. *[7]*

MacLennan DH, Rice WJ, Green NM: The mechanism of Ca²⁺ transport by sarco(endo)plasmic reticulum Ca²⁺-ATPases. *J Biol Chem.* 272:28815-28818, **1997**. *[7]*

MacLeod KT, Bers DM: The effects of rest duration and ryanodine on extracellular calcium concentration in cardiac muscle from rabbits. *Am J Physiol.* 253:C398-C407, **1987**. *[7,9]*

Mahaney JE, Autry JM, Jones LR: Kinetics studies of the cardiac Ca-ATPase expressed in Sf21 cells: New insights on Ca-ATPase regulation by phospholamban. *Biophys J.* 78:1306-1323, **2000**. *[7]*

Mahony L, Jones LR: Developmental changes in cardiac sarcoplasmic reticulum in sheep. *J Biol Chem.* 261:15257-15265, **1986**. *[9]*

Maier LS, Pieske B, Allen DG: Influence of stimulation frequency on [Na⁺]ᵢ and contractile function in Langendorff-perfused rat heart. *Am J Physiol.* 273:H1246-H1254, **1997a**. *[9]*

Maier LS, Hasenfuss G, Pieske B: Frequency-dependent changes in intracellular Na⁺-concentration in isolated human myocardium. *Circulation.* 96:I-178, **1997b**. *[10]*

Maier LS, Bers DM, Pieske B: Differences in Ca²⁺-handling and sarcoplasmic reticulum Ca²⁺-content in isolated rat and rabbit myocardium. *J Mol Cell Cardiol.* 32:2249-2258, **2000**. *[9]*

Mak IT, Weglicki WB: Protection by β-blocking agents against free radical-mediated sarcolemmal lipid peroxidation. *Circ Res.* 63:262-266, **1988**. *[10]*

Makowski L, Caspar DLD, Phillips WC, Goodenough DA: Gap junction structures II. Analysis of the x-ray diffraction data. *J Cell Biol.* 74:629-645, **1977**. *[1]*

Malécot CO, Katzung BG: Use-dependence of ryanodine effects on postrest contraction in ferret cardiac muscle. *Circ Res.* 60:560-567, **1987**. *[7,9]*

Malécot CO, Bers DM, Katzung BG: Biphasic contractions induced by milrinone at low temperature in ferret ventricular muscle: Role of the sarcoplasmic reticulum and transmembrane calcium influx. *Circ Res.* 59:151-162, **1986**. *[9]*

Maltsev VA, Sabbah HN, Higgins RS, Silverman N, Lesch M, Undrovinas AI: Novel, ultraslow inactivating sodium current in human ventricular cardiomyocytes. *Circulation.* 98:2545-2552, **1998**. *[4,10]*

Malviya AN, Rogue PJ: "Tell me where is calcium bred": Clarifying the roles of nuclear calcium. *Cell.* 92:17-23, **1998**. *[8]*

Mandel F, Kranias EG, Grassi de Gende A, Sumida M, Schwartz A: The effect of pH on the transient-state kinetics of Ca²⁺-Mg²⁺-ATPase of cardiac sarcoplasmic reticulum. A comparison with skeletal sarcoplasmic reticulum. *Circ Res.* 50:310-317, **1982**. *[10]*

Manjunath CK, Page E: Cell biology and protein composition of cardiac gap junctions. *Am J Physiol.* 248:H783-H791, **1985**. *[1]*

Manjunath CK, Goings GE, Page E: Isolation and protein composition of gap junctions from rabbit hearts. *Biochem J.* 205:189-194, **1982**. *[1]*

Mannuzzu LM, Moronne MM, Isacoff EY: Direct physical measure of conformational rearrangement underlying potassium channel gating. *Science.* 271:213-216, **1996**. *[4]*

Mansier P, Bers DM: Evaluation of the role of potential dependent sarcolemmal Ca binding in cardiac E-C coupling. *Circulation.* 70:II-75, **1984**. *[3]*

Marbán E: Myocardial stunning and hibernation. The physiology behind the colloquialisms. *Circulation.* 83:681-688, **1991**. *[10]*

Marbán E, Tsien RW: Enhancement of calcium current during digitalis inotropy in mammalian heart: Positive feedback regulation by intracellular calcium? *J Physiol.* 329:589-614, **1982**. *[10]*

Marbán E, Rink TJ, Tsien RW, Tsien RY: Free calcium in heart muscle at rest and during contraction measured with Ca²⁺-sensitive microelectrodes. *Nature.* 286:845-850, **1980**. *[10]*

Marber MS, Mestril R, Chi SH, Sayen MR, Yellon DM, Dillmann WH: Overexpression of the rat inducible 70-kD heat stress protein in a transgenic mouse increases the resistance of the heart to ischemic injury. *J Clin Invest.* 95:1446-1456, **1995**. *[10]*

Margreth A, Damiani E, Tobaldin G: Ratio of dihydropyridine to ryanodine receptors in mammalian and frog twitch muscles in relation to the mechanical hypothesis of excitation-contraction coupling. *Biochem Biophys Res Commun.* 197:1303-1311, **1993**. *[8]*

Marks AR: Cellular functions of immunophilins. *Physiol Rev.* 76:631-649, **1996**. *[7]*

Marks AR: Cardiac intracellular calcium release channels - Role in heart failure. *Circ Res.* 87:8-11, **2000**. *[7]*

Marks AR, Tempst P, Hwang KS, Taubman MB, Inui M, Chadwick C, Fleischer S, Nadal-Ginard B: Molecular cloning and characterization of the ryanodine receptor/junctional channel complex cDNA from skeletal muscle sarcoplasmic reticulum. *Proc Natl Acad Sci USA.* 86:8683-8687, **1989**. *[7]*

Martin AF, Ball K, Gao LZ, Kumar P, Solaro RJ: Identification and functional significance of troponin I isoforms in neonatal rat heart myofibrils. *Circ Res.* 69:1244-1252, **1991**. *[2]*

Martin JL, Mestril R, Hilal-Dandan R, Brunton LL, Dillmann WH: Small heat shock proteins and protection against ischemic injury in cardiac myocytes. *Circulation.* 96:4343-4348, **1997**. *[10]*

Martínez ML, Heredia MP, Delgado C: Expression of T-type Ca^{2+} channels in ventricular cells from hypertrophied rat hearts. *J Mol Cell Cardiol.* 31:1617-1625, **1999**. *[5]*

Marx SO, Ondrias K, Marks AR: Coupled gating between individual skeletal muscle Ca^{2+} release channels (ryanodine receptors). *Science.* 281:818-821, **1998a**. *[7,8]*

Marx SO, Ondrias K, Gaburjakova M, Marks AR: Activation and inactivation of the skeletal muscle ryanodine receptor by peptides from the II-II loop of the dihydropyridine receptor. *Circulation.* 98:I-822, **1998b**. *[8]*

Marx SO, Reiken S, Hisamatsu Y, Jayaraman T, Burkhoff D, Rosemblit N, Marks AR: PKA phosphorylation dissociates FKBP12.6 from the calcium release channel (ryanodine receptor): Defective regulation in failing hearts. *Cell.* 101:365-376, **2000**. *[7,10]*

Mascher D, Peper K: Two components of inward current in myocardial muscle fibers. *Pflügers Arch.* 307:190-203, **1969**. *[5]*

Mason CA, Ferrier GR: Tetracaine can inhibit contractions initiated by a voltage-sensitive release mechanism in guinea-pig ventricular myocytes. *J Physiol.* 519:851-865, **1999**. *[8]*

Matlib MA, Zhou Z, Knight S, Ahmed S, Choi KM, Krause-Bauer J, Phillips R, Altschuld R, Katsube Y, Sperelakis N, Bers DM: Oxygen-bridged dinuclear ruthenium amine complex specifically inhibits Ca^{2+} uptake into mitochondria in vitro and in situ in single cardiac myocytes. *J Biol Chem.* 273:10223-10231, **1998**. *[3]*

Matsuda N, Hagiwara N, Shoda M, Kasanuki H, Hosoda S: Enhancement of the L-type Ca^{2+} current by mechanical stimulation in single rabbit cardiac myocytes. *Circ Res.* 78:650-659, **1996**. *[4]*

Matsuoka S, Hilgemann DW: Steady-state and dynamic properties of cardiac sodium-calcium exchange. Ion and voltage dependencies of the transport cycle. *J Gen Physiol.* 100:963-1001, **1992**. *[6]*

Matsuoka S, Nicoll DA, Reilly RF, Hilgemann DW, Philipson KD: Initial localization of regulatory regions of the cardiac sarcolemmal Na$^+$-Ca^{2+} exchanger. *Proc Natl Acad Sci USA.* 90:3870-3874, **1993**. *[6]*

Matsuoka S, Nicoll DA, Hryshko LV, Levitsky DO, Weiss JN, Philipson KD: Regulation of the cardiac Na$^+$-Ca^{2+} exchanger by Ca^{2+}. Mutational analysis of the Ca^{2+}-binding domain. *J Gen Physiol.* 105:403-420, **1995**. *[6]*

Matsuoka S, Nicoll DA, He ZP, Philipson KD: Regulation of the cardiac Na$^+$-Ca^{2+} exchanger by the endogenous XIP region. *J Gen Physiol.* 109:273-286, **1997**. *[6]*

Matsuura H, Ehara T: Activation of chloride current by purinergic stimulation in guinea pig heart cells. *Circ Res.* 70:851-855, **1992**. *[4]*

Matsuura H, Ehara T: Modulation of the muscarinic K$^+$ channel by P2-purinoceptors in guinea-pig atrial myocytes. *J Physiol.* 497:379-393, **1996**. *[4]*

Matsuura H, Shattock MJ: Membrane potential fluctuations and transient inward currents induced by reactive oxygen intermediates in isolated rabbit ventricular cells. *Circ Res.* 68:319-329, **1991**. *[10]*

Mattiazzi A: Positive inotropic effect of angiotensin II. Increases in intracellular Ca^{2+} or changes in myofilament Ca^{2+} responsiveness? *J Pharmacol Toxicol Methods.* 37:205-214, **1997**. *[8]*

Mattiazzi A, Hove-Madsen L, Bers DM: Protein kinase inhibitors reduce SR Ca transport in permeabilized cardiac myocytes. *Am J Physiol.* 267:H812-H820, **1994**. *[3,7]*

Maurice JP, Shah AS, Kypson AP, Hata JA, White DC, Glower DD, Koch WJ: Molecular β-adrenergic signaling abnormalities in failing rabbit hearts after infarction. *Am J Physiol.* 276:H1853-H1860, **1999**. *[10]*

Maxwell K, Scott J, Omelchenko A, Lukas A, Lu L, Lu Y, Hnatowich M, Philipson KD, Hryshko LV: Functional role of ionic regulation of Na$^+$/Ca^{2+} exchange assessed in transgenic mouse hearts. *Am J Physiol.* 277:H2212-H2221, **1999**. *[6]*

Maylie JG: Excitation-contraction coupling in neonatal and adult myocardium of cat. *Am J Physiol.* 242:H834-H843, **1982**. *[9]*

Maylie J, Morad M: A transient outward current related to calcium release and development of tension in elephant seal atrial fibres. *J Physiol.* 357:267-292, **1984**. *[8]*

Mazzanti M, DiFrancesco D: Intracellular Ca modulates K-inward rectification in cardiac myocytes. *Pflügers Arch.* 413:322-324, **1989**. *[4]*

McCall E, Bers DM: BAY K 8644 depresses excitation-contraction coupling in cardiac muscle. *Am J Physiol.* 270:C878-C884, **1996**. *[8]*

McCall E, Harrison SM, Boyett MR, Orchard CH: Intracellular sodium activity, intracellular pH and contractility in isolated rat ventricular myocytes during respiratory acidosis. *J Physiol.* 429:17P, **1990**. *[10]*

McCall E, Li L, Satoh H, Shannon TR, Blatter LA, Bers DM: Effects of FK-506 on contraction and Ca^{2+} transients in rat cardiac myocytes. *Circ Res.* 79:1110-1121, **1996a**. *[7,10]*

McCall E, Hryshko LV, Stiffel VM, Christensen DM, Bers DM: Possible functional linkage between the cardiac dihydropyridine and ryanodine receptor: Acceleration of rest decay by Bay K 8644. *J Mol Cell Cardiol.* 28:79-93, **1996b**. *[8]*

McCall E, Ginsburg KS, Bassani RA, Shannon TR, Qi M, Samarel AM, Bers DM: Ca flux, contractility, and excitation-contraction coupling in hypertrophic rat ventricular myocytes. *Am J Physiol.* 274:H1348-H1360, **1998**. *[10]*

McClellan GB, Winegrad S: The regulation of the calcium sensitivity of the contractile system in mammalian cardiac muscle. *J Gen Physiol.* 72:737-764, **1978**. *[2]*

McCleskey EW: Perspective - Calcium channel permeation: A field in flux. *J Gen Physiol.* 113:765-772, **1999**. *[5]*

McCleskey EW, Almers W: The Ca channel in skeletal muscle is a large pore. *Proc Natl Acad Sci USA.* 82:7149-7153, **1985**. *[5,8]*

McCleskey EW, Fox AP, Feldman DH, Cruz LJ, Olivera BM, Tsien RW, Yoshikami D: ω-Conotoxin: Direct and persistent blockade of specific types of calcium channels in neurons but not muscle. *Proc Natl Acad Sci USA*. 84:4327-4331, **1987**. *[5]*

McCord JM: Free radicals and inflammation: Protection of synovial fluid by superoxide dismutase. *Science*. 185:529-531, **1974**. *[10]*

McCormack JG, Browne HM, Dawes NJ: Studies on mitochondrial Ca^{2+}-transport and matrix Ca^{2+} using fura-2-loaded rat heart mitochondria. *Biochim Biophys Acta*. 973:420-427, **1989**. *[3]*

McDonald KS, Moss RL: Osmotic compression of single cardiac myocytes eliminates the reduction in Ca^{2+} sensitivity of tension at short sarcomere length. *Circ Res*. 77:199-205, **1995**. *[2]*

McDonald TF, Nawrath H, Trautwein W: Membrane currents and tension in cat ventricular muscle treated with cardiac glycosides. *Circ Res*. 37:674-682, **1975**. *[8]*

McDonald TF, Cavalie A, Trautwein W, Pelzer D: Voltage-dependent properties of macroscopic and elementary calcium channel currents in guinea pig ventricular myocytes. *Pflügers Arch*. 406:437-448, **1986**. *[5]*

McDonald TF, Pelzer S, Trautwein W, Pelzer DJ: Regulation and modulation of calcium channels in cardiac, skeletal, and smooth muscle cells. *Physiol Rev*. 74:365-507, **1994**. *[4,5]*

McDonald KS, Field LJ, Parmacek MS, Soonpaa M, Leiden JM, Moss RL: Length dependence of Ca^{2+} sensitivity of tension in mouse cardiac myocytes expressing skeletal troponin C. *J Physiol*. 483:131-139, **1995a**. *[2]*

McDonald KS, Mammen PPA, Strang KT, Moss RL, Miller WP: Isometric and dynamic contractile properties of porcine skinned cardiac myocytes after stunning. *Circ Res*. 77:964-972, **1995b**. *[10]*

McDonald TV, Yu ZH, Ming Z, Palma E, Meyers MB, Wang KW, Goldstein SAN, Fishman GI: A minK-HERG complex regulates the cardiac potassium current I_{Kr}. *Nature*. 388:289-292, **1997**. *[4]*

McDonald KS, Moss RL, Miller WP: Incorporation of the troponin regulatory complex of post-ischemic stunned porcine myocardium reduces myofilament calcium sensitivity in rabbit psoas skeletal muscle fibers. *J Mol Cell Cardiol*. 30:285-296, **1998**. *[10]*

McDonough AA, Geering K, Farley RA: The sodium pump needs its β subunit. *FASEB J*. 4:1598-1605, **1990**. *[4]*

McDonough AA, Zhang YB, Shin V, Frank JS: Subcellular distribution of sodium pump isoform subunits in mammalian cardiac myocytes. *Am J Physiol*. 270:C1221-C1227, **1996**. *[4,10]*

McGarry SJ, Williams AJ: Digoxin activates sarcoplasmic reticulum Ca^{2+}-release channels: A possible role in cardiac inotropy. *Br J Pharmacol*. 108:1043-1050, **1993**. *[10]*

McIvor ME, Orchard CH, Lakatta EG: Dissociation of changes in apparent myofibrillar Ca^{2+} sensitivity and twitch relaxation induced by adrenergic and cholinergic stimulation in isolated ferret cardiac muscle. *J Gen Physiol*. 92:509-529, **1988**. *[2,7,10]*

McLaughlin S: Electrostatic potentials at membrane-solution interfaces, in Curr Top Memb and Transp. Vol. 9. Bonner F, Kleinzeller A (eds). *New York, NY, Academic Press*. 71-144, **1977**. *[5]*

McLaughlin S: The electrostatic properties of membranes. *Ann Rev Biophys Biophys Chem*. 18:113-135, **1989**. *[5]*

McLaughlin S, Mulrine N, Gresalfi T, Vaio G, McLaughlin A: Absorption of divalent cations to bilayer membranes containing phosphatidylserine. *J Gen Physiol*. 77:445-473, **1981**. *[5]*

Mechmann S, Pott L: Identification of Na-Ca exchange current in single cardiac myocytes. *Nature*. 319:597-599, **1986**. *[6]*

Meissner G: Isolation and characterization of two types of sarcoplasmic reticulum vesicles. *Biochim Biophys Acta*. 389:51-68, **1975**. *[1,7]*

Meissner G: Ryanodine activation and inhibition of the Ca^{2+} release channel of sarcoplasmic reticulum. *J Biol Chem*. 261:6300-6306, **1986a**. *[7]*

Meissner G: Permeability of sarcoplasmic reticulum to monovalent ions, in Sarcoplasmic Reticulum in Muscle Physiology. Entman ML, van Winkle WB (eds). *Boca Raton, FL, CRC Press, Inc*. Vol. 1 21-30, **1986b**. *[7,8]*

Meissner G: Ryanodine receptor/Ca^{2+} release channels and their regulation by endogenous effectors. *Annu Rev Physiol*. 56:485-508, **1994**. *[7]*

Meissner G, Henderson JS: Rapid calcium release from cardiac sarcoplasmic reticulum vesicles is dependent on Ca^{2+} and is modulated by Mg^{2+}, adenine nucleotide, and calmodulin. *J Biol Chem*. 262:3065-3073, **1987**. *[7]*

Mejia-Alvarez R, Kettlun C, Ríos E, Stern M, Fill M: Unitary Ca^{2+} current through cardiac ryanodine receptor channels under quasi-physiological ionic conditions. *J Gen Physiol*. 113:177-186, **1999**. *[7]*

Mela L: Inhibition and activation of calcium transport in mitochondria. Effect of lanthanides and local anesthetic drugs. *Biochemistry*. 8:2481-2486, **1969**. *[3]*

Melzer W, Ríos E, Schneider MF: A general procedure for determining the rate of calcium release from the sarcoplasmic reticulum in skeletal muscle fibers. *Biophys J*. 51:849-863, **1987**. *[8]*

Mentrard D, Vassort G, Fischmeister R: Changes in external sodium induce a membrane current related to the sodium-calcium exchange in cesium-loaded frog heart cells. *J Gen Physiol*. 84:201-220, **1984**. *[6]*

Mercadier JJ, Lompre AM, Duc P, Boheler KR, Fraysse JB, Wisnewsky C, Allen PD, Komajda M, Schwartz K: Altered sarcoplasmic reticulum Ca^{2+} ATPase gene expression in the human ventricle during end-stage heart failure. *J Clin Invest*. 85:305-309, **1990**. *[10]*

Méry PF, Pavoine C, Belhassen L, Pecker F, Fischmeister R: Nitric oxide regulates cardiac Ca^{2+} current. Involvement of cGMP-inhibited and cGMP-stimulated phosphodiesterases through guanylyl cyclase activation. *J Biol Chem*. 268:26286-26295, **1993**. *[5,10]*

Mestril R, Giordano FJ, Conde AG, Dillmann WH: Adenovirus-mediated gene transfer of a heat shock protein 70 (hsp 70i) protects against simulated ischemia. *J Mol Cell Cardiol*. 28:2351-2358, **1996**. *[10]*

Meszaros LG, Bak J, Chu A: Cyclic ADP-ribose as an endogenous regulator of the non-skeletal type ryanodine receptor Ca^{2+} channel. *Nature*. 364:76-79, **1993**. *[7]*

Metzger JM, Parmacek MS, Barr E, Pasyk K, Lin WI, Cochrane KL, Field LJ, Leiden JM: Skeletal troponin C reduces contractile sensitivity to acidosis in cardiac myocytes from transgenic mice. *Proc Natl Acad Sci USA*. 90:9036-9040, **1993**. *[2]*

Mewes T, Ravens U: L-type calcium currents of human myocytes from ventricle of non-failing and failing hearts and from atrium. *J Mol Cell Cardiol.* 26:1307-1320, **1994**. *[10]*

Meyer M, Schillinger W, Pieske B, Holubarsch C, Heilmann C, Posival H, Kuwajima G, Mikoshiba K, Just H, Hasenfuss G: Alterations of sarcoplasmic reticulum proteins in failing human dilated cardiomyopathy. *Circulation.* 92:778-784, **1995**. *[10]*

Meyers MB, Pickel VM, Sheu SS, Sharma VK, Scotto KW, Fishman GI: Association of sorcin with the cardiac ryanodine receptor. *J Biol Chem.* 270:26411-26418, **1995**. *[7,8]*

Meyers MB, Puri TS, Chien AJ, Gao TY, Hsu PH, Hosey MM, Fishman GI: Sorcin associates with the pore-forming subunit of voltage-dependent L-type Ca^{2+} channels. *J Biol Chem.* 273:18930-18935, **1998**. *[7,8]*

Michaelis ML, Michaelis EK: Alcohol and local anesthetic effects on sodium-dependent calcium fluxes in brain synaptic membrane vesicles. *Biochem Pharmacol.* 32:963-969, **1983**. *[6]*

Michaelis ML, Michaelis EK, Nunley EW, Galton N: Effects of chronic alcohol administration on synaptic membrane sodium-calcium exchange activity. *Brain Res.* 414:239-244, **1987**. *[6]*

Michel MC, Knowlton KU, Gross G, Chien KR: α$_1$-adrenergic receptor subtypes mediate distinct functions in adult and neonatal rat heart. *Circulation.* 82:III-561, **1990**. *[10]*

Michikawa T, Hamanaka H, Otsu H, Yamamoto A, Miyawaki A, Furuichi T, Tashiro Y, Mikoshiba K: Transmembrane topology and sites of N-glycosylation of inositol 1,4,5-trisphosphate receptor. *J Biol Chem.* 269:9184-9189, **1994**. *[7]*

Michikawa T, Hirota J, Kawano S, Hiraoka M, Yamada M, Furuichi T, Mikoshiba K: Calmodulin mediates calcium-dependent inactivation of the cerebellar type 1 inositol 1,4,5-trisphosphate receptor. *Neuron.* 23:799-808, **1999**. *[7]*

Mickelson JR, Louis CF: Malignant hyperthermia: Excitation-contraction coupling, Ca^{2+} release channel, and cell Ca^{2+} regulation defects. *Physiol Rev.* 76:537-592, **1996**. *[7]*

Mickelson JR, Gallant EM, Litterer LA, Johnson KM, Rempel WE, Louis CF: Abnormal sarcoplasmic reticulum ryanodine receptor in malignant hyperthermia. *J Biol Chem.* 263:9310-9315, **1988**. *[7]*

Mickelson JR, Litterer LA, Jacobson BA, Louis CF: Stimulation and inhibition of [3H]ryanodine binding to sarcoplasmic reticulum from malignant hyperthermia susceptible pigs. *Arch Biochem Biophys.* 278:251-257, **1990**. *[7]*

Mignery GA, Südhof TC: The ligand binding site and transduction mechanism in the inositol-1,4,5-triphosphate receptor. *EMBO J.* 9:3893-3898, **1990**. *[7]*

Mignery GA, Südhof TC, Takei K, De Camilli P: Putative receptor for inositol 1,4,5-triphosphate similar to ryanodine receptor. *Nature.* 342:192-195, **1989**. *[7]*

Mikami A, Imoto K, Tanabe T, Niidome T, More Y, Takeshima H, Narumiya S, Numa S: Primary structure and functional expression of the cardiac dihydropyridine-sensitive calcium channel. *Nature.* 340:230-233, **1989**. *[5]*

Mikos GJ, Snow TR: Failure of inositol 1,4,5-triphosphate to elicit or potentiate Ca^{2+} release from isolated skeletal muscle sarcoplasmic reticulum. *Biochim Biophys Acta.* 927:256-260, **1987**. *[8]*

Milano CA, Allen LF, Rockman HA, Dolber PC, McMinn TR, Chien KR, Johnson TD, Bond RA, Lefkowitz RJ: Enhanced myocardial function in transgenic mice overexpressing the β$_2$-adrenergic receptor. *Science.* 264:582-586, **1994**. *[10]*

Miledi R, Parker I, Schalow G: Measurement of calcium transients in frog muscle by the use of arsenazo III. *Proc R Soc Lond B Biol Sci.* 198:201-210, **1977**. *[8]*

Miller DJ, Smith GL: EGTA purity and the buffering of calcium ions in physiological solutions. *Am J Physiol.* 246:C160-C166, **1984**. *[2]*

Miller WP, McDonald KS, Moss RL: Onset of reduced Ca^{2+} sensitivity of tension during stunning in porcine myocardium. *J Mol Cell Cardiol.* 28:689-697, **1996**. *[10]*

Miller MS, Frieman WF, Wetzel GT: Caffeine-induced contractions in developing rabbit heart. *Pediatr Res.* 42:287-292, **1997**. *[9]*

Milner RE, Famulski KS, Michalak M: Calcium binding proteins in the sarcoplasmic/endoplasmic reticulum of muscle and nonmuscle cells. *Mol Cell Biochem.* 112:1-13, **1992**. *[7]*

Minamisawa S, Hoshijima M, Chu G, Ward CA, Frank K, Gu Y, Martone ME, Wang Y, Ross J Jr, Kranias EG, Giles WR, Chien KR: Chronic phospholamban-sarcoplasmic reticulum calcium ATPase interaction is the critical calcium cycling defect in dilated cardiomyopathy. *Cell.* 99:313-322, **1999**. *[10]*

Minneman KP: α$_1$-Adrenergic receptor subtypes, inositol phosphates, and sources of cell Ca^{2+}. *Pharmacol Rev.* 40:87-119, **1988**. *[10]*

Minneman KP, Han C, Abel PW: Comparison of α$_1$-adrenergic receptor subtypes distinguished by chloroethylclonindine and WB 4101. *Mol Pharmacol.* 33:509-514, **1988**. *[10]*

Mintz E, Guillain F: Ca^{2+} transport by the sarcoplasmic reticulum ATPase. *Biochim Biophys Acta.* 1318:52-70, **1997**. *[7]*

Missiaen L, Declerck I, Droogmans G, Plessers L, De Smedt H, Raeymaekers L, Casteels R: Agonist-dependent Ca^{2+} and Mn^{2+} entry dependent on state of filling of Ca^{2+} stores in aortic smooth muscle cells of the rat. *J Physiol.* 427:171-186, **1990**. *[8]*

Missiaen L, de Smedt H, Parys JB, Casteels R: Co-activation of inositol trisphosphate-induced Ca^{2+} release by cytosolic Ca^{2+} is loading-dependent. *J Biol Chem.* 269:7238-7242, **1994**. *[8]*

Mitchell P, Moyle J: Respiration-driven proton translocation in rat liver mitochondria. *Biochem J.* 105:1147-1162, **1967**. *[3]*

Mitchell RD, Simmerman HKB, Jones LR: Ca^{2+} binding effects on protein conformation and protein interactions of canine cardiac calsequestrin. *J Biol Chem.* 263:1376-1381, **1988**. *[7]*

Mitra R, Morad M: Two types of calcium channels in guinea-pig venricular myocytes. *Proc Natl Acad Sci USA.* 83:5340-5344, **1986**. *[5]*

Mitterdorfer J, Froschmayr M, Grabner M, Striessnig J, Glossmann H: Calcium channels: The β-subunit increases the affinity of dihydropyridine and Ca^{2+} binding sites of the α$_1$- subunit. *FEBS Lett.* 352:141-145, **1994**. *[5]*

Mitterdorfer J, Grabner M, Kraus RL, Hering S, Prinz H, Glossmann H, Striessnig J: Molecular basis of drug interaction with L-type Ca^{2+} channels. *J Bioenerg Biomembr.* 30:319-334, **1998**. *[5]*

Miura Y, Kimura J: Sodium-calcium exchange current. *J Gen Physiol.* 93:1129-1145, **1989**. *[6]*

Miyamoto MI, del Monte F, Schmidt U, DiSalvo TS, Kang ZB, Matsui T, Guerrero JL, Gwathmey JK, Rosenzweig A, Hajjar RJ: Adenoviral gene transfer of SERCA2a improves left-ventricular function in aortic-banded rats in transition to heart failure. *Proc Natl Acad Sci USA.* 97:793-798, **2000**. *[10]*

Miyata H, Silverman HS, Sollott SJ, Lakatta EG, Stern MD, Hansford RG: Measurement of mitochondrial free Ca^{2+} concentration in living single rat cardiac myocytes. *Am J Physiol.* 261:H1123-H1134, **1991**. *[3]*

Miyata S, Minobe W, Bristow MR, Leinwand LA: Myosin heavy chain isoform expression in the failing and nonfailing human heart. *Circ Res.* 86:386-390, **2000**. *[10]*

Mobley BA, Eisenberg BR: Sizes of components in frog skeletal muscle measured by methods of stereology. *J Gen Physiol.* 66:31-45, **1975**. *[1]*

Mobley BA, Page E: The surface area of sheep cardiac Purkinje fibres. *J Physiol.* 220:547-563, **1972**. *[1]*

Molkentin JD: Calcineurin and beyond - Cardiac hypertrophic signaling. *Circ Res.* 87:731-738, **2000**. *[10]*

Molkentin JD, Dorn GW II: Cytoplasmic signaling pathways that regulate cardiac hypertrophy. *Annu Rev Physiol.* 63:391-426, **2001**. *[10]*

Molkentin JD, Lu JR, Antos CL, Markham B, Richardson J, Robbins J, Grant SR, Olson EN: A calcineurin-dependent transcriptional pathway for cardiac hypertrophy. *Cell.* 93:215-228, **1998**. *[10]*

Molloy JE, Burns JE, Kendrick-Jones J, Tregear RT, White DC: Movement and force produced by a single myosin head. *Nature.* 378:209-212, **1995**. *[2]*

Moore CL: Specific inhibition of mitochondrial Ca^{2+} transport by ruthenium red. *Biochem Biophys Res Commun.* 42:298-305, **1971**. *[3]*

Mope L, McClellan GB, Winegrad S: Calcium sensitivity of the contractile system and phosphorylation of troponin in hyperpermeable cardiac cells. *J Gen Physiol.* 75:271-282, **1980**. *[2]*

Morad M, Cleemann L: Role of Ca^{2+} channel in development of tension in heart muscle. *J Mol Cell Cardiol.* 19:527-553, **1987**. *[9]*

Morad M, Goldman Y: Excitation-contraction coupling in heart muscle: Membrane control of development of tension. *Prog Biophys Molec Biol.* 27:257-313, **1973**. *[8]*

Morad M, Trautwein W: The effect of the duration of the action potential on contraction in the mammalian heart muscle. *Pflügers Arch.* 299:66-82, **1968**. *[9]*

Morales MJ, Castellino RC, Crews AL, Rasmusson RL, Strauss HC: A novel β subunit increases rate of inactivation of specific voltage-gated potassium channel α subunits. *J Biol Chem.* 270:6272-6277, **1995**. *[4]*

Morano I, Hofmann F, Zimmer M, Rüegg JC: The influence of P-light chain phosphorylation by myosin light chain kinase on the calcium sensitivity of chemically skinned heart fibres. *FEBS Lett.* 189:221-224, **1985**. *[2]*

Morano I, Ritter O, Bonz A, Timek T, Vahl CF, Michel G: Myosin light chain-actin interaction regulates cardiac contractility. *Circ Res.* 76:720-725, **1995**. *[2]*

Moravec CS, Bond M: X-ray microanalysis of subcellular calcium distribution in contracted and relaxed cardiac muscle. *Biophys J.* 57:503a, 1990.

Moreno-Sanchez R, Hansford RG: Dependence of cardiac mitochondrial pyruvate dehydrogenase activity on intramitochondrial free Ca^{2+} concentration. *Biochem J.* 256:403-412, **1988**. *[3]*

Morgan JP: The effects of digitalis on intracellular calcium transients in mammalian working myocardium as detected with aequorin. *J Mol Cell Cardiol.* 17:1065-1075, **1985**. *[10]*

Morkin E: Chronic adaptions in contractile proteins: Genetic regulation. *Annu Rev Physiol.* 49:545-554, **1987**. *[2]*

Mosca SM, Cingolani HE: Comparison of the protective effects of ischemic preconditioning and the Na^+/H^+ exchanger blockade. *Naunyn Schmiedebergs Arch Pharmacol.* 362:7-13, **2000**. *[10]*

Moschella MC, Marks AR: Inositol 1,4,5-trisphosphate receptor expression in cardiac myocytes. *J Cell Biol.* 120:1137-1146, **1993**. *[7]*

Moss RL, Buck SH: Regulation of cardiac contraction by Ca^{2+}, in <u>Handbook of Physiology</u>. Page E, Fozzard HA, Solaro RJ (eds). *New York, NY, Oxford University Press.* In press, **2001**. *[2]*

Moss RL, Nwoye LO, Greaser ML: Substitution of cardiac troponin C into rabbit muscle does not alter the length dependence of Ca^{2+} sensitivity of tension. *J Physiol.* 440:273-289, **1991**. *[2]*

Movsesian MA, Nishikawa M, Adelstein RS: Phosphorylation of phospholamban by Ca^{2+}-activated, phospholipid- dependent protein kinase. Stimulation of cardiac sarcoplasmic reticulum Ca^{2+} uptake. *J Biol Chem.* 259:8029-8032, **1984**. *[7]*

Movsesian MA, Thomas AP, Selak M, Williamson JR: Inositol trisphosphate does not release Ca^{2+} from permeabilized cardiac myocytes and sarcoplasmic reticulum. *FEBS Lett.* 185:328-332, **1985**. *[8]*

Movsesian MA, Karimi M, Green K, Jones LR: Ca^{2+}-transporting ATPase, phospholamban, and calsequestrin levels in nonfailing and failing human myocardium. *Circulation.* 90:653-657, **1994**. *[10]*

Mukai M, Terada H, Sugiyama S, Satoh H, Hayashi H: Effects of a selective inhibitor of Na^+/Ca^{2+} exchange, KB-R7943, on reoxygenation-induced injuries in guinea pig papillary muscles. *J Cardiovasc Pharmacol.* 35:121-128, **2000**. *[10]*

Mukherjee R, Spinale FG: L-type calcium channel abundance and function with cardiac hypertrophy and failure: A review. *J Mol Cell Cardiol.* 30:1899-1916, **1998**. *[10]*

Mulder BJM, de Tombe PP, ter Keurs HEDJ: Spontaneous and propagated contractions in rat cardiac trabeculae. *J Gen Physiol.* 93:943-961, **1989**. *[8,10]*

Mulieri LA, Hasenfuss G, Leavitt B, Allen PD, Alpert NR: Altered myocardial force-frequency relation in human heart failure. *Circulation.* 87:199-212, **1992**. *[10]*

Mullins LJ: The generation of electric currents in cardiac fibers by Na/Ca exchange. *Am J Physiol.* 236:C103-C110, **1979**. *[6]*

Mundina-Weilenmann C, Vittone L, Ortale M, de Cingolani GC, Mattiazzi A: Immunodetection of phosphorylation sites gives new insights into the mechanisms underlying phospholamban phosphorylation in the intact heart. *J Biol Chem.* 271:33561-33567, **1996**. *[7]*

Muramatsu H, Zou AR, Berkowitz GA, Nathan RD: Characterization of a TTX-sensitive Na^+ current in pacemaker cells isolated from rabbit sinoatrial node. *Am J Physiol.* 270:H2108-H2119, **1996**. *[4]*

Murphy E, Freundenrich CC, Levy LA, London RE, Lieberman M: Monitoring cytosolic free magnesium in cultured chicken heart cells by use of the fluorescent indicator furaptra. *Proc Natl Acad Sci USA.* 86:2981-2984, **1989a.** *[3]*

Murphy E, Steenbergen C, Levy LA, Raju B, London RE: Cytosolic free magnesium levels in ischemic rat heart. *J Biol Chem.* 264:5622-5627, **1989b.** *[3,7,10]*

Murphy E, Perlman M, London RE, Steenbergen C: Amiloride delays the ischemia-induced rise in cytosolic free calcium. *Circ Res.* 68:1250-1258, **1991.** *[10]*

Murphy BJ, Rossie S, De JK, Catterall WA: Identification of the sites of selective phosphorylation and dephosphorylation of the rat brain Na$^+$ channel α subunit by cAMP-dependent protein kinase and phosphoprotein phosphatases. *J Biol Chem.* 268:27355-27362, **1993.** *[4]*

Murphy AM, Kögler H, Georgakopoulos D, McDonough JL, Kass DA, Van Eyk JE, Marbán E: Transgenic mouse model of stunned myocardium. *Science.* 287:488-491, **2000.** *[10]*

Murray BE, Ohlendieck K: Cross-linking analysis of the ryanodine receptor and α_1-dihydropyridine receptor in rabbit skeletal muscle triads. *Biochem J.* 324:689-696, **1997.** *[8]*

Murray KT, Fahrig SA, Deal KK, Po SS, Hu NN, Snyders DJ, Tamkun MM, Bennett PB: Modulation of an inactivating human cardiac K$^+$ channel by protein kinase C. *Circ Res.* 75:999-1005, **1994.** *[4]*

Murrell-Lagnado RD, Aldrich RW: Interactions of amino terminal domains of *Shaker* K channels with a pore blocking site studied with synthetic peptides. *J Gen Physiol.* 102:949-975, **1993.** *[4]*

Murry CE, Jennings RB, Reimer KA: Preconditioning with ischemia: A delay of lethal cell injury in ischemic myocardium. *Circulation.* 74:1124-1136, **1986.** *[10]*

Musser B, Morgan ME, Leid M, Murray TF, Linden J, Vestal RE: Species comparison of adenosine and β-adrenoceptors in mammalian atrial and ventricular myocardium. *Eur J Pharmacol Mol Pharmacol.* 246:105-111, **1993.** *[10]*

Näbauer M, Kääb S: Potassium channel down-regulation in heart failure. *Cardiovasc Res.* 37:324-334, **1998.** *[4,10]*

Näbauer M, Morad M: Ca^{2+}-induced Ca^{2+} release as examined by photolysis of caged Ca^{2+} in single ventricular myocytes. *Am J Physiol.* 258:C189-C193, **1990.** *[8]*

Näbauer M, Callewart G, Cleemann L, Morad M: Regulation of calcium release is gated by calcium current, not gating charge, in cardiac myocytes. *Science.* 244:800-803, **1989.** *[3,8]*

Näbauer M, Beuckelmann DJ, Überfuhr P, Steinbeck G: Regional differences in current density and rate-dependent properties of the transient outward current in subepicardial and subendocardial myocytes of human left ventricle. *Circulation.* 93:168-177, **1996.** *[4,10]*

Nagasaki K, Fleischer S: Modulation of the calcium release channel of sarcoplasmic reticulum by adriamycin and other drugs. *Cell Calcium.* 10:63-70, **1989.** *[7]*

Nakade S, Rhee SK, Hamanaka H, Mikoshiba K: Cyclic AMP-dependent phosphorylation of an immunoaffinity-purified homotetrameric inositol 1,4,5-trisphosphate receptor (type I) increases Ca^{2+} flux in reconstituted lipid vesicles. *J Biol Chem.* 269:6735-6742, **1994.** *[7]*

Nakai J, Imagawa T, Hakamata Y, Shigekawa M, Takeshima H, Numa S: Primary structure and functional expression from cDNA of cardiac muscle ryanodine receptor/calcium release channel. *FEBS Lett.* 271:169-177, **1990.** *[7]*

Nakai J, Dirksen RT, Nguyen HT, Pessah IN, Beam KG, Allen PD: Enhanced dihydropyridine receptor channel activity in the presence of ryanodine receptor. *Nature.* 380:72-75, **1996.** *[8]*

Nakai J, Ogura T, Protasi F, Franzini-Armstrong C, Allen PD, Beam KG: Functional nonequality of the cardiac and skeletal ryanodine receptors. *Proc Natl Acad Sci USA.* 94:1019-1022, **1997.** *[8]*

Nakai J, Sekiguchi N, Rando TA, Allen PD, Beam KG: Two regions of the ryanodine receptor involved in coupling with L-type Ca^{2+} channels. *J Biol Chem.* 273:13403-13406, **1998a.** *[7,8]*

Nakai J, Tanabe T, Konno T, Adams B, Beam KG: Localization in the II-III loop of the dihydropyridine receptor of a sequence critical for excitation-contraction coupling. *J Biol Chem.* 273:24983-24986, **1998b.** *[8]*

Nakajima Y, Endo M: Release of calcium induced by "depolarisation" of the sarcoplasmic reticulum membrane. *Nature New Biol.* 246:216-218, **1973.** *[8]*

Nakamura Y, Schwartz A: The influence of hydrogen ion concentration on calcium binding and release by skeletal muscle sarcoplasmic reticulum. *J Gen Physiol.* 59:22-32, **1972.** *[8]*

Nakamura Y, Kobayashi J, Gilmore J, Mascal M, Rinehart KL Jr, Nakamura H, Ohizumi Y: Bromo-eudistomin D, a novel inducer of calcium release from fragmented sarcoplasmic reticulum that causes contractions of skinned muscle fibers. *J Biol Chem.* 261:4139-4142, **1986.** *[7]*

Nakamura H, Nakasaki Y, Matsuda N, Shigekawa M: Inhibition of sarcoplasmic reticulum Ca^{2+}-ATPase by 2,5-di(*tert*-butyl)-1,4-benzohydroquinone. *J Biochem (Tokyo).* 112:750-755, **1992.** *[7]*

Nakamura TY, Coetzee WA, de Miera EV, Artman M, Rudy B: Modulation of Kv4 channels, key components of rat ventricular transient outward K$^+$ current, by PKC. *Am J Physiol.* 273:H1775-H1786, **1997.** *[4]*

Nakanishi T, Jarmakani JM: Developmental changes in myocardial mechanical function and subcellular organelles. *Am J Physiol.* 246:H615-H625, **1984.** *[9]*

Nakanishi T, Seguchi M, Tsuchiya T, Yasukouchi S, Takao A: Effect of acidosis on intracellular pH and calcium concentration in the newborn and adult rabbit myocardium. *Circ Res.* 67:111-123, **1990.** *[10]*

Nakano A, Baines CP, Kim SO, Pelech SL, Downey JM, Cohen MV, Critz SD: Ischemic preconditioning activates MAPKAPK2 in the isolated rabbit heart: Evidence for involvement of p38 MAPK. *Circ Res.* 86:144-151, **2000.** *[10]*

Nakao M, Gadsby DC: Voltage dependence of Na translocation by the Na/K pump. *Nature.* 323:628-630, **1986.** *[4]*

Nakayama H, Taki M, Striessnig J, Glossmann H, Catterall WA, Kanaoka Y: Identification of 1,4-dihydropyridine binding regions within the α_1 subunit of skeletal muscle Ca^{2+} channels by photoaffinity labeling with diazipine. *Proc Natl Acad Sci USA.* 88:9203-9207, **1991.** *[5]*

Napolitano R, Vittone L, Mundiña C, Chiappe de Cingolani G, Mattiazzi A: Phosphorylation of phospholamban in the intact heart. A study on the physiological role of the Ca^{2+}-calmodulin- dependent protein kinase system. *J Mol Cell Cardiol.* 24:387-396, **1992.** *[7]*

Nargeot J, Nerbonne JM, Engels J, Lester HA: Time course of the increase in myocardial slow inward current after a photochemically generated concentration jump of intracellular cyclic AMP. *Proc Natl Acad Sci USA*. 80:2395-2399, **1983**. *[5]*

Nastainczyk W, Röhrkasten A, Sieber M, Rudolph C, Schächtele C, Marmè D, Hofmann F: Phosphorylation of the purified receptor for calcium channel blockers by cAMP kinase and protein kinase C. *Eur J Biochem*. 169:137-142, **1987**. *[5]*

Nawrath H: Adrenoceptor-mediated changes in excitation and contraction in isolated heart muscle preparations. *J Cardiovasc Pharmacol*. 14:S1-S10, **1989**. *[10]*

Nayler WG, Fassold E: Calcium accumulation and ATPase activity of cardiac sarcoplasmic reticulum before and after birth. *Cardiovasc Res*. 11:231-237, **1977**. *[9]*

Nayler WG, Daile P, Chipperfield D, Gan K: Effect of ryanodine on calcium in cardiac muscle. *Am J Physiol*. 219:1620-1626, **1970**. *[7]*

Neely A, Wei X, Olcese R, Birnbaumer L, Stefani E: Potentiation by the β subunit of the ratio of the ionic current to the charge movement in the cardiac calcium channel. *Science*. 262:575-578, **1993**. *[5]*

Negretti N, O'Neill SC, Eisner DA: The relative contributions of different intracellular and sarcolemmal systems to relaxation in rat ventricular myocytes. *Cardiovasc Res*. 27:1826-1830, **1993**. *[3,9]*

Nelson TE: Abnormality in calcium release from skeletal sarcoplasmic reticulum of pigs susceptible to malignant hyperthermia. *J Clin Invest*. 72:862-870, **1983**. *[7]*

Nelson MT, Cheng H, Rubart M, Santana LF, Bonev AD, Knot HJ, Lederer WJ: Relaxation of arterial smooth muscle by calcium sparks. *Science*. 270:633-637, **1995**. *[8]*

Nerbonne JM: Molecular basis of functional voltage-gated K+ channel diversity in the mammalian myocardium. *J Physiol*. 525:285-298, **2000**. *[4]*

Nerbonne JM: Molecular mechanisms controlling functional voltage-gated K+ channel diversity and expression in the mammalian heart, in Potassium Channels in Cardiovascular Biology. Rusch NJ, Archer SL (eds). In press, **2001**. *[4]*

Neubauer S, Horn M, Naumann A, Tian R, Hu K, Laser M, Friedrich J, Gaudron P, Schnackerz K, Ingwall JS, Ertl G: Impairment of energy metabolism in intact residual myocardium of rat hearts with chronic myocardial infarction. *J Clin Invest*. 95:1092-1100, **1995**. *[10]*

Neumann J, Schmitz W, von Meyerinck I, Scholz H, Döring V, Kalmar P: Increase in myocardial Gi proteins in heart failure. *Lancet*. 2:936-937, **1988**. *[10]*

Neumann J, Gupta RC, Schmitz W, Scholz H, Nairn AC, Watanabe AM: Evidence for isoproterenol-induced phosphorylation of phosphatase inhibitor-1 in the intact heart. *Circ Res*. 69:1450-1457, **1991**. *[7]*

Neumann J, Eschenhagen T, Grupp IL, Haverich A, Herzig JW, Hirt S, Kalmár P, Schmitz W, Scholz H, Stein B, Wenzlaff H, Zimmermann N: Positive inotropic effects of the calcium sensitizer CGP 48506 in failing human myocardium. *J Pharmacol Exp Ther*. 277:1579-1585, **1996**. *[10]*

Neumann J, Eschenhagen T, Jones LR, Linck B, Schmitz W, Scholz H, Zimmermann N: Increased expression of cardiac phosphatases in patients with end-stage heart failure. *J Mol Cell Cardiol*. 29:265-272, **1997**. *[10]*

Nicholls DG, Akerman KEO: Mitochondrial calcium transport. *Biochim Biophys Acta*. 683:57-88, **1982**. *[3]*

Nichols CG, Lederer WJ: The regulation of ATP-sensitive K+ channel activity in intact and permeabilized rat ventricular myocytes. *J Physiol*. 423:91-110, **1990**. *[10]*

Nichols CG, Ripoll C, Lederer WJ: ATP-sensitive potassium channel modulation of the guinea pig ventricular action potential and contraction. *Circ Res*. 68:280-287, **1991**. *[4,10]*

Nicoll DA, Longoni S, Philipson KD: Molecular cloning and functional expression of the cardiac sarcolemmal Na+-Ca2+ exchanger. *Science*. 250:562-565, **1990**. *[6]*

Nicoll DA, Quednau BD, Qui ZY, Xia YR, Lusis AJ, Philipson KD: Cloning of a third mammalian Na+-Ca 2+ exchanger, NCX3. *J Biol Chem*. 271:24914-24921, **1996**. *[6]*

Nicoll DA, Ottolia M, Lu LY, Lu YJ, Philipson KD: A new topological model of the cardiac sarcolemmal Na+-Ca2+ exchanger. *J Biol Chem*. 274:910-917, **1999**. *[6]*

Niggli E: Localized intracellular calcium signaling in muscle: Calcium sparks and calcium quarks. *Annu Rev Physiol*. 61:311-335, **1999**. *[8]*

Niggli E, Lederer WJ: Voltage-independent calcium release in heart muscle. *Science*. 250:565-568, **1990**. *[8]*

Niggli E, Lipp P: Voltage dependence of Na-Ca exchanger conformational currents. *Biophys J*. 67:1516-1524, **1994**. *[6]*

Niggli V, Adunyah ES, Penniston JT, Carafoli E: Purified (Ca2+-Mg2+)-ATPase of the erythrocyte membrane. *J Biol Chem*. 256:395-401, **1981a**. *[6]*

Niggli V, Adunyah ES, Carafoli E: Acidic phospholipids, unsaturated fatty acids, and limited proteolysis mimic the effect of calmodulin on the purified erythrocyte Ca2+-ATPase. *J Biol Chem*. 256:8588-8592, **1981b**. *[6]*

Nilius B: Calcium block of guinea-pig heart sodium channels with and without modification by the piperazinylindole DPI 201-106. *J Physiol*. 399:537-558, **1988**. *[4]*

Nilius B, Hess P, Lansman JB, Tsien RW: A novel type of cardiac calcium channel in ventricular cells. *Nature*. 316:443-446, **1985**. *[5]*

Nimer LR, Needleman DH, Hamilton SL, Krall J, Movsesian MA: Effect of ryanodine on sarcoplasmic reticulum Ca2+ accumulation in nonfailing and failing human myocardium. *Circulation*. 92:2504-2510, **1995**. *[10]*

Nixon GF, Mignery GA, Somlyo AV: Immunogold localization of inositol 1,4,5-trisphosphate receptors and characterization of ultrastructural features of the sarcoplasmic reticulum in phasic and tonic smooth muscle. *J Muscle Res Cell Motil*. 15:682-700, **1994**. *[8]*

Noble D: Mechanism of action of therapeutic levels of cardiac glycosides. *Cardiovasc Res*. 14:495-514, **1980**. *[10]*

Noble D: Ionic bases of rhythmic activity in the heart, in Cardiac Electrophysiology and Arrhythmias. Zipes DJ, Jalife J (eds). Grune and Stratton. 3-11, **1985**. *[10]*

Noceti F, Baldelli P, Wei X, Qin N, Toro L, Birnbaumer L, Stefani E: Effective gating charges per channel in voltage-dependent K+ and Ca2+ channels. *J Gen Physiol*. 108:143-155, **1996**. *[4]*

Noda M, Simizu S, Tanabe T, Takai T, Kayano T, Ikeda T, Takahashi H, Nakayama H, Kanaoka Y, Minamino N, Kangawa K, Matsuo H, Raftery M, Hirose T, Inayama S, Hayashida H, Miyata T, Numa S: Primary structure of Electrophorus electricus sodium channel deduced from cDNA sequence. *Nature*. 312:121-127, **1984**. *[4]*

Noland TA Jr, Guo XD, Raynor RL, Jideama NM, Averyhart-Fullard V, Solaro RJ, Kuo JF: Cardiac troponin I mutants - Phosphorylation by protein kinases C and A and regulation of Ca²⁺-stimulated MgATPase of reconstituted actomyosin S-1. *J Biol Chem.* 270:25445-25454, **1995**. *[10]*

Noland TA Jr, Raynor RL, Jideama NM, Guo XD, Kazanietz MG, Blumberg PM, Solaro RJ, Kuo JF: Differential regulation of cardiac actomyosin S-1 MgATPase by protein kinase C isozyme-specific phosphorylation of specific sites in cardiac troponin I and its phosphorylation site mutants. *Biochemistry.* 35:14923-14931, **1996**. *[10]*

Noma A: ATP-regulated K⁺ channels in cardiac muscle. *Nature.* 305:147-148, **1983**. *[4,10]*

Noma A: Ionic mechanisms of the cardiac pacemaker potential. *Jpn Heart J.* 37:673-682, **1996**. *[4,10]*

Nomura N, Satoh H, Terada H, Hayashi H: CAMKII is responsible for reactivation of SR Ca uptake and contractile recovery during intracellular acidosis. *J Mol Cell Cardiol.* 32:A98, **2000**. *[10]*

Nonner W, Eisenberg B: Ion permeation and glutamate residues linked by Poisson-Nernst-Planck theory in L-type calcium channels. *Biophys J.* 75:1287-1305, **1998**. *[5]*

Nordin C: Computer model of membrane current and intracellular Ca²⁺ flux in the isolated guinea pig ventricular myocyte. *Am J Physiol.* 265:H2117-H2136, **1993**. *[4]*

Nørgaard A, Bagger JP, Bjerregaard P, Baandrup U, Kjeldsen K, Thomsen PE: Relation of left ventricular function and Na,K-pump concentration in suspected idiopathic dilated cardiomyopathy. *Am J Cardiol.* 61:1312-1215, **1988**. *[10]*

Nosek TM, Williams MF, Ziegler ST, Godt RE: Inositol trisphosphate enhances calcium release in skinned cardiac and skeletal muscle. *Am J Physiol.* 250:C807-C811, **1986**. *[8]*

Nosek TM, Fender KY, Godt RE: It is diprotonated inorganic phosphate that depresses force in skinned skeletal muscle fibers. *Science.* 236:191-193, **1987**. *[10]*

Nowycky MC, Fox AP, Tsien RW: Three types of neuronal calcium channel with different calcium agonist sensitivity. *Nature.* 316:440-443, **1985**. *[5]*

Nozawa Y, Haruno A, Oda N, Yamasaki Y, Matsuura N, Yamada S, Inabe K, Kimura R, Suzuki H, Hoshino T: Angiotensin II receptor subtypes in bovine and human ventricular myocardium. *J Pharmacol Exp Ther.* 270:566-571, **1994**. *[10]*

Nuss HB, Houser SR: T-type Ca²⁺ current is expressed in hypertrophied adult feline left ventricular myocytes. *Circ Res.* 73:777-782, **1993**. *[5]*

Nuss HB, Marbán E: Whether "slip-mode conductance" occurs - Technical Comments. *Science.* 284:711a, **1999**. *[4,8]*

Nuss HB, Kääb S, Kass DA, Tomaselli GF, Marbán E: Cellular basis of ventricular arrhythmias and abnormal automaticity in heart failure. *Am J Physiol.* 277:H80-H91, **1999**. *[4]*

Obermann WM, Plessmann U, Weber K, Furst DO: Purification and biochemical characterization of myomesin, a myosin-binding and titin-binding protein, from bovine skeletal muscle. *Eur J Biochem.* 233:110-115, **1995**. *[1]*

O'Callahan CM, Ptasienski J, Hosey MM: Phosphorylation of the 165-kDa dihydro-pyridine/phenylalkylamine receptor from skeletal muscle by protein kinase C. *J Biol Chem.* 263:17342-17349, **1988**. *[5]*

Ochi R: The slow inward current and the action of manganese ions in guinea-pig's myocardium. *Pflügers Arch.* 316:81-84, **1970**. *[5]*

Odermatt A, Kurzydlowski K, MacLennan DH: The Vmax of the Ca²⁺-ATPase of cardiac sarcoplasmic reticulum (SERCA2a) is not altered by Ca²⁺/calmodulin dependent phosphorylation or by interaction with phospholamban. *J Biol Chem.* 271:14206-14213, **1996**. *[7,9]*

O'Dowd JJ, Robins DJ, Miller DJ: Detection, characterisation, and quantification of carnosine and other histidyl derivatives in cardiac and skeletal muscle. *Biochim Biophys Acta.* 967:241-249, **1988**. *[2]*

Offer G: C-protein and periodicity in the thick filaments of vertebrate skeletal muscle. *Cold Spring Harbor Symp Quant Biol.* 37:87-93, **1972**. *[1].*

Ogura T, Shuba LM, McDonald TF: L-type Ca²⁺ current in guinea pig ventricular myocytes treated with modulators of tyrosine phosphorylation *Am J Physiol.* 276:H1724-H1733, **1999**. *[5]*

Ohnishi ST: A method for studying the depolarization-induced calcium release from fragmented sarcoplasmic reticulum. *J Biochem.* 86:1147-1150, **1979**. *[7]*

Ohte N, Cheng CP, Suzuki M, Little WC: The cardiac effects of pimobendan (but not amrinone) are preserved at rest and during exercise in conscious dogs with pacing-induced heart failure. *J Pharmacol Exp Ther.* 282:23-31, **1997**. *[10]*

Ohtsuki I: Molecular arrangement of troponin T in the thin filament. *J Biochem.* 86:491-497, **1979**. *[2]*

Ojamaa K, Kenessey A, Shenoy R, Klein I: Thyroid hormone metabolism and cardiac gene expression after acute myocardial infarction in the rat. *Am J Physiol Endocrinol Metab.* 279:E1319-E1324, **2000**. *[10]*

Okazaki O, Suda N, Hongo K, Konishi M, Kurihara S: Modulation of Ca²⁺ transients and contractile properties by β adrenoceptor stimulation in ferret ventricular myocytes. *J Physiol.* 423:221-240, **1990**. *[2]*

Okubo S, Xi L, Bernardo NL, Yoshida K, Kukreja RC: Myocardial preconditioning: basic concepts and potential mechanisms. *Mol Cell Biochem.* 196:3-12, **1999**. *[10]*

Olcese R, Qin N, Schneider T, Neely A, Wei X, Stefani E, Birnbaumer L: The amino terminus of a calcium channel β subunit sets rates of channel inactivation independently of the subunit's effect on activation. *Neuron.* 13:1433-1438, **1994**. *[5]*

Olivera BM, Miljanich GP, Ramachandran J, Adams ME: Calcium channel diversity and neurotransmitter release: The ω-conotoxins and ω-agatoxins. *Annu Rev Biochem.* 63:823-867, **1994**. *[9]*

Olivetti G, Anversa P, Loud AV: Morphometric study of early postnatal development in the left and right ventricular myocardium of the rat. II. Tissue composition, capillary growth, and sarcoplasmic alterations. *Circ Res.* 46:503-512, **1980**. *[9]*

Olson EN, Molkentin JD: Prevention of cardiac hypertrophy by calcineurin inhibition - Hope or hype? *Circ Res.* 84:623-632, **1999**. *[10]*

Ondrias K, Borgatta L, Kim DH, Ehrlich BE: Biphasic effects of doxorubicin on the calcium release channel from sarcoplasmic reticulum of cardiac muscle. *Circ Res.* 67:1167-1174, **1990**. *[7]*

O'Neill SC, Donoso P, Eisner DA: The role of [Ca²⁺]i and [Ca²⁺]-sensitization in the caffeine contracture of rat myocytes: measurement of [Ca²⁺]i and [caffeine]i. *J Physiol.* 425:55-70, **1990a**. *[7,9]*

O'Neill SC, Mill JG, Eisner DA: Local activation of contraction in isolated rat ventricular myocytes. *Am J Physiol.* 258:C1165-C1168, **1990b.** *[8]*

Ono K, Trautwein W: Potentiation by cyclic GMP of β-adrenergic effect on Ca^{2+} current in guinea-pig ventricular cells. *J Physiol.* 443:387-404, **1991.** *[5]*

Ono K, Fozzard HA, Hanck DA: Mechanism of cAMP-dependent modulation of cardiac sodium channel current kinetics. *Circ Res.* 72:807-815, **1993.** *[4]*

Opie LH: The Heart Physiology: From Cell to Circulation. 3rd ed. Philadelphia, PA, Lippincott-Raven, 1-637, **1998.** *[10]*

Orchard CH: The role of the sarcoplasmic reticulum in the response of ferret and rat heart muscle to acidosis. *J Physiol.* 384:431-449, **1987.** *[10]*

Orchard CH, Kentish JC: Effects of changes of pH on the contractile function of cardiac muscle. *Am J Physiol.* 258:C967-C981, **1990.** *[8,10]*

Orchard CH, Eisner DA, Allen DG: Oscillations of intracellular Ca^{2+} in mammalian cardiac muscle. *Nature.* 304:735-738, **1983.** *[8]*

O'Rourke B: Myocardial K_{ATP} channels in preconditioning. *Circ Res.* 87:845-855, **2000.** *[10]*

O'Rourke B, Backx PH, Marbán E: Phosphorylation-independent modulation of L-type calcium channels by magnesium-nucleotide complexes. *Science.* 257:245-248, **1992.** *[5]*

O'Rourke B, Kass DA, Tomaselli GF, Kääb S, Tunin R, Marbán E: Mechanisms of altered excitation-contraction coupling in canine tachycardia-induced heart failure, I - Experimental studies. *Circ Res.* 84:562-570, **1999.** *[6,10]*

Osaka T, Joyner RW: Developmental changes in calcium currents of rabbit ventricular cells. *Circ Res.* 68:788-796, **1991.** *[9]*

Osterrieder W, Brum G, Hescheler J, Trautwein W, Flockerzi V, Hofmann F: Injection of subunits of cyclic AMP-dependent protein kinase into cardiac myocytes modulates Ca^{2+} current. *Nature.* 298:576-578, **1982.** *[5]*

Ostwald TJ, MacLennan DH: Isolation of a high affinity calcium-binding protein from sarcoplasmic reticulum. *J Biol Chem.* 249:974-979, **1974.** *[1,7]*

Otani H, Das DK: $α_1$-Adrenoreceptor-mediated phosphoinositide breakdown and inotropic response in rat left ventricular papillary muscles. *Circ Res.* 62:8-17, **1988.** *[8,10]*

Otsu K, Willard HF, Khana VJ, Zorzato F, Green NM, MacLennan DH: Molecular cloning of cDNA encoding the Ca^{2+} release channel (ryanodine receptor) of rabbit cardiac muscle sarcoplasmic reticulum. *J Biol Chem.* 265:13713-13720, **1990.** *[7]*

Ouadid H, Albat B, Nargeot J: Calcium currents in diseased human cardiac cells. *J Cardiovasc Pharmacol.* 25:282-291, **1995.** *[10]*

Overend CL, Eisner DA, O'Neill SC: The effect of tetracaine on spontaneous Ca^{2+} release and sarcoplasmic reticulum calcium content in rat ventricular myocytes. *J Physiol.* 502:471-479, **1997.** *[9]*

Overend CL, O'Neill SC, Eisner DA: The effect of tetracaine on stimulated contractions, sarcoplasmic reticulum Ca^{2+} content and membrane current in isolated rat ventricular myocytes. *J Physiol.* 507:759-769, **1998.** *[7,9]*

Overholt JL, Hobert ME, Harvey RD: On the mechanism of rectification of the isoproterenol-activated chloride current in guinea-pig ventricular myocytes. *J Gen Physiol.* 102:871-895, **1993.** *[4]*

Pacaud P, Loirand G, Gregoire G, Mironneau C, Mironneau J: Calcium-dependence of the calcium-activated chloride current in smooth muscle cells of rat portal vein. *Pflügers Arch.* 421:125-130, **1992.** *[8]*

Page E: Quantitative ultrastructural analysis in cardiac membrane physiology. *Am J Physiol.* 235:C147-C158, **1978.** *[1]*

Page E, Buecker JL: Development of dyadic junctional complexes between sarcoplasmic reticulum and plasmalemma in rabbit left ventricular myocardial cells. *Circ Res.* 48:519-522, **1981.** *[9]*

Page SG, Niedergerke R: Structures of physiological interest in the frog heart ventricle. *J Cell Sci.* 11:179-203, **1972.** *[1]*

Page E, Shibata Y: Permeable junctions between cardiac cells. *Annu Rev Physiol.* 43:431-441, **1981.** *[1]*

Page E, Surdyk-Droske M: Distribution, surface density, and membrane area of diadic junctional contacts between plasma membrane and terminal cisterns in mammalian ventricle. *Circ Res.* 45:260-267, **1979.** *[1]*

Page E, McCallister LP, Power B: Stereological measurements of cardiac ultrastructures implicated in excitation-contraction coupling. *Proc Natl Acad Sci USA.* 68:1465-1466, **1971.** *[1]*

Palade P: Drug-induced Ca^{2+} release from isolated sarcoplasmic reticulum. I. Use of pyrophosphate to study caffeine-induced Ca^{2+} release. *J Biol Chem.* 262:6135-6141, **1987a.** *[7]*

Palade P: Drug-induced Ca^{2+} release from isolated sarcoplasmic reticulum. II. Releases involving a Ca^{2+}-induced Ca^{2+} release channel. *J Biol Chem.* 262:6142-6148, **1987b.** *[7]*

Palade P: Drug-induced Ca^{2+} release from isolated sarcoplasmic reticulum. III. Block of Ca^{2+}-induced Ca^{2+} release by inorganic polyamines. *J Biol Chem.* 262:6149-6154, **1987c.** *[7,8]*

Palade P, Dettbarn C, Brunder D, Stein P, Hals G: Pharmacology of calcium release from sarcoplasmic reticulum. *J Bioenerg Biomemb.* 21:295-320, **1989.** *[7]*

Palmer S, Kentish JC: Roles of Ca^{2+} and crossbridge kinetics in determining the maximum rates of Ca^{2+} activation and relaxation in rat and guinea pig skinned trabeculae. *Circ Res.* 83:179-186, **1998.** *[2]*

Palmer RF, Posey VA: Ion effects on calcium accumulation by cardiac sarcoplasmic reticulum. *J Gen Physiol.* 50:2085-2095, **1967.** *[8]*

Pan BS, Solaro J: Calcium-binding properties of troponin C in detergent-skinned heart muscle fibers. *J Biol Chem.* 262:7839-7849, **1987.** *[2,3]*

Papazian DM, Shao XM, Seoh SA, Mock AF, Huang Y, Wainstock DH: Electrostatic interactions of S4 voltage sensor in Shaker K^+ channel. *Neuron.* 14:1293-1301, **1995.** *[4]*

Pape PC, Konishi M, Baylor SM, Somlyo AP: Excitation-contraction coupling in skeletal muscle fibers injected with the InsP3 blocker, heparin. *FEBS Lett.* 235:57-62, **1988.** *[8]*

Papp Z, Sipido KR, Callewaert G, Carmeliet E: Two components of $[Ca^{2+}]_i$-activated Cl^- current during large $[Ca^{2+}]_i$ transients in single rabbit heart Purkinje cells. *J Physiol.* 483:319-330, **1995**. *[10]*

Park YB, Herrington J, Babcock DF, Hille B: Ca²⁺ clearance mechanisms in isolated rat adrenal chromaffin cells. *J Physiol.* 492:329-346, **1996**. *[3]*

Parker I, Zang WJ, Wier WG: Ca²⁺ sparks involving multiple Ca²⁺ release sites along Z-lines in rat heart cells. *J Physiol.* 497:31-38, **1996**. *[7,8]*

Passier R, Zeng H, Frey N, Naya FJ, Nicol RL, McKinsey TA, Overbeek P, Richardson JA, Grant SR, Olson EN: CaM kinase signaling induces cardiac hypertrophy and activates the MEF2 transcription factor in vivo. *J Clin Invest.* 105:1395-1406, **2000**. *[10]*

Patlak J: Molecular kinetics of voltage-dependent Na⁺ channels. *Physiol Rev.* 71:1047-1080, **1991**. *[4]*

Peachey LD: The sarcoplasmic reticulum and transverse tubules of the frog's sartorius. *J Cell Biol.* 25:209-231, **1965**. *[1]*

Peachey LL, Porter KR: Intracellular impulse conduction in muscle cells. *Science.* 129:721-722, **1959**. *[8]*

Pegg W, Michalak M: Differentiation of sarcoplasmic reticulum during cardiac myogenesis. *Am J Physiol.* 21:H22-H31, **1987**. *[9]*

Pelzer D, Pelzer S, McDonald TF: Properties and regulation of calcium channels in muscle cells. *Rev Physiol Biochem Pharmacol.* 114:107-207, **1990**. *[5]*

Penefsky ZJ: Studies on the mechanism of inhibition of cardiac muscle contractile tension by ryanodine. *Pflügers Arch.* 347:173-184, **1974**. *[9]*

Penefsky ZJ: Perinatal development of cardiac mechanisms, in Perinatal Cardiovascular Function. Gootman N, Gootman PM (eds). *New York, NY, M. Dekker.* 109-200, **1983**. *[6,9]*

Perez PJ, Ramos-Franco J, Fill M, Mignery GA: Identification and functional reconstitution of the type 2 inositol 1,4,5-trisphosphate receptor from ventricular cardiac myocytes. *J Biol Chem.* 272:23961-23969, **1997**. *[7,8]*

Pérez NG, Hashimoto K, McCune S, Altschuld RA, Marbán E: Origin of contractile dysfunction in heart failure: Calcium cycling versus myofilaments. *Circulation.* 99:1077-1083, **1999**. *[10]*

Perez-Reyes E, Schneider T: Molecular biology of calcium channels. *Kidney Int.* 48:1111-1124, **1995**. *[5]*

Perez-Reyes E, Kim HS, Lacerda AE, Horne W, Wei X, Rampe D, Campbell KP, Brown AM, Birnbaumer L: Induction of calcium currents by the expression of the α₁- subunit of the dihydropyridine receptor from skeletal muscle. *Nature.* 340:233-236, **1989**. *[5]*

Perez-Reyes E, Castellano A, Kim HS, Bertrand P, Baggstrom E, Lacerda AE, Wei X, Birnbaumer L: Cloning and expression of a cardiac/brain β subunit of the L-type calcium channel. *J Biol Chem.* 267:1792-1797, **1992**. *[5]*

Perez-Reyes E, Yuan W, Wei X, Bers DM: Regulation of the cloned L-type cardiac calcium channel by cyclic-AMP-dependent protein kinase. *FEBS Lett.* 342:119-123, **1994**. *[5]*

Perez-Reyes E, Cribbs LL, Daud A, Lacerda AE, Barclay J, Williamson MP, Fox M, Rees M, Lee JH: Molecular characterization of a neuronal low-voltage-activated T-type calcium channel. *Nature.* 391:896-900, **1998**. *[5]*

Perozo E, Cortes DM, Cuello LG: Structural rearrangements underlying K⁺-channel activation gating. *Science.* 285:73-78, **1999**. *[4]*

Perreault CL, Bing OH, Brooks WW, Ransil BJ, Morgan JP: Differential effects of cardiac hypertrophy and failure on right versus left ventricular calcium activation. *Circ Res.* 67:707-712, **1990**. *[10]*

Peskoff A, Bers DM: Electrodiffusion of ions approaching the mouth of a conducting membrane channel. *Biophys J.* 53:863-875, **1988**. *[5]*

Pessah IN, Waterhouse AL, Casida JE: The calcium-ryanodine receptor complex of skeletal and cardiac muscle. *Biochem Biophys Res Commun.* 128:449-456, **1985**. *[7]*

Peterson BZ, Tanada TN, Catterall WA: Molecular determinants of high affinity dihydropyridine binding in L-type calcium channels. *J Biol Chem.* 271:5293-5296, **1996**. *[5]*

Peterson BZ, Johnson BD, Hockerman GH, Acheson M, Scheuer T, Catterall WA: Analysis of the dihydropyridine receptor site of L-type calcium channels by alanine-scanning mutagenesis. *J Biol Chem.* 272:18752-18758, **1997**. *[5]*

Peterson BZ, DeMaria CD, Yue DT: Calmodulin is the Ca²⁺ sensor for Ca²⁺-dependent inactivation of L-type calcium channels. *Neuron.* 22:549-558, **1999**. *[5]*

Petit-Jacques J, Hartzell HC: Effect of arachidonic acid on the L-type calcium current in frog cardiac myocytes. *J Physiol.* 493:67-81, **1996**. *[5]*

Pfitzer G, Rüegg JC, Flockerzi V, Hofmann F: cGMP-dependent protein kinase decreases calcium sensitivity of skinned cardiac fibers. *FEBS Lett.* 149:171-175, **1982**. *[10]*

Philipson KD: Interaction of charged amphiphiles with Na⁺-Ca²⁺ exchange in cardiac sarcolemmal vesicles. *J Biol Chem.* 259:12999-14002, **1984**. *[6]*

Philipson KD: Symmetry properties of the Na⁺-Ca²⁺ exchange mechanism in cardiac sarcolemmal vesicles. *Biochim Biophys Acta.* 821:367-376, **1985**. *[6]*

Philipson KD, Nicoll DA: Sodium-Calcium Exchange: A molecular perspective. *Annu Rev Physiol.* 62:111-133, **2000**. *[6]*

Philipson KD, Nishimoto AY: Na⁺-Ca²⁺ exchange is affected by membrane potential in cardiac sarcolemmal vesicles. *J Biol Chem.* 255:6880-6882, **1980**. *[6]*

Philipson KD, Nishimoto AY: Efflux of Ca²⁺ from cardiac sarcolemmal vesicles. Influence of external Ca²⁺ and Na⁺. *J Biol Chem.* 256:3698-3702, **1981**. *[6]*

Philipson KD, Nishimoto AY: Na⁺-Ca²⁺ exchange in inside-out cardiac sarcolemmal vesicles. *J Biol Chem.* 257:5111-5117, **1982a**. *[6]*

Philipson KD, Nishimoto AY: Stimulation of Na⁺-Ca²⁺ exchange in cardiac sarcolemmal vesicles by proteinase pretreatment. *Am J Physiol.* 243:C191-C195, **1982b**. *[6]*

Philipson KD, Nishimoto AY: Stimulation of Na⁺-Ca²⁺ exchange in cardiac sarcolemmal vesicles by phospholipase D. *J Biol Chem.* 259:16-19, **1984**. *[6]*

Philipson KD, Ward R: Effects of fatty acids on Na⁺-Ca²⁺ exchange and Ca²⁺ permeability of cardiac sarcolemmal vesicles. *J Biol Chem.* 260:9666-9671, **1985**. *[6]*

Philipson KD, Ward R: Ca²⁺ transport capacity of sarcolemmal Na⁺-Ca²⁺ exchange. Extrapolation of vesicle data to invivo conditions. *J Mol Cell Cardiol.* 18:943-951, **1986**. *[6]*

Philipson KD, Ward R: Modulation of Na⁺-Ca²⁺ exchange and Ca²⁺ permeability in cardiac sarcolemmal vesicles by doxylstearic acids. *Biochim Biophys Acta.* 897:152-158, **1987**. *[6]*

Philipson KD, Bers DM, Nishimoto AY: The role of phospholipids in Ca^{2+} binding of isolated cardiac sarcolemma. *J Mol Cell Cardiol.* 12:1159-1173, **1980**. *[3]*

Philipson KD, Bersohn MM, Nishimoto AY: Effects of pH on Na^+-Ca^{2+} exchange in canine cardiac sarcolemmal vesicles. *Circ Res.* 50:287-293, **1982**. *[6,10]*

Philipson KD, Langer GA, Rich TL: Charged amphiphiles regulate heart contractility and sarcolemma-Ca^{2+} interactions. *Am J Physiol.* 248:H147-H150, **1985**. *[6]*

Philipson KD, Longoni S, Ward R: Purification of the cardiac Na^+-Ca^{2+} exchange protein. *Biochim Biophys Acta.* 945:298-306, **1988**. *[6]*

Phillips RM, Narayan P, Gómez AM, Dilly K, Jones LR, Lederer WJ, Altschuld RA: Sarcoplasmic reticulum in heart failure: central player or bystander? *Cardiovasc Res.* 37:346-351, **1998**. *[10]*

Piacentino V III, Dipla K, Gaughan JP, Houser SR: Voltage-dependent Ca^{2+} release from the SR of feline ventricular myocytes is explained by Ca^{2+}-induced Ca^{2+} release. *J Physiol.* 523:533-548, **2000**. *[8]*

Piedras-Rentería ES, Chen CC, Best PM: Antisense oligonucleotides against rat brain α_{1E} DNA and its atrial homologue decrease T-type calcium current in atrial myocytes. *Proc Natl Acad Sci USA.* 94:14936-14941, **1997**. *[5]*

Pierce GN, Philipson KD, Langer GA: Passive calcium-buffering capacity of a rabbit ventricular homogenate preparation. *Am J Physiol.* 249:C248-C255, **1985**. *[3]*

Pierce GN, Rich TL, Langer GA: Trans-sarcolemmal Ca^{2+} movements associated with contraction of the rabbit right ventricular wall. *Circ Res.* 61:805-814, **1987**. *[7]*

Pieske B, Kretschmann B, Meyer M, Holubarsch C, Weirich J, Posival H, Minami K, Just H, Hasenfuss G: Alterations in intracellular calcium handling associated with the inverse force-frequency relation in human dilated cardiomyopathy. *Circulation.* 92:1169-1178, **1995**. *[9,10]*

Pieske B, Maier LS, Bers DM, Hasenfuss G: Ca^{2+} handling and sarcoplasmic reticulum Ca^{2+} content in isolated failing and nonfailing human myocardium. *Circ Res.* 85:38-46, **1999a**. *[9,10]*

Pieske B, Beyermann B, Breu V, Loffler BM, Schlotthauer K, Maier LS, Schmidt-Schweda S, Just H, Hasenfuss G. Functional effects of endothelin and regulation of endothelin receptors in isolated human nonfailing and failing myocardium. *Circulation.* 99:1802-1809, **1999b**. *[10]*

Pietrobon D, Hess P: Modal gating of L-type calcium channels. *Biophys J.* 57:24a, **1990**. *[5]*

Pinçon-Raymond M, Rieger F, Fosset M, Lazdunski M: Abnormal transverse tubule system and abnormal amount of receptors for Ca^{2+} channel inhibitors of the dihydropyridine family in skeletal muscle from mice with embryonic muscular dysgenesis. *Dev Biol.* 112:458-466, **1985**. *[8]*

Ping P, Zhang J, Zheng YT, Li RC, Dawn B, Tang XL, Takano H, Balafanova Z, Bolli R: Demonstration of selective protein kinase C-dependent activation of Src and Lck tyrosine kinases during ischemic preconditioning in conscious rabbits. *Circ Res.* 85:542-550, **1999a**. *[10]*

Ping P, Takano H, Zhang J, Tang XL, Qiu Y, Li RC, Banerjee S, Dawn B, Balafonova Z, Bolli R: Isoform-selective activation of protein kinase C by nitric oxide in the heart of conscious rabbits: a signaling mechanism for both nitric oxide- induced

and ischemia-induced preconditioning. *Circ Res.* 84:587-604, **1999b**. *[10]*

Ping P, Zhang J, Cao X, Li RC, Kong D, Tang XL, Qiu Y, Manchikalapudi S, Auchampach JA, Black RG, Bolli R: PKC-dependent activation of p44/p42 MAPKs during myocardial ischemia-reperfusion in conscious rabbits. *Am J Physiol.* 276:H1468-H1481, **1999c**. *[10]*

Ping P, Zhang J, Zheng Y, Li R, Guo Y, Bao W, Bolli R: Cardiac targeted transgenesis of active PKCε renders the heart resistant to infarction. *Circulation.* 102:II-24, **2000**. *[10]*

Piot C, Lemaire S, Albat B, Seguin J, Nargeot J, Richard S: High frequency-induced upregulation of human cardiac calcium currents. *Circulation.* 93:120-128, **1996**. *[10]*

Pires E, Perry SV, Thomas M: Myosin light chain kinase, a new enzyme from striated muscle. *FEBS Lett.* 41:292-296, **1974**. *[2]*

Pitts BJR: Stoichiometry of sodium-calcium exchange in cardiac sarcolemmal vesicles. *J Biol Chem.* 254:6232-6235, **1979**. *[6]*

Piwnica-Worms D, Jacob R, Horres CR, Lieberman M: Na^+-H^+ exchange in cultured chick heart cells. *J Gen Physiol.* 85:43-64, **1985**. *[10]*

Pizarró G, Cleemann L, Morad M: Optical measurement of voltage-dependent Ca^{2+} influx in frog heart. *Proc Natl Acad Sci USA.* 82:1864-1868, **1985**. *[7,10]*

Pizarró G, Fitts R, Uribe I, Ríos E: The voltage sensor of excitation-contraction coupling in skeletal muscle. *J Gen Physiol.* 94:405-428, **1989**. *[8]*

Pizarró G, Csernoch L, Uribe I, Ríos E: Differential effects of tetracaine on two kinetic components of calcium release in frog skeletal muscle fibres. *J Physiol.* 457:525-538, **1992**. *[8]*

Plank B, Wyskovsky W, Hohenegger M, Hellmann G, Suko J: Inhibition of calcium release from skeletal muscle sarcoplasmic reticulum by calmodulin. *Biochim Biophys Acta.* 938:79-88, **1988**. *[7]*

Poggioli J, Sulpice JC, Vassort G: Inositol phosphate production following α_1-adrenergic, muscarinic, or electrical stimulation in isolated rat heart. *FEBS Lett.* 206:292-298, **1986**. *[8,10]*

Pogwizd SM: Focal mechanisms underlying ventricular tachycardia during prolonged ischemic cardiomyopathy. *Circulation.* 90:1441-1458, **1994**. *[10]*

Pogwizd SM: Nonreentrant mechanisms underlying spontaneous ventricular arrhythmias in a model of nonischemic heart failure in rabbits. *Circulation.* 92:1034-1048, **1995**. *[10]*

Pogwizd SM, Hoyt RH, Saffitz JE, Corr PB, Cox JL, Cain ME: Reentrant and focal mechanisms underlying ventricular tachycardia in the human heart. *Circulation.* 86:1872-1887, **1992**. *[4,10]*

Pogwizd SM, Chung MK, Cain ME: Termination of ventricular tachycardia in the human heart. Insights from three-dimensional mapping of nonsustained and sustained ventricular tachycardias. *Circulation.* 95:2528-2540, **1997**. *[4]*

Pogwizd SM, McKenzie JP, Cain ME: Mechanisms underlying spontaneous and induced ventricular arrhythmias in patients with idiopathic dilated cardiomyopathy. *Circulation.* 98:2404-2414, **1998**. *[4,10]*

Pogwizd SM, Qi M, Yuan W, Samarel AM, Bers DM: Upregulation of Na^+/Ca^{2+} exchanger expression and function in an arrhythmogenic rabbit model of heart failure. *Circ Res.* 85:1009-1019, **1999**. *[3,4,9,10]*

Pogwizd SM, Schlotthauer K, Li L, Yuan W, Bers DM: Arrhythmogenesis and contractile dysfunction in heart failure: Roles of sodium-calcium exchange, inward rectifier potassium current and residual β-adrenergic responsiveness. *Circ Res*. In press. **2001**. *[10]*

Pond AL, Scheve BK, Benedict AT, Petrecca K, Van Wagoner DR, Shrier A, Nerbonne JM: Expression of distinct ERG proteins in rat, mouse, and human heart. Relation to functional I_{Kr} channels. *J Biol Chem*. 275:5997-6006, **2000**. *[4]*

Pongs O: Molecular biology of voltage-dependent potassium channels. *Physiol Rev*. 72:S69-S88, **1992**. *[4]*

Post JA, Langer GA: Sarcolemmal calcium binding sites in heart: I. Molecular origin in "gas-dissected" sarcolemma. *J Membr Biol*. 129:49-57, **1992**. *[3]*

Post JA, Langer GA, Op den Kamp JAF, Verkleij AJ: Phospholipid asymmetry in cardiac sarcolemma. Analysis of intact cells and "gas-dissected" membranes. *Biochim Biophys Acta*. 943:256-266, **1988**. *[3,5]*

Post SR, Hammond HK, Insel PA: β-adrenergic receptors and receptor signaling in heart failure. *Annu Rev Pharmacol Toxicol*. 39:343-360, **1999**. *[10]*

Potter JD, Johnson JD: Troponin, in Calcium and Function. Cheung W (ed). *New York, NY, Academic Press*. Vol II. 145-173, **1982**. *[2]*

Powers FM, Solaro RJ: Caffeine alters cardiac myofilament activity and regulation independently of Ca^{2+} binding to troponin C. *Am J Physiol*. 268:C1348-C1353, **1995**. *[2,10]*

Prabhu SD, Salama G: The heavy metal ions Ag^+ and Hg^{2+} trigger calcium release from cardiac sarcoplasmic reticulum. *Arch Biochem Biophys*. 277:47-55, **1990**. *[7,8]*

Pragnell M, de Waard M, Mori Y, Tanabe T, Snutch TP, Campbell KP: Calcium channel β-subunit binds to a conserved motif in the I-II cytoplasmic linker of the α_1-subunit. *Nature*. 368:67-70, **1994**. *[5]*

Prestle J, Janssen PML, Janssen AP, Zeitz O, Lehnart SE, Bruce L, Smith GL, Hasenfuss G: Overexpression of FK506-binding protein FKBP12.6 in cardiomyocytes reduces ryanodine receptor-mediated Ca^{2+} leak from the sarcoplasmic reticulum and increases contractility. *Circ Res*. 88:188-194, **2001**. *[10]*

Price MG: Striated muscle endosarcomeric and exosarcomeric lattices. *Adv Struct Biol*. 1:175-207, **1991**. *[1,2]*

Price MG, Sanger JW: Intermediate filaments in striated muscle. A review of structural studies in embryonic and adult skeletal and cardiac muscle, in Cell and Muscle Motility. Dowben RM, Shay JW (eds). *New York, NY, Plenum Press*. 1-40, **1983**. *[1]*

Priebe L, Beuckelmann DJ: Simulation study of cellular electric properties in heart failure. *Circ Res*. 82:1206-1223, **1998**. *[10]*

Prod'hom B, Pietrobon D, Hess P: Direct measurement of proton transfer rates to a group controlling the dihydropyridine-sensitive Ca^{2+} channel. *Nature*. 329:243-246, **1987**. *[5]*

Proenza C, Wilkens CM, Beam KG: Excitation-contraction coupling is not affected by scrambled sequence in residues 681-690 of the dihydropyridine receptor II-III loop. *J Biol Chem*. 275:29935-29937, **2000**. *[8]*

Przyklenk K, Kloner RA: Effect of superoxide dismutase plus catalase given at the time of reperfusion on myocardial blood flow. *Circ Res*. 64:86-96, **1989**. *[10]*

Pucéat M: pH_i regulatory ion transporters: An update on structure, regulation and cell function. *Cell Mol Life Sci*. 55:1216-1229, **1999**. *[10]*

Puett DW, Forman MB, Cates CU, Wilson BH, Hande KR, Friesinger GC, Virmani R: Oxypurinol limits myocardial stunning but does not reduce infarct size after reperfusion. *Circulation*. 76:678-686, **1987**. *[10]*

Puglisi JL, Bassani RA, Bassani JWM, Amin JN, Bers DM: Temperature and relative contributions of Ca transport systems in cardiac myocyte relaxation. *Am J Physiol*. 270:H1772-H1778, **1996**. *[3,10]*

Puglisi JL, Yuan W, Bassani JWM, Bers DM: Ca^{2+} influx through Ca^{2+} channels in rabbit ventricular myocytes during action potential clamp: influence of temperature. *Circ Res*. 85:e7-e16, **1999**. *[4,5,8,10]*

Puglisi JL, Pogwizd SM, Yuan W, Bers DM: Increased Na/Ca exchange and reduced I_{K1} facilitate triggered action potentials in a rabbit model of heart failure. *Biophys J*. 78:55A, 2000 *[10]*

Puri TS, Gerhardstein BL, Zhao XL, Ladner MB, Hosey MM: Differential effects of subunit interactions on protein kinase A- and C-mediated phosphorylation of L-type calcium channels. *Biochem*. 36:9605-9615, **1997**. *[5]*

Putney JW Jr: A model for receptor-regulated calcium entry. *Cell Calcium*. 7:1-12, **1986**. *[8]*

Putney JW Jr: Capacitative Calcium Entry. *Austin, TX, Landes Biomedical Publishing*. **1997**. *[7]*

Putney JW Jr, Ribeiro CMP: Signaling pathways between the plasma membrane and endoplasmic reticulum calcium stores. *Cell Mol Life Sci*. 57:1272-1286, **2000**. *[8]*

Pytkowski B: Rest-and stimulation-dependent changes in exchangeable calcium content in rabbit ventricular myocardium. *Bas Res Cardiol*. 84:22-29, **1989**. *[7]*

Pytkowski B, Lewartowski B, Prokopczuk A, Zdanowski K, Lewandowska K: Excitation- and rate-dependent shifts of Ca in guinea-pig ventricular myocardium. *Pflügers Arch*. 398:103-113, **1983**. *[7]*

Qin N, Olcese R, Zhou JM, Cabello OA, Birnbaumer L, Stefani E: Identification of a second region of the β-subunit involved in regulation of calcium channel inactivation. *Am J Physiol*. 271:C1539-C1545, **1996**. *[5]*

Qin N, Platano D, Olcese R, Costantin JL, Stefani E, Birnbaumer L: Unique regulatory properties of the type 2a Ca^{2+} channel β subunit caused by palmitoylation. *Proc Natl Acad Sci USA*. 95:4690-4695, **1998**. *[5]*

Qin N, Olcese R, Bransby M, Lin T, Birnbaumer L: Ca^{2+}-induced inhibition of the cardiac Ca^{2+} channel depends on calmodulin. *Proc Natl Acad Sci USA*. 96:2435-2438, **1999**. *[5]*

Qiu Y, Ping P, Tang XL, Manchikalapudi S, Rizvi A, Zhang J, Takano H, Wu WJ, Teschner S, Bolli R: Direct evidence that protein kinase C plays an essential role in the development of late preconditioning against myocardial stunning in conscious rabbits and that ε is the isoform involved. *J Clin Invest*. 101:2182-2198, **1998**. *[10]*

Qu Y, Himmel HM, Campbell DL, Strauss HC: Effects of extracellular ATP on I_{Ca}, $[Ca^{2+}]_i$, and contraction in isolated ferret ventricular myocytes. Am J Physiol. 264:C702-C708, **1993**. [5]

Quednau BD, Nicoll DA, Philipson KD: Tissue specificity and alternative splicing of the Na$^+$/Ca^{2+} exchanger isoforms NCX1, NCX2, and NCX3 in rat. Am J Physiol. 272:C1250-C1261, **1997**. [6]

Raffaeli S, Capogrossi MC, Spurgeon HA, Stern MD, Lakatta EG: Isoproterenol abolishes negative staircase of Ca^{2+} transient and twitch in single rat cardiac myocytes. Circulation. 76:IV-212, **1987**. [10]

Ragsdale DS, McPhee JC, Scheuer T, Catterall WA: Molecular determinants of state-dependent block of Na$^+$ channels by local anesthetics. Science. 265:1724-1728, **1994**. [4]

Rakowski RF, Gadsby DC, De Weer P: Voltage dependence of the Na/K pump. J Membr Biol. 155:105-112, **1997**. [4]

Ramirez MT, Zhao XL, Schulman H, Brown JH: The nuclear δ_B isoform of Ca^{2+}/calmodulin-dependent protein kinase II regulates atrial natriuretic factor gene expression in ventricular myocytes. J Biol Chem. 272:31203-31208, **1997**. [8,10]

Ramos-Franco J, Fill M, Mignery GA: Isoform-specific function of single inositol 1,4,5-trisphosphate receptor channels. Biophys J. 75:834-839, **1998**. [7]

Ramos-Franco J, Galvan D, Mignery GA, Fill M: Location of the permeation pathway in the recombinant type I inositol 1,4,5-trisphosphate receptor. J Gen Physiol. 114:243-250, **1999**. [7]

Rampe D, Lacerda AE: A new site for the activation of cardiac calcium channels defined by the nondihydropyridine FPL 64176. J Pharmacol Exp Ther. 259:982-987, **1991**. [5]

Rapundalo ST, Grupp I, Grupp G, Matlib MA, Solaro RJ, Schwartz A: Myocardial actions of milrinone: Characterization of its mechanism of action. Circulation. 73:134-144, **1986**. [9,10]

Rardon DP, Wasserstrom JA: Cardiotonic steroids activate cardiac sarcoplasmic reticulum calcium release channels. Circulation. 82:Suppl: III-342, **1990**. [10]

Rasmussen RP, Minobe W, Bristow MR: Calcium antagonist binding sites in failing and nonfailing human ventricular myocardium. Biochem Pharmacol. 39:691-696, **1990**. [10]

Ravens U, Wang XL, Wettwer E: α-Adrenoceptor stimulation reduces outward currents in rat ventricular myocytes. J Pharmacol Exp Ther. 250:364-370, **1989**. [10]

Ray KP, England PJ: Phosphorylation of the inhibitory subunit of troponin and its effect on the calcium dependence of cardiac myofibril adenosine triphosphatase. FEBS Lett. 70:11-16, **1976**. [2]

Rayment I, Holden HM, Whittaker M, Yohn CB, Lorenz M, Holmes KC, Milligan RA: Structure of the actin-myosin complex and its implications for muscle contraction. Science. 261:58-65, **1993a**. [2]

Rayment I, Rypniewski WR, Schmidt-Base K, Smith R, Tomchick DR, Benning MM, Winkelmann DA, Wesenberg G, Holden HM: Three-dimensional structure of myosin subfragment-1: A molecular motor. Science. 261:50-58, **1993b**. [2]

Reber WR, Weingart R: Ungulate cardiac Purkinje fibres: The influence of intracellular pH on the electrical cell-to-cell coupling. J Physiol. 328:87-104, **1982**. [1]

Reddy LG, Jones LR, Cala SE, O'Brian JJ, Tatulian SA, Stokes DL: Functional reconstitution of recombinant phospholamban

with rabbit skeletal Ca^{2+}-ATPase. J Biol Chem. 270:9390-9397, **1995**. [7]

Reddy LG, Jones LR, Pace RC, Stokes DL: Purified, reconstituted cardiac Ca^{2+}-ATPase is regulated by phospholamban but not by direct phosphorylation with Ca^{2+}/calmodulin-dependent protein kinase. J Biol Chem. 271:14964-14970, **1996**. [7,9]

Reed KC, Bygrave FL: A kinetic study of mitochondrial calcium transport. Eur J Biochem. 55:497-503, **1975**. [3]

Reeves JP: Na$^+$/Ca^{2+} exchange and cellular Ca^{2+} homeostasis. J Bioenerg Biomembr . 30:151-160, **1998**. [6]

Reeves JP, Hale CC: The stoichiometry of the cardiac sodium-calcium exchange system. J Biol Chem. 259:7733-7739, **1984**. [6]

Reeves JP, Philipson KD: Sodium-calcium exchange activity in plasma membrane vesicles, in Sodium Calcium Exchange. Allen TJA, Noble D, Reuter H (eds). Oxford, UK, Oxford University Press. 27-53, **1989**. [6]

Reeves JP, Poronnik P: Modulation of Na$^+$-Ca^{2+} exchange in sarcolemmal vesicles by intravesicular Ca^{2+}. Am J Physiol. 252:C17-C23, **1987**. [6]

Reeves JP, Sutko JL: Sodium-calcium exchange in cardiac membrane vesicles. Proc Natl Acad Sci USA. 76:590-594, **1979**. [6]

Reeves JP, Sutko JL: Sodium-calcium exchange activity generates a current in cardiac membrane vesicles. Science. 208:1461-1464, **1980**. [6]

Reeves JP, Bailey CA, Hale CC: Redox modification of sodium-calcium exchange activity in cardiac sarcolemmal vesicles. J Biol Chem. 261:4948-4955, **1986**. [6,10]

Rega AF, Garrahan PJ: The Ca^{2+}-Pump of Plasma Membranes. Boca Raton, FL, CRC Press, Inc. 1-173, **1986**. [6]

Regitz-Zagrosek V, Friedel N, Heymann A, Bauer P, Neuss M, Rolfs A, Steffen C, Hildebrandt A, Hetzer R, Fleck E: Regulation, chamber localization, and subtype distribution of angiotensin II receptors in human hearts. Circulation. 91:1461-1471, **1995**. [10]

Reiländer H, Achilles A, Friedel U, Maul G, Lottspeich F, Cook NJ: Primary structure and functional expression of the Na/Ca,K-exchanger from bovine rod photoreceptors. EMBO J. 11:1689-1695, **1992**. [6]

Reimer KA, Jennings RB: Myocardial ischemia, hypoxia, and infarction, in The Heart and Cardiovascular System. Fozzard HA et al. (eds). 2nd ed. New York, NY, Raven Press. 1875-1973, **1992**. [3,10]

Reinecke H, Studer R, Vetter R, Holtz J, Drexler H: Cardiac Na/Ca exchange activity in patients with end-stage heart failure. Cardiovasc Res. 31:48-54, **1996**. [10]

Reiter M, Vierling W, Seibel K: Excitation-contraction coupling in rested-state contractions of guinea-pig ventricular myocardium. Arch Pharmacol. 325:159-169, **1984**. [9]

Repke K: Über den biochemischen Wirkungsmodus von Digitalis. Klin Wochenschr. 42:157-165, **1964**. [6,10]

Rettig J, Heinemann SH, Wunder F, Lorra C, Parcej DN, Dolly JO, Pongs O: Inactivation properties of voltage-gated K$^+$ channels altered by presence of beta-subunit. Nature. 369:289-294, **1994**. [4]

Reuben JP, Brandt PW, Berman M, Grundfest H: Regulation of tension in the skinned crayfish muscle fiber. J Gen Physiol. 57:385-407, **1971**. [2]

Reuter H: The dependence of the slow inward current on external calcium concentration in Purkinje fibres. *J Physiol.* 192:479-492, **1967**. *[5]*

Reuter H, Seitz N: The dependence of calcium efflux from cardiac muscle on temperature and external ion composition. *J Physiol.* 195:45-70, **1968**. *[6,10]*

Reuter H, Stevens CF, Tsien RW, Yellen G: Properties of single calcium channels in cultured cardiac cells. *Nature.* 297:501-504, **1982**. *[5]*

Reuveny E, Slesinger PA, Inglese J, Morales JM, Iñiguez-Lluhi JA, Lefkowitz RJ, Bourne HR, Jan YN, Jan LY: Activation of the cloned muscarinic potassium channel by G protein beta gamma subunits. *Nature.* 370:143-146, **1994**. *[4]*

Revel JP, Karnovsky MJ: Hexagonal array of subunits in intercellular junctions of the mouse heart and liver. *J Cell Biol.* 33:C7-C12, **1967**. *[1]*

Rich TL, Langer GA, Klassen MG: Two components of coupling calcium in single ventricular cell of rabbits and rats. *Am J Physiol.* 254:H937-H946, **1988**. *[3,8]*

Richard S, Leclercq F, Lemaire S, Piot C, Nargeot J: Ca²⁺ currents in compensated hypertrophy and heart failure. *Cardiovasc Res.* 37:300-311, **1998**. *[10]*

Ringer S: A further contribution regarding the influence of the different constituents of the blood on the contraction of the heart. *J Physiol.* 4:29-42, **1883**. *[5,8]*

Ríos E, Brum G: Involvement of dihydropyridine receptors in excitation- contraction coupling in skeletal muscle. *Nature.* 325:717-720, **1987**. *[8]*

Ríos E, Pizarró G: Voltage sensors and calcium channels of excitation-contraction coupling. *News Physiol Sci.* 3:223-227, **1988**. *[8]*

Ríos E, Pizarró G: Voltage sensor of excitation-contraction coupling in skeletal muscle. *Physiol Rev.* 71:849-908, **1991**. *[8]*

Ríos E, Pizarró G, Stefani E: Charge movement and the nature of signal transduction in skeletal muscle excitation-contraction coupling. *Annu Rev Physiol.* 54:109-133, **1992**. *[8]*

Rizzuto R, Simpson AW, Brini M, Pozzan T: Rapid changes of mitochondrial Ca²⁺ revealed by specifically targeted recombinant aequorin. *Nature.* 358:325-327, **1992**. *[3]*

Rizzuto R, Brini M, Murgia M, Pozzan T: Microdomains with high Ca²⁺ close to IP₃-sensitive channels that are sensed by neighboring mitochondria. *Science.* 262:744-747, **1993**. *[3]*

Rizzuto R, Pinton P, Carrington W, Fay FS, Fogarty KE, Lifshitz LM, Tuft RA, Pozzan T: Close contacts with the endoplasmic reticulum as determinants of mitochondrial Ca²⁺ responses. *Science.* 280:1763-1766, **1998**. *[3]*

Robertson SP, Johnson JD, Potter JD: The time-course of Ca²⁺ exchange with calmodulin, troponin, parvalbumin, and myosin in response to transient increases in Ca²⁺. *Biophys J.* 34:559-569, **1981**. *[3]*

Roden DM, George AL Jr: Structure and function of cardiac sodium and potassium channels. *Am J Physiol.* 273:H511-H525, **1997**. *[4]*

Roeper J, Lorra C, Pongs O: Frequency-dependent inactivation of mammalian A-type K⁺ channel KV1.4 regulated by Ca²⁺/calmodulin-dependent protein kinase. *J Neurosci.* 17:3379-3391, **1997**. *[4]*

Rogart RB, Cribbs LL, Muglia LK, Kephart DD, Kaiser MW: Molecular cloning of a putative tetrodotoxin-resistant rat heart Na⁺ channel isoform. *Proc Natl Acad Sci USA.* 86:8170-8174, **1989**. *[4]*

Rogers TB, Gaa ST, Massey C, Dosemeci A: Protein kinase C inhibits Ca²⁺ accumulation in cardiac sarcoplasmic reticulum. *J Biol Chem.* 265:4302-4308, **1990**. *[7]*

Rohde S, Sabri A, Kamasamudran R, Steinberg SF: The α₁-adrenoceptor subtype- and protein kinase C isoform-dependence of norepinephrine's actions in cardiomyocytes. *J Mol Cell Cardiol.* 32:1193-1209, **2000**. *[10]*

Rohrer D, Desai KH, Jasper JR, Stevens ME, Regula DP, Barsh GS, Bernstein D, Kobilka BK: Targeted disruption of the mouse β₁-adrenergic receptor gene: Developmental and cardiovascular effects. *Proc Natl Acad Sci USA.* 93:7375-7380, **1996**. *[10]*

Rolett EL: Adrenergic mechanisms in mammalian myocardium, in The Mammalian Myocardium. Langer GA, Brady AJ (eds). *New York, NY, John Wiley & Sons.* 219-250, **1974**. *[10]*

Roos KP: Mechanics and force production, in The Myocardium. Langer GA (ed). 2ⁿᵈ ed. *San Diego, CA, Academic Press.* 235-323, **1997**. *[2]*

Rosen MR, Gelband H, Merker C, Hoffman BF: Mechanisms of digitalis toxicity. Effects of ouabain on phase four of canine Purkinje fiber transmembrane potentials. *Circulation.* 47:681-689, **1973a**. *[4,10]*

Rosen MR, Gelband H, Hoffman BF: Correlation between effects of ouabain on the canine electrocardiogram and transmembrane potentials of isolated Purkinje fibers. *Circulation.* 47:65-72, **1973b**. *[10]*

Rosenberg RL, Hess P, Reeves JP, Smilowitz H, Tsien RW: Calcium channels in planar lipid bilayers: insights into mechanisms of ion permeation and gating. *Science.* 231:1564-1566, **1986**. *[5]*

Rothermel BA, McKinsey TA, Vega RB, Nicol RL, Mammen P, Yang J, Antos CL, Shelton JM, Bassel-Duby R, Olson EN, Williams RS: Myocyte-enriched calcineurin-interacting protein, MCIP1, inhibits cardiac hypertrophy in vivo. *Proc Natl Acad Sci USA .* 98:3328-3333, **2001**. *[10]*

Rougier O, Gargouil YM, Coraboeuf E: Existence and role of a slow inward current during the frog atrial action potential. *Pflügers Arch.* 308:91-110, **1969**. *[5]*

Rousseau E, Meissner G: Single cardiac sarcoplasmic reticulum Ca²⁺-release channel: Activation by caffeine. *Am J Physiol.* 256:H328-H333, **1989**. *[7]*

Rousseau E, Pinkos J: pH modulates conducting and gating behaviour of single calcium release channels. *Pflügers Arch.* 415:645-647, **1990**. *[7,10]*

Rousseau E, Smith JS, Henderson JS, Meissner G: Single channel and ⁴⁵Ca²⁺ flux measurements of the cardiac sarcoplasmic reticulum calcium channel. *Biophys J.* 50:1009-1014, **1986**. *[7]*

Rousseau E, Smith JS, Meissner G: Ryanodine modifies conductance and gating behavior of single Ca²⁺ release channel. *Am J Physiol.* 253:C364-C368, **1987**. *[7]*

Rousseau E, Ladine J, Liu QY, Meissner G: Activation of the Ca²⁺ release channel of skeletal muscle sarcoplasmic reticulum by caffeine and related compounds. *Arch Biochem Biophys.* 267:75-86, **1988**. *[7,8]*

Rousseau E, Michaud C, Lefebvre D, Proteau S, Decrouy A: Reconstitution of ionic channels from inner and outer membranes of mammalian cardiac nuclei. *Biophys J.* 70:703-714, **1996**. *[8]*

Rousseau MF, Massart PE, van Eyll C, Etienne J, Ahn S, Schaefer HG, Mueck W, Bornemann M, Pouleur H: Dose-related hemodynamic and electrocardiographic effects of the calcium promoter BAY y 5959 in the presence or absence of congestive heart failure. *J Am Coll Cardiol*. 30:1751-1757, **1997**. *[10]*

Rowe GT, Eaton LR, Hess ML: Neutrophil-derived, oxygen free radical-mediated cardiovascular dysfunction. *J Mol Cell Cardiol*. 16:1075-1079, **1984**. *[10]*

Rüegg JC: Effects of new inotropic agents on Ca^{2+} sensitivity of contractile proteins. *Circulation*. 73:III-73, **1986**. *[2]*

Rüegg JC, Brewer S, Zeugner C, Trayer IP: Peptides from the myosin heavy chain are calcium sensitizers of skinned skeletal muscle fibres. *J Muscle Res Cell Motil*. 10:152, **1989**. *[10]*

Ruth P, Röhrkasten A, Biel M, Bosse E, Regulla S, Meyer HE, Flockerzi V, Hofmann F: Primary structure of the β subunit of the DHP-sensitive calcium channel from skeletal muscle. *Science*. 245:1115-1118, **1989**. *[5]*

Rybin VO, Xu X, Steinberg SF: Activated protein kinase C isoforms target to cardiomyocyte caveolae: stimulation of local protein phosphorylation. *Circ Res*. 84:980-988, **1999**. *[1]*

Südhof TC, Newton CL, Archer BT III, Ushkaryov YA, Mignery GA: Structure of a novel InsP3 receptor. *EMBO J*. 10:3199-3206, **1991**. *[7]*

Sadoshima J, Izumo S: Mechanical stretch rapidly activates multiple signal transduction pathways in cardiac myocytes: Potential involvement of an autocrine/paracrine mechanism. *EMBO J*. 12:1681-1692, **1993**. *[10]*

Sadoshima J, Izumo S: The cellular and molecular response of cardiac myocytes to mechanical stress. *Annu Rev Physiol*. 59:551-571, **1997**. *[10]*

Sadoshima J, Takahashi T, Jahn L, Izumo S: Roles of mechano-sensitive ion channels, cytoskeleton, and contractile activity in stretch-induced immediate-early gene expression and hypertrophy of cardiac myocytes. *Proc Natl Acad Sci USA*. 89:9905-9909, **1992**. *[10]*

Sadoshima J, Xu Y, Slayter HS, Izumo S: Autocrine release of angiotensin II mediates stretch-induced hypertrophy of cardiac myocytes in vitro. *Cell*. 75:977-984, **1993**. *[10]*

Sagara Y, Inesi G: Inhibition of the sarcoplasmic reticulum Ca^{2+} transport ATP-ase by thapsigargin at subnanomolar concentrations. *J Biol Chem*. 266:13503-13506, **1991**. *[3,7]*

Saida K: Intracellular Ca release in skinned smooth muscle. *J Gen Physiol*. 80:191-202, **1982**. *[8]*

Saida K, van Breemen C: GTP requirement for inositol-1,4,5-trisphosphate-induced Ca^{2+} release from sarcoplasmic reticulum in smooth muscle. *Biochem Biophys Res Commun*. 144:1313-1316, **1987**. *[8]*

Saiki Y, el-Hayek R, Ikemoto N: Involvement of the Glu^{724}-Pro^{760} region of the dihydropyridine receptor II-III loop in skeletal muscle-type excitation-contraction coupling. *J Biol Chem*. 274:7825-7832, **1999**. *[8]*

Saint DA, Ju YK, Gage PW: A persistent sodium current in rat ventricular myocytes. *J Physiol*. 453:219-231, **1992**. *[4,10]*

Sainte Beuve C, Allen PD, Dambrin G, Rannou F, Marty I, Trouve P, Bors V, Pavie A, Gandgjbakch I, Charlemagne D: Cardiac calcium release channel (ryanodine receptor) in control and cardiomyopathic human hearts: mRNA and protein contents are differentially regulated. *J Mol Cell Cardiol*. 29:1237-1246, **1997**. *[10]*

Saito A, Seiler S, Chu A, Fleischer S: Preparation and morphology of SR terminal cisternae from rabbit skeletal muscle. *J Cell Biol*. 99:875-885, **1984**. *[7]*

Saito A, Inui M, Radermacher M, Frank J, Fleischer S: Ultrastructure of the calcium release channel of sarcoplasmic reticulum. *J Cell Biol*. 107:211-219, **1988**. *[1,7]*

Sakai T: The effect of temperature and caffeine on the action of the contractile mechanism in striated muscle fibres. *Jikeikea Med J*. 12:88-102, **1965**. *[7,8]*

Salama G, Abramson J: Silver ions trigger Ca^{2+} release by acting at the apparent physiological release site in sarcoplasmic reticulum. *J Biol Chem*. 259:13363-13360, **1984**. *[7,8]*

Salata JJ, Jurkiewicz NK, Jow B, Folander K, Guinosso PJJ, Raynor B, Swanson R, Fermini B: I_K of rabbit ventricle is composed of two currents: Evidence for I_{Ks}. *Am J Physiol*. 271:H2477-H2489, **1996**. *[4]*

Sallés J, Gascon S, Ivorra D, Badia A: In vivo recovery of α_1-adrenoceptors in rat myocardial tissue after alkylation with phenoxybenzamine. *Eur J Pharmacol*. 266:35-42, **1994**. *[10]*

Samsó M, Wagenknecht T: Contributions of electron microscopy and single-particle techniques to the determination of the ryanodine receptor three-dimensional structure. *J Struct Biol*. 121:172-180, **1998**. *[7]*

Samsó M, Trujillo R, Gurrola GB, Valdivia HH, Wagenknecht T: Three-dimensional location of the imperatoxin A binding site on the ryanodine receptor. *J Cell Biol*. 146:493-499, **1999**. *[1,7]*

Sanchez JA, Stefani E: Inward calcium current in twitch muscle fibres of the frog. *J Physiol*. 283:197-209, **1978**. *[8]*

Sanchez JA, Stefani E: Kinetic properties of calcium channels of twitch muscle fibres of the frog. *J Physiol*. 337:1-17, **1983**. *[8]*

Sanchez-Chapula J, Elizalde A, Navarro-Polanco R, Barajas H: Differences in outward currents between neonatal and adult rabbit ventricular cells. *Am J Physiol*. 266:H1184-H1194, **1994**. *[4]*

Sanguinetti MC, Jurkiewicz NK: Two components of cardiac delayed rectifier K^+ current. Differential sensitivity to block by class III antiarrhythmic agents. *J Gen Physiol*. 96:195-215, **1990**. *[4]*

Sanguinetti MC, Jurkiewicz NK: Delayed rectifier outward K^+ current is composed of two currents in guinea pig atrial cells. *Am J Physiol*. 260:H393-H399, **1991**. *[4]*

Sanguinetti MC, Kass RS: Voltage-dependent block of calcium channel current in the calf cardiac Purkinje fiber by dihydropyridine calcium channel antagonists. *Circ Res*. 55:336-348, **1984**. *[5]*

Sanguinetti MC, Jiang C, Curran ME, Keating MT: A mechanistic link between an inherited and an acquired cardiac arrhythmia: HERG encodes the I_{Kr} potassium channel. *Cell*. 81:299-307, **1995**. *[4]*

Sanguinetti MC, Curran ME, Spector PS, Keating MT: Spectrum of HERG K^+-channel dysfunction in an inherited cardiac arrhythmia. *Proc Natl Acad Sci USA*. 93:2208-2212, **1996a**. *[4]*

Sanguinetti MC, Curran ME, Zou A, Shen J, Spector PS, Atkinson DL, Keating MT: Coassembly of KvLQT1 and minK (IsK) proteins to form cardiac I_{Ks} potassium channel. *Nature*. 384:80-83, **1996b**. *[4]*

Santana LF, Cheng H, Gómez AM, Cannell MB, Lederer WJ: Relation between the sarcolemmal Ca²⁺ current and Ca²⁺ sparks and local control theories for cardiac excitation-contraction coupling. *Circ Res.* 78:166-171, **1996**. *[8]*

Santana LF, Kranias EG, Lederer WJ: Calcium sparks and excitation-contraction coupling in phospholamban-deficient mouse ventricular myocytes. *J Physiol.* 503:21-29, **1997**. *[10]*

Santana LF, Gómez AM, Lederer WJ: Ca²⁺ flux through promiscuous cardiac Na⁺ channels: Slip-mode conductance. *Science.* 279:1027-1033, **1998**. *[4,8,10]*

Santoro B, Liu DT, Yao H, Bartsch D, Kandel ER, Siegelbaum SA, Tibbs GR: Identification of a gene encoding a hyperpolarization-activated pacemaker channel of brain. *Cell.* 93:717-729, **1998**. *[4]*

Sarkadi B, Shubert A, Gardos G: Effect of Ca-EGTA buffers on active calcium transport in inside-out red cell membrane vesicles. *Experientia.* 35:1045-1047, **1979**. *[6]*

Sasaguri T, Hirata M, Kuriyama H: Dependence on Ca²⁺ of the activities of phosphatidylinositol 4,5-bisphosphate phosphodiesterase and inositol 1,4,5-trisphosphate phosphatase in smooth muscles of the porcine coronary artery. *Biochem J.* 231:497-503, **1985**. *[8]*

Sasaki T, Inui M, Kimura Y, Kuzuya T, Tada M: Molecular mechanism of regulation of Ca²⁺ pump ATPase by phospholamban in cardiac sarcoplasmic reticulum. Effects of synthetic phospholamban peptides on Ca²⁺ pump ATPase. *J Biol Chem.* 267:1674-1679, **1992**. *[7]*

Sasaki N, Sato T, Ohler A, O'Rourke B, Marbán E: Activation of mitochondrial ATP-dependent potassium channels by nitric oxide. *Circulation.* 101:439-445, **2000**. *[10]*

Satin J, Kyle JW, Chen M, Bell P, Cribbs LL, Fozzard HA, Rogart RB: A mutant of TTX-resistant cardiac sodium channels with TTX-sensitive properties. *Science.* 256:1202-1205, **1992a**. *[4]*

Satin J, Kyle JW, Chen M, Rogart RB, Fozzard HA: The cloned cardiac Na channel α-subunit expressed in Xenopus oocytes show gating and blocking properties of native channels. *J Membr Biol.* 130:11-22, **1992b**. *[4]*

Sato R, Noma A, Kurachi Y, Irisawa H: Effects of intracellular acidification on membrane currents in ventricular cells of the guinea-pig. *Circ Res.* 57:553-561, **1985**. *[10]*

Sato N, Uechi M, Asai K, Patrick T, Kudej RK, Vatner SF: Effects of a novel inotropic agent, BAY y 5959, in conscious dogs: Comparison with dobutamine and milrinone. *Am J Physiol.* 272:H753-H759, **1997**. *[10]*

Sato T, O'Rourke B, Marbán E: Modulation of mitochondrial ATP-dependent K⁺ channels by protein kinase C. *Circ Res.* 83:110-114, **1998a**. *[4,10]*

Sato Y, Ferguson DG, Sako H, Dorn GW II, Kadambi VJ, Yatani A, Hoit BD, Walsh RA, Kranias EG: Cardiac-specific overexpression of mouse cardiac calsequestrin is associated with depressed cardiovascular function and hypertrophy in transgenic mice. *J Biol Chem.* 273:28470-28477, **1998b**. *[7]*

Sato T, Sasaki N, Seharaseyon J, O'Rourke B, Marbán E: Selective pharmacological agents implicate mitochondrial but not sarcolemmal K_ATP channels in ischemic cardioprotection. *Circulation.* 101:2418-2423, **2000a**. *[10]*

Sato T, Sasaki N, O'Rourke B, Marbán E: Adenosine primes the opening of mitochondrial ATP-sensitive potassium channels: A key step in ischemic preconditioning? *Circulation.* 102:800-805, **2000b**. *[10]*

Satoh H, Delbridge LM, Blatter LA, Bers DM: Surface:volume relationship in cardiac myocytes studied with confocal microscopy and membrane capacitance measurements: species-dependence and developmental effects. *Biophys J.* 70:1494-1504, **1996**. *[1,3]*

Satoh H, Blatter LA, Bers DM: Effects of [Ca²⁺]ᵢ, SR Ca²⁺ load, and rest on Ca²⁺ spark frequency in ventricular myocytes. *Am J Physiol.* 272:H657-H668, **1997**. *[4,7,8,9,10]*

Satoh H, Katoh H, Velez P, Fill M, Bers DM: Bay K 8644 increases resting Ca²⁺ spark frequency in ferret ventricular myocytes independent of Ca influx: contrast with caffeine and ryanodine effects. *Circ Res.* 83:1192-1204, **1998**. *[8]*

Satoh H, Ginsburg KS, Qing K, Terada H, Hayashi H, Bers DM. KB-R7943 block of Ca²⁺ influx via Na⁺/Ca²⁺ exchange does not alter twitches or glycoside inotropy, but prevents Ca²⁺ overload in rat ventricular myocytes. *Circulation.* 101:1441-1446, **2000**. *[6,10]*

Scamps F, Rybin V, Puceat M, Tkachuk V, Vassort G: A Gs protein couples P₂-purinergic stimulation to cardiac Ca channels without cyclic AMP production. *J Gen Physiol.* 100:675-701, **1992**. *[5]*

Scarpa A, Graziotti P: Mechanisms for intracellular calcium regulation in heart. *J Gen Physiol.* 62:756-772, **1973**. *[3]*

Schatzmann HJ: ATP dependent Ca²⁺ extrusion from human red cells. *Experientia.* 22:364-368, **1966**. *[6]*

Schatzmann HJ: Dependence on calcium concentrations and stoichiometry of the calcium pump in human red cells. *J Physiol.* 235:551-569, **1973**. *[6]*

Schatzmann HJ: The plasma membrane calcium pump of erythrocytes and other animal cells, in Membrane Transport of Calcium. Carafoli E (ed). *London, UK, Academic Press.* 41-108, **1982**. *[6]*

Schatzmann HJ: The calcium pump of the surface membrane and of the sarcoplasmic reticulum. *Annu Rev Physiol.* 51:473-485, **1989**. *[6,7]*

Scherer NM, Ferguson JE: Inositol 1,4,5-triphosphate is not effective in releasing calcium from skeletal sarcoplasmic reticulum microsomes. *Biochem Biophys Res Commun.* 128:1064-1070, **1985**. *[8]*

Schiebler T, Wolff HH: Electron microscopic studies on the rat myocardium during its development. *Z Zellforsch Mikrosk Anat*. 69:22-40, **1962**. *[9]*

Schiefer A, Meissner G, Isenberg G: Ca²⁺ activation and Ca²⁺ inactivation of canine reconstituted cardiac sarcoplasmic reticulum Ca²⁺-release channels. *J Physiol.* 489:337-348, **1995**. *[7]*

Schilling WP, Drewe JA: Voltage-sensitive nitrendipine binding in an isolated cardiac sarcolemma preparation. *J Biol Chem.* 261:2750-2758, **1986**. *[5]*

Schillinger W, Meyer M, Kuwajima G, Mikoshiba K, Just H, Hasenfuss G: Unaltered ryanodine receptor protein levels in ischemic cardiomyopathy. *Mol Cell Biochem.* 160-161:297-302, **1996**. *[10]*

Schillinger W, Janssen PML, Emami S, Henderson SA, Ross RS, Teucher N, Zeitz O, Philipson KD, Prestle J, Hasenfuss G: Impaired contractile performance of cultured rabbit ventricular myocytes after adenoviral gene transfer of Na⁺-Ca²⁺ exchanger. *Circ Res.* 87:581-587, **2000**. *[10]*

Schlaepfer DD, Hauck CR, Sieg DJ: Signaling through focal adhesion kinase. *Prog Biophys Mol Biol.* 71:435-478, **1999**. *[1]*

Schlotthauer K, Bers DM: Sarcoplasmic reticulum Ca²⁺ release causes myocyte depolarization: Underlying mechanism and threshold for triggered action potentials. *Circ Res.* 87:774-780, **2000**. *[4,10]*

Schlotthauer K, Schattmann J, Bers DM, Maier LS, Schütt U, Minami K, Just H, Hasenfuss G, Pieske B: Frequency-dependent changes in contribution of SR Ca²⁺ to Ca²⁺ transients in failing human myocardium assessed with ryanodine. *J Mol Cell Cardiol.* 30:1285-1294, **1998**. *[9]*

Schlotthauer K, Pogwizd SM, Bers DM: Myocytes from failing hearts need less sarcoplasmic reticulum Ca release to trigger an action potential (AP). *Circulation.* 102:II-4-II-5, **2000**. *[4,10]*

Schmidt TA, Allen PD, Colucci WS, Marsh JD, Kjeldsen K: No adaptation to digitalization as evaluated by digitalis receptor (Na,K-ATPase) quantification in explanted hearts from donors without heart disease and from digitalized recipients with end-stage heart failure. *Am J Cardiol.* 71:110-114, **1993**. *[10]*

Schmidt U, Hajjar RJ, Helm PA, Kim CS, Doye AA, Gwathmey JK: Contribution of abnormal sarcoplasmic reticulum ATPase activity to systolic and diastolic dysfunction in human heart failure. *J Mol Cell Cardiol.* 30:1929-1937, **1998**. *[10]*

Schmitz W, von der Leyen H, Meyer W, Neumann J, Scholz H: Phosphodiesterase inhibition and positive inotropic effects. *J Cardiovasc Pharmacol.* 14:S11-S14, **1989**. *[10]*

Schneider MF, Chandler WK: Voltage dependence charge movement in skeletal muscle: A possible step in excitation-contraction coupling. *Nature.* 242:244-246, **1973**. *[8]*

Schneider MF, Simon BJ: Inactivation of calcium release from the sarcoplasmic reticulum in frog skeletal muscle. *J Physiol* . 405:727-745, **1988**. *[8]*

Schnetkamp PPM, Basu DK, Szerencsei RT: Na⁺-Ca²⁺ exchange in bovine rod outer segments requires and transports K⁺. *Am J Physiol.* 257:C153-C157, **1989**. *[6]*

Scholtysik G, Salzmann R, Berthold R, Quast JW, Markstein R: DPI 201-106, a novel cardiotonic agent. Combination of cAMP- independent positive inotropic, negative chronotropic, action potential prolonging and coronary dilatory properties. *Naunyn Schmiedebergs Arch Pharmacol.* 329:316-325, **1985**. *[2,10]*

Scholtysik G, Salzmann R, Gerber W: Interaction of DPI 201-106 with cardiac glycosides. *J Cardiovasc Pharmacol.* 13:342-347, **1989**. *[10]*

Scholz J, Schaeffer B, Schmitz W, Scholz H, Steinfath M, Lohse M, Schwabe U, Puurunen J: α₁-Adrenoreceptor-mediated positive inotropic effect and inositol trisphosphate increase in mammalian heart. *J Pharmacol Exp Ther.* 245:337-345, **1988**. *[8,10]*

Scholz W, Albus U, Lang HJ, Linz W, Martorana PA, Englert HC, Schölkens BA: Hoe 694, a new Na⁺/H⁺ exchange inhibitor and its effects in cardiac ischaemia. *Br J Pharmacol.* 109:562-568, **1993**. *[10]*

Scholz W, Albus U, Counillon L, Gogelein H, Lang HJ, Linz W, Weichert A, Scholkens BA: Protective effects of HOE642, a selective sodium-hydrogen exchange subtype 1 inhibitor, on cardiac ischaemia and reperfusion. *Cardiovasc Res.* 29:260-268, **1995**. *[10]*

Schoppa NE, McCormack K, Tanouye MA, Sigworth FJ: The size of gating charge in wild-type and mutant *Shaker* potassium channels. *Science.* 255:1712-1715, **1992**. *[4]*

Schouten JA: Interval dependence of force and twitch duration in rat heart explained by Ca²⁺ pump inactivation in sarcoplasmic reticulum. *J Physiol.* 431:427-444, **1990**. *[9]*

Schouten VJ, ter Keurs HEDJ: The slow repolarization phase of the action potential in rat heart. *J Physiol.* 360:13-25, **1985**. *[9]*

Schouten VJ, ter Keurs HEDJ: The force-frequency relationship in rat myocardium. The influence of muscle dimensions. *Pflügers Arch.* 407:14-17, **1986**. *[9]*

Schouten VJA, van Deen JK, de Tombe PP, Verveen AA: Force-interval relationship in heart muscle of mammals. A calcium compartment model. *Biophys J.* 51:13-26, **1987**. *[9]*

Schramm M, Thomas G, Towart R, Franckowiak G: Novel dihydropyridines with positive inotropic action through activation of Ca channel. *Nature.* 303:535-537, **1983**. *[10]*

Schramm M, Klieber HG, Daut J: The energy expenditure of actomyosin-ATPase, Ca²⁺-ATPase and Na⁺,K⁺-ATPase in guinea-pig cardiac ventricular muscle. *J Physiol.* 481:647-662, **1994**. *[7]*

Schreiber SL, Crabtree GR: The mechanism of action of cyclosporin A and FK506. *Immunol Today.* 13:136-142, **1992**. *[7]*

Schümann HJ, Endoh M, Wagner J: Positive inotropic effects of phenylephrine in the isolated rabbit papillary muscle mediated both by α- and β-adrenoceptors. *Arch Pharmacol.* 284:133-148, **1974**. *[10]*

Schümann HJ, Endoh M, Brodde OE: The time course of the effects of β- and α-adrenoceptor stimulation by isoprenaline and methoxamine on the contractile force and cAMP level of the isolated rabbit papillary muscle. *Arch Pharmacol.* 289:291-302, **1975**. *[10]*

Schuster A, Lacinová L, Klugbauer N, Ito H, Birnbaumer L, Hofmann F: The IVS6 segment of the L-type calcium channel is critical for the action of dihydropyridines and phenylalkylamines. *EMBO J.* 15:2365-2370, **1996**. *[5]*

Schwartz LM, McCleskey EW, Almers W: Dihydropyridine receptors in muscle are voltage-dependent but most are not functional calcium channels. *Nature.* 314:747-751, **1985**. *[5]*

Schwinger RHG, Böhm M, Schmidt U, Karczewski P, Bavendiek U, Flesch M, Krause EG, Erdmann E: Unchanged protein levels of SERCA II and phospholamban but reduced Ca²⁺ uptake and Ca²⁺-ATPase activity of cardiac sarcoplasmic reticulum from dilated cardiomyopathy patients compared with patients with nonfailing hearts. *Circulation.* 92:3220-3228, **1995**. *[10]*

Schwinger RHG, Hoischen S, Reuter H, Hullin R: Regional expression and functional characterization of the L-type Ca²⁺-channel in myocardium from patients with end-stage heart failure and in non-failing human hearts. *J Mol Cell Cardiol.* 31:283-296, **1999a**. *[10]*

Schwinger RHG, Wang J, Frank K, Müller-Ehmsen J, Brixius K, McDonough AA, Erdmann E: Reduced sodium pump α₁, α₃, and β₁-isoform protein levels and Na⁺,K⁺-ATPase activity but unchanged Na⁺-Ca²⁺ exchanger protein levels in human heart failure. *Circulation.* 99:2105-2112, **1999b**. *[4,10]*

Schwinger RHG, Münch G, Bolck B, Karczewski P, Krause EG, Erdmann E: Reduced Ca²⁺-sensitivity of SERCA 2a in failing human myocardium due to reduced serin-16 phospholamban phosphorylation. *J Mol Cell Cardiol.* 3:479-491, **1999c**. *[10]*

Scott BT, Simmerman HKB, Collins JH, Nadal-Ginard B, Jones LR: Complete amino acid sequence of canine cardiac calsequestrin deduced by cDNA cloning. *J Biol Chem.* 263:8958-8964, **1988**. *[7]*

Scriven DRL, Dan P, Moore EDW: Distribution of proteins implicated in excitation-contraction coupling in rat ventricular myocytes. *Biophys J.* 79:2682-2691, **2000**. *[1]*

Sculptoreanu A, Scheuer T, Catterall WA: Voltage-dependent potentiation of L-type Ca^{2+} channels due to phosphorylation by cAMP-dependent protein kinase. *Nature.* 364:240-243, **1993a**. *[5]*

Sculptoreanu A, Rotman E, Takahashi M, Scheuer T, Catterall WA: Voltage-dependent potentiation of the activity of cardiac L-type calcium channel α_1 subunits due to phosphorylation by cAMP-dependent protein kinase. *Proc Natl Acad Sci USA.* 90:10135-10139, **1993b**. *[5]*

Sedarat F, Xu L, Moore ED, Tibbits GF: Colocalization of dihydropyridine and ryanodine receptors in neonate rabbit heart using confocal microscopy. *Am J Physiol.* 279:H202-H209, **2000**. *[9]*

Seguchi M, Harding JA, Jarmakani JM: Developmental change in the function of sarcoplasmic reticulum. *J Mol Cell Cardiol.* 18:189-195, **1986**. *[9]*

Seibel K, Karema E, Takeya K, Reiter M: Effect of noradrenaline on an early and a late component of the myocardial contraction. *Arch Pharmacol.* 305:65-74, **1978**. *[9]*

Seidler NW, Jona I, Vegh M, Martonosi A: Cyclopiazonic acid is a specific inhibitor of the Ca^{2+}-ATPase of sarcoplasmic reticulum. *J Biol Chem.* 264:17816-17823, **1989**. *[7]*

Seidman CE, Seidman JG: Molecular genetic studies of familial hypertrophic cardiomyopathy. *Basic Res Cardiol.* 93:III13-III16, **1998**. *[10]*

Seino A, Kobayashi M, Kobayashi J, Fang YI, Ishibashi M, Nakamura H, Momose K, Ohizumi Y: 9-methyl-7-bromoeudistomin D, a powerful radio-labelable Ca^{2+} releaser having caffeine-like properties, acts on Ca^{2+}-induced Ca^{2+} release channels of sarcoplasmic reticulum. *J Pharmacol Exp Ther.* 256:861-867, **1991**. *[7]*

Semb SO, Lunde PK, Holt E, Tonnessen T, Christensen G, Sejersted OM: Reduced myocardial Na$^+$, K$^+$-pump capacity in congestive heart failure following myocardial infarction in rats. *J Mol Cell Cardiol.* 30:1311-1328, **1998**. *[10]*

Senzaki H, Isoda T, Paolocci N, Ekelund U, Hare JM, Kass DA: Improved mechanoenergetics and cardiac rest and reserve function of in vivo failing heart by calcium sensitizer EMD-57033. *Circulation.* 101:1040-1048, **2000**. *[10]*

Serysheva II, Orlova EV, Chiu W, Sherman MB, Hamilton SL, van Heel M: Electron cryomicroscopy and angular reconstitution used to visualize the skeletal muscle calcium release channel. *Nat Struct Biol.* 2:18-24, **1995**. *[1,7]*

Serysheva II, Schatz M, van Heel M, Chiu W, Hamilton SL: Structure of the skeletal muscle calcium release channel activated with Ca^{2+} and AMP-PCP. *Biophys J.* 77:1936-1944, **1999**. *[1,7]*

Severs NJ: The cardiac gap junction and intercalated disc. *Int J Cardiol.* 26:137-173, **1990**. *[1]*

Severs NJ: Functional microanatomy of the cardiac muscle cell and its gap junctions, in Recent Advances in Microscopy of Cell, Tissues, and Organs. Motta PM (ed). *Rome, Italy, Antonio Delfino Editore.* 281-290, **1997**. *[1]*

Shacklock PS, Wier WG, Balke CW: Local Ca^{2+} transients (Ca^{2+} sparks) originate at transverse tubules in rat heart cells. *J Physiol.* 487:601-608, **1995**. *[8]*

Shah AM, Spurgeon HA, Sollott SJ, Talo A, Lakatta EG: 8-bromo-cGMP reduces the myofilament response to Ca^{2+} in intact cardiac myocytes. *Circ Res.* 74:970-978, **1994**. *[10]*

Sham JSK, Jones LR, Morad M: Phospholamban mediates the β-adrenergic-enhanced Ca^{2+} uptake in mammalian ventricular myocytes. *Am J Physiol.* 261:H1344-H1349, **1991**. *[7]*

Sham JSK, Cleemann L, Morad M: Gating of the cardiac Ca^{2+} release channel: the role of Na$^+$ current and Na$^+$-Ca^{2+} exchange. *Science.* 255:850-853, **1992**. *[8]*

Sham JSK, Cleemann L, Morad M: Functional coupling of Ca^{2+} channels and ryanodine receptors in cardiac myocytes. *Proc Natl Acad Sci USA.* 92:121-125, **1995a**. *[5]*

Sham JSK, Hatem SN, Morad M: Species differences in the activity of the Na$^+$-Ca^{2+} exchanger in mammalian cardiac myocytes. *J Physiol.* 488:623-631, **1995b**. *[6]*

Sham JSK, Song LS, Chen Y, Deng LH, Stern MD, Lakatta EG, Cheng HP: Termination of Ca^{2+} release by a local inactivation of ryanodine receptors in cardiac myocytes. *Proc Natl Acad Sci USA.* 95:15096-15101, **1998**. *[8]*

Shanne FAX, Kane AB, Young EE, Farber JL: Calcium dependence of toxic cell death: A final common pathway. *Science.* 206:700-702, **1979**. *[3]*

Shannon TR, Bers DM: Assessment of intra-SR free [Ca] and buffering in rat heart. *Biophys J.* 73:1524-1531, **1997**. *[3,7]*

Shannon TR, Ginsburg KS, Bers DM: Reverse mode of the SR Ca-pump and load-dependent cytosolic Ca decline in voltage clamped cardiac ventricular myocytes. *Biophys J.* 78:322-333, **2000a**. *[3,7]*

Shannon TR, Ginsburg KS, Bers DM: Potentiation of fractional SR Ca release by total and free intra-SR Ca concentration. *Biophys J.* 78:334-343, **2000b**. *[3,7,8]*

Shannon TR, Chu G, Kranias EG, Bers DM: Phospholamban decreases the energetic efficiency of the SR Ca pump. *J Biol Chem.* 276:7195-7201, **2001**. *[7,10]*

Sharp AH, Imagawa T, Leung AT, Campbell KP: Identification and characterization of the dihydropyridine-binding subunit of the skeletal muscle dihydropyridine receptor. *J Biol Chem.* 262:12309-12315, **1987**. *[5]*

Shattock MJ: Studies on the isolated papillary muscle preparation with particular emphasis on the effects of hypothermia. *Ph.D. thesis, University of London, UK.* **1984**. *[10]*

Shattock MJ, Bers DM: Inotropic response to hypothermia and the temperature-dependence of ryanodine action in isolated rabbit and rat ventricular muscle: Implications for excitation-contraction coupling. *Circ Res.* 61:761-771, **1987**. *[9,10]*

Shattock MJ, Bers DM: Rat vs. rabbit ventricle: Ca flux and intracellular Na assessed by ion-selective microelectrodes. *Am J Physiol.* 256:C813-C822, **1989**. *[4,6,7,9,10]*

Shattock MJ, Matsuura H: Measurement of Na$^+$-K$^+$ pump current in isolated rabbit ventricular myocytes using the whole-cell voltage-clamp technique: Inhibition of the pump by oxidant stress. *Circ Res.* 72:91-101, **1993**. *[10]*

Shepherd N, McDonough HB: Ionic diffusion in transverse tubules of cardiac ventricular myocytes. *Am J Physiol.* 275:H852-H860, **1998**. *[1]*

Sheu SS, Fozzard HA: Transmembrane Na and Ca electrochemical gradients in cardiac muscle and their relation to force development. *J Gen Physiol.* 80:325-351, **1982**. *[10]*

Shi W, Wymore R, Yu H, Wu J, Wymore RT, Pan Z, Robinson RB, Dixon JE, McKinnon D, Cohen IS: Distribution and prevalence of hyperpolarization-activated cation channel (HCN) mRNA expression in cardiac tissues. *Circ Res*. 85:e1-e6, **1999**. *[4]*

Shigekawa M, Finegan JAM, Katz AM: Calcium transport ATPase of canine cardiac sarcoplasmic reticulum. *J Biol Chem*. 251:6894-6900, **1976**. *[7,10]*

Shimahara T, Bournaud R, Inoue I, Strube C: Reduced intramembrane charge movement in the dysgenic skeletal muscle cell. *Pflügers Arch*. 417:111-113, **1990**. *[8]*

Shipolini AR, Yokoyama H, Galiñanes M, Edmondson SJ, Hearse DJ, Avkiran M: Na+/H+ exchanger activity does not contribute to protection by ischemic preconditioning in the isolated rat heart. *Circulation*. 96:3617-3625, **1997**. *[10]*

Shirokova N, Ríos E: Small event Ca2+ release: a probable precursor of Ca2+ sparks in frog skeletal muscle. *J Physiol*. 502:3-11, **1997**. *[8]*

Shirokova N, García J, Pizarró G, Ríos E: Ca2+ release from the sarcoplasmic reticulum compared in amphibian and mammalian skeletal muscle. *J Gen Physiol*. 107:1-18, **1996**. *[8]*

Shirokova N, Shirokov R, Rossi D, González A, Kirsch WG, García J, Sorrentino V, Ríos E: Spatially segregated control of Ca2+ release in developing skeletal muscle of mice. *J Physiol*. 521:483-495, **1999**. *[8]*

Shivkumar K, Deutsch NA, Lamp ST, Khuu K, Goldhaber JI, Weiss JN: Mechanism of hypoxic K loss in rabbit ventricle. *J Clin Invest*. 100:1782-1788, **1997**. *[10]*

Shlafer M, Myers CL, Adkins S: Mitochondrial hydrogen peroxide generation and activities of glutathione peroxidase and superoxide dismutase following global ischemia. *J Mol Cell Cardiol*. 19:1195-1206, **1987**. *[10]*

Shorofsky SR, January CT: L- and T-type Ca2+ channels in canine cardiac Purkinje cells: single-channel demonstration of L-type Ca2+ window current. *Circ Res*. 70:456-464, **1992**. *[4]*

Shoshan-Barmatz V, Ashley RH: The structure, function, and cellular regulation of ryanodine-sensitive Ca2+ release channels. *Int Rev Cytol*. 183:185-270, **1998**. *[7]*

Shtifman A, Ward CW, Wang J, Valdivia HH, Schneider MF: Effects of imperatoxin A on local sarcoplasmic reticulum Ca2+ release in frog skeletal muscle. *Biophys J*. 79:814-827, **2000**. *[8]*

Shuba YM, Iwata T, Naidenov VG, Oz M, Sandberg K, Kraev A, Carafoli E, Morad M: A novel molecular determinant for cAMP-dependent regulation of the frog heart Na+-Ca2+ exchanger. *J Biol Chem*. 273:18819-18825, **1998**. *[6]*

Shull GE, Greeb J: Molecular cloning of two isoforms of the plasma membrane Ca2+-transporting ATPase from rat brain. Structural and functional domains exhibit similarity to Na+,K+- and other cation transport ATPases. *J Biol Chem*. 263:8646-8657, **1988**. *[6]*

Shull GE, Schwartz A, Lingrel JB: Amino-acid sequence of the catalytic subunit of the (Na+,K+)ATPase deduced from a complementary DNA. *Nature*. 316:691-695, **1985**. *[4]*

Sicouri S, Antzelevitch C: A subpopulation of cells with unique electrophysiological properties in the deep subepicardium of the canine ventricle. The M cell. *Circ Res*. 68:1729-1741, **1991**. *[4]*

Sieber M, Nastainczyk W, Zubor V, Wernet W, Hofmann F: The 165-kDa peptide of the purified skeletal muscle dihydropyridine receptor contains the known regulatory sites of the calcium channel. *Eur J Biochem*. 167:117-122, **1987**. *[5]*

Siegl PKS, Garcia ML, King VF, Scott AL, Morgan G, Kaczorowski GJ: Interactions of DPI 201-106, a novel cardiotonic agent, with cardiac calcium channels. *Arch Pharmacol*. 338:684-691, **1988**. *[10]*

Siemankowski RF, Wiseman MO, White HD: ADP dissociation from actomyosin subfragment 1 is sufficiently slow to limit the unloaded shortening velocity in vertebrate muscle. *Proc Natl Acad Sci USA*. 82:658-662, **1985**. *[2]*

Silver PJ, Buja LM, Stull JT: Frequency-dependent myosin light chain phosphorylation in isolated myocardium. *J Mol Cell Cardiol*. 18:31-37, **1986**. *[2]*

Silver PJ, Pinto PB, Dachiw J: Modulation of vascular and cardiac contractile protein regulatory mechanisms by calmodulin inhibitors and related compounds. *Biochem Pharmacol*. 35:3545-3551, **1987**. *[2]*

Simmerman HKB, Jones LR: Phospholamban: protein structure, mechanism of action, and role in cardiac function. *Physiol Rev*. 78:921-947, **1998**. *[7]*

Simmerman HKB, Collins JH, Theibert JL, Wegener AD, Jones LR: Sequence analysis of phospholamban. Identification of phosphorylation sites and two major structural domains. *J Biol Chem*. 261:13333-13341, **1986**. *[7]*

Simmerman HKB, Kobayashi YM, Autry JM, Jones LR: A leucine zipper stabilizes the pentameric membrane domain of phospholamban and forms a coiled-coil pore structure. *J Biol Chem*. 271:5941-5946, **1996**. *[7]*

Simon BJ, Klein MG, Schneider MF: Caffeine slows turn-off of calcium release in voltage clamped skeletal muscle fibers. *Biophys J*. 55:793-797, **1989**. *[8]*

Simpson PC, Cuenco RG, Panaingbatan MO, Murphy MD: An α1-receptor subtype sensitive to WB-4101 transduces cardiac myocyte growth. *Circulation*. 82:III-561, **2000**. *[10]*

Singer D, Biel M, Lotan I, Flockerzi V, Hofmann F, Dascal N: The roles of the subunits in the function of the calcium channel. *Science*. 253:1553-1557, **1991**. *[5]*

Sinnegger MJ, Wang ZY, Grabner M, Hering S, Striessnig J, Glossmann H, Mitterdorfer J: Nine L-type amino acid residues confer full 1,4-dihydropyridine sensitivity to the neuronal calcium channel α1A subunit - Role of L-type MET. *J Biol Chem*. 272:27686-27693, **1997**. *[5]*

Sipido KR, Wier WG: Flux of Ca2+ across the sarcoplasmic reticulum of guinea-pig cardiac cells during excitation-contraction coupling. *J Physiol*. 435:605-630, **1991**. *[3,8]*

Sipido KR, Callewaert G, Carmeliet E: [Ca2+]i transients and [Ca2+]i-dependent chloride current in single Purkinje cells from rabbit heart. *J Physiol*. 468:641-667, **1993**. *[4]*

Sipido KR, Callewaert G, Carmeliet E: Inhibition and rapid recovery of Ca2+ current during Ca2+ release from sarcoplasmic reticulum in guinea pig ventricular myocytes. *Circ Res*. 76:102-109, **1995a**. *[4,5]*

Sipido KR, Carmeliet E, Pappano A: Na+ current and Ca2+ release from the sarcoplasmic reticulum during action potentials in guinea-pig ventricular myocytes. *J Physiol*. 489:1-17, **1995b**. *[8]*

Sipido KR, Maes M, van de Werf F: Low efficiency of Ca2+ entry through the Na+-Ca2+ exchanger as trigger for Ca2+ release from the sarcoplasmic reticulum - A comparison between L-type Ca^{2+} current and reverse-mode Na^+-Ca^{2+} exchange. *Circ Res.* 81:1034-1044, **1997**. *[8]*

Sipido KR, Carmeliet E, van de Werf F: T-type Ca^{2+} current as a trigger for Ca^{2+} release from the sarcoplasmic reticulum in guinea-pig ventricular myocytes. *J Physiol.* 508:439-451, **1998a**. *[8]*

Sipido KR, Stankovicova T, Flameng W, Vanhaecke J, Verdonck F: Frequency dependence of Ca^{2+} release from the sarcoplasmic reticulum in human ventricular myocytes from end-stage heart failure. *Cardiovasc Res.* 37:478-488, **1998b**. *[10]*

Sipido KR, Volders PGA, de Groot SHM, Verdonck F, van de Werf F, Wellens HJJ, Vos MA: Enhanced Ca^{2+} release and Na/Ca exchange activity in hypertrophied canine ventricular myocytes - Potential link between contractile adaptation and arrhythmogenesis. *Circulation.* 102:2137-2144, **2000**. *[10]*

Sitsapesan R, Williams AJ: Regulation of the gating of the sheep cardiac sarcoplasmic reticulum Ca^{2+}-release channel by luminal Ca^{2+}. *J Membr Biol.* 137:215-226, **1994**. *[7]*

Sitsapesan R, Williams AJ: Modification of the conductance and gating properties of ryanodine receptors by suramin. *J Membr Biol.* 153:93-103, **1996**. *[7]*

Sitsapesan R, Williams AJ: Regulation of current flow through ryanodine receptors by luminal Ca^{2+}. *J Membr Biol.* 159:179-185, **1997**. *[7]*

Sitsapesan R, Williams AJ: The Structure and Function of Ryanodine Receptors. *London, UK, Imperial College Press.* 1-325, **1998**. *[7]*

Sitsapesan R, Montgomery RAP, MacLeod KT, Williams AJ: Sheep cardiac sarcoplasmic reticulum calcium-release channels: Modification of conductance and gating by temperature. *J Physiol.* 434:469-488, **1991**. *[7,10]*

Sitsapesan R, McGarry SJ, Williams AJ: Cyclic ADP-ribose competes with ATP for the adenine nucleotide binding site on the cardiac ryanodine receptor Ca^{2+}-release channel. *Circ Res.* 75:596-600, **1994**. *[7]*

Sitsapesan R, Montgomery RAP, Williams AJ: New insights into the gating mechanisms of cardiac ryanodine receptors revealed by rapid changes in ligand concentration. *Circ Res.* 77:765-772, **1995**. *[7]*

Sjöstrand FS, Andersson-Cedergren E, Dewey MM: The ultrastructure of the intercalated disc of frog, mouse and guinea pig cardiac muscle. *J Ultrastruct Res.* 1:271-287, **1958**. *[1]*

Skou JC: Enzymatic basis for active transport of Na^+ and K^+ across cell membrane. *Physiol Rev.* 45:596-617, **1965**. *[10]*

Slaughter RS, Sutko JL, Reeves JP: Equilibrium calcium-calcium exchange in cardiac sarcolemmal vesicles. *J Biol Chem.* 258:3183-3190, **1983**. *[6]*

Slaughter RS, Shevell JL, Felix JP, Garcia ML, Kaczorowski GJ: High levels of sodium-calcium exchange in vascular smooth muscle sarcolemmal membrane vesicles. *Biochemistry.* 28:3995-4002, **1989**. *[6]*

Slavik KJ, Wang JP, Aghdasi B, Zhang JZ, Mandel F, Malouf N, Hamilton SL: A carboxy-terminal peptide of the α_1-subunit of the dihydropyridine receptor inhibits Ca^{2+}-release channels. *Am J Physiol.* 272:C1475-C1481, **1997**. *[8]*

Slodzinski MK, Blaustein MP: Physiological effects of Na^+/Ca^{2+} exchanger knockdown by antisense oligodeoxynucleotides in arterial myocytes. *Am J Physiol.* 275:C251-C259, **1998a**. *[6]*

Slodzinski MK, Blaustein MP: Na^+/Ca^{2+} exchange in neonatal rat heart cells: antisense inhibition and protein half-life. *Am J Physiol.* 275:C459-C467, **1998b**. *[6]*

Smith SJ, England PJ: The effects of reported Ca^{2+} sensitisers on the rates of Ca^{2+} release from cardiac troponin C and the troponin-tropomyosin complex. *Br J Pharmacol.* 100:779-785, **1990**. *[10]*

Smith JS, Coronado R, Meissner G: Sarcoplasmic reticulum contains adenine nucleotide-activated calcium channels. *Nature.* 316:446-449, **1985a**. *[7]*

Smith JB, Smith L, Higgins BL: Temperature and nucleotide dependence of calcium release by myo-inositol 1,4,5-trisphosphate in cultured vascular smooth muscle cells. *J Biol Chem.* 259:14413-14416, **1985b**. *[8]*

Smith JS, Coronado R, Meissner G: Single channel measurements of the calcium release channel from skeletal muscle sarcoplasmic reticulum. *J Gen Physiol.* 88:573-588, **1986**. *[7]*

Smith JS, Imagawa T, Ma J, Foll M, Campbell KP, Coronado R: Purified ryanodine receptor from rabbit skeletal muscle is the calcium-release channel of sarcoplasmic reticulum. *J Gen Physiol.* 92:1-26, **1988**. *[7]*

Smith JS, Rousseau E, Meissner G: Calmodulin modulation of single sarcoplasmic reticulum Ca release channels from cardiac and skeletal muscle. *Circ Res.* 64:352-359, **1989**. *[7]*

Smith PL, Baukrowitz T, Yellen G: The inward rectification mechanism of the HERG cardiac potassium channel. *Nature.* 379:833-836, **1996**. *[4]*

Snabaitis AK, Yokoyama H, Avkiran M: Roles of mitogen-activated protein kinases and protein kinase C in α_{1A}-adrenoceptor-mediated stimulation of the sarcolemmal Na^+-H^+ exchanger. *Circ Res.* 86:214-220, **2000**. *[10]*

Soeller C, Cannell MB: Numerical simulation of local calcium movements during L-type calcium channel gating in the cardiac diad. *Biophys J.* 73:97-111, **1997**. *[8]*

Soeller C, Cannell MB: Examination of the transverse tubular system in living cardiac rat myocytes by 2-photon microscopy and digital image-processing techniques. *Circ Res.* 84:266-275, **1999**. *[1]*

Solaro RJ: Modulation of cardiac myofilament activity by protein phosphorylation, in Handbook of Physiology. Page E, Fozzard HA, Solaro RJ (eds). *New York, NY, Oxford University Press.* In press. **2001**. *[2,10]*

Solaro RJ, Briggs FN: Estimating the functional capabilities of sarcoplasmic reticulum in cardiac muscle. *Circ Res.* 34:531-540, **1974**. *[3,7]*

Solaro RJ, Rarick HM: Troponin and tropomyosin - Proteins that switch on and tune in the activity of cardiac myofilaments. *Circ Res.* 83:471-480, **1998**. *[2]*

Solaro RJ, Rüegg JC: Stimulation of Ca^{2+} binding and ATPase activity of dog cardiac myofibrils by AR-L115 BS, a novel cardiotonic agent. *Circ Res.* 51:290-294, **1982**. *[2,10]*

Solaro RJ, Wise RM, Shiner JS, Briggs FN: Calcium requirements for cardiac myofibrillar activation. *Circ Res.* 34:525-530, **1974**. *[2]*

Solaro RJ, Moir AJG, Perry SV: Phosphorylation of a troponin I and the inotropic effect of adrenaline in perfused rabbit heart. *Nature.* 262:615-617, **1976**. *[2]*

Solaro RJ, Kumar P, Blanchard EM, Martin AF: Differential effects of pH on calcium activation of myofilaments of adult and perinatal dog hearts. *Circ Res.* 58:721-729, **1986**. *[2,10]*

Solaro RJ, Rapundalo ST, Garvey JL, Karnias EG: Mechanics of cardiac contraction and the phosphorylation of sarcotubular and myofilament proteins, in Mechanics of the Circulation. ter Keurs HEDJ, Tyberg JV (eds). *Martinus Nijhoff Publishers.* 135-152, **1987**. *[2]*

Solaro RJ, Lee JA, Kentish JC, Allen DG: Effects of acidosis on ventricular muscle from adult and neonatal rats. *Circ Res.* 63:779-787, **1988**. *[2,10]*

Solaro RJ, el-Saleh SC, Kentish JC: Ca²⁺, pH and the regulation of cardiac myofilament force and ATPase activity. *Mol Cell Biochem.* 89:163-167, **1989**. *[10]*

Solaro RJ, Gambassi G, Warshaw DM, Keller MR, Spurgeon HA, Beier N, Lakatta EG: Stereoselective actions of thiadiazinones on canine cardiac myocytes and myofilaments. *Circ Res.* 73:981-990, **1993**. *[2,10]*

Sollott SJ, Ziman BD, Warshaw DM, Spurgeon HA, Lakatta EG: Actomyosin interaction modulates resting length of unstimulated cardiac ventricular cells. *Am J Physiol.* 271:H896-H905, **1996**. *[2]*

Somlyo AP, Himpens B: Cell calcium and its regulation in smooth muscle. *FASEB J.* 3:2266-2276, **1989**. *[8,10]*

Somlyo AV, Somlyo AP: Electron optical studies of calcium and other ion movements in the sarcoplasmic reticulum in situ, in Sarcoplasmic Reticulum in Muscle Physiology. Entman ML, van Winkle WB (eds). *Boca Raton, FL, CRC Press, Inc.* Vol. 1. 31-50, **1986**. *[7,8]*

Somlyo AP, Somlyo AV: Flash photolysis studies of excitation-contraction coupling, regulation, and contraction in smooth muscle. *Annu Rev Physiol.* 52:857-874, **1990**. *[8]*

Somlyo AP, Somlyo AV: Signal transduction and regulation in smooth muscle. *Nature.* 372:231-236, **1994**. *[8]*

Somlyo AV, Shuman H, Somlyo AP: Composition of sarcoplasmic reticulum in situ by electron probe X-ray microanalysis. *Nature.* 268:556-558, **1977a**. *[7,8]*

Somlyo AV, Shuman H, Somlyo AP: Elemental distribution in striated muscle and the effects of hypertonicity. Electron probe analysis of cryosections. *J Cell Biol.* 74:828-857, **1977b**. *[7,8]*

Somlyo AV, Bond M, Somlyo AP, Scarpa A: Inositol trisphosphate-induced calcium release and contraction in vascular smooth muscle. *Proc Natl Acad Sci USA.* 85:5231-5235, **1985**. *[8]*

Somlyo AP, Walker JW, Goldman YE, Trentham DR, Kobayashi S, Kitazawa T, Somlyo AV: Inositol trisphosphate, calcium and muscle contraction. *Phil Trans Roy Soc London B.* 320:399-414, **1988**. *[8]*

Sommer JR, Johnson EA: Cardiac muscle. A comparative study of Purkinje fibers and ventricular fibers. *J Cell Biol.* 36:497-526, **1968**. *[1]*

Sommer JR, Johnson EA: Ultrastructure of cardiac muscle, in Handbook of Physiology. Section 2. The Cardiovascular System. Berne RM (ed). *Bethesda, MD, Am Physiol Soc.* Vol. 1. 113-186, **1979**. *[1]*

Sommer JR, Waugh RA: The ultrastructure of the mammalian cardiac muscle cell with special emphasis on the tubular membrane systems. A review. *Am J Pathol.* 82:192-232, **1976**. *[1]*

Song KS, Scherer PE, Tang Z, Okamoto T, Li S, Chafel M, Chu C, Kohtz DS, Lisanti MP: Expression of caveolin-3 in skeletal, cardiac, and smooth muscle cells. Caveolin-3 is a component of the sarcolemma and co-fractionates with dystrophin and dystrophin-associated glycoproteins. *J Biol Chem.* 271:15160-15165, **1996**. *[1]*

Song LS, Stern MD, Lakatta EG, Cheng HP: Partial depletion of sarcoplasmic reticulum calcium does not prevent calcium sparks in rat ventricular myocytes. *J Physiol.* 505:665-675, **1997**. *[8]*

Song LS, Sham JS, Stern MD, Lakatta EG, Cheng HP: Direct measurement of SR release flux by tracking 'Ca²⁺ spikes' in rat cardiac myocytes. *J Physiol.* 512:677-691, **1998**. *[8]*

Soonpaa MH, Field LJ: Survey of studies examining mammalian cardiomyocyte DNA synthesis. *Circ Res.* 83:15-26, **1998**. *[10]*

Sordahl LA: Effects of magnesium, ruthenium red and the antibiotic ionophore A-23187 on initial rates of calcium uptake and release by heart mitochondria. *Arch Biochem Biophys.* 167:104-115, **1975**. *[3]*

Sorota S: Swelling-induced chloride-sensitive current in canine atrial cells revealed by whole-cell patch-clamp method. *Circ Res.* 70:679-687, **1992**. *[4]*

Sorota S: Tyrosine protein kinase inhibitors prevent activation of cardiac swelling-induced chloride current. *Pflügers Arch.* 431:178-185, **1995**. *[4]*

Sorota S: Insights into the structure, distribution and function of the cardiac chloride channels. *Cardiovasc Res.* 42:361-376, **1999**. *[4]*

Spaetgens RL, Zamponi GW: Multiple structural domains contribute to voltage-dependent inactivation of rat brain α₁ₑ calcium channels. *J Biol Chem.* 274:22428-22436, **1999**. *[5]*

Sparagna GC, Gunter KK, Sheu SS, Gunter TE: Mitochondrial calcium uptake from physiological-type pulses of calcium. A description of the rapid uptake mode. *J Biol Chem.* 270:27510-27515, **1995**. *[3]*

Spencer CI, Berlin JR: Control of sarcoplasmic reticulum calcium release during calcium loading in isolated rat ventricular myocytes. *J Physiol.* 488:267-279, **1995**. *[8]*

Sperelakis N, Lee EC: Characterization of Na⁺,K⁺-ATPase isolated from embryonic chick hearts and cultured chick heart cells. *Biochim Biophys Acta.* 233:562-579, **1971**. *[10]*

Sperelakis N, Katsube Y, Yokoshiki H, Sada H, Sumii K: Regulation of the slow Ca²⁺ channels of myocardial cells. *Mol Cell Biochem.* 163-164:85-98, **1996**. *[5]*

Spray DC: Gap junction proteins: Where they live and how they die. *Circ Res.* 83:679-681, **1998**. *[1]*

Spray DC, Burt JM: Structure-activity relations of the cardiac gap junction channel. *Am J Physiol.* 258:C195-C205, **1990**. *[1]*

Spray TL, Waugh RA, Sommer JR: Peripheral couplings in adult vertebrate skeletal muscle. Anatomical observations and functional implications. *J Cell Biol.* 62:223-227, **1974**. *[1]*

Spray DC, Stern JH, Harris AL, Bennett MVL: Comparison of sensitivities of gap junctional conductance to H and Ca ions. *Proc Natl Acad Sci USA.* 79:441-445, **1982**. *[1]*

Spurgeon HA, Isenberg G, Talo A, Stern MD, Capogrossi MC, Lakatta EG: Negative staircase in cytosolic Ca²⁺ in rat myocytes is modulated by depolarization duration. *Biophys J.* 53:601a, **1988**. *[9]*

Spurgeon HA, Stern MD, Baartz G, Raffaeli S, Hansford RG, Talo A, Lakatta EG, Capogrossi MC: Simultaneous measurement of Ca²⁺, contraction, and potential in cardiac myocytes. *Am J Physiol.* 258:H574-H586, **1990**. *[10]*

Spurgeon HA, duBell WH, Stern MD, Sollott SJ, Ziman BD, Silverman HS, Capogrossi MC, Talo A, Lakatta EG : Cytosolic calcium and myofilaments in single rat cardiac myocytes achieve a dynamic equilibrium during twitch relaxation. *J Physiol.* 447:83-102, **1992**. *[10]*

Stehno-Bittel L, Luckhoff A, Clapham DE: Calcium release from the nucleus by InsP₃ receptor channels. *Neuron.* 14:163-167, **1995**. *[8]*

Steinfath M, Chen YY, Lavicky J, Magnussen O, Nose M, Rosswag S, Schmitz W, Scholz H: Cardiac α₁-adrenoceptor densities in different mammalian species. *Br J Pharmacol.* 107:185-188, **1992**. *[10]*

Stephenson EW: Excitation of skinned muscle fibers by imposed ion gradients. I. Stimulation of ⁴⁵Ca efflux at constant [K][Cl] product. *J Gen Physiol.* 86:813-832, **1985**. *[8]*

Stephenson DG, Williams DA: Calcium-activated force-responses in fast and slow-twitch skinned muscle fibres from the rat. *J Physiol.* 317:281-302, **1981**. *[2]*

Stephenson DG, Williams DA: Temperature-dependent calcium sensitivity changes in skinned muscle fibres of the rat and toad. *J Physiol.* 360:1-12, **1985**. *[2]*

Stern MD: Theory of excitation-contraction coupling in cardiac muscle. *Biophys J.* 63:497-517, **1992**. *[8]*

Stern MD, Kort AA, Bhatnagar GM, Lakatta EG: Scattered-light intensity fluctuations in diastolic rat cardiac muscle caused by spontaneous Ca²⁺-dependent cellular mechanical oscillations. *J Gen Physiol.* 82:119-153, **1983**. *[8]*

Stern MD, Song LS, Cheng HP, Sham JS, Yang HT, Boheler KR, Ríos E: Local control models of cardiac excitation-contraction coupling - A possible role for allosteric interactions between ryanodine receptors. *J Gen Physiol.* 113:469-489, **1999**. *[7,8]*

Stewart PS, MacLennan DH: Surface particles of sarcoplasmic reticulum membranes. Structural features of the adenosine triphosphatase. *J Biol Chem.* 249:985-993, **1974**. *[1]*

Stiles GL, Caron MG, Lefkowitz RJ: β-Adrenergic receptors: Biochemical mechanisms of physiologic regulation. *Physiol Rev.* 64:661-743, **1984**. *[10]*

Stokes DL, Green NM: Modeling a dehalogenase fold into the 8-Å density map for Ca²⁺-ATPase defines a new domain structure. *Biophys J.* 78:1765-1776, **2000**. *[7]*

Strang KT, Moss RL: α₁-adrenergic receptor stimulation decreases maximum shortening velocity of skinned single ventricular myocytes from rats. *Circ Res.* 77:114-120, **1995**. *[10]*

Striessnig J, Scheffauer F, Mitterdorfer J, Schirmer M, Glossmann H: Identification of the benzothiazepine-binding polypeptide of skeletal muscle calcium channels with (+)-cis-azidodiltiazem and anti-ligand antibodies. *J Biol Chem.* 265:363-370, **1990a**. *[5]*

Striessnig J, Glossmann H, Catterall WA: Identification of a phenylalkylamine binding region within the α₁ subunit of skeletal muscle Ca²⁺ channels. *Proc Natl Acad Sci USA.* 87:9108-9112, **1990b**. *[5]*

Striessnig J, Murphy BJ, Catterall WA: Dihydropyridine receptor of L-type Ca²⁺ channels: identification of binding domains for [3H](+)-PN200-110 and [3H]azidopine within the α₁ subunit. *Proc Natl Acad Sci USA.* 88:10769-10773, **1991**. *[5]*

Stromer H, de Groot MC, Horn M, Faul C, Leupold A, Morgan JP, Scholz W, Neubauer S: Na⁺/H⁺ exchange inhibition with HOE642 improves postischemic recovery due to attenuation of Ca²⁺ overload and prolonged acidosis on reperfusion. *Circulation.* 101:2749-2755, **2000**. *[10]*

Strübing C, Hering S, Glossmann H: Evidence for an external location of the dihydropyridine agonist receptor site on smooth muscle and skeletal muscle calcium channels. *Br J Pharmacol.* 108:884-891, **1993**. *[5]*

Studer R, Reinecke H, Bilger J, Eschenhagen T, Böhm M, Hasenfuss G, Just H, Holtz J, Drexler H: Gene expression of the cardiac Na⁺-Ca²⁺ exchanger in end-stage human heart failure. *Circ Res.* 75:443-453, **1994**. *[4,10]*

Stühmer W, Conti F, Suzuki H, Wang XD, Noda M, Yahagi N, Kubo H, Numa S: Structural parts involved in activation and inactivation of the sodium channel. *Nature.* 339:597-603, **1989**. *[4]*

Stuyvers BDMY, Miura M, ter Keurs HEDJ: Dynamics of viscoelastic properties of rat cardiac sarcomeres during the diastolic interval: Involvement of Ca²⁺. *J Physiol.* 502:661-677, **1997**. *[2]*

Su JH, Kerrick WGL: Effects of halothane on caffeine-induced tension transients in functionally skinned myocardial fibers. *Pflügers Arch.* 380:29-34, **1979**. *[7]*

Su Z, Bridge JH, Philipson KD, Spitzer KW, Barry WH: Quantitation of Na Ca exchanger function in single ventricular myocytes. *J Mol Cell Cardiol.* 31:1125-1135, **1999**. *[6]*

Su Z, Sugishita K, Ritter M, Li F, Spitzer KW, Barry WH: The sodium pump modulates the influence of Iₙₐ on [Ca²⁺]ᵢ transients in mouse ventricular myocytes. *Biophys J.* 80:1230-1237, **2001**. *[10]*

Suárez-Isla BA, Irribarra V, Oberhauser A, Larralde L, Bull R, Hidalgo C, Jaimovich E: Inositol(1,4,5)-trisphosphate activates a calcium channel in isolated sarcoplasmic reticulum membranes. *Biophys J.* 54:737-741, **1988**. *[8]*

Suematsu E, Hirata M, Hashimoto T, Kuriyama H: Inositol 1,4,5-trisphosphate releases Ca²⁺ from intracellular store sites in skinned single cells of porcine coronary artery. *Biochem Biophys Res Commun.* 120:481-485, **1984**. *[8]*

Sugden PH: Signaling in myocardial hypertrophy - Life after calcineurin? *Circ Res.* 84:633-646, **1999**. *[10]*

Sugden PH, Clerk A: Cellular mechanisms of cardiac hypertrophy. *J Mol Med.* 76:725-746, **1998**. *[10]*

Sugden PH, Clerk A: Activation of the small GTP-binding protein Ras in the heart by hypertrophic agonists. *Trends Cardiovasc Med.* 10:1-8, **2000**. *[10]*

Suh-Kim H, Wei X, Klos A, Pan S, Ruth P, Flockerzi V, Hofmann F, Perez-Reyes E, Birnbaumer L: Reconstitution of the skeletal muscle dihydropyridine receptor. Functional interaction among α₁, β, γ and α₂δ subunits. *Receptors Channels.* 4:217-225, **1996**. *[5]*

Suleiman MS, Reeves JP: Inhibition of Na⁺-Ca²⁺ exchange mechanism in cardiac sarcolemmal vesicles by harmaline. *Comp Biochem Physiol C.* 88:197-200, **1987**. *[6]*

Sumbera J, Kruta V, Braveny P: Influence of a rapid change of temperature on the mechanical response of mammalian myocardium. *Arch Int Physiol Biochem.* 74:627-641, **1966**. *[10]*

Sumii K, Sperelakis N: cGMP-dependent protein kinase regulation of the L-type Ca²⁺ current in rat ventricular myocytes. *Circ Res.* 77:803-812, **1995**. *[10]*

Sun XH, Protasi F, Takahashi M, Takeshima H, Ferguson DG, Franzini-Armstrong C: Molecular architecture of membranes involved in excitation-contraction coupling of cardiac muscle. *J Cell Biol.* 129:659-671, **1995**. *[1]*

Supattapone S, Worley PF, Baraban JM, Snyder SH: Solubilization, purification, and characterization of an inositol triphosphate receptor. *J Biol Chem.* 263:1530-1534, **1988**. *[7]*

Sussman MA, Sakhi S, Barrientos P, Ito M, Kedes L: Tropomodulin in rat cardiac muscle. Localization of protein is independent of messenger RNA distribution during myofibrillar development. *Circ Res.* 75:221-232, **1994**. *[1]*

Sussman MA, Lim HW, Gude N, Taigen T, Olson EN, Robbins J, Colbert MC, Gualberto A, Wieczorek DF, Molkentin JD: Prevention of cardiac hypertrophy in mice by calcineurin inhibition. *Science.* 281:1690-1693, **1998**. *[10]*

Sutko JL, Airey JA: Ryanodine receptor Ca²⁺ release channels: Does diversity in form equal diversity in function. *Physiol Rev.* 76:1027-1071, **1996**. *[7,8]*

Sutko JL, Kenyon JL: Ryanodine modification of cardiac muscle responses to potassium free solutions. Evidence for inhibition of sarcoplasmic reticulum calcium release. *J Gen Physiol.* 82:385-404, **1983**. *[9]*

Sutko JL, Willerson JT: Ryanodine alteration of the contractile state of rat ventricular myocardium. Comparison with dog, cat and rabbit ventricular tissues. *Circ Res.* 46:332-343, **1980**. *[7,9]*

Sutko JL, Ito K, Kenyon JL: Ryanodine: A modifier of sarcoplasmic-reticulum calcium release. Biochemical and functional consequences of its actions on striated muscle. *Fed Proc.* 44:2984-2988, **1985**. *[7,9]*

Sutko JL, Bers DM, Reeves JP: Postrest inotropy in rabbit ventricle: Na⁺-Ca²⁺ exchange determines sarcoplasmic reticulum Ca²⁺ content. *Am J Physiol.* 250:H654-H661, **1986**. *[9]*

Sutko JL, Airey JA, Welch W, Ruest L: The pharmacology of ryanodine and related compounds. *Pharmacol Rev.* 49:53-98, **1997**. *[7]*

Suzuki K: The structure of calpains and the calpain gene, in Intracellular Calcium-Dependent Proteolysis. Mellgren RL, Murachi T (eds). *Boca Raton, FL, CRC, Inc.* 26-35, **1990**. *[10]*

Suzuki T, Wang JH: Stimulation of bovine cardiac sarcoplasmic reticulum Ca²⁺ pump and blocking of phospholamban phosphorylation and dephosphorylation by a phospholamban monoclonal antibody. *J Biol Chem.* 261:7018-7023, **1986**. *[7]*

Swartz DR, Moss RL: Influence of a strong-binding myosin analogue on calcium-sensitive mechanical properties of skinned skeletal muscle fibers. *J Biol Chem.* 267:20497-20506, **1992**. *[2]*

Swynghedauw B: Developmental and functional adaptation of contractile proteins in cardiac and skeletal muscles. *Physiol Rev.* 66:710-771, **1986**. *[2]*

Szigeti G, Rusznak Z, Kovacs L, Papp Z: Calcium-activated transient membrane currents are carried mainly by chloride ions in isolated atrial, ventricular and Purkinje cells of rabbit heart. *Exp Physiol.* 83:137-153, **1998**. *[10]*

Tada M: The sarcoplasmic reticulum Ca²⁺ pump, in Handbook of Physiology. Page E, Fozzard HA, Solaro RJ (eds). *New York, NY, Oxford University Press.* In press. **2001**. *[7]*

Tada M, Katz AM: Phosphorylation of the sarcoplasmic reticulum and sarcolemma. *Annu Rev Physiol.* 44:401-423, **1982**. *[7]*

Tada M, Kirchberger MA, Repke DI, Katz AM: The stimulation of calcium transport in cardiac sarcoplasmic reticulum by adenosine 3':5'-monophosphate-dependent protein kinase. *J Biol Chem.* 249:6174-6180, **1974**. *[2,7]*

Tada M, Yamaamoto T, Tonomura Y: Molecular mechanism of active calcium transport by sarcoplasmic reticulum. *Physiol Rev.* 58:1-79, **1978**. *[7]*

Tada M, Yamada M, Kadoma M, Inui M, Ohmori F: Calcium transport by cardiac sarcoplasmic reticulum and phosphorylation of phospholamban. *Mol Cell Biochem.* 46:74-95, **1982**. *[7]*

Tada M, Inui M, Yamada M, Kadoma M, Kuzuya T, Abe H, Kakiuchi S: Effects of phospholamban phosphorylation catalyzed by adenosine 3':5'-monophosphate- and calmodulin-dependent protein kinases on calcium transport ATPase of cardiac sarcoplasmic reticulum. *J Mol Cell Cardiol.* 15:335-346, **1983**. *[7]*

Tada M, Yabuki M, Toyofuku T: Molecular regulation of phospholamban function and gene expression. *Ann NY Acad Sci.* 853:116-129, **1998**. *[7]*

Tagawa H, Koide M, Sato H, Zile MR, Carabello BA, Cooper G: Cytoskeletal role in the transition from compensated to decompensated hypertrophy during adult canine left ventricular pressure overloading. *Circ Res.* 82:751-761, **1998**. *[1]*

Takahashi T, Allen PD, Lacro RV, Marks AR, Dennis AR, Schoen FJ, Grossman W, Marsh JD, Izumo S: Expression of dihydropyridine receptor (Ca²⁺ channel) and calsequestrin genes in the myocardium of patients with end-stage heart failure. *J Clin Invest.* 90:927-935, **1992**. *[10]*

Takamatsu T, Wier WG: Calcium waves in mammalian heart: Quantification of origin, magnitude, waveform, and velocity. *FASEB J.* 4:1519-1525, **1990**. *[8,10]*

Takanashi M, Norota I, Endoh M: Potent inhibitory action of chlorethylclonidine on the positive inotropic effect and phosphoinositide hydrolysis mediated via myocardial α₁-adrenoceptors in the rabbit ventricular myocardium. *Naunyn Schmiedebergs Arch Pharmacol.* 343:669-673, **1991**. *[10]*

Takano H, Tang XL, Qiu Y, Guo Y, French BA , Bolli R: Nitric oxide donors induce late preconditioning against myocardial stunning and infarction in conscious rabbits via an antioxidant- sensitive mechanism. *Circ Res.* 83:73-84, **1998**. *[10]*

Takasago T, Imagawa T, Furukawa K, Ogurusu T, Shigekawa M: Regulation of the cardiac ryanodine receptor by protein kinase- dependent phosphorylation. *J Biochem (Tokyo).* 109:163-170, **1991**. *[7]*

Takashi E, Wang YG, Ashraf M: Activation of mitochondrial K_ATP channel elicits late preconditioning against myocardial infarction via protein kinase C signaling pathway. *Circ Res.* 85:1146-1153, **1999**. *[4,10]*

Takekura H, Bennett L, Tanabe T, Beam KG, Franzini-Armstrong C: Restoration of junctional tetrads in dysgenic myotubes by dihydropyridine receptor cDNA. *Biophys J.* 67:793-803, **1994**. *[8]*

Takenaka H, Adler PN, Katz AM: Calcium fluxes across the membrane of sarcoplasmic reticulum vesicles. *J Biol Chem.* 257:12649-12656, **1982**. *[7]*

Takeshima H, Hishimura S, Matsumoto T, Ishida H, Kangawa K, Minamino N, Matsuo H, Ueda M, Hanaoka M, Hirose T, Numa S: Primary structure and expression from complementary DNA of skeletal muscle ryanodine receptor. *Nature.* 339:439-445, **1989.** *[1,7]*

Takeshima H, Iino M, Takekura H, Nishi M, Kuno J, Minowa O, Takano H, Noda T: Excitation-contraction uncoupling and muscular degeneration in mice lacking functional skeletal muscle ryanodine-receptor gene. *Nature.* 369:556-559, **1994.** *[7,8]*

Takeshima H, Ikemoto T, Nishi M, Nishiyama N, Shimuta M, Sugitani Y, Kuno J, Saito I, Saito H, Endo M, Iino M, Noda T: Generation and characterization of mutant mice lacking ryanodine receptor type 3. *J Biol Chem.* 271:19649-19652, **1996.** *[7]*

Takeshima H, Komazaki S, Hirose K, Nishi M, Noda T, Lino M: Embryonic lethality and abnormal cardiac myocytes in mice lacking ryanodine receptor type 2. *EMBO J.* 17:3309-3316, **1998.** *[7]*

Takimoto K, Li D, Nerbonne JM, Levitan ES: Distribution, splicing and glucocorticoid-induced expression of cardiac α_{1C} and α_{1D} voltage-gated Ca^{2+} channel mRNAs. *J Mol Cell Cardiol.* 29:3035-3042, **1997.** *[5]*

Talosi L, Edes I, Kranias EG: Intracellular mechanisms mediating reversal of β-adrenergic stimulation in intact beating hearts. *Am J Physiol.* 264:H791-H797, **1993.** *[7]*

Tanabe T, Takeshima H, Mikami A, Flockerzi V, Takahashi H, Kangawa K, Kojima M, Matsuo H, Hirose T, Numa S: Primary structure of the receptor for calcium channel blockers from skeletal muscle. *Nature.* 328:313-318, **1987.** *[5]*

Tanabe T, Beam KG, Powell JA, Numa S: Restoration of excitation-contraction coupling and slow calcium current in dysgenic muscle by dihydropyridine receptor complementary DNA. *Nature.* 336:134-139, **1988.** *[8]*

Tanabe T, Mikami A, Numa S, Beam KG: Cardiac-type excitation-contraction coupling in dysgenic skeletal muscle injected with cardiac dihydropyridine receptor cDNA. *Nature.* 344:451-453, **1990a.** *[8]*

Tanabe T, Beam KG, Adams BA, Niidome T, Numa S: Regions of the skeletal muscle dihydropyridine receptor critical for excitation-contraction coupling. *Nature.* 356:567-569, **1990b.** *[8]*

Tanabe T, Adams BA, Numa S, Beam KG: Repeat I of the dihydropyridine receptor is critical in determining calcium channel activation kinetics. *Nature.* 352:800-803, **1991.** *[5]*

Tanna B, Welch W, Ruest L, Sutko JL, Williams AJ: Interactions of a reversible ryanoid (21-amino-9α-hydroxy-ryanodine) with single sheep cardiac ryanodine receptor channels. *J Gen Physiol.* 112:55-69, **1998.** *[7]*

Tanna B, Welch W, Ruest L, Sutko JL, Williams AJ: The interaction of a neutral ryanoid with the ryanodine receptor channel provides insights into the mechanisms by which ryanoid binding is modulated by voltage. *J Gen Physiol.* 116:1-9, **2000.** *[7]*

Tarroni P, Rossi D, Conti A, Sorrentino V: Expression of the ryanodine receptor type 3 calcium release channel during development and differentiation of mammalian skeletal muscle cells. *J Biol Chem.* 272:19808-19813, **1997.** *[8]*

Tate CA, Bick RJ, Chu A, van Winkle WB, Entman ML: Nucleotide specificity of canine cardiac sarcoplasmic reticulum. GTP-induced calcium accumulation and GTPase activity. *J Biol Chem.* 260:9618-9623, **1985.** *[7]*

Tate CA, Bick RJ, Blaylock SL, Youker KA, Scherer NM, Entman ML: Nucleotide specificity of canine cardiac sarcoplasmic reticulum. Differential alteration of enzyme properties by detergent treatment. *J Biol Chem.* 264:7809-7813, **1989.** *[7]*

Terracciano CMN, MacLeod KT: Reloading of Ca^{2+}-depleted sarcoplasmic reticulum during rest in guinea pig ventricular myocytes. *Am J Physiol.* 271:H1814-H1822, **1996.** *[9]*

Terracciano CMN, MacLeod KT: Measurements of Ca^{2+} entry and sarcoplasmic reticulum Ca^{2+} content during the cardiac cycle in guinea pig and rat ventricular myocytes. *Biophys J.* 72:1319-1326, **1997.** *[5,7,9]*

Terracciano CMN, Naqvi RU, MacLeod KT: Effects of rest interval on the release of calcium from the sarcoplasmic reticulum in isolated guinea pig ventricular myocytes. *Circ Res.* 77:354-360, **1995.** *[7]*

Terracciano CMN, de Souza AI, Philipson KD, MacLeod KT: Na^+-Ca^{2+} exchange and sarcoplasmic reticular Ca^{2+} regulation in ventricular myocytes from transgenic mice overexpressing the Na^+-Ca^{2+} exchanger. *J Physiol.* 512:651-667, **1998.** *[6]*

Thastrup O, Cullen PJ, Drobak BK, Hanley MR, Dawson AP: Thapsigargin, a tumor promoter, discharges intracellular Ca^{2+} stores by specific inhibition of the endoplasmic reticulum Ca^{2+}-ATPase. *Proc Natl Acad Sci USA.* 87:2466-2470, **1990.** *[7]*

Thieleczek R, Mayr GW, Brandt NR: Inositol polyphosphate-mediated repartitioning of aldolase in skeletal muscle triads and myofibrils. *J Biol Chem.* 264:7449-7456, **1989.** *[8]*

Thomas AP, Bird GSJ, Hajnóczky G, Robb-Gaspers LD, Putney JW Jr: Spatial and temporal aspects of cellular calcium signaling. *FASEB J.* 10:1505-1517, **1996.** *[7]*

Thomas GP, Sims SM, Karmazyn M: Differential effects of endothelin-1 on basal and isoprenaline-enhanced Ca^{2+} current in guinea-pig ventricular myocytes. *J Physiol.* 503:55-65, **1997.** *[5]*

Tiaho F, Richard S, Lory P, Nerbonne JM, Nargeot J: Cyclic-AMP-dependent phosphorylation modulates the stereospecific activation of cardiac Ca channels by Bay K 8644. *Pflügers Arch.* 417:58-66, **1990.** *[5]*

Tian R, Ingwall JS: Energetic basis for reduced contractile reserve in isolated rat hearts. *Am J Physiol.* 270:H1207-H1216, **1996.** *[10]*

Tian R, Nascimben L, Ingwall JS, Lorell BH: Failure to maintain a low ADP concentration impairs diastolic function in hypertrophied rat hearts. *Circulation.* 96:1313-1319, **1997.** *[10]*

Tian R, Halow JM, Meyer M, Dillmann WH, Figueredo VM, Ingwall JS, Camacho SA: Thermodynamic limitation for Ca^{2+} handling contributes to decreased contractile reserve in rat hearts. *Am J Physiol.* 275:H2064-H2071, **1998.** *[7,10]*

Tibbits GF, Philipson KD: Na^+-dependent alkaline earth metal uptake in cardiac sarcolemmal vesicles. *Biochim Biophys Acta.* 817:327-332, **1985.** *[6]*

Tidball JG, Cederdahl JE, Bers DM: Quantitative analysis of regional variability in the distribution of transverse tubules in rabbit myocardium. *Cell Tissue Res.* 264:293-298, **1991.** *[1]*

Timerman AP, Ogunbumni E, Freund E, Wiederrecht G, Marks AR, Fleischer S: The calcium release channel of sarcoplasmic reticulum is modulated by FK-506-binding protein. Dissociation and reconstitution of FKBP-12 to the calcium release channel of skeletal muscle sarcoplasmic reticulum. *J Biol Chem.* 268:22992-22999, **1993**. *[7]*

Timerman AP, Jayaraman T, Wiederrecht G, Onoue H, Marks AR, Fleischer S: The ryanodine receptor from canine heart sarcoplasmic reticulum is associated with a novel FK-506 binding protein. *Biochem Biophys Res Commun.* 198:701-706, **1994**. *[7]*

Timerman AP, Onoue H, Xin HB, Barg S, Copello J, Wiederrecht G, Fleischer S: Selective binding of FKBP12.6 by the cardiac ryanodine receptor. *J Biol Chem.* 271:20385-20391, **1996**. *[7]*

Tinker A, Williams AJ: Using large organic cations to probe the nature of ryanodine modification in the sheep cardiac sarcoplasmic reticulum calcium release channel. *Biophys J.* 65:1678-1683, **1993**. *[7]*

Tinker A, Williams AJ: Measuring the length of the pore of the sheep cardiac sarcoplasmic reticulum calcium-release channel using related trimethylammonium ions as molecular calipers. *Biophys J.* 68:111-120, **1995**. *[7]*

Tinker A, Lindsay AR, Williams AJ: Cation conduction in the calcium release channel of the cardiac sarcoplasmic reticulum under physiological and pathophysiological conditions. *Cardiovasc Res.* 27:1820-1825, **1993**. *[7]*

Tiwari-Woodruff SK, Schulteis CT, Mock AF, Papazian DM: Electrostatic interactions between transmembrane segments mediate folding of Shaker K+ channel subunits. *Biophys J.* 72:1489-1500, **1997**. *[4]*

Tohse N, Kameyama M, Irisawa H: Intracellular Ca^{2+} and protein kinase C modulate K+ current in guinea pig heart cells. *Am J Physiol.* 253:H1321-H1324, **1987**. *[4]*

Tohse N, Hattori Y, Nakaya H, Endou M, Kanno M: Inability of endothelin to increase Ca^{2+} current in guinea-pig heart cells. *Br J Pharmacol.* 99:437-438, **1990**. *[5]*

Tomita F, Bassett AL, Myerburg RJ, Kimura S: Diminished transient outward currents in rat hypertrophied ventricular myocytes. *Circ Res.* 75:296-303, **1994**. *[4]*

Toyofuku T, Kurzydlowski K, Tada M, MacLennan DH: Identification of regions in the Ca^{2+}-ATPase of sarcoplasmic reticulum that affect functional association with phospholamban. *J Biol Chem.* 268:2809-2815, **1993**. *[7]*

Toyofuku T, Kurzydlowski K, Tada M, MacLennan DH: Amino acids Glu2 to Ile18 in the cytoplasmic domain of phospholamban are essential for functional association with the Ca^{2+}-ATPase of sarcoplasmic reticulum. *J Biol Chem.* 269:3088-3094, **1994a**. *[7]*

Toyofuku T, Kurzydlowski K, Tada M, MacLennan DH: Amino acids Lys-Asp-Asp-Lys-Pro-Val402 in the Ca^{2+}-ATPase of cardiac sarcoplasmic reticulum are critical for functional association with phospholamban. *J Biol Chem.* 269:22929-22932, **1994b**. *[7]*

Toyofuku T, Curotto KK, Narayanan N, MacLennan DH: Identification of Ser38 as the site in cardiac sarcoplasmic reticulum Ca^{2+}-ATPase that is phosphorylated by Ca^{2+}/calmodulin-dependent protein kinase. *J Biol Chem.* 269:26492-26496, **1994c**. *[7]*

Toyoshima C, Nakasako M, Nomura H, Ogawa H: Crystal structure of the calcium pump of sarcoplasmic reticulum at 2.6 Å resolution. *Nature.* 405:647-655, **2000**. *[7]*

Trafford AW, Díaz ME, O'Neill SC, Eisner DA: Comparison of subsarcolemmal and bulk calcium concentration during spontaneous calcium release in rat ventricular myocytes. *J Physiol.* 488:577-586, **1995**. *[6]*

Trafford AW, Díaz ME, Negretti N, Eisner DA: Enhanced Ca^{2+} current and decreased Ca^{2+} efflux restore sarcoplasmic reticulum Ca^{2+} content after depletion. *Circ Res.* 81:477-484, **1997**. *[5,6,7,9]*

Trafford AW, Díaz ME, Eisner DA: Ca-activated chloride current and Na-Ca exchange have different timecourses during sarcoplasmic reticulum Ca release in ferret ventricular myocytes. *Pflügers Arch.* 435:743-745, **1998**. *[4]*

Trafford AW, Díaz ME, Eisner DA: A novel, rapid and reversible method to measure Ca buffering and time-course of total sarcoplasmic reticulum Ca content in cardiac ventricular myocytes. *Pflügers Arch.* 437:501-503, **1999**. *[3,7]*

Trafford AW, Díaz ME, Sibbring GC, Eisner DA: Modulation of CICR has no maintained effect on systolic Ca^{2+}: Simultaneous measurements of sarcoplasmic reticulum and sarcolemmal Ca^{2+} fluxes in rat ventricular myocytes. *J Physiol.* 522:259-270, **2000**. *[9]*

Trimm JL, Salama G, Abramson J: Sulfhydryl oxidation induces rapid calcium release from sarcoplasmic reticulum vesicles. *J Biol Chem.* 261:16092-16098, **1986**. *[7,8]*

Trinick J: Titin and nebulin: Protein rulers in muscle? *Trends Biochem Sci.* 19:405-409, **1994**. *[1]*

Tripathy A, Meissner G: Sarcoplasmic reticulum lumenal Ca^{2+} has access to cytosolic activation and inactivation sites of skeletal muscle Ca^{2+} release channel. *Biophys J.* 70:2600-2615, **1996**. *[7]*

Tripathy A, Xu L, Mann G, Meissner G: Calmodulin activation and inhibition of skeletal muscle Ca^{2+} release channel (ryanodine receptor). *Biophys J.* 69:106-119, **1995**. *[7]*

Tripathy A, Resch W, Xu L, Valdivia HH, Meissner G: Imperatoxin A induces subconductance states in Ca^{2+} release channels (ryanodine receptors) of cardiac and skeletal muscle. *J Gen Physiol.* 111:679-690, **1998**. *[7]*

Trosper TL, Philipson KD: Effects of divalent and trivalent cations on Na^+-Ca^{2+} exchange in cardiac sarcolemmal vesicles. *Biochim Biophys Acta.* 731:63-68, **1983**. *[6]*

Trosper TL, Philipson KD: Stimulatory effect of calcium chelators on Na^+-Ca^{2+} exchange in cardiac sarcolemmal vesicles. *Cell Calcium.* 5:211-222, **1984**. *[6]*

Tse J, Huang MW, Leone RJ, Weiss HR, He YQ, Scholz PM: Down regulation of myocardial β1-adrenoceptor signal transduction system in pacing-induced failure in dogs with aortic stenosis-induced left ventricular hypertrophy. *Mol Cell Biochem.* 205:67-73, **2000**. *[10]*

Tseng GN: Calcium current restitution in mammalian ventricular myocytes is modulated by intracellular calcium. *Circ Res.* 63:468-482, **1988**. *[5,8,9]*

Tseng GN: Cell swelling increases membrane conductance of canine cardiac cells: Evidence for a volume-sensitive Cl channel. *Am J Physiol.* 262:C1056-C1068, **1992**. *[4]*

Tseng GN, Boyden PA: Different effects of intracellular Ca and protein kinase C on cardiac T and L Ca currents. *Am J Physiol.* 261:H364-H379, **1991**. *[5]*

Tsien RW: Adrenaline-like effects of intracellular iontophoresis of cyclic AMP in cardiac Purkinje fibres. *Nature New Biol.* 245:120-122, **1973**. *[5]*

Tsien RW: Cyclic AMP and contractile activity in heart. *Adv Cyclic Nucl Res.* 8:363-420, **1977**. *[10]*

Tsien RW, Giles W, Greengard P: Cyclic AMP mediates the action of adrenaline on the action potential plateau of cardiac Purkinje fibres. *Nature.* 140:181-183, **1972.** *[5]*

Tsien RW, Bean BP, Hess P, Nowycky M: Calcium channels: mechanisms of β-adrenergic modulation and ion permeation. *Cold Spring Harbor Symp Quant Biol.* 48:201-211, **1983.** *[5]*

Tsien RW, Bean BP, Hess P, Lansman JB, Nilius B, Nowycky MC: Mechanisms of calcium channel modulation by β-adrenergic agents and dihydropyridine calcium agonists. *J Mol Cell Cardiol.* 18:691-710, **1986.** *[5,10]*

Tsien RW, Hess P, McCleskey EW, Rosenberg RL: Calcium channels: Mechanisms of selectivity, permeation and block. *Ann Rev Biophys Chem.* 16:265-290, **1987.** *[4,5]*

Tsugorka A, Ríos E, Blatter LA: Imaging elementary events of calcium release in skeletal muscle cells. *Science.* 269:1723-1726, **1995.** *[8]*

Tu Q, Vélez P, Brodwick M, Fill M: Streaming potentials reveal a short ryanodine-sensitive selectivity filter in cardiac Ca^{2+} release channel. *Biophys J.* 67:2280-2285, **1994.** *[7]*

Tyska MJ, Dupuis DE, Guilford WH, Patlak JB, Waller GS, Trybus KM, Warshaw DM, Lowey S: Two heads of myosin are better than one for generating force and motion. *Proc Natl Acad Sci USA.* 96:4402-4407, **1999.** *[2]*

Undrovinas AI, Fleidervish IA, Makielski JC: Inward sodium current at resting potentials in single cardiac myocytes induced by the ischemic metabolite lysophosphatidylcholine. *Circ Res.* 71:1231-1241, **1992.** *[4,10]*

Undrovinas AI, Maltsev VA, Sabbah HN: Repolarization abnormalities in cardiomyocytes of dogs with chronic heart failure: Role of sustained inward current. *Cell Mol Life Sci.* 55:494-505, **1998.** *[10]*

Unwin PNT, Zampighi G: Structure of the junction between communicating cells. *Nature.* 283:545-549, **1980.** *[1]*

Vaghy PL, Striessnig J, Miwa K, Knaus HG, Itagaki K, McKenna E, Glossmann H, Schwartz A: Identification of a novel 1,4-dihydrodpyridine- and phenylalkylamine-binding polypeptide in calcium channel preparations. *J Biol Chem.* 262:14337-14342, **1987.** *[5]*

Valdeolmillos M, O'Neill SC, Smith GL, Eisner DA: Calcium-induced calcium release activates contraction in intact cardiac cells. *Pflügers Arch.* 413:676-678, **1989.** *[8]*

Valdivia HH: Modulation of intracellular Ca^{2+} levels in the heart by sorcin and FKBP12, two accessory proteins of ryanodine receptors. *Trends Pharmacol Sci.* 19:479-482, **1998.** *[7]*

Valdivia HH, Coronado R: Pharmacological profile of skeletal muscle calcium channels in lipid bilayers. *Biophys J.* 53:555a, **1988.** *[5]*

Valdivia HH, Kirby MS, Lederer WJ, Coronado R: Scorpion toxins targeted against the sarcoplasmic reticulum Ca^{2+}-release channel of skeletal and cardiac muscle. *Proc Natl Acad Sci USA.* 89:12185-12189, **1992.** *[7]*

Valdivia HH, Kaplan JH, Ellis-Davies GCR, Lederer WJ: Rapid adaptation of cardiac ryanodine receptors: Modulation by Mg^{2+} and phosphorylation. *Science.* 267:1997-2000, **1995.** *[7,10]*

van Amsterdam FTHM, Zaagsma J: Modulation of ATP-dependent calcium extrusion and sodium-calcium exchange across rat cardiac sarcolemma by calcium antagonists. *Eur J Pharmacol.* 123:441-449, **1986.** *[6]*

van Breemen C, Saida K: Cellular mechanisms regulating $[Ca^{2+}]_i$ in smooth muscle. *Annu Rev Physiol.* 51:315-329, **1989.** *[8]*

van Breemen C, Chen Q, Laher I: Superficial buffer barrier function of smooth muscle sarcoplasmic reticulum. *Trends Pharmacol Sci.* 16:98-105, **1995.** *[8]*

van Eyk JE, Powers F, Law W, Larue C, Hedges RS, Solaro RJ: Breakdown and release of myofilament proteins during ischemia and ischemia/reperfusion in rat hearts - Identification of degradation products and effects on the pCa-force relation. *Circ Res.* 82:261-271, **1998.** *[10]*

van Wagoner DR: Mechanosensitive gating of atrial ATP-sensitive potassium channels. *Circ Res.* 72:973-983, **1993.** *[4]*

van Winkle WB: Calcium release from skeletal muscle sarcoplasmic reticulum: Site of action of dantrolene sodium? *Science.* 193:1130-1131, **1976.** *[7]*

van Wylen DG, Willis J, Sodhi J, Weiss R, Lasley RD, Mentzer RM: Cardiac microdialysis to estimate interstitial adenosine and coronary bloow flow. *Am J Physiol.* 258:H1642-H1649, **1990.** *[10]*

Vandenberg CA: Inward rectification of a potassium channel in cardiac ventricular cells depends on internal magnesium ions. *Proc Natl Acad Sci USA.* 84:2560-2564, **1987.** *[4]*

Vandenberg JI, Yoshida A, Kirk K, Powell T: Swelling-activated and isoprenaline-activated chloride currents in guinea pig cardiac myocytes have distinct electrophysiology and pharmacology. *J Gen Physiol.* 104:997-1017, **1994.** *[4]*

Vandenberg JI, Bett GCL, Powell T: Contribution of a swelling-activated chloride current to changes in the cardiac action potential. *Am J Physiol.* 273:C541-C547, **1997.** *[4]*

Vannier C, Lakomkine V, Vassort G: Tension response of the cardiotonic agent (+)-EMD-57033 at the single cell level. *Am J Physiol.* 272:C1586-C1593, **1997.** *[2]*

Varadi G, Strobeck M, Koch S, Caglioti L, Zucchi C, Palyi G: Molecular elements of ion permeation and selectivity within calcium channels. *Crit Rev Biochem Mol Biol.* 34:181-214, **1999.** *[5]*

Varghese P, Harrison RW, Lofthouse RA, Georgakopoulos D, Berkowitz DE, Hare JM: β3-Adrenoceptor deficiency blocks nitric oxide-dependent inhibition of myocardial contractility. *J Clin Invest.* 106:697-703, **2000.** *[10]*

Varnum MD, Busch AE, Bond CT, Maylie J, Adelman JP: The min K channel underlies the cardiac potassium current I_{Ks} and mediates species-specific responses to protein kinase C. *Proc Natl Acad Sci USA.* 90:11528-11532, **1993.** *[4]*

Varro A, Negretti N, Hester SB, Eisner DA: An estimate of the calcium content of the sarcoplasmic reticulum in rat ventricular myocytes. *Pflügers Arch.* 423:158-160, **1993.** *[3,7]*

Varsanyi M, Messer M, Brandt NR: Intracellular localization of inositol-phospholipid-metabolizing enzymes in rabbit fast-twitch muscle. *Eur J Biochem.* 179:473-479, **1989.** *[8]*

Vassalle M: The pacemaker current (I_f) does not play an important role in regulating SA node pacemaker activity. *Cardiovasc Res.* 30:309-310, **1995.** *[4]*

Vassort G: Influence of sodium ions on the regulation of frog myocardiac contractility. *Pflügers Arch.* 339:225-246, **1973.** *[8]*

Vatner DE, Lee DL, Schwarz KR, Longabaugh JP, Fujii AM, Vatner SF, Homcy CJ: Impaired cardiac muscarinic receptor function in dogs with heart failure. *J Clin Invest.* 81:1836-1842, **1988.** *[10]*

Vatner DE, Sato N, Kiuchi K, Shannon RP, Vatner SF: Decrease in myocardial ryanodine receptors and altered excitation-contraction coupling early in the development of heart failure. *Circulation.* 90:1423-1430, **1994**. *[10]*

Vaughan-Jones RD: Chloride-bicarbonate exchange in the sheep cardiac purkinje fiber, in Intracellular pH, its Measurement, Regulation and Utilization in Cellular Functions. *New York, NY, Alan R. Liss, Inc.* 239-252, **1982**. *[10]*

Vaughan-Jones RD, Lederer WJ, Eisner DA: Ca^{2+} ions can affect intracellular pH in mammalian cardiac muscle. *Nature.* 301:522-524, **1983**. *[3,10]*

Veldkamp MW, Van Ginneken ACG, Bouman LN: Single delayed rectifier channels in the membrane of rabbit ventricular myocytes. *Circ Res.* 72:865-878, **1993**. *[4]*

Vemuri R, Philipson KD: Phospholipid composition modulates the Na^+-Ca^{2+} exchange activity of cardiac sarcolemma in reconstituted vesicles. *Biochim Biophys Acta.* 937:258-268, **1988a**. *[6]*

Vemuri R, Philipson KD: Protein methylation inhibits Na^+-Ca^{2+} exchange activity in cardiac sarcolemmal vesicles. *Biochim Biophys Acta.* 939:503-508, **1988b**. *[6]*

Venosa RA, Horowicz P: Density and apparent location of the sodium pump in frog sartorius muscle. *J Memb Biol.* 59:225-232, **1981**. *[1]*

Verboomen H, Wuytack F, van den Bosch L, Mertens L, Casteels R: The functional importance of the extreme C-terminal tail in the gene 2 organellar Ca^{2+}-transport ATPase (SERCA2a/b). *Biochem J.* 303:979-984, **1994**. *[7]*

Vercesi A, Reynafarje B, Lehninger AL: Stoichiometry of H^+ ejection and Ca^{2+} uptake coupled to electron transfer in rat heart mitochondria. *J Biol Chem.* 253:6379-6385, **1978**. *[3]*

Verdonck F, Volders PGA, Vos MA, Sipido KR: Cardiac hypertrophy is associated with an increase in subsarcolemmal Na^+. *Biophys J.* 80: 598A, **2001**. *[10]*

Vergara J, Tsien RW, Delay M: Inositol 1,4,5-triphosphate: A possible chemical link in excitation-contraction coupling in muscle. *Proc Natl Acad Sci USA.* 82:6352-6356, **1985**. *[8]*

Vergara J, Astora K, Delay M: A chemical link in excitation-contraction coupling in skeletal muscle, in Cell Calcium and Control of Membrane Transport. Mandel LJ, Eaton DC (eds). *New York, NY, Rockefeller University Press.* 133-151, **1987**. *[7]*

Verjovski-Almeida S, Inesi G: Fast-kinetic evidence for an activating effect of ATP on the Ca^{2+} transport of sarcoplasmic reticulum ATPase. *J Biol Chem.* 254:18-21, **1979**. *[7]*

Verma AK, Filoteo A, Stanford DR, Wieben ED, Penniston JT, Strehler EE, Fischer R, Heim R, Vogel G, Mathews S, Strehler-Page MA, James P, Vorherr T, Krebbs J, Carafoli E: Complete primary structure of a human plasma membrane Ca^{2+} pump. *J Biol Chem.* 263:14152-14159, **1988**. *[6]*

Vermeulen JT, McGuire MA, Opthof T, Coronel R, de Bakker JM, Klopping C, Janse MJ: Triggered activity and automaticity in ventricular trabeculae of failing human and rabbit hearts. *Cardiovasc Res.* 28:1547-1554, **1994**. *[10]*

Vites AM, Pappano A: Inositol 1,4,5-trisphosphate releases intracellular Ca^{2+} in permeabilized chick atria. *Am J Physiol.* 258:H1745-H1752, **1990**. *[8]*

Vites AM, Wasserstrom JA: Fast sodium influx provides an initial step to trigger contractions in cat ventricle. *Am J Physiol.* 271:H674-H686, **1996**. *[8]*

Vittone L, Mundina C, Chiappe de Cingolani G, Mattiazzi A: Role of Ca^{2+}-calmodulin dependent phospholamban phosphorylation on the relaxant effect of β-adrenergic agonists. *Mol Cell Biochem.* 124:33-42, **1993**. *[7]*

Vittone L, Mundiña-Weilenmann C, Said M, Mattiazzi A: Mechanisms involved in the acidosis enhancement of the isoproterenol-induced phosphorylation of phospholamban in the intact heart. *J Biol Chem.* 273:9804-9811, **1998**. *[7,10]*

Vogel S, Sperelakis N: Induction of slow action potentials by microiontophoresis of cyclic AMP into heart cells. *J Mol Cell Cardiol.* 13:51-64, **1981**. *[5]*

Volders PG, Sipido KR, Vos MA, Spatjens RL, Leunissen JD, Carmeliet E, Wellens HJ: Downregulation of delayed rectifier K^+ currents in dogs with chronic complete atrioventricular block and acquired torsades de pointes. *Circulation.* 100:2455-2461, **1999**. *[10]*

Volpe P, Stephenson EW: Ca^{2+} dependence of transverse tubule-mediated calcium release in skinned skeletal muscle fibers. *J Gen Physiol.* 87:271-288, **1986**. *[8]*

Volpe P, Salviati G, Di Virgilio F, Pozzan T: Inositol 1,4,5-triphosphate induces calcium release from sarcoplasmic reticulum of skeletal muscle. *Nature.* 316:347-349, **1985**. *[7,8]*

Volpe P, Di Virgilio F, Pozzan T, Salviati G: Role of inositol-1,4,5-trisphosphate in excitation-contraction-coupling in skeletal muscle. *FEBS Lett.* 197:1-4, **1986**. *[8]*

von der Leyen H, Colberg H, Meyer W, Scholz H, Wenzlaff H: Phosphodiesterase III inhibition by new cardiotonic agents in failing human heart. *Arch Pharmacol.* 338:R40, **1988**. *[10]*

von Wilbrandt W, Koller H: Die Calciumwirkung am Froschherzen als Funktion des lonengleichgewichts zwischen Zellmembran und Umgebung. *Helv Physiol Pharmacol Acta.* 6:208-221, **1948**. *[6]*

Wagenknecht T, Radermacher M: Three-dimensional architecture of the skeletal muscle ryanodine receptor. *FEBS Lett.* 369:43-46, **1995**. *[1]*

Wagenknecht T, Grassucci R, Frank J, Saito A, Inui M, Fleischer S: Three-dimensional architecture of the calcium channel/foot structure of sarcoplasmic reticulum. *Nature.* 338:167-170, **1989**. *[1,7]*

Wagenknecht T, Berkowitz J, Grassucci R, Timerman AP, Fleischer S: Localization of calmodulin binding sites on the ryanodine receptor from skeletal muscle by electron microscopy. *Biophys J.* 67:2286-2295, **1994**. *[1,7]*

Wagenknecht T, Grassucci R, Berkowitz J, Wiederrecht GJ, Xin HB, Fleischer S: Cryoelectron microscopy resolves FK506-binding protein sites on the skeletal muscle ryanodine receptor. *Biophys J.* 70:1709-1715, **1996**. *[7]*

Wagenknecht T, Radermacher M, Grassucci R, Berkowitz J, Xin HB, Fleischer S: Locations of calmodulin and FK506-binding protein on the three-dimensional architecture of the skeletal muscle ryanodine receptor. *J Biol Chem.* 272:32463-32471, **1997**. *[7]*

Wahler GM, Sperelakis N: Intracellular injection of cyclic GMP depresses cardiac slow action potentials. *J Cyclic Nucl Prot Phosphor Res.* 10:83-95, **1985**. *[5]*

Wahler GM, Rusch NJ, Sperelakis N: 8-Bromo-cyclic GMP inhibits the calcium channel current in embryonic chick ventricular myocytes. *Can J Physiol Pharmacol.* 68:531-534, **1990**. *[5]*

Wahler GM, Dollinger SJ: Nitric oxide donor SIN-1 inhibits mammalian cardiac calcium current through cGMP-dependent protein kinase. *Am J Physiol.* 268:C45-C54, **1995**. *[10]*

Walker JW, Somlyo AV, Goldman YE, Somlyo AP, Trentham DR: Kinetics of smooth and skeletal muscle activation by laser pulse photolysis of caged inositol 1,4,5-triphosphate. *Nature.* 327:249-252, **1987**. *[7,8]*

Wallert MA, Fröhlich O: Na^+-H^+ exchange in isolated myocytes from adult rat heart. *Am J Physiol.* 257:C207-C213, **1989**. *[3]*

Wallert MA, Fröhlich O: α_1-Adrenergic stimulation of Na-H exchange in cardiac myocytes. *Am J Physiol.* 263:C1096-C1102, **1992**. *[10]*

Walseth TF, Aarhus R, Zeleznikar RJ Jr, Lee HC: Determination of endogenous levels of cyclic ADP-ribose in rat tissues. *Biochim Biophys Acta.* 1094:113-120, **1991**. *[7]*

Walsh KB, Kass RS: Regulation of a heart potassium channel by protein kinase A and C. *Science.* 242:67-69, **1988**. *[4,5,10]*

Walsh KB, Kass RS: Distinct voltage-dependent regulation of a heart-delayed k by protein kinases A and C. *Am J Physiol.* 261:C1081-C1090, **1991**. *[4,10]*

Walsh M, Bridenbaugh R, Kerrick WG, Hartshorne D: Gizzard Ca-dependent myosin light chain kinase: evidence in favor of the phosphorylation theory. *Fed Proc.* 42:45-50, **1983**. *[2]*

Wang J, Best PM: Inactivation of the sarcoplasmic reticulum calcium channel by protein kinase. *Nature.* 359:739-741, **1992**. *[7]*

Wang YP, Fuchs F: Length, force, and Ca^{2+}-troponin C affinity in cardiac and slow skeletal muscle. *Am J Physiol.* 266:C1077-C1082, **1994**. *[2]*

Wang YP, Fuchs F: Osmotic compression of skinned cardiac and skeletal muscle bundles: Effects on force generation, Ca^{2+} sensitivity and Ca^{2+} binding. *J Mol Cell Cardiol.* 27:1235-1244, **1995**. *[2]*

Wang YG, Lipsius SL: Acetylcholine activates a glibenclamide-sensitive K^+ current in cat atrial myocytes. *Am J Physiol.* 268:H1322-H1334, **1995a**. *[4]*

Wang YG, Lipsius SL: Acetylcholine elicits a rebound stimulation of Ca^{2+} current mediated by pertussis toxin-sensitive G protein and cAMP-dependent protein kinase A in atrial myocytes. *Circ Res.* 76:634-644, **1995b**. *[5]*

Wang YG, Lipsius SL: A cellular mechanism contributing to postvagal tachycardia studied in isolated pacemaker cells from cat right atrium. *Circ Res.* 79:109-114, **1996**. *[5]*

Wang YG, Lipsius SL: Genistein elicits biphasic effects on L-type Ca^{2+} current in feline atrial myocytes *Am J Physiol.* 275:H204-H212, **1998**. *[5]*

Wang K, Wright LC, Madian CL, Allen BG, Conigrave AD, Roufogalis BD: Protein kinase C phosphorylates the carboxyl terminus of the plasma membrane Ca^{2+}-ATPase from human erythrocytes. *J Biol Chem.* 266:9078-9085, **1991**. *[6]*

Wang Z, Fermini B, Nattel S: Sustained depolarization-induced outward current in human atrial myocytes: evidence for a novel delayed rectifier K^+ current similar to Kv1.5 cloned channel currents. *Circ Res.* 73:1061-1076, **1993a**. *[4]*

Wang Z, Fermini B, Nattel S: Delayed rectifier outward current and repolarization in human atrial myocytes. *Circ Res.* 73:276-285, **1993b**. *[4]*

Wang Q, Shen JX, Li ZZ, Timothy K, Vincent GM, Priori SG, Schwartz PJ, Keating MT: Cardiac sodium channel mutations in patients with long QT syndrome, an inherited cardiac arrhythmia. *Hum Mol Genet.* 4:1603-1607, **1995a**. *[4]*

Wang SY, Clague JR, Langer GA: Increase in calcium leak channel activity by metabolic inhibition or hydrogen peroxide in rat ventricular myocytes and its inhibition by polycation. *J Mol Cell Cardiol.* 27:211-222, **1995b**. *[10]*

Wang DW, Yazawa K, George AL Jr, Bennett PB: Characterization of human cardiac Na^+ channel mutations in the congenital long QT syndrome. *Proc Natl Acad Sci USA.* 93:13200-13205, **1996a**. *[4]*

Wang Q, Curran ME, Splawski I, Burn TC, Millholland JM, VanRaay TJ, Shen J, Timothy KW, Vincent GM, de Jager T, Schwartz PJ, Toubin JA, Moss AJ, Atkinson DL, Landes GM, Connors TD, Keating MT: Positional cloning of a novel potassium channel gene: KVLQT1 mutations cause cardiac arrhythmias. *Nat Genet.* 12:17-23, **1996b**. *[4]*

Wang JN, Schwinger RHG, Frank K, Müller-Ehmsen J, Martin-Vasallo P, Pressley TA, Xiang A, Erdmann E, McDonough AA: Regional expression of sodium pump subunit isoforms and Na^+-Ca^{2+} exchanger in the human heart. *J Clin Invest.* 98:1650-1658, **1996c**. *[4]*

Wang Y, Gao J, Mathias RT, Cohen IS, Sun X, Baldo GJ: α-adrenergic effects on Na^+-K^+ pump current in guinea-pig ventricular myocytes. *J Physiol.* 509:117-128, **1998a**. *[4]*

Wang S, Trumble WR, Liao H, Wesson CR, Dunker AK, Kang CH: Crystal structure of calsequestrin from rabbit skeletal muscle sarcoplasmic reticulum. *Nat Struct Biol.* 5:476-483, **1998b**. *[7]*

Wang ZG, Feng JL, Shi H, Pond A, Nerbonne JM, Nattel S: Potential molecular basis of different physiological properties of the transient outward K^+ current in rabbit and human atrial myocytes. *Circ Res.* 84:551-561, **1999**. *[4]*

Warber KD, Potter JD: Contractile proteins and phosphorylation, in The Heart and Cardiovascular System. Fozzard HA (ed). *New York, NY, Raven Press.* 779-788, **1986**. *[2]*

Ward CW, Schneider MF, Castillo D, Protasi F, Wang YM, Chen SRW, Allen PD: Expression of ryanodine receptor RyR3 produces Ca^{2+} sparks in dyspedic myotubes. *J Physiol.* 525:91-103, **2000**. *[8]*

Warshaw DM: The in vitro motility assay: A window into the myosin molecular motor. *News Physiol Sci.* 11:1-7, **1996**. *[2]*

Wasserstrom JA, Vites AM: The role of Na^+-Ca^{2+} exchange in activation of excitation-contraction coupling in rat ventricular myocytes. *J Physiol.* 493:529-542, **1996**. *[8]*

Wasserstrom JA, Schwartz DJ, Fozzard HA: Catecholamine effects on intracellular sodium activity and tension in dog heart. *Am J Physiol.* 243:H670-H675, **1982**. *[10]*

Wasserstrom JA, Schwartz DJ, Fozzard HA: Relation between intracellular sodium and twitch tension in sheep cardiac Purkinje strands exposed to cardiac glycosides. *Circ Res.* 52:697-705, **1983**. *[10]*

Watanabe AM, Jones LR, Manalan AS, Besch HR Jr: Cardiac autonomic receptors: Recent concepts from radiolabelled ligand studies. *Circ Res.* 50:161-174, **1982**. *[10]*

Watano T, Kimura J: Calcium-dependent inhibition of the sodium-calcium exchange current by KB-R7943. *Can J Cardiol.* 14:259-262, **1998**. *[6]*

Watano T, Kimura J, Morita T, Nakanishi H: A novel antagonist, No 7943, of the Na^+/Ca^{2+} exchange current in guinea-pig cardiac ventricular cells. *Br J Pharmacol.* 119:555-563, **1996**. *[6]*

Watras J, Benevolensky D: Inositol 1,4,5-triphosphate-induced calcium release from canine aortic sarcoplasmic reticulum vesicles. *Biochim Biophys Acta.* 931:354-363, **1987**. *[8]*

Wattanapermpool J, Reiser PJ, Solaro RJ: Troponin I isoforms and differential effects of acidic pH on soleus and cardiac myofilaments. *Am J Physiol.* 268:C323-C330, **1995a**. *[2]*

Wattanapermpool J, Guo X, Solaro RJ: The unique amino-terminal peptide of cardiac troponin I regulates myofibrillar activity only when it is phosphorylated. *J Mol Cell Cardiol.* 27:1383-1391, **1995b**. *[2]*

Weber A, Herz R: The relationship between caffeine contracture of intact muscle and the effect of caffeine on reticulum. *J Gen Physiol.* 52:750-759, **1968**. *[9]*

Weber CR, Ginsburg KS, Philipson KD, Shannon TR, Bers DM. Allosteric regulation of Na/Ca exchange current by cytosolic Ca in intact cardiac myocytes. *J Gen Physiol.* 117:119-131, **2001**. *[6]*

Wegener AD, Simmerman HKB, Lindemann JP, Jones LR: Phospholamban phosphorylation in intact ventricles. Phosphorylation of serine 16 and threonine 17 in response to β-adrenergic stimulation. *J Biol Chem.* 264:11468-11474, **1989**. *[7]*

Wei XY, Pan S, Lang WH, Kim HY, Schneider T, Perez-Reyes E, Birnbaumer L: Molecular determinants of cardiac Ca^{2+} channel pharmacology - Subunit requirement for the high affinity and allosteric regulation of dihydropyridine binding. *J Biol Chem.* 270:27106-27111, **1995**. *[5]*

Weingart R: The actions of ouabain on intercellular coupling and conduction velocity in mammalian ventricular muscle. *J Physiol.* 264:341-365, **1977**. *[1]*

Weingart R, Hess P: Free calcium in sheep cardiac tissue and frog skeletal muscle measured with Ca^{2+}-selective microelectrodes. *Pflügers Arch.* 402:1-9, **1984**. *[10]*

Weisberg A, Winegrad S: Alteration of myosin cross bridges by phosphorylation of myosin-binding protein C in cardiac muscle. *Proc Natl Acad Sci USA.* 93:8999-9003, **1996**. *[2]*

Weishaar RE, Kobylarz-Singer DC, Quade MM, Steffen RP, Kaplan HR: Role of cyclic AMP in regulating cardiac muscle contractility: Novel pharmacological approaches to modulating cyclic AMP degradation by phosphodiesterase. *Drug Develop Res.* 12:119-129, **1988**. *[10]*

Weiss JN: Ion Channels in Cardiac Muscle, in <u>The Myocardium</u>. Langer GA (ed). 2nd ed. *San Diego, CA, Academic Press.* 81-142, **1997**. *[4]*

Weiss JN, Lamp ST: Glycolysis preferentially inhibits ATP-sensitive K^+ channels in isolated guinea pig cardiac myocytes. *Science.* 238:67-69, **1987**. *[10]*

Weiss JN, Lamp ST: Cardiac ATP-sensitive K^+ channels. Evidence for preferential regulation by glycolysis. *J Gen Physiol.* 94:911-935, **1989**. *[4,10]*

Weiss J, Couper GS, Hiltbrand B, Shine KI: Role of acidosis in early contractile dysfunction during ischemia: Evidence from pH_o measurements. *Am J Physiol.* 247:H760-H767, **1984**. *[2]*

Weiss JN, Venkatesh N, Lamp ST: ATP-sensitive K^+ channels and cellular K^+ loss in hypoxic and ischaemic mammalian ventricle. *J Physiol.* 447:649-673, **1992**. *[4,10]*

Weiss JN, Garfinkel A, Karagueuzian HS, Qu Z, Chen PS: Chaos and the transition to ventricular fibrillation: a new approach to antiarrhythmic drug evaluation. *Circulation.* 99:2819-2826, **1999**. *[4]*

Wendt IR, Stephenson DG: Effects of caffeine on Ca-activated force production in skinned cardiac and skeletal muscle fibres of the rat. *Pflügers Arch.* 398:210-216, **1983**. *[2,7,9]*

Wendt-Gallitelli MS, Isenberg G: X-ray microanalysis of single cardiac myocytes frozen under voltage-clamp conditions. *Am J Physiol.* 256:H574-H583, **1989**. *[7]*

Werns SW, Shea MJ, Driscoll EM, Cohen C, Abrams GD, Pitt B, Lucchesi BR: The independent effects of oxygen radical scavengers on canine infarct size. Reduction by superoxide dismutase but not catalase. *Circ Res.* 56:895-898, **1985**. *[10]*

West GA, Isenberg G, Belardinelli L: Antagonism of forskolin effects of adenosine in isolated hearts and ventricular myocytes. *Am J Physiol.* 250:H769-H777, **1986**. *[5]*

West JW, Patton DE, Scheuer T, Wang Y, Goldin AL, Catterall WA: A cluster of hydrophobic amino acid residues required for fast Na^+-channel inactivation. *Proc Natl Acad Sci USA.* 89:10910-10914, **1992**. *[4]*

Westfall MV, Solaro RJ: Alterations in myofibrillar function and protein profiles after complete global ischemia in rat hearts. *Circ Res.* 70:302-313, **1992**. *[10]*

Wettwer E, Amos GJ, Posival H, Ravens U: Transient outward current in human ventricular myocytes of subepicardial and subendocardial origin. *Circ Res.* 75:473-482, **1994**. *[10]*

Wetzel GT, Chen F, Klitzner TS: L- and T-type calcium channels in acutely isolated neonatal and adult cardiac myocytes. *Pediatr Res.* 30:89-94, **1991**. *[9]*

Wetzel GT, Chen F, Klitzner TS: Ca^{2+} channel kinetics in acutely isolated fetal, neonatal, and adult rabbit cardiac myocytes. *Circ Res.* 72:1065-1074, **1993**. *[9]*

Wetzel GT, Chen F, Klitzner TS: Na^+/Ca^{2+} exchange and cell contraction in isolated neonatal and adult rabbit cardiac myocytes. *Am J Physiol.* 268: H1723-H1733, **1995**. *[9]*

Wheeler-Clark ES, Tormey JMD: Electron probe X-ray microanalysis of sarcolemma and junctional sarcoplasmic reticulum in rabbit papillary muscles: low sodium-induced calcium alterations. *Circ Res.* 60:246-250, **1987**. *[7]*

White J, Lee JA, Shah N, Orchard CH: Differential effects of the optical isomers of EMD 53998 on contraction and cytoplasmic Ca^{2+} in isolated ferret cardiac muscle. *Circ Res.* 73:61-70, **1993**. *[2,10]*

Wibo M, Godfraind T: Comparative localization of inositol 1,4,5-trisphosphate and ryanodine receptors in intestinal smooth muscle: An analytical subfractionation study. *Biochem J.* 297:415-423, **1994**. *[8]*

Wibo M, Bravo G, Godfraind T: Postnatal maturation of excitation-contraction coupling in rat ventricle in relation to the subcellular localization and surface density of 1,4-dihydropyridine and ryanodine receptors. *Circ Res.* 68:662-673, **1991**. *[1]*

Wickenden AD, Kaprielian R, Parker TG, Jones OT, Backx PH: Effects of development and thyroid hormone on K^+ currents and K^+ channel gene expression in rat ventricle. *J Physiol.* 504:271-286, **1997**. *[4]*

Wickenden AD, Kaprielian R, Kassiri Z, Tsoporis JN, Tsushima R, Fishman GI, Backx PH: The role of action potential prolongation and altered intracellular calcium handling in the pathogenesis of heart failure. *Cardiovasc Res.* 37:312-323, **1998**. *[10]*

Wickman K, Clapham DE: Ion channel regulation by G proteins. *Physiol Rev.* 75:865-885, **1995**. *[4]*

Wickman K, Nemec J, Gendler SJ, Clapham DE: Abnormal heart rate regulation in GIRK4 knockout mice. *Neuron.* 20:103-114, **1998**. *[4]*

Wier WG, Balke CW: Ca²⁺ release mechanisms, Ca²⁺ sparks, and local control of excitation-contraction coupling in normal heart muscle. *Circ Res.* 85:770-776, **1999**. *[8]*

Wier WG, Hess P: Excitation-contraction coupling in cardiac Purkinje Fibers. Effects of cardiotonic steroids on the intracellular [Ca²⁺] transient, membrane potential, and contraction. *J Gen Physiol.* 83:395-415, **1984**. *[10]*

Wier WG, Yue DT: Intracellular calcium transients underlying the short-term force-interval relationship in ferret ventricular myocardium. *J Physiol.* 376:507-530, **1986**. *[8]*

Wier WG, Kort AA, Stern MD, Lakatta EG, Marbán E: Cellular calcium fluctuations in mammalian heart: direct evidence from noise analysis of aequorin signals in Purkinje fibers. *Proc Natl Acad Sci USA.* 80:7367-7371, **1983**. *[8]*

Wier WG, Egan TM, López-López JR, Balke CW: Local control of excitation-contraction coupling in rat heart cells. *J Physiol.* 474:463-471, **1994**. *[3,7,8]*

Wier WG, ter Keurs HEDJ, Marbán E, Gao WD, Balke CW : Ca²⁺ 'sparks' and waves in intact ventricular muscle resolved by confocal imaging. *Circ Res.* 81:462-469, **1997**. *[10]*

Williams AJ: Ryanodine Receptor Ion Conduction and Selectivity, in <u>The Structure and Function of Ryanodine Receptors</u>. Sitsapesan R, Williams AJ (eds). *London, UK, Imperial College Press.* 75-93, **1998**. *[7]*

Williams AJ, Holmberg SRM: Sulmazole (AR-L 115BS) activates the sheep cardiac muscle sarcoplasmic reticulum calcium-release channel in the presence and absence of calcium. *J Memb Biol.* 115:167-178, **1990**. *[7,10]*

Williams JS, Grupp IL, Grupp G, Vaghy PL, Dumont L, Schwartz A: Profile of the oppositely acting enantiomers of the dihydropyridine 202-791 in cardiac preparations: receptor binding, electrophysiological, and pharmacological studies. *Biochem Biophys Res Commun.* 131:13-21, **1985**. *[5]*

Williams ME, Feldman DH, McCue AF, Brenner R, Velicelebi G, Ellis SB, Harpold MM: Structure and functional expression of α₁, α₂, and β- subunits of a novel human neuronal calcium channel subtype. *Neuron.* 8:71-84, **1992**. *[5]*

Williamson AP, Seifen E, Lindemann JP, Kennedy RH: The positive inotropic effect of α₁A-adrenoceptor stimulation is inhibited by 4-aminopyridine. *Eur J Pharmacol.* 304:73-80, **1996**. *[10]*

Wilson DL, Morimoto K, Tsuda Y, Brown AM: Interaction between calcium ions and surface charge as it relates to calcium currents. *J Memb Biol.* 72:117-130, **1983**. *[5]*

Wimsatt DK, Hohl CM, Brierly GP, Altschuld RA: Calcium accumulation and release by the sarcoplasmic reticulum of digitonin-lysed adult mammalian ventricular cardiomyocytes. *J Biol Chem.* 265:14849-14875, **1990**. *[7]*

Winegrad S: Autoradiographic studies of intracellular calcium in frog skeletal muscle. *J Gen Physiol.* 48:455-479, **1965**. *[1]*

Winegrad S: Cardiac myosin binding protein C. *Circ Res.* 84:1117-1126, **1999**. *[2]*

Winfree A: Spiral waves of chemical activity. *Science.* 175:634-636, **1972**. *[4]*

Winslow RL, Rice J, Jafri S, Marbán E, O'Rourke B: Mechanisms of altered excitation-contraction coupling in canine tachycardia-induced heart failure, II: Model studies. *Circ Res.* 84:571-586, **1999**. *[4]*

Wit AL, Rosen MR: Afterdepolarizations and triggered activity: Distinction from automaticity as an arrhythmogenic mechanism, in <u>Heart and Cardiovascular System: Scientific Foundations</u>. Fozzard HA, Habert E, Jennings RB, Katz AM, Morgan HE (eds). 2ⁿᵈ ed. *New York, NY, Raven Press.* 2113-2163, **1992**. *[10]*

Witcher DR, Kovacs RJ, Schulman H, Cefali DC, Jones LR: Unique phosphorylation site on the cardiac ryanodine receptor regulates calcium channel activity. *J Biol Chem.* 266:11144-11152, **1991**. *[7]*

Withering W: <u>An Account of the Foxglove, and some of its Medicinal Uses: With Practical Remarks on Dropsy and other Diseases.</u> *London, UK, G.G.J. & J. Robinson.* **1785**. *[10]*

Wohlfart B: Relationship between peak force, action potential duration and stimulus interval in rabbit myocardium. *Acta Physiol Scand.* 106:395-409, **1979**. *[8]*

Wohlfart B: Analysis of mechanical alternans in rabbit papillary muscle. *Acta Physiol Scand.* 115:405-414, **1982**. *[9]*

Wohlfart B, Noble MIM: The cardiac excitation-contraction cycle. *Pharmacol Ther.* 16:1-43, **1982**. *[9]*

Wolff MR, McDonald KS, Moss RL: Rate of tension development in cardiac muscle varies with level of activator calcium. *Circ Res.* 76:154-160, **1995a**. *[2]*

Wolff MR, Whitesell LF, Moss RL: Calcium sensitivity of isometric tension is increased in canine experimental heart failure. *Circ Res.* 76:781-789, **1995b**. *[10]*

Wolff MR, Buck SH, Stoker SW, Greaser ML, Mentzer RM: Myofibrillar calcium sensitivity of isometric tension is increased in human dilated cardiomyopathies - Role of altered β-adrenergically mediated protein phosphorylation. *J Clin Invest.* 98:167-176, **1996**. *[10]*

Wolff DW, Dang HK, Liu MF, Jeffries WB, Scofield MA: Distribution of α₁-adrenergic receptor mRNA species in rat heart. *J Cardiovasc Pharmacol.* 32:117-122, **1998**. *[10]*

Wolska BM, Kitada Y, Palmiter KA, Westfall MV, Johnson MD, Solaro RJ: CGP-48506 increases contractility of ventricular myocytes and myofilaments by effects on actin-myosin reaction. *Am J Physiol.* 270:H24-H32, **1996a**. *[2,10]*

Wolska BM, Stojanovic MO, Luo W, Kranias EG, Solaro RJ: Effect of ablation of phospholamban on dynamics of cardiac myocyte contraction and intracellular Ca²⁺. *Am J Physiol.* 271:C391-C397, **1996b**. *[10]*

Wood EH, Heppner RL, Weidman S: Inotropic effects of electric currents. *Circ Res.* 24:409-445, **1969**. *[9]*

Woodworth RS: Maximal contraction, "staircase" contraction, refractory period, and compensatory pause, of the heart. *Am J Physiol.* 8:213-249, **1902**. *[9]*

Worley PF, Barban JM, Surachai S, Wilson VS, Snyder SH: Characterization of inositol trisphosphate receptor binding in brain. *J Biol Chem.* 262:12132-12136, **1987**. *[8]*

Wu JY, Lipsius SL: Effects of extracellular Mg²⁺ on T- and L-type Ca²⁺ currents in single atrial myocytes. *Am J Physiol.* 259:H1842-H1850, **1990**. *[5]*

Wyatt CN, Campbell V, Brodbeck J, Brice NL, Page KM, Berrow NS, Brickley K, Terracciano CMN, Naqvi RU, MacLeod KT, Dolphin AC: Voltage-dependent binding and calcium channel current inhibition by an anti-α₁D subunit antibody in rat dorsal root ganglion neurones and guinea-pig myocytes. *J Physiol.* 502:307-319, **1997**. *[5]*

Xiao XH, Allen DG: Role of Na$^+$/H$^+$ exchanger during ischemia and preconditioning in the isolated rat heart. *Circ Res.* 85:723-730, **1999**. *[10]*

Xiao RP, Lakatta EG: β_1-Adrenoceptor stimulation and β_2-adrenoceptor stimulation differ in their effects on contraction, cytosolic Ca^{2+}, and Ca^{2+} current in single rat ventricular cells. *Circ Res.* 73:286-300, **1993**. *[5]*

Xiao RP, Cheng H, Lederer WJ, Suzuki T, Lakatta EG: Dual regulation of Ca^{2+}/calmodulin-dependent kinase II activity by membrane voltage and by calcium influx. *Proc Natl Acad Sci USA.* 91:9659-9663, **1994a**. *[5]*

Xiao RP, Hohl C, Altschuld R, Jones L, Livingston B, Ziman B, Tantini B, Lakatta EG: β_2-Adrenergic receptor-stimulated increase in cAMP in rat heart cells is not coupled to changes in Ca^{2+} dynamics, contractility, or phospholamban phosphorylation. *J Biol Chem.* 269:19151-19156, **1994b**. *[5]*

Xiao RP, Ji X, Lakatta EG: Functional coupling of the β_2-adrenoceptor to a pertussis toxin-sensitive G protein in cardiac myocytes. *Mol Pharmacol.* 47:322-329, **1995**. *[10]*

Xiao RP, Valdivia HH, Bogdanov K, Valdivia C, Lakatta EG, Cheng HP: The immunophilin FK506-binding protein modulates Ca^{2+} release channel closure in rat heart. *J Physiol.* 500:343-354, **1997**. *[7]*

Xiao RP, Avdonin P, Zhou YY, Chen HP, Akhter SA, Eschenhagen T, Lefkowitz RJ, Koch WJ, Lakatta EG: Coupling of β_2-adrenoceptor to G$_i$ proteins and its physiological relevance in murine cardiac myocytes. *Circ Res.* 84:43-52, **1999**. *[10]*

Xu KY, Becker LC: Ultrastructural localization of glycolytic enzymes on sarcoplasmic reticulum vesicles. *J Histochem Cytochem.* 46:419-427, **1998**. *[7]*

Xu L, Meissner G: Regulation of cardiac muscle Ca^{2+} release channel by sarcoplasmic reticulum lumenal Ca^{2+}. *Biophys J.* 75:2302-2312, **1998**. *[7]*

Xu A, Hawkins C, Narayanan N: Phosphorylation and activation of the Ca^{2+}-pumping ATPase of cardiac sarcoplasmic reticulum by Ca^{2+}/calmodulin-dependent protein kinase. *J Biol Chem.* 268:8394-8397, **1993**. *[7,9]*

Xu KY, Zweier JL, Becker LC: Functional coupling between glycolysis and sarcoplasmic reticulum Ca^{2+} transport. *Circ Res.* 77:88-97, **1995**. *[7]*

Xu L, Mann G, Meissner G: Regulation of cardiac Ca^{2+} release channel (ryanodine receptor) by Ca^{2+}, H$^+$, Mg^{2+}, and adenine nucleotides under normal and simulated ischemic conditions. *Circ Res.* 79:1100-1109, **1996**. *[7,10]*

Xu L, Tripathy A, Pasek DA, Meissner G: Potential for pharmacology of ryanodine receptor calcium release channels. *Ann NY Acad Sci.* 853:130-148, **1998a**. *[7]*

Xu L, Eu JP, Meissner G, Stamler JS: Activation of the cardiac calcium release channel (ryanodine receptor) by poly-S-nitrosylation. *Science.* 279:234-237, **1998b**. *[7]*

Xu HD, Guo WN, Nerbonne JM: Four kinetically distinct depolarization-activated K$^+$ currents in adult mouse ventricular myocytes. *J Gen Physiol.* 113:661-677, **1999a**. *[4]*

Xu HD, Li HL, Nerbonne JM: Elimination of the transient outward current and action potential prolongation in mouse atrial myocytes expressing a dominant negative Kv4 α subunit. *J Physiol.* 519:11-21, **1999b**. *[4]*

Xu H, Barry DM, Li H, Brunet S, Guo W, Nerbonne JM. Attenuation of the slow component of delayed rectification, action potential prolongation, and triggered activity in mice expressing a dominant-negative Kv2 α subunit. *Circ Res.* 85:623-633, **1999c**. *[4]*

Xu X, Rials SJ, Wu Y, Salata JJ, Liu T, Bharucha DB, Marinchak RA, Kowey PR. Left ventricular hypertrophy decreases slowly but not rapidly activating delayed rectifier potassium currents of epicardial and endocardial myocytes in rabbits. *Circulation.* 103:1585-1590, **2001**. *[10]*

Xue YX, Aye NN, Hashimoto K: Antiarrhythmic effects of HOE642, a novel Na$^+$-H$^+$ exchange inhibitor, on ventricular arrhythmias in animal hearts. *Eur J Pharmacol.* 317:309-316, **1996**. *[10]*

Yamada M, Miyawaki A, Saito K, Nakajima T, Yamamoto-Hino M, Ryo Y, Furuichi T, Mikoshiba K: The calmodulin-binding domain in the mouse type 1 inositol 1,4,5-trisphosphate receptor. *Biochem J.* 308:83-88, **1995**. *[7]*

Yamaguchi H, Hara M, Strobeck M, Fukasawa K, Schwartz A, Varadi G: Multiple modulation pathways of calcium channel activity by a β subunit - Direct evidence of β subunit participation in membrane trafficking of the α_{1c} subunit. *J Biol Chem.* 273:19348-19356, **1998**. *[5]*

Yamamoto H, Van Breemen C: Inositol 1,4,5-trisphosphate releases calcium from skinned cultured smooth muscle cells. *Biochem Biophys Res Commun.* 130:270-274, **1985**. *[8]*

Yamazaki J, Hume JR: Inhibitory effects of glibenclamide on cystic fibrosis transmembrane regulator, swelling-activated, and Ca^{2+}-activated Cl$^-$ channels in mammalian cardiac myocytes. *Circ Res.* 81:101-109, **1997**. *[4]*

Yamazaki T, Komuro I, Kudoh S, Zou YZ, Shiojima I, Hiroi Y, Mizuno T, Maemura K, Kurihara H, Aikawa R, Takano H, Yazaki Y: Endothelin-1 is involved in mechanical stress-induced cardiomyocyte hypertrophy. *J Biol Chem.* 271:3221-3228, **1996**. *[10]*

Yan GX, Kléber AG: Changes in extracellular and intracellular pH in ischemic rabbit papillary muscle. *Circ Res.* 71:460-470, **1992**. *[10]*

Yang HT, Endoh M: Pharmacological evidence for α_{1D}-adrenoceptors in the rabbit ventricular myocardium: analysis with BMY 7378. *Br J Pharmacol.* 122:1541-1550, **1997**. *[10]*

Yang J, Ellinor PT, Sather WA, Zhang JF, Tsien RW: Molecular determinants of Ca^{2+} selectivity and ion permeation in L-type Ca^{2+} channels. *Nature.* 366:158-161, **1993**. *[4,5]*

Yang J, Jan YN, Jan LY: Control of rectification and permeation by residues in two distinct domains in an inward rectifier K$^+$ channel. *Neuron.* 14:1047-1054, **1995**. *[4]*

Yang NB, George AL Jr, Horn R: Molecular basis of charge movement in voltage-gated sodium channels. *Neuron.* 16:113-122, **1996**. *[4]*

Yang Z, Stull JT, Levine RJ, Sweeney HL: Changes in interfilament spacing mimic the effects of myosin regulatory light chain phosphorylation in rabbit psoas fibers. *J Struct Biol.* 122:139-148, **1998**. *[2]*

Yano M, Ono K, Ohkusa T, Suetsugu M, Kohno M, Hisaoka T, Kobayashi S, Hisamatsu Y, Yamamoto T, Kohno M, Noguchi N, Takasawa S, Okamoto H, Matsuzaki M: Altered stoichiometry of FKBP12.6 versus ryanodine receptor as a cause of abnormal Ca^{2+} leak through ryanodine receptor in heart failure. *Circulation.* 102:2131-2136, **2000**. *[10]*

Yao Z, Gross GJ: Effects of the KATP channel opener bimakalim on coronary blood flow, monophasic action potential duration, and infarct size in dogs. *Circulation.* 89:1769-1775, **1994**. *[4,10]*

Yao AS, Su Z, Nonaka A, Zubair I, Lu LY, Philipson KD, Bridge JH, Barry WH: Effects of overexpression of the Na$^+$-Ca^{2+} exchanger on [Ca^{2+}] transients in murine ventricular myocytes. *Circ Res.* 82:657-665, **1998**. *[6,9]*

Yasutake M, Ibuki C, Hearse DJ, Avkiran M: Na$^+$/H$^+$ exchange and reperfusion arrhythmias: Protection by intracoronary infusion of a novel inhibitor. *Am J Physiol.* 267:H2430-H2440, **1994**. *[10]*

Yatani A, Brown AM: Rapid ß-adrenergic modulation of cardiac calcium channel currents by a fast G protein pathway. *Science.* 245:71-74, **1989**. *[5]*

Yatani A, Codina J, Imoto Y, Reeves JP, Birmbaumer L, Brown AM: A G protein directly regulates mammalian cardiac calcium channels. *Science.* 238:1288-1292, **1987**. *[5]*

Yeh JZ, Narahashi T: Kinetic analysis of pancuronium interaction with sodium channels in squid axon membranes. *J Gen Physiol.* 69:293-323, **1977**. *[4]*

Yellen G: The moving parts of voltage-gated ion channels. *Q Rev Biophys.* 31:239-295, **1998**. *[4]*

Ying WL, Emerson J, Clarke MJ, Sanadi DR: Inhibition of mitochondrial calcium ion transport by an oxo-bridged dinuclear ruthenium ammine complex. *Biochemistry.* 30:4949-4952, **1991**. *[3]*

Yoshida K, Sorimachi Y, Fujiwara M, Hironaka K: Calpain is implicated in rat myocardial injury after ischemia or reperfusion. *Jpn Circ J.* 59:40-48, **1995**. *[10]*

Yu H, Chang F, Cohen IS: Pacemaker current exists in ventricular myocytes. *Circ Res.* 72:232-236, **1993**. *[4]*

Yu H, Chang F, Cohen IS: Pacemaker current I$_f$ in adult canine cardiac ventricular myocytes. *J Physiol.* 485:469-483, **1995**. *[4]*

Yuan W, Bers DM: Ca-dependent facilitation of cardiac Ca current is due to Ca-calmodulin-dependent protein kinase. *Am J Physiol.* 267:H982-H993, **1994**. *[5]*

Yuan W, Bers DM: Protein kinase inhibitor H-89 reverses forskolin stimulation of cardiac L-type calcium current. *Am J Physiol.* 268:C651-C659, **1995**. *[5]*

Yuan W, Ginsburg KS, Bers DM: Comparison of sarcolemmal calcium channel current in rabbit and rat ventricular myocytes. *J Physiol.* 493:733-746, **1996**. *[3,5,9]*

Yue DT, Marbán E: Single Ca channel currents carried by Ca and Ba in heart cells: No anomalous mole fraction effect. *Circulation.* 76:IV-330, **1987**. *[4]*

Yue DT, Marbán E: Permeation in the dihyropyridine-sensitive calcium channel: Multi-ion occupancy but non anomalous mole-fraction effect between Ba^{2+} and Ca^{2+}. *J Gen Physiol.* 95:911-939, **1990**. *[5]*

Yue DT, Burkoff D, Franz MR, Hunter WC, Sagawa K: Postextrasystolic potentiation of the isolated canine left ventricle. *Circ Res.* 56:340-350, **1985**. *[8]*

Yue DT, Marbán E, Wier WG: Relationship between force and intracellular[Ca^{2+}] in tetanized mammalian heart muscle. *J Gen Physiol.* 87:223-242, **1986**. *[2,3]*

Yue DT, Herzig S, Marbán E: ß-Adrenergic stimulation of calcium channels occurs by potentiation of high-activity gating modes. *Proc Natl Acad Sci USA.* 87:753-757, **1990**. *[5]*

Zagotta WN, Hoshi T, Aldrich RW: Restoration of inactivation in mutants of Shaker potassium channels by a peptide derived from ShB. *Science.* 250:568-571, **1990**. *[4]*

Zahradníková A, Zahradník I, Györke I, Györke S: Rapid activation of the cardiac ryanodine receptor by submillisecond calcium stimuli. *J Gen Physiol.* 114:787-798, **1999a**. *[7,8]*

Zahradníková A, Dura M, Györke S: Modal gating transitions in cardiac ryanodine receptors during increases of Ca^{2+} concentration produced by photolysis of caged Ca^{2+}. *Pflügers Arch.* 438:283-288, **1999b**. *[7,8]*

Zang WJ, Yu XJ, Honjo H, Kirby MS, Boyett MR: On the role of G protein activation and phosphorylation in desensitization to acetylcholine in guinea-pig atrial cells. *J Physiol.* 464:649-679, **1993**. *[4]*

Zeng J, Laurita KR, Rosenbaum DS, Rudy Y: Two components of the delayed rectifier K$^+$ current in ventricular myocytes of the guinea pig type: Theoretical formulation and their role in repolarization. *Circ Res.* 77:140-152, **1995**. *[4]*

Zhai J, Schmidt AG, Hoit BD, Kimura Y, MacLennan DH, Kranias EG: Cardiac-specific overexpression of a superinhibitory pentameric phospholamban mutant enhances inhibition of cardiac function in vivo. *J Biol Chem.* 275:10538-10544, **2000**. *[7]*

Zhang R, Zhao J, Mandveno A, Potter JD: Cardiac troponin I phosphorylation increases the rate of cardiac muscle relaxation. *Circ Res.* 76:1028-1035, **1995a**. *[2]*

Zhang R, Zhao JJ, Potter JD: Phosphorylation of both serine residues in cardiac troponin is required to decrease the Ca^{2+} affinity of cardiac troponin C. *J Biol Chem.* 270:30773-30780, **1995b**. *[2]*

Zhang ZH, Johnson JA, Chen L, el-Sherif N, Mochly-Rosen D, Boutjdir M: C2 region-derived peptides of p-protein kinase C regulate cardiac Ca^{2+} channels. *Circ Res.* 80:720-729, **1997a**. *[5]*

Zhang L, Kelley J, Schmeisser G, Kobayashi YM, Jones LR: Complex formation between junctin, triadin, calsequestrin, and the ryanodine receptor. Proteins of the cardiac junctional sarcoplasmic reticulum membrane. *J Biol Chem.* 272:23389-23397, **1997b**. *[7]*

Zhang ST, Hiraoka M, Hirano Y: Effects of α$_1$-adrenergic stimulation on L-type Ca^{2+} current in rat ventricular myocytes. *J Mol Cell Cardiol.* 30:1955-1965, **1998**. *[5]*

Zhong HY, Minneman KP: α$_1$-adrenoceptor subtypes. *Eur J Pharmacol.* 375:261-276, **1999**. *[10]*

Zhou Z, Bers DM: Ca^{2+} influx via the L-type Ca^{2+} channel during tail current and above current reversal potential in ferret ventricular myocytes. *J Physiol.* 523:57-66, **2000**. *[5]*

Zhou ZF, January CT: Both T- and L-type Ca^{2+} channels can contribute to excitation-contraction coupling in cardiac Purkinje cells. *Biophys J.* 74:1830-1839, **1998**. *[8]*

Zhou Z, Lipsius SL: Na$^+$-Ca^{2+} exchange current in latent pacemaker cells isolated from cat right atrium. *J Physiol.* 466:263-285, **1993**. *[4]*

Zhou Z, Lipsius SL: T-type calcium current in latent pacemaker cells isolated from cat right atrium. *J Mol Cell Cardiol.* 26:1211-1219, **1994**. *[4]*

Zhou JM, Olcese R, Qin N, Noceti F, Birnbaumer L, Stefani E: Feedback inhibition of Ca^{2+} channels by Ca^{2+} depends on a short sequence of the C terminus that does not include the Ca^{2+}-binding function of a motif with similarity to Ca^{2+}-binding domains. *Proc Natl Acad Sci USA.* 94:2301-2305, **1997**. *[5]*

Zhou Z, Matlib MA, Bers DM: Cytosolic and mitochondrial Ca^{2+} signals in patch clamped mammalian ventricular myocytes. *J Physiol.* 507:379-403, **1998**. *[3]*

Zhou YY, Cheng HP, Song LS, Wang DJ, Lakatta EG, Xiao RP: Spontaneous β_2-adrenergic signaling fails to modulate L-type Ca^{2+} current in mouse ventricular myocytes. *Mol Pharmacol.* 56:485-493, **1999**. *[5]*

Zhu XS, Gurrola G, Jiang MT, Walker JW, Valdivia HH: Conversion of an inactive cardiac dihydropyridine receptor II-III loop segment into forms that activate skeletal ryanodine receptors. *FEBS Lett.* 450:221-226, **1999**. *[8]*

Zhu W, Zou Y, Shiojima I, Kudoh S, Aikawa R, Hayashi D, Mizukami M, Toko H, Shibasaki F, Yazaki Y, Nagai R, Komuro I: Ca^{2+}/calmodulin-dependent kinase II and calcineurin play critical roles in endothelin-1-induced cardiomyocyte hypertrophy. *J Biol Chem.* 275:15239-15245, **2000**. *[10]*

ZhuGe RH, Sims SM, Tuft RA, Fogarty KE, Walsh JV Jr: Ca^{2+} sparks activate K^+ and Cl^- channels, resulting in spontaneous transient currents in guinea-pig tracheal myocytes. *J Physiol.* 513:711-718, **1998**. *[8]*

ZhuGe RH, Tuft RA, Fogarty KE, Bellve K, Fay FS, Walsh JV Jr: The influence of sarcoplasmic reticulum Ca^{2+} concentration on Ca^{2+} sparks and spontaneous transient outward currents in single smooth muscle cells. *J Gen Physiol.* 113:215-228, **1999**. *[8]*

Zilberter YI, Starmer CF, Starobin J, Grant AO: Late Na channels in cardiac cells: The physiological role of background Na channels. *Biophys J.* 67:153-160, **1994**. *[4]*

Zile MR, Koide M, Sato H, Ishiguro Y, Conrad CH, Buckley JM, Morgan JP, Cooper G: Role of microtubules in the contractile dysfunction of hypertrophied myocardium. *J Am Coll Cardiol.* 33:250-260, **1999**. *[1]*

Zimmerman ANE, Hülsmann WC: Paradoxical influence of calcium ions in the permeability of the cell membranes of the isolated rat heart. *Nature.* 211:646-647, **1966**. *[1]*

Zong X, Schreieck J, Mehrke G, Welling A, Schuster A, Bosse E, Flockerzi V, Hofmann F: On the regulation of the expressed L-type calcium channel by cAMP-dependent phosphorylation. *Pflügers Arch.* 430:340-347, **1995**. *[5]*

Zoratti M, Szabo I: The mitochondrial permeability transition. *Biochim Biophys Acta.* 1241:139-176, **1995**. *[3]*

Zorzato F, Salviati G, Facchinetti T, Volpe P: Doxorubicin induces calcium release from terminal cisternae of skeletal muscle. *J Biol Chem.* 260:7349-7355, **1985**. *[7]*

Zorzato F, Fujii J, Otsu K, Phillips M, Green NM, Lai FA, Meissner G, MacLennan DH: Molecular cloning of cDNA encoding human and rabbit forms of the Ca^{2+} release channel (ryanodine receptor) of skeletal muscle sarcoplasmic reticulum. *J Biol Chem.* 265:2244-2256, **1990**. *[7]*

Zot AS, Potter JD: Structural aspects of troponin-tropomyosin regulation of skeletal muscle contraction. *Ann Rev Biophys Biophys Chem.* 16:535-559, **1987**. *[2]*

Zucchi R, Ronca-Testoni S: The sarcoplasmic reticulum Ca^{2+} channel/ryanodine receptor: Modulation by endogenous effectors, drugs and disease states. *Pharmacol Rev.* 49:1-51, **1997**. *[7]*

Zühlke RD, Reuter H: Ca^{2+}-sensitive inactivation of L-type Ca^{2+} channels depends on multiple cytoplasmic amino acid sequences of the α_{1C} subunit. *Proc Natl Acad Sci USA.* 95:3287-3294, **1998**. *[5]*

Zühlke RD, Pitt GS, Deisseroth K, Tsien RW, Reuter H: Calmodulin supports both inactivation and facilitation of L-type calcium channels. *Nature.* 399:159-162, **1999**. *[5]*

Zygmunt AC: Intracellular calcium activates a chloride current in canine ventricular myocytes. *Am J Physiol.* 267:H1984-H1995, **1994**. *[4]*

Zygmunt AC, Maylie J: Stimulation-dependent facilitation of the high threshold calcium current in guinea-pig ventricular myocytes. *J Physiol.* 428:653-671, **1990**. *[5]*

Zygmunt AC, Gibbons WR: Calcium-activated chloride current in rabbit ventricular myocytes. *Circ Res.* 68:424-437, **1991**. *[4,10]*

Zygmunt AC, Gibbons WR: Properties of the calcium-activated chloride current in heart. *J Gen Physiol.* 99:391-414, **1992**. *[4]*

Zygmunt AC, Goodrow RJ, Weigel CM: I_{NaCa} and $I_{Cl(Ca)}$ contribute to isoproterenol-induced delayed afterdepolarizations in midmyocardial cells. *Am J Physiol.* 275:H1979-H1992, **1998**. *[4,10]*

INDEX

Bold entries refer to key illustrations & tables